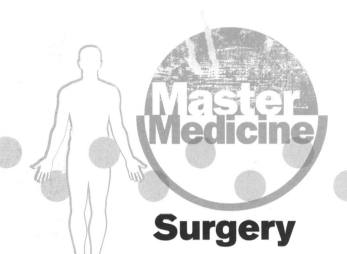

Master Medicine

Surgery

Commissioning Editor: Laurence Hunter
Development Editor: Barbara Simmons
Project Manager: Jess Thompson
Designer: Stewart Larking
Illustration Manager: Merlyn Harvey

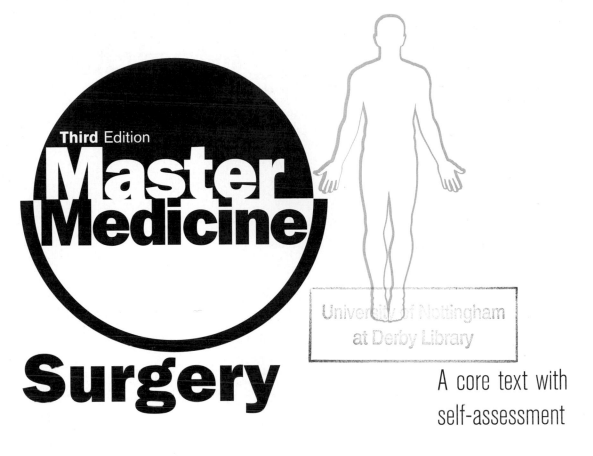

Third Edition

Master Medicine

Surgery

A core text with
self-assessment

EDITED BY

Michael Lavelle-Jones
MBChB FRCS FRCS (Edinburgh) MD
Consultant Surgeon and Honorary Senior
Lecturer,
Ninewells Hospital and Medical School,
Dundee, UK

John A. Dent
MMEd MD FHEA FRCS (Edinburgh)
Reader and Honorary Consultant in
Orthopaedic and Trauma Surgery,
University of Dundee,
Ninewells Hospital and Medical School,
Dundee, UK

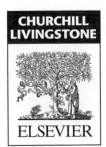

Edinburgh London New York Oxford Philadelphia St Louis Sydney Toronto 2008

CHURCHILL
LIVINGSTONE
ELSEVIER

An imprint of Elsevier Limited

© Pearson Professional Limited 1997
© Harcourt Publishers Limited 2002
© 2008, Elsevier Limited. All rights reserved.

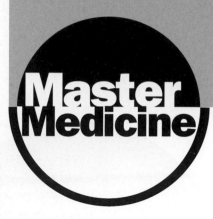

First edition 1997
Second edition 2002
Third edition 2008
Previously published as 'Surgery 1': Lavelle-Jones and 'Surgery 2': Dent

ISBN-13: 978-0-443-10333-9   1005 346044

British Library Cataloguing in Publication Data
A catalogue record for this book is available from the British Library

Library of Congress Cataloging in Publication Data
A catalog record for this book is available from the Library of Congress

Note
Neither the Publisher nor the Author assumes any responsibility for any loss or injury and/or damage to persons or property arising out of or related to any use of the material contained in this book. It is the responsibility of the treating practitioner, relying on independent expertise and knowledge of the patient, to determine the best treatment and method of application for the patient.

The Publisher

 ELSEVIER your source for books, journals and multimedia in the health sciences

www.elsevierhealth.com

The publisher's policy is to use paper manufactured from sustainable forests

Working together to grow
libraries in developing countries

www.elsevier.com | www.bookaid.org | www.sabre.org

ELSEVIER   BOOK AID International   Sabre Foundation

Printed in China

Contributors

Paul Allcock FRCS (Tr & Orth)
Consultant Orthopaedic Surgeon, Royal Alexandra Hospital, Paisley

Eric Ballantyne BSc MBChB FRCS (Edinburgh) (SN) MD
Consultant Neurosurgeon, Ninewells Hospital and Medical School, Dundee

Robin L. Blair FRCS
Professor of Otolaryngology, University of Dundee, Dundee

John A. Dent MMEd MD FHEA FRCS (Edinburgh)
Reader and Honorary Consultant in Orthopaedic and Trauma Surgery, Ninewells Hospital and Medical School, University of Dundee, Dundee

Quentin Gardiner FRCS FRCS (Edinburgh) FRCS(ORL)
Consultant Otolaryngologist, Ninewells Hospital and Medical School, Dundee

Douglas Gentleman BSc MBChB FRCS FRCS (Glasgow)
Consultant in Charge of the Brain Injury Rehabilitation Service and Honorary Consultant Neurosurgeon, Royal Victoria and Ninewells Hospitals, Dundee

Chris M. Goodman MD FRCS (Edinburgh)
Consultant Urologist, Ninewells Hospital and Medical School, Dundee

Gareth D. Griffiths MD FRCS
Consultant Vascular Surgeon, Ninewells Hospital, Dundee

Paul A. Johnstone BSc MBChB MRCOphth DipMedEd
Specialist Registrar, Department of Ophthalmology, Ninewells Hospital, Dundee

Syed A. Kazmi MBBS (Punjab) MCPS (Pakistan) FRCS (Edinburgh)
Associate Specialist, Department of Surgery, Ninewells Hospital, Dundee

Michael Lavelle-Jones MBChB FRCS FRCS (Edinburgh) MD
Consultant Surgeon and Honorary Senior Lecturer, Ninewells Hospital and Medical School, Dundee

Caroline J. MacEwen MD FRCS FRCOphth FFSEM
Consultant Ophthalmologist, Ninewells Hospital and Head of Department of Ophthalmology, University of Dundee

Peter T. McCollum MCh FRCS (Ireland) FRCS (Edinburgh)
Professor of Vascular Surgery, University of Hull; Honorary Consultant Vascular Surgeon & Associate Medical Director, Hull & East Yorkshire Hospitals NHS Trust

Simon Phipps BM MS MRCS (England) DM
Specialist Registrar in Urology, Department of Urology, Ninewells Hospital, Dundee

David Smith FRCS
Consultant Endocrine and General Surgeon, Ninewells Hospital and Medical School, Dundee

J. Howard Stevenson MD FRCS (Edinburgh)
Consultant Plastic Surgeon, Ninewells Hospital and Medical School; Senior Lecturer, University of Dundee, Dundee

Alastair M. Thompson BSc MBChB MD FRCS (Edinburgh)
Professor of Surgical Oncology, University of Dundee, Dundee

William S. Walker MA MB BChir FRCS FRCS (Edinburgh)
Consultant Cardiothoracic Surgeon, Royal Infirmary of Edinburgh, Edinburgh

Contents

Contents

Using this book

'What do I need to know about surgery in general and the surgical specialties?'

'Do I know the right things?'

'Can I remember the key points in the management of . . . ?'

These are the sort of questions which haunt us as exams approach but by then, unfortunately, there is seldom time to go back to extensive textbooks or sketchy lecture notes for the answers.

This is just the time when this new revision textbook comes in useful. In it you will find the 'core' information you require presented in a concise and systematic fashion, which highlights the key facts you should know about any topic in a way that will help you remember them. But, rather than simply giving you lots of facts to memorise, the principles of diagnosis and management are explained so that it becomes easier for you to work out the answers for yourself. The book does not aim to offer a complete 'syllabus'. It is impossible to draw boundaries around medical knowledge and learning as this is really a continuous process carried out throughout your medical career. With this in mind, you should aim to develop the ability to discern knowledge which you *need to know* from that which it is *nice to know*.

The aims of this introductory chapter are:

- to help plan your learning
- to show you how to use this book to increase your understanding as well as knowledge
- to realise how self-assessment can make learning easier and more enjoyable.

Layout and contents

The main part of the text describes topics considered to be of 'core' importance to the major subject areas. Within each chapter, essential information is presented in a set order with explanations and logical 'links' between topics. Where relevant, key facts about basic sciences, aetiology and pathological features are outlined. Where it is possible the clinical features are described under key headings. Differential diagnosis and an approach to investigation are then described. Finally, the principles of management and the prognosis are presented. It is recognised that at the level of an undergraduate or newly qualified doctor a detailed knowledge is not required, but an ability to understand basic principles is expected.

You will need to be sure that you are reaching the required standards, so in the final section of each chapter there are opportunities for you to check your knowledge

and understanding. This self-assessment is in the form of multiple choice questions (MCQs), extended matching items questions (EMIs), constructed response questions (CRQs), objective structured clinical examination questions (OSCEs) and best of 5 questions. All of these are centred around common clinical problems, which are important in judging your performance as a doctor. Detailed answers are given. These answers will also contain some information and explanations that you will not find elsewhere, so you must do the assessment to get the most out of this book!

Using this book

If you are using this book as part of your exam preparations, we suggest that your first task should be to map out on a sheet of paper three lists dividing the major subjects (corresponding to the chapter headings) into your strong, reasonable and weak areas. This will give you a rough outline of your revision schedule, which you must then fit in with the time available. Clearly, if your exams are looming large you will have to be ruthless in the time allocated to your strong areas. The major subjects should be further classified into individual topics. Encouragement to store information and to test your ongoing improvement is by the use of the self-assessment sections – you must not just read passively. It is important to keep checking your current level of knowledge, both strengths and weaknesses. This should be assessed objectively – self-rating in the absence of testing can be misleading. You may consider yourself strong in a particular area whereas it is more a reflection on how much you enjoy and are stimulated by the subject. Conversely, you may be stronger in a subject than you would expect simply because the topic does not appeal to you.

It is a good idea to discuss topics and problems with colleagues/friends; the areas which you understand least well will soon become apparent when you try to explain them to someone else.

Approaching the examinations

The discipline of learning is closely linked to preparation for examinations. Many of us opt for a process of superficial learning that is directed towards retention of facts and recall under exam conditions because full understanding is often not required. It is much better if you try to acquire a deeper knowledge and understanding, combining the necessity of passing exams with longer-term needs.

First, you need to know how you will be examined. Does the examination involve clinical assessment such as history taking and clinical examination? If you are sitting a written examination, what are the length and types of question? How many must you answer and how much choice will you have?

Now you have to choose what sources you are going to use for your learning and revision. Textbooks come in different forms. At one extreme, there is the large reference book. This type of book should be avoided at this stage of revision and used only (if at all) for reference, when answers to questions cannot be found in smaller books. At the other end of the spectrum is the condensed 'lecture note' format, which often relies heavily on lists. Facts of this nature on their own are difficult to remember if they are not supported by understanding. In the middle of the range are the medium-sized textbooks. These are often of the most use, whether you are approaching final university examinations or the first part of professional examinations. Our advice is to choose one of the several medium-sized books on offer on the basis of which one you find the most readable. The best approach is to combine your lecture notes, textbooks (appropriate to the level of study) and past examination papers as a framework for your preparation.

Armed with information about the format of the exams, a rough syllabus, your own lecture notes and some books that you feel comfortable in using, your next step is to map out the time available for preparation. You must be realistic, allow time for breaks and work *steadily*, not cramming. If you do attempt to cram, you have to realise that only a certain amount of information can be retained in your short-term memory, so as the classification of one condition moves in, the treatment of another moves out! Cramming simply retains facts. If the examination requires understanding you will be in trouble.

It is often a good idea to begin by outlining the topics to be covered and then attempt to summarise your knowledge about each in note form. In this way your existing knowledge will be activated and any gaps will become apparent. Self-assessment also helps determine the time to be allocated to each subject for exam preparation. If you are consistently scoring excellent marks in a particular subject, it is not cost-effective to spend a lot of time trying to achieve the 'perfect' mark.

In an essay it is many times easier to obtain the first mark (try writing your name) than the last. You should also try to decide on the amount of time assigned to each subject based on the likelihood of it appearing in the exam! Commonest things are usually commonest!

The main types of examination

Multiple choice questions (MCQs)

Unless very sophisticated, MCQs test your recall of information. The aim is to gain the maximum marks from the knowledge that you can remember. The stem statement must be read with great care highlighting the 'little' words such as *only, rarely, usually, never* and *always*. Overlooking

negatives, such as *not, unusual* and *unsuccessful* often cause marks to be lost. *May occur* has an entirely different connotation from *characteristic*. The latter may mean a feature that should be there and the absence of which would make you question the correctness of the diagnosis.

Remember to check the marking method before starting. Most multiple choice papers employ a negative system in which marks are lost for incorrect answers. The temptation is to adopt a cautious approach answering a relatively small number of questions. However, this can lead to problems as we all make simple mistakes or even disagree vehemently with the answer in the computer! Caution may lead you to answer too few questions to obtain a pass after the marks have been deducted for incorrect answers.

Extended matching item questions (EMIs)

EMIs begin by stating the theme to which they relate. Usually ten possible answers are then listed. A number of questions in the form of statements or clinical scenarios follows and you have to select the correct or most appropriate answer from the previous list. There should be only one correct answer for each of these questions, but, unlike MCQs, it is more difficult to guess the right one.

Constructed response questions (CRQs)

A more sophisticated form of exam question is an evolving case history with information being presented sequentially and you being asked to give a response at each stage. CRQs are constructed so that a wrong response in the first part of the questions does not mean that no more marks can be obtained from the subsequent parts. Each part should stand on its own. Patient management problems are designed to test the recall and application of knowledge through an understanding of the principles involved.

Objective structured clinical examination questions (OSCEs)

The objective structured clinical examination (OSCE) is now extensively used to examine clinical competencies. The questions may relate to a patient, a simulated patient or a mannikin or to a clinical photograph, radiograph, pathology specimen or laboratory report. Good questions test clinical skills, practical procedures and clinical reasoning rather than factual recall.

Best of 5 questions

In this format there are five possible answers supplied but only one is the best correct answer. Although some answers are obviously incorrect, there will be others which are possible or reasonably good. Be careful to read the questions and the answers carefully to select the best possible answer available.

Conclusions

You should amend your framework for using this book according to your own needs and the examinations you are facing. Whatever approach you adopt, your aim should be for an understanding of the principles involved rather than rote learning of a large number of poorly connected facts.

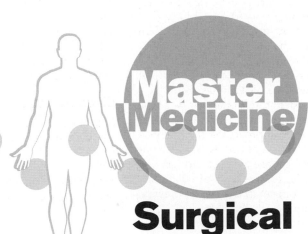

Master Medicine

Surgical principles

Surgical principles

Chapter

1

Chapter overview

This chapter outlines the principles of management that are common to all patients requiring surgical intervention. Surgical disease and its treatment cannot be considered in isolation. Take account of any coexisting medical conditions or previous surgical intervention which may affect the patient's management. Many surgical procedures disturb the gastrointestinal tract and all patients undergoing general anaesthesia will require a period of starvation. A thorough understanding of the theory and practice of fluid balance is essential. Most surgical procedures will cause pain. Effective postoperative pain management is vital and assists recovery during the postoperative period. Although most patients will recover uneventfully after surgery a few will develop complications which may range from a minor wound infection to a life-threatening pulmonary embolus. The management of postoperative complications that are common to all surgical procedures is also described.

1.1 Pre- and postoperative management

Learning objectives

You should:
- be able to recognise any risk factors in patients undergoing surgery and instigate a management plan
- understand the principles and importance of careful fluid balance in surgical patients
- be able to choose an analgesic of appropriate strength and route of delivery according to a patient's needs.

Preoperative preparation

History and physical examination

A thorough history and physical examination are the key initial steps in the preoperative work-up of any surgical patient. Although the presenting complaint is of prime importance, any previous medical or surgical history, drug history or allergies must be sought as they

may influence the choice of operation, anaesthetic or perioperative care.

Laboratory investigations

Baseline haematology, biochemistry and a coagulation profile are important in all patients undergoing major surgery and in older patients undergoing minor surgery. These tests can detect an unsuspected anaemia, metabolic abnormality or a coagulopathy that would require investigation or correction prior to surgery.

Diagnostic radiology

Many patients will have undergone diagnostic radiology prior to surgery and often prior to hospital admission. These films must be available and have been reviewed prior to operation.

Preoperative chest radiography and ECG

Patients over 50 years of age and younger patients with respiratory or cardiovascular abnormalities detected on history and examination should have a preoperative chest radiograph and/or ECG.

Blood cross-match

Blood samples either for grouping and serum saving or for cross-matching should be taken according to the magnitude of the intended operation.

Informed consent

Obtaining consent should not be delegated to the most junior member of the surgical team. Instead, a careful, logical explanation of the planned operation and any alternatives should be given to the patient, preferably by the surgeon who is to perform the operation.

Medical problems in surgical patients

Many medical disorders can influence the management of the surgical patient. The three most commonly encountered groups of problems are:

- respiratory disease
- cardiovascular disease
- diabetes mellitus.

Respiratory disease

Upper respiratory tract infection

Any patient with evidence of an upper respiratory tract infection should have *elective* surgery postponed until the infection has cleared. Although most of these infections are viral in origin, manipulation of the airway during induction and maintenance of anaesthesia render these patients prone to a serious secondary bacterial respiratory tract infection in the postoperative period.

Chronic obstructive airways disease and asthma

Patients known preoperatively to have chronic pulmonary disease must stop smoking 1–2 weeks prior to surgery and should be admitted in advance of their operation to enable the following measures to be undertaken:

- full evaluation of respiratory system: both pulmonary function testing and arterial blood gases
- preoperative physiotherapy
- sputum culture and treatment of any infection
- anaethestic consultation: regional anaesthesia (spinal or epidural) may be more appropriate than general anaesthesia in certain cases.

Cardiovascular disease

Patients with cardiovascular disease are at risk during surgery and in the immediate postoperative period, when fluctuations in blood pressure and fluid balance can compromise a limited cardiac reserve. The decision to operate in this group of patients is a balance of risks which requires close cooperation between surgeon, cardiologist and anaesthetist.

Myocardial infarction and angina

The risks of reinfarction are minimised if surgery can be delayed until at least 6 months after a previous myocardial infarction. Patients with angina should be symptomatically well controlled before undergoing surgery.

Hypertension

Medical therapy and control should be optimised before surgery.

Congestive heart failure

Surgery is likely to aggravate heart failure in these patients when they lie flat on the operating table, particularly if intravenous fluid therapy is needed. Diuretic therapy and cardiac inotropic support should be optimised prior to surgery.

Valvular heart disease

These patients require special precautions to prevent fluid overload as their cardiac reserve may be limited. Many patients will be taking long-term anticoagulation therapy, which will need to be temporarily withdrawn or reduced, and the patient will need to be closely monitored to allow surgery to be undertaken without risk of major bleeding. Antibiotic prophylaxis is essential to prevent endocarditis.

Diabetes mellitus

Glucose, potassium (K^+) and insulin (GKI) continuous infusion regimens have revolutionised the management of diabetic patients undergoing surgery. The amount of insulin added to the 10% dextrose (glucose) solution is varied depending upon the patient's blood sugar level, which is regularly monitored. An insulin-induced hypokalaemia is prevented by continuous potassium supplementation.

This regimen is established on the morning of surgery for insulin-dependent diabetics and also for those non-insulin-dependent diabetics who usually use oral hypoglycaemic agents. It is continued until patients resume their normal diet after surgery. Special measures are rarely required for diabetics who are normally adequately controlled by dietary measures alone.

Fluid balance and nutrition

Surgery profoundly affects the whole body balance and distribution of fluids and electrolytes. The principles of fluid management in the surgical patient depend upon an understanding of the baseline daily fluid requirements plus a knowledge of the effects of surgical procedures and disease on normal metabolism.

Fluid and electrolyte balance in the surgical patient

The three most important components are water, sodium and potassium. The normal water and electrolyte turnover in a healthy individual is summarised in Table 1. Fluid and electrolyte therapy depends upon:

- maintenance of daily requirements
- replacement of ongoing fluid losses
- replacement of long-standing fluid deficits.

Maintenance of daily requirements

A healthy 70-kg person needs 2500 ml water plus 100 mmol sodium plus 40 mmol potassium each day. This is equivalent to 2 l of 5% dextrose with 40 mmol added potassium plus 500 ml of 0.9% (normal) saline solution. This fluid regimen will maintain the baseline fluid requirements in most patients.

Table 1 Normal daily turnover of water and electrolytes

	Intake		Output	
Water (ml)	Food and liquid	2000	Urine	1500
	Internal metabolism	500	Sweat	500
			Expired air	250
			Stools	250
Total water (ml)		2500		2500
Sodium (mmol)	Diet	100	Urine	100
Potassium (mmol)	Diet	100	Urine	60
			Internal metabolism	40

Replacement of ongoing losses

A daily fluid balance chart has a central role to play in managing each patient's fluid requirements. It is especially important to record fluid losses from:

- nasogastric aspiration
- vomit
- stoma output
- fistula output
- drain output
- urine output.

These volumes should be considered together with the daily urine, stool and insensible losses (see Table 1) and should be replaced volume for volume in the following 24 h with either normal saline or a balanced salt solution (Ringer's solution or Hartmann's solution).

Insensible losses If a patient is febrile, excess water will be lost through sweating and evaporation and this should be replaced with an extra 500 ml of 5% dextrose solution.

Replacement of long-standing fluid deficits

This is a difficult concept to grasp. In patients who, for example, have had a long-standing bowel obstruction or who have had severe burns, large volumes of fluid will be sequestered either in the intestinal lumen or in the interstitial fluid. This fluid, which has been 'lost' from the circulation and from the intracellular and extracellular fluid spaces, can amount to several litres and if replaced too rapidly would overexpand the circulating plasma volume causing heart failure and gross oedema.

Complex formulae exist that help estimate these losses, which should be replaced slowly over a period of days. As a general rule, not more than one-half of the long-standing fluid deficit should be replaced in any 24-h period.

Surgical nutrition

A good nutritional status is vital to ensure repair and healing after surgery. Wherever possible, elective surgery should be postponed until nutritional deficiencies have been corrected.

The key factors that determine a patient's nutritional status are:

- dietary history
- weight loss (>5 kg is significant)
- anthropomorphic measurements of muscle and fat stores
- serum albumin level.

The optimum diet includes an adequate number of calories, protein, fat, minerals and vitamins to meet the energy and growth and repair demands of daily activities. These requirements are summarised in Table 2. Calories and nitrogen should be given simultaneously to achieve a positive nitrogen balance (a net synthesis of protein). The optimum ratio is 150 kcal for every gram of nitrogen. At least one-half of the calories must be given as glucose (in order to stimulate insulin secretion which in turn facilitates protein synthesis). The remaining calories can be given as fat, which will have the added

Table 2 Essential dietary components

- 2500 kcal/day caloric intake for a 70 kg human
- 1 g/kg protein to supply essential amino acids
- Fat-soluble vitamins: vitamins A, D, K, E
- Water-soluble vitamins: vitamin B group, vitamin C
- Essential fatty acids
- Trace elements: copper, zinc, iron, manganese

benefit of providing the essential fatty acids necessary for a balanced diet.

The two main forms of surgical nutrition are:

- enteral nutrition
- parenteral nutrition.

Enteral nutrition, which uses the patient's own gastrointestinal tract for nutrient absorption, is preferable to the parenteral (intravenous route), which is prone to serious complication and is more expensive.

Enteral nutrition There are three main types of enteral nutrition:

- oral supplementation: using high-calorie/high-protein drinks to supplement oral intake
- nasogastric or nasojejunal tube feeding: using finebore silastic tubes to deliver enteral nutrition direct to the small bowel
- feeding gastrostomy or jejunostomy: exteriorising part of the stomach or proximal jejunum as a conduit for feeding.

Enteral nutrition is most useful in patients who have an intact, functioning full-length gastrointestinal tract or at least 300 cm of small bowel. Abdominal cramps, diarrhoea and vomiting are the major side effects and are caused by the delivery of hypertonic enteral feeds directly to the small intestine.

Parenteral nutrition The composition of parenteral nutrition can be individualised to the nutritional requirements of each patient. Each pharmacy-prepared nutrition bag contains enough nutrients for a 24-h period and consists of:

- amino acids
- dextrose
- lipids
- vitamins, minerals and trace elements.

This solution is thrombogenic and has to be administered via a large central vein to avoid thrombosis. The catheter tip should lie in the superior vena cava just above the right atrium. For long-term feeding, silastic catheters are used which are tunnelled subcutaneously from the subclavian vein or internal jugular vein to an exit point on the chest wall. In the short term (2–3 weeks) peripherally inserted central venous catheters (PICC), which are threaded into the central veins from the antecubital fossa, are used to deliver nutrition. Strict aseptic technique must be used when changing the nutrition bag to prevent introducing sepsis.

One

Parenteral nutrition is best restricted to those patients whose intestinal tract cannot cope with enteral nutrition. Typically this includes:

- patients with Crohn's disease
- patients with high small bowel fistulae
- patients with short gut syndrome following major small bowel resection
- catabolic postoperative patients with septic complications.

Analgesia

Adequate pain control is vital to allay anxiety pre- and postoperatively and to allow patients to rest, recuperate and sleep. Three groups of drugs are used:

- opioids (usually morphine)
- oral or intravenous non-opioid analgesics
- non-steroidal anti-inflammatory drugs (NSAIDs).

Opioids

These drugs are the most potent analgesics and form the cornerstone of treatment in postoperative analgesia. Newer methods of delivery have supplanted intramuscular and subcutaneous routes, which are prone to unpredictable absorption and should not be used as they may cause patients to overdose, causing respiratory depression, or underdose, causing inadequate pain control.

Epidural opioids

This is the optimum technique for pain management after major surgery. Opioids or local anaesthetic agents (e.g. bupivacaine) are infused into the epidural space through a suitably postioned catheter. This technique blocks the afferent nerves and effectively controls pain. It is a type of regional anaesthesia. Respiratory depression is less in comparison with opiates which have been administered systemically. Because the vasomotor nerves are also blocked, epidural analgesia can cause severe orthostatic hypotension and these patients require careful monitoring of their blood pressure.

Patient-controlled analgesia

This technique enables patients to manage their own pain control. A predetermined bolus of morphine is delivered intravenously from a special pump that is activated by the patient. Overdosage is prevented by a 'lock-out' mechanism that prevents the patient reactivating the pump until a set time has elapsed. In each case, the bolus dose and lock-out time can be adjusted to suit the individual patient's needs.

Oral or intravenous non-opioid analgesics

Many of these non-opioid analgesics can only be delivered by the oral route and require a functioning gastrointestinal tract to ensure absorption. Paracetamol is an exception and can be given intravenously or rectally. These drugs should be given on a regular rather than 'as required' basis to provide maximum benefit. If this regime is ineffective, weak opioid analgesics such as dihydrocodeine should be used either alone or as a compound analgesic preparation with paracetamol.

Non-steroidal anti-inflammatory drugs

These agents can be administered by intramuscular, rectal or oral routes. They are effective in relieving pain after minor surgery or for patients who have had major surgery and no longer require opioid therapy. Like paracetamol and other non-opioid analgesics they can be used in combination with opioids to reduce the dose of opioid required to relieve pain. NSAIDs are contraindicated in patients with a history of asthma or peptic ulcer disease and also in patients who are at risk of perioperative or postoperative bleeding as they interfere with platelet function.

Postoperative monitoring

Close observation of a patient's vital signs (pulse/blood pressure/temperature/respiration rate) and careful fluid balance will optimise recovery and enable early detection of impending complications.

In most surgical units there are three levels of postoperative monitoring activity and care:

- general surgical ward
- high dependency unit
- intensive care unit.

The majority of patients undergoing routine elective surgery will be recovered satisfactorily in an ordinary surgical ward. Others with intercurrent medical problems (see p. 3), undergoing epidural anaesthetic techniques (see p. 6) or who have undergone emergency major surgery may require more intensive monitoring. Many of these patients can be effectively managed on a high dependency surgical unit, which provides continuous pulse, blood pressure and oximetry measurements together with hourly fluid balance. The high dependency unit also provides a higher nurse/patient ratio than the general surgical ward.

Intensive care is reserved for those patients who require ventilation after surgery or who develop serious respiratory, cardiac or septic complications.

1.2 Postoperative complications

(see p. 3), (see p. 6)

Learning objectives

You should:

- recognise that prevention is better than cure. Many postoperative complications can be *avoided* by meticulous pre- and perioperative care.
- be able to diagnose and initiate primary treatment in any of the common postoperative surgical complications. Remember, prompt diagnosis and early intervention can prevent minor complications becoming catastrophes.

For most patients, postoperative recovery is uneventful and is characterised by a systematic return to normal function. Any deviation from this predicted course is a postoperative complication. Complications are sometimes unavoidable in critically ill patients who undergo urgent surgery. In healthy patients who undergo elective surgery, complications should be rare and may be avoided with careful pre- and perioperative care.

Pulmonary problems

Respiratory complications are the most frequent and are common to all surgical procedures. Suspect a respiratory complication in any patient with:

- respiratory rate <10 or >25 breaths/min
- pulse rate >100 beats/min
- reduced conscious level
- SpO$_2$ <92% measured by pulse oximetery.

Atelectasis and pneumonia

Inadequate ventilation of small pulmonary airways plus retention of respiratory secretions leads to alveolar collapse and atelectasis. If untreated, a secondary bacterial infection will supervene causing lobar or broncho-pneumonia. The most important predisposing factors are:

- smoking
- chronic obstructive airways disease (COAD)
- postoperative pain (inhibits respiratory effort and coughing).

Onset of these complications can be prevented preoperatively by:

- stopping smoking before surgery
- preoperative physiotherapy for patients with COAD
- deferring elective surgery for at least 2 weeks in patients with a chest infection.

An important intraoperative measure is the choice of incision. Respiratory complications are more frequent after vertical midline abdominal incisions than after transverse abdominal incisions.

Important postoperative measures are:

- adequate pain relief
- intensive physiotherapy.

Diagnosis and treatment

An early postoperative fever is caused by a respiratory complication until proved otherwise. After physical examination these patients should have arterial blood gas analysis, a sputum culture and ECG (to exclude an underlying cardiac event) plus a chest radiograph.

Oxygen therapy is the cornerstone of management and should be delivered via a nasal cannula or a face mask to maintain an oxygen saturation of >92% as measured by a pulse oximeter.

Pulmonary aspiration Supine posture and the absence of the normal protective reflexes during general anaesthesia predispose surgical patients to pulmonary aspiration. Regurgitated gastric contents usually enter the right main bronchus. Three groups are especially at risk:

- pregnant women
- patients with bowel obstruction
- non-fasted patients requiring urgent surgery.

The most important preventative measures are:

- preoperative nasogastric drainage
- an adequately fasted patient
- anaesthetic care using cricoid pressure to prevent aspiration during intubation and use of a cuffed endotracheal tube to prevent aspiration while the patient is paralysed and ventilated.

Postoperative respiratory depression

A respiratory rate less than 10 breaths/min is the hallmark of respiratory depression.

Immediate respiratory depression is caused by the persistent action of opiates or muscular relaxants administered during surgery, or by a massive pulmonary collapse. Respiratory depression later on in the postoperative period is usually caused by oversedation with opioid analgesic agents.

These complications can be prevented by careful prescribing practice and close monitoring of the conscious level and postoperative respiratory effort. A pulse oximeter will give an early indication of arterial desaturation.

Postoperative respiratory failure

Patients with severe intra-abdominal sepsis, fat embolus or those who have had a massive blood transfusion are at risk of developing adult respiratory distress syndrome (ARDS). Untreated, arterial hypoxaemia and carbon dioxide retention will be accompanied by a progressive radiological opacification of the lung fields (Figure 1). Without treatment these patients will develop irreversible pulmonary failure and will die. Their management is complex and depends upon:

- identifying and eliminating any treatable underlying cause
- intubation and mechanical ventilatory support.

Postoperative shock

Shock is defined as a failure to maintain adequate tissue perfusion. Hypotension, tachycardia, sweating, pallor and peripheral vasoconstriction are the hallmarks of hypovolaemic and cardiogenic shock. Without treatment, oliguria and multisystem organ failure develop and lead to death.

The precise clinical picture (Table 3) will depend on the underlying cause. The three main types of postoperative shock are:

- hypovolaemic
- septic
- cardiogenic.

Hypovolaemic shock

This is the most common type of postoperative shock. It may be caused by:

- inadequate replacement of pre- or perioperative fluid losses
- continued haemorrhage in the postoperative period.

Treatment

Careful fluid balance will prevent most cases of hypovolaemic shock. Ongoing haemorrhage may be obvious from

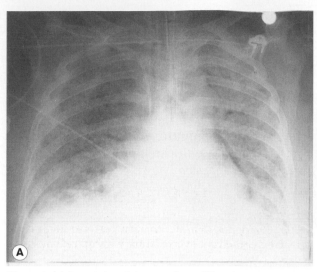
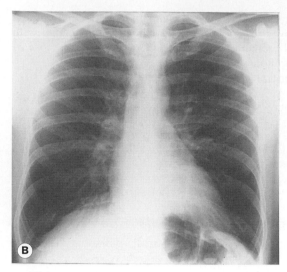

Figure 1 Adult respiratory distress syndrome (**A**); and a normal chest radiograph (**B**) for comparison.

Table 3 A comparison of the key clinical features in hypovolaemic, cardiogenic and septic shock

	Normal	Hypovolaemic shock	Cardiogenic shock	Septic shock	
				Early	Late
Pulse rate (beats/min)	72	>100	40–120, regular or irregular	>100	>100
Jugular venous pressure (cmH₂O)	5–10	0–5 or negative	>10	0–5 or negative	0–5 or negative
Skin	–	Cold, clammy	Cold, clammy	Warm	Cold, clammy
Blood pressure (mmHg)	120/80	<100 systolic	<100 systolic	Normal, or <100 systolic	<100 systolic
Urine output (ml/h)	30	<30	<30	30	<30

a chest drain but is less clear after abdominal surgery, when large volumes of blood can collect unnoticed in the abdomen. A careful judgement may be required by the surgeon with regard to the need for reoperation.

The essential management points are:

Replacement Replace the circulating volume and extracellular fluid losses with a combination of whole blood and a balanced salt solution.

Monitor Monitor the response:

- blood pressure and pulse rate (aim to restore preoperative values)
- urine output (keep at 30 ml/h; 0.5–1 ml/kg/h)
- establish central venous pressure measurement (aim for values between 5 and 10 cm water).

Appraisal Think about re-operation if ongoing haemorrhage is suspected.

Septic shock

The most frequent causes of septic shock in the postoperative patient are listed in Table 4. Early septic shock is characterised by a hyperdynamic circulation with fevers, rigors, a warm vasodilated periphery and a bounding pulse. Untreated, late septic shock supervenes with hypotension, peripheral vasoconstriction and anuria.

Table 4 Major causes of postoperative fever and sepsis

Day 1	Atelectasis, chest infection
Day 5	Wound infection
Days 7–10	Intra-abdominal sepsis, thromboembolism
Any day	Catheter or i.v. line sepsis

The essential points of management are:

Assessment Identify and remedy any underlying cause: this may involve anything from changing an infected central venous line to re-operation for intra-abdominal sepsis.

Antibiotic therapy Implement broad-spectrum aerobic and anaerobic antibiotic therapy after an infection screen and blood/sputum/urine culture.

Monitor and support Instigate intensive monitoring plus fluid therapy and respiratory and renal function support to prevent multisystem organ failure.

Cardiogenic shock

This is usually secondary to acute myocardial ischaemia or infarction causing left ventricular failure or a rhythm disturbance. In patients with pre-existing cardiac disease, fluid overload may induce cardiac failure.

In addition to poor peripheral perfusion, these patients will have an elevated jugular venous pressure, basal crepitations and a gallop cardiac rhythm plus acute electrocardiographic changes.

The essential management points are:

Control fluid overload Establish a diuresis to remove fluid overload.

Monitor Instigate invasive monitoring of cardiac function (CVP or Swann–Ganz catheter).

Drug therapy Use vasoactive or inotropic drugs to optimise myocardial efficiency.

Oxygen therapy Maintain an oxygen saturation above 92%.

Wound complications

The two most important wound complications are:

- wound infection
- wound dehiscence.

Wound infection

This is one of the most frequent surgical postoperative complications. It is seen least in clean elective surgical wounds (e.g. inguinal hernia repair) and most often in contaminated wounds (e.g. perforated diverticular disease).

The main factors in reducing the risk of wound infection are surgical technique and aseptic care.

Meticulous surgical technique:
- minimise tissue trauma
- preserve wound blood supply
- prevent wound haematoma.

Prevention of wound contamination:
- perioperative antibiotic prophylaxis
- good surgical technique.

Wound infections present with a fever on about the fifth postoperative day. Inspection of the wound site reveals tenderness, erythema and induration. An infected wound should be opened widely to enable release of any contained pus and the wound packed loosely with gauze to ensure adequate drainage. Antibiotics have only a secondary role in wound sepsis and are not a substitute for surgical drainage. After treatment, these wounds should be left to heal by secondary intention.

Wound dehiscence

A wound dehiscence is a failure of wound healing. Although any wound can dehisce, it usually affects abdominal wounds (burst abdomen), which disrupt usually 7–10 days after surgery, leaking serosanguinous fluid and then revealing the viscera.

The two most important groups of factors predisposing to wound dehiscence are poor surgical technique and impaired wound healing.

Iatrogenic (poor surgical technique):
- tight sutures causing wound ischaemia
- suture breakage.

Patient-related (poor wound healing)
This occurs more often in patients at increased risk:

- malnourished patients
- septic patients
- patients with inoperable malignancy
- morbidly obese patients
- jaundiced patients.

Treatment Re-exploration and resuture of the wound under general anaesthesia is essential. Dehiscence rarely recurs.

Urinary problems and postoperative renal failure

Acute urinary retention and urinary tract infection are the most common postoperative urinary complications.

Acute urinary retention

There are three major predisposing factors:

- preoperative history of symptoms of bladder outflow obstruction
- postoperative immobility
- postoperative pain.

Retention may be prevented by selective perioperative catheterisation of at-risk patients, e.g. those with symptoms of prostatic outflow obstruction or who are undergoing major abdominal or perineal surgery.

Urinary tract infection

Postcatheterisation urinary tract infection is usually caused by:

- a breakdown in sterile technique during catheter insertion
- contamination of the catheter drainage system.

Infection can be difficult to eradicate. The choice of antibiotics is dictated by the results of urine culture. Prompt removal of the catheter as soon as the patient is ambulant will reduce the frequency of infection.

Postoperative renal failure

Acute renal failure can be:

- prerenal
- renal
- postrenal.

Prerenal failure
Underperfusion of the kidneys is the final common pathway. This is usually caused by inadequate fluid balance during the pre- and perioperative period or by continued haemorrhage and fluid losses that have been overlooked. The management is outlined on p. 4.

Renal failure
Uncorrected prerenal failure will eventually cause acute parenchymal renal failure. Other important causes are:

- incompatible blood transfusion
- myoglobinuria from a soft tissue crush injury

One

- septic shock
- hepatorenal syndrome (renal failure associated with obstructive jaundice).

Treatment Wherever possible, any underlying cause is treated. Haemodialysis may be necessary until renal function recovers.

Postrenal failure

The two most important causes of postrenal failure are:

- catheter blockage
- ureteric ligation.

Catheter blockage is easily treated. Unilateral ureteric ligation is usually silent and the remaining kidney compensates. Bilateral ligation is rare but may occur in patients who have undergone a difficult surgical dissection in the pelvis. Surgical reintervention will be required.

Thromboembolic disorders

The pathogenesis of venous thrombosis involves stasis, increased blood coagulability and damage to the blood vessel wall (Virchow's triad). Prevention of deep vein thrombosis or early detection of an established thrombosis is essential in order to prevent death from pulmonary embolus. Despite all current measures, 1 in 200 patients undergoing major surgery will die from pulmonary embolus.

Deep vein thrombosis

Most deep vein thromboses start in an area of venous stasis, usually in the calf veins. Local vascular damage and hypercoagulability caused by surgical stress also contribute. The following factors increase the risk of thrombosis:

- patient-related factors
  - increasing age, obesity
  - oral contraception
  - prolonged postoperative immobility
  - smoking
  - pregnancy
- disease-related factors
  - malignancy
  - recent myocardial infarction
- procedure-related factors
  - long operation time
  - limb or hip surgery
  - intra-abdominal pelvic dissection.

Diagnosis

A deep vein thrombosis may be clinically silent or present with a painful, tender swollen calf. It may be a cause of postoperative fever. The diagnosis is confirmed by:

- Doppler ultrasonography
- venography.

Prophylaxis

Stopping smoking before surgery and losing weight, if appropriate, will help reduce the risk of deep vein thrombosis. Each patient's prophylaxis regime should be optimised to minimise their risk of developing a thrombosis. A combination of graduated full-length elastic calf compression stockings plus pre- and perioperative cover with low-dose subcutaneous heparin injections effectively reduces the incidence of deep vein thrombosis *and* fatal pulmonary embolus. During surgery, pneumatic calf compression devices or foot pumps can be used to prevent venous stasis in patients at high risk of thrombosis.

Treatment

An established deep vein thrombosis is treated by immediate full anticoagulation using a continuous intravenous heparin infusion and simultaneous oral anticoagulation with warfarin. Heparin therapy is stopped once the patient is on full oral anticoagulation, which is then continued for 3–6 months.

Pulmonary embolism

Most pulmonary emboli arise from a propagated clot which detaches and embolises from the iliac or femoral veins. The clinical presentation depends on the size of the embolus:

- massive embolus: circulatory collapse, cardiac arrest and death
- small embolus: pleuritic chest pain, haemoptysis, cyanosis, pleural friction rub, tachycardia, tachypnoea, right heart failure
- recurrent embolus: progressive dyspnoea.

Diagnosis

Confirming the diagnosis, particularly if the embolus is small, can be difficult. The following features are usually present either alone or in combination:

- arterial hypoxia
- electrocardiographic changes (S waves, lead 1; Q waves and T wave inversion in lead 3)
- chest radiograph may be normal or show reduced pulmonary vascular markings
- a mismatched defect on isotope ventilation/perfusion scanning
- computed tomography (CT) angiography will demonstrate the embolus in the pulmonary artery.

Treatment

The key steps in the treatment of pulmonary emboli are:

- supplemental oxygen therapy
- systemic anticoagulation

Most pulmonary emboli will be satisfactorily treated by these measures.

- surgery: although urgent thoracotomy and open embolectomy for a massive embolus may be lifesaving, it is rarely feasible; transvenous embolectomy using a special suction catheter introduced via the femoral vein is sometimes successful. Filters can be placed into the inferior vena cava using radiological techniques to prevent recurrent emboli.

Postoperative intra-abdominal sepsis

Postoperative sepsis is usually caused by anastomotic breakdown or a failure to eradicate infection at the original laparotomy. The infection is either generalised (peritonitis) or localised (intra-abdominal abscess) and can be extremely difficult to diagnose. It should be suspected in any patient who develops signs of sepsis 7–10 days after a laparotomy.

Diagnosis

Investigations include:

- contrast radiology: using a water soluble contrast agent (gastrograffin) to detect any anastomotic leak
- ultrasound or CT scan: to detect any abnormal intra-abdominal fluid collections or abscess
- laparotomy: should be undertaken if doubt remains despite negative radiology.

Treatment

Postoperative intra-abdominal abscess can be drained percutaneously using interventional radiology techniques under antibiotic cover. If infection is widespread, causing generalised peritonitis, laparotomy and drainage is usually required with exteriorisation of any disrupted anastomosis. Overall mortality rates are high (up to 50%) for this serious complication.

Self-assessment: questions

Extended matching items questions (EMIs)

EMI 1

Theme: Postoperative complications – respiratory

A. pleural effusion

B. pulmonary embolus

C. aspiration pneumonia

D. tension pneumothorax

E. narcotic overdose

F. adult respiratory distress syndrome (ARDS)

G. empyema thoracis

For each patient described below select the most likely diagnosis from the list above.

1. A 47-year-old woman who is morbidly obese suddenly becomes breathless 6 days after an emergency open cholecystectomy and common bile duct exploration. She looks cyanosed and has bloodstained sputum.

2. An 83-year-old man undergoes an urgent laparotomy for large bowel obstruction. The following day he is febrile with a temperature of 39.5°C. The only abnormality you can detect is reduced air entry and percussion dullness in the right hemithorax.

3. You are asked to review a 21-year-old man who is 12 h post laparotomy for a perforated duodenal ulcer. The nursing staff are concerned because he has a respiratory rate of 8. On examination he has reduced air entry in both lung fields and is poorly responsive.

EMI 2

Theme: Surgical principles – nutrition

A. high-protein, high-calorie drink supplements

B. feeding gastrostomy

C. light diet and fluid restriction

D. feeding jejunostomy

E. nasogastric tube feeding

F. total parenteral nutrition

G. elemental/low residue diet

Select the most appropriate option from the list above for nutritional support in the following patients.

1. A patient with long-standing Crohn's disease who has recently developed a low output distal small bowel enterocutaneous fistula.

2. A 45-year-old man who has sustained multiple trauma after a road traffic accident. He has a major head and chest injury in addition to a fractured femur. He is admitted to the intensive care unit and judged to require a 7–10-day period of nutritional support.

3. A 70-year-old man who has an oesophagectomy which is complicated by an anastomotic leak.

EMI 3

Theme: Postoperative management – oliguria/anuria

A. add 2 l 5% dextrose to the daily intravenous fluid regime

B. add 2 l normal saline or Hartmann's solution to the daily intravenous fluid regime

C. urinary catheterisation

D. intravenous frusemide

E. administer desmopressin

F. commence renal dose dopamine infusion

From the list above select the most appropriate management for the following surgical patients with oliguria/anuria after surgery.

1. A 74-year-old man has passed only a small quantity of urine 24 h after an inguinal hernia repair. He has a tender suprapubic mass on abdominal examination.

2. A 70-year-old woman is 4 days post right hemicolectomy. She appears breathless and has bilateral basal crepitations on auscultation. Reviewing her fluid charts you see that her urine output for the last 24 h was less than 1000 ml. She has a 3-l positive fluid balance over the last 3 days.

3. A 61-year-old man has undergone an elective aorto-bifemoral bypass graft for severe claudication. He develops a postoperative ileus which is treated conservatively. His nasogastric aspirate is approximately 2 l each 24 h. He has passed only 500 ml urine in the last 12 h.

EMI 4

Theme: Fluid balance

	5% dextrose (ml)	0.9% normal saline (ml)	Added potassium (mmol/l)
A.	2000	500	20
B.	500	2000	40
C.	2000	500	40
D.	2500	500	40
E.	2000	500	80
F.	2000	2000	20
G.	2000	2000	60
H.	3500	500	60

Select the most appropriate fluid regime for the following patients.

1. A febrile patient with a chest infection after an appendicectomy.
2. A previously healthy 40-year-old male requiring starvation for an elective orthopaedic procedure.
3. A patient on the second postoperative day after elective colonic surgery whose serum potassium is 2.9 mmol/l.
4. A 57-year-old woman admitted with a 2-day history of vomiting. You make a clinical diagnosis of adhesive small bowel obstruction. She looks dehydrated and has a serum potassium level of 3.1 mmol/l.

EMI 5

Theme: Pain control

A. epidural analgesia
B. wound infiltration with local anaesthetic
C. patient-controlled analgesia
D. ring block
E. intravenous paracetamol
F. rectal non-steroidal analgesics
G. oral paracetamol
H. oral non-steroidal analgesics

For each of the scenarios described below, select the most suitable method of pain control from the list above. Each option may be used once, more than once or not at all.

1. A previously fit 46-year-old woman who has just undergone an open cholecystectomy for acute cholecystitis. The surgeons were unable to perform the procedure using the laparoscope because of the severity of the inflammation.
2. A 76-year-old man who has undergone a Whipple's resection for pancreatic cancer. He has a previous history of chronic obstructive airways disease.
3. A 60-year-old woman who is recovering from an oesophagectomy and has not yet resumed her oral intake. She has a previous history of peptic ulcer disease. She is using a patient-controlled analgesic pump but is still complaining of abdominal pain.

Constructed response questions (CRQs)

CRQ 1

You are called to see a patient in the middle of the night. He is a 72-year-old man who had an emergency partial gastrectomy for a bleeding gastric ulcer 6 h previously. The nursing staff are concerned because he has not passed any urine for 2 h.

a. On the way to the ward you consider the most likely causes. Name two of these.

When you reach the patient you note that he has a systolic blood pressure of 90 mmHg.

b. The patient has a history of angina. What two important physical signs would support a diagnosis of cardiac failure?

Your physical examination does not support this diagnosis. You think the patient might be hypovolaemic.

c. List three important physical signs in keeping with this diagnosis.
d. What are the two most likely causes of hypovolaemia in this patient?
e. How would you manage this patient? List three important steps.
f. List three parameters you would use to assess the effectiveness of your resuscitation. What values would you be aiming for?

CRQ 2

You are asked to see a 61-year-old man who has developed a fever of 38.4°C 7 days after an anterior resection.

a. On your way to the patient you consider the possible causes. List the three that are most likely.

The patient looks quite unwell. You take a history from him and he describes a sudden onset of severe lower abdominal pain several hours ago. It is worse when he moves. Up until this point his recovery had been uneventful.

b. Describe two physical signs you would look for on abdominal examination.

In addition to abdominal signs you think the patient might be septic.

c. Name three other physical signs you would look for in addition to fever.
d. Outline four key steps in the initial management of this patient.
e. How would you confirm your suspected diagnosis?

CRQ 3

You are asked to review a 67-year-old woman the day after a hip replacement. The nursing staff are concerned because she has an oxygen saturation of 87% measured by pulse oximetry.

a. What is the significance of this reading?

When you reach the bedside you notice that the patient appears confused and has a respiratory rate of 30 breaths/min.

b. List three possible causes for this patient's symptoms.

Your physical examination records a reduced air entry in the left lung base and mid zone. You notice she has a temperature of 38.5°C. You decide to organise a chest radiograph.

c. What other key investigations would you arrange for this patient? List three.

The chest radiograph shows extensive shadowing in both lung bases and mid zones.

d. Outline four important steps in this patient's management.

Objective structured clinical examination questions (OSCEs)

OSCE 1

Compare ECG tracing A and B (Figure 2). Tracing A is from a preoperative ECG in a 52-year-old man undergoing a right hemicolectomy for Crohn's disease. He makes a good recovery until postoperative day 8 when he is found collapsed in the bathroom. Tracing B was taken from the same patient shortly after the syncopal episode.

a. What are the abnormalities on tracing B?
b. What is the most likely diagnosis?
c. What physical signs might you find?
d. How would you confirm the diagnosis?
e. How would you treat this patient?

OSCE 2

Examine this postoperative monitoring chart (Figure 3). It records a male patient's progress on postoperative day 8 following repair of a fractured neck of femur.

a. Describe the abnormalities recorded at 07.00 hours.
b. Name two possible causes for these changes.
c. What bedside test might help you to confirm the diagnosis?
d. What investigations would you organise?

OSCE 3

Look at this chest radiograph (Figure 4), which has been taken three days after a major laparotomy.

a. What is the key abnormality?
b. What is the radiological diagnosis?

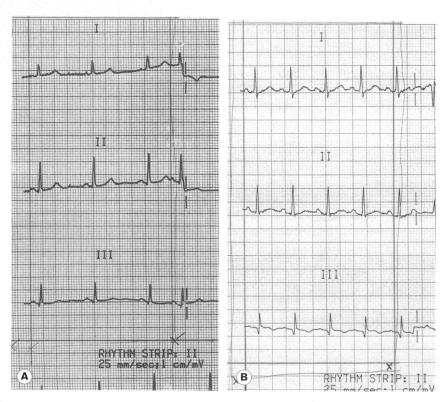

Figure 2 ECG tracing.

c. What blood gas abnormalities might this patient have?

d. Name three causes of this condition.

e. How should this patient be managed?

Best of 5s questions

1. A 28-year-old man presents with recurrent Crohn's disease. He has previously had multiple small bowel resections and has 150 cm of small intestine left. On this occasion he has been admitted with an enterocutaneous fistula. Which of the following options would provide the most suitable nutritional support?

   a. naso-jejunal tube feeding

   b. parenteral nutrition delivered via a standard grey cannula

   c. a feeding jejunostomy

   d. oral supplementation using high-protein high-calorie drinks

   e. parenteral nutrition delivered via a tunnelled central venous catheter

2. You have been asked to review a male patient who, 1 h ago, underwent a difficult urethral catheterisation. You are concerned that he might be developing septic shock after this traumatic procedure. Which set of clinical features outlined in the table below are most in keeping with a diagnosis of early septic shock?

Multiple choice questions

1. The following are contraindications to major elective surgery requiring general anaesthesia:

   a. a myocardial infarction 12 months ago

   b. a preoperative serum potassium of 2.6 mmol/l in a patient on diuretic therapy

   c. previous mitral valve replacement

   d. a resolving upper respiratory tract infection

   e. unsuspected glycosuria on routine ward urine testing

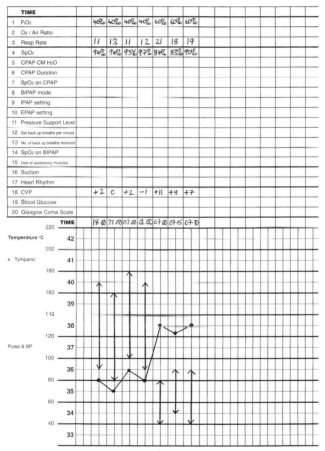

Figure 3

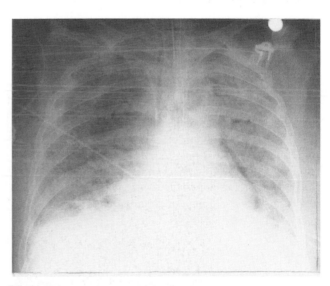

Figure 4

	Pulse rate (beats/min)	Jugular venous pressure (cmH$_2$0)	Skin	Blood pressure (mm Hg)	Urine output (ml/h)
a.	>100	0–5 or negative	Cold, clammy	<100 systolic	<30
b.	70	5–10	Normal	120/80	30
c.	120	>10	Cold, clammy	<100 systolic	<30
d.	>100	0–5 or negative	Warm	Normal or <100	30
e.	>100	0–5 or negative	Cold, clammy	<100 systolic	<30

2. The following statements concerning fluid and electrolyte balance are correct:
   a. nasogastric aspirates should be replaced volume for volume with 5% dextrose solution
   b. 100 mmol potassium are required each day to replace baseline losses
   c. long-standing fluid deficits should be replaced within the first 24 h
   d. insensible losses are unchanged by fever
   e. a total daily intravenous fluid intake of 1500 ml will maintain baseline fluid requirements in a normal individual

3. Enteral nutrition is:
   a. highly thrombogenic
   b. used in patients with the short gut syndrome
   c. a potential cause of abdominal cramps and diarrhoea
   d. more likely to cause septic complications than parenteral nutrition
   e. contraindicated in patients after a cerebrovascular accident

4. The following features are in keeping with a postoperative opiate overdose:
   a. hyperventilation
   b. mydriasis
   c. hypotension
   d. tachycardia
   e. hypoxaemia

5. Venous thromboembolism prophylaxis is required in:
   a. a 24-year-old woman undergoing appendicectomy who uses oral contraception
   b. a 50-year-old woman with rectal cancer requiring anterior resection
   c. an 80-year-old man requiring hip replacement
   d. a 50-year-old woman undergoing palliative bypass for inoperable pancreatic cancer
   e. a 40-year-old man undergoing inguinal hernia repair

6. The following statements concern cardiogenic shock:
   a. it can be distinguished from hypovolaemic shock by central venous blood pressure measurements
   b. it can be distinguished from hypovolaemic shock by systemic blood pressure recordings
   c. it responds to a fluid challenge
   d. it responds to inotropic support
   e. it is a cause of postoperative oliguria

7. The following features are in keeping with a major pulmonary embolus:
   a. a matched defect on isotopic ventilation/perfusion scanning
   b. pleuritic pain and haemoptysis
   c. peripheral but not central cyanosis
   d. tachypnoea
   e. ECG evidence of left ventricular strain

8. An abdominal wound dehiscence:
   a. usually occurs before the fifth postoperative day
   b. frequently recurs
   c. is often fatal
   d. is more common in jaundiced patients
   e. is increased in patients on steroid therapy

9. Aspiration pneumonia:
   a. most commonly affects the left upper lobe
   b. is more frequent following emergency than elective surgery
   c. is less likely if cricoid pressure is used during intubation
   d. is aggravated by gastric acidity
   e. is less common in patients with reflux oesophagitis

10. Postoperative atelectasis is more common in:
    a. smokers
    b. patients undergoing lower abdominal surgery
    c. obstructed patients
    d. the period between the fifth and tenth postoperative days
    e. oversedated patients

Self-assessment: answers

EMI answers

EMI 1

Theme: Postoperative complications – respiratory

1. B. Pulmonary embolus.

This patient presents many of the classic features of a pulmonary embolus – sudden onset dyspnoea, cyanosis and bloodstained sputum. In addition the timing is 'right' – about a week after major surgery. The patient also has at least one risk factor for a pulmonary embolus: she is obese.

2. C. Aspiration pneumonia.

Postoperative chest infections are common. Anaesthesia, postoperative pain, pre-existing lung disease and smoking are all important risk factors and are common to many patients. This patient has an additional risk factor: he has undergone emergency surgery for an intestinal obstruction. In these patients there is always a risk of regurgitation of gastric contents during the perioperative period despite anaesthetic precautions and the use of a nasogastric tube. The right lung is more susceptible because the anatomy of the right main bronchus (almost vertical) will direct aspirated material preferentially into that lung field. Always think of aspiration in an obstructed patient with an early postoperative pneumonia.

3. E. Narcotic overdose.

The low respiratory rate and depressed conscious state are the hallmarks of a narcotic overdose. Look for other signs such as constricted pupils. It can be difficult to titrate the correct dose of opiate that will relieve pain and not cause oversedation.

EMI 2

Theme: Surgical principles – nutrition

1. G. Elemental/low residue diet.

Wherever possible the patient's own gastrointestinal tract should be used for nutrition. An elemental/low-residue diet should be almost completely absorbed by the time the distal small bowel is reached. Provided there is no intestinal obstruction beyond the fistula site (which would prevent the fistula from healing) this diet should provide optimum conditions for the fistula to heal without surgery by reducing the output of the fistula and providing nutritional support for the patient.

2. E. Nasogastric tube feeding.

In this patient there has been no disturbance to the gastrointestinal tract and this route should be used for nutrition delivery. A nasogastric tube is an ideal short-term delivery system under these circumstances and can be used until the patient is well enough to feed himself. A feeding gastrostomy would be useful in this type of patient if long-term nutritional support was required.

3. F. Total parenteral nutrition.

This is the most obvious choice. Total restriction of oral intake is a key step in the management of a patient with an oesophageal leak in order to 'rest' the anastomosis and prevent further contamination of the mediastinum with food debris. Any attempt to pass a nasogastric tube risks further damage to the oesophageal anastomosis and must be avoided.

EMI 3

Theme: Postoperative management – oliguria/anuria

1. C. Urinary catheterisation.

Until proven otherwise this patient has developed urinary retention. It is especially common in elderly men after hernia repair. The combination of postoperative discomfort plus any pre-existing bladder outflow obstruction which is frequent in this age group will be sufficient to precipitate urinary retention.

2. D. Intravenous frusemide.

The clinical features suggest cardiac failure with pulmonary oedema. Look for other signs as well, for example ankle and sacral pitting oedema. In this case the cause would appear to be fluid overload.

3. B. Add 2 l normal saline or Hartmann's solution to the daily intravenous fluid regime.

A postoperative ileus interferes with the absorptive function of the small intestine. As a result large volumes of fluid can be sequestered in the small intestine or lost through vomit or nasogastric aspirate. These patients can become severely fluid depleted and as a consequence have a poor urine output. The intestinal fluid that is lost is rich in electrolytes and should be replaced volume for volume by normal saline or Hartmann's solution to maintain fluid balance. If 5% dextrose is used these patients will become hyponatraemic.

EMI 4

Theme: Fluid balance

1. D. 2500 ml 5% dextrose/500 ml 0.9% normal saline/40 mmol potassium.

This regime incorporates an extra 500 ml of 5% dextrose over the normal 24-h daily requirements. This will make up for the extra evaporative losses through the skin caused by fever.

2. C. 2000 ml 5% dextrose/500 ml 0.9% normal saline/40 mmol potassium.

This is the baseline daily fluid requirement for a fit individual who is not allowed any oral fluid intake.

3. E. 2000 ml 5% dextrose/500 ml 0.9% normal saline/80 mmol potassium.

This fluid regime incorporates the baseline daily fluid requirements plus an extra 40 mmol potassium to replace this patient's depleted extracellular potassium.

4. G. 2000 ml 5% dextrose/2000 ml 0.9% normal saline/60 mmol potassium.

This fluid regime incorporates the baseline daily requirements plus an allowance (an extra 1500 ml of normal saline) to make up this patient's fluid depletion caused by obstruction together with an extra 20 mmol potassium to correct the hypokalaemia.

EMI 5

Theme: Pain control

1. C. Patient-controlled analgesia.

In a fit healthy patient who has undergone a laparotomy a patient-controlled analgesic system will provide adequate pain control. This can be supplemented, where necessary, by non-opioid analgesics or non-steroidal type drugs.

2. A. Epidural analgesia.

An elderly patient with pre-existing lung disease who undergoes major surgery is at high risk of developing postoperative respiratory complication. Epidural delivered postoperative analgesia provides optimum pain relief and reduces the incidence of postoperative respiratory complications because these patients are able to cough and expectorate and expand their lung bases fully to avoid atelectasis.

3. E. Intravenous paracetamol.

Non-opioid drugs and non-steroidal drugs can be used to augment analgesia in patients already using opiates. This patient has a history of peptic ulcer disease and non-steroidal agents are contraindicated. As her oral intake is restricted intravenous paracetamol would be the ideal choice.

CRQ answers

CRQ 1

a. Hypovolaemia.

  Blocked catheter.

Poor urine output in the early postoperative period is a frequent indicator of inadequate fluid replacement. Hypovolaemia should be your first thought; always consider ongoing haemorrhage as a possibility. Don't forget that simple problems such as a blocked catheter can confuse the picture.

b. Elevated jugular venous pressure.

  Symmetrical basal crepitations.

These are the most obvious and often the easiest physical signs of cardiac failure to detect. Look also for sacral or ankle oedema. The patient may also have a gallop cardiac rhythm.

c. Pallor.

  Poor capillary return.

  Tachycardia, thready pulse.

  Cold, clammy patient.

  External signs of ongoing blood loss (e.g. fresh blood from a nasogastric tube or drain).

Any three responses from this list would score marks.

These are all features of hypovolaemia. Don't forget to look for obvious evidence of ongoing blood loss (e.g. from a nasogastric tube) and remember that the peritoneal cavity can sequester several litres of blood without any obvious external sign.

d. Ongoing haemorrhage.

  Under-replacement of blood/crystalloid in the perioperative fluid regime.

These are the most likely causes. If there is ongoing bleeding, the response to resuscitation is likely to be temporary and definitive surgical intervention will be required.

e. Fluid resuscitation using colloid or whole blood.

  Call early for senior help if you suspect ongoing blood loss.

  Consider the need for CVP measurement.

In the early postoperative period, hypovolaemia usually responds best to replacement with colloid or whole blood. If the patient does not respond to simple measures or if you suspect ongoing blood loss call your seniors early for help. A central venous line will enable you to monitor the response to treatment and is best inserted once fluid resuscitation is under way. In this way resuscitation is not delayed and placement of the line is often easier once the central veins have begun to distend in response to volume replacement.

f. Pulse and blood pressure, aim to restore preoperative values.

  Urine output, greater than 30 ml/h.

  CVP readings, between 5 and 10 cm water.

These are the key parameters. Failure to respond or reach these values after 1–2 l of fluid resuscitation may be an indication of internal bleeding requiring reoperation.

CRQ 2

a. Wound infection.

  Anastomotic leak.

  Chest infection.

  DVT.

  Intravenous line or catheter sepsis.

Any three of these responses would score marks. This list incorporates the major causes of sepsis in any postoperative patient. All should be considered and discarded in each patient as appropriate.

b. Evidence of peritonism – percussion or rebound tenderness.

  Guarding and rigidity.

  Reduced or absent bowel sounds.

Any two of these responses would score marks.

  This patient's history points to a sudden catastrophic postoperative intra-abdominal event. Aggravation of his pain by movement suggests he may have peritonitis. Percussion or rebound tenderness, guarding and rigidity would support this diagnosis. Bowel sounds are frequently reduced or absent in this condition, but *occasionally* they may be normal. If all the features on clinical examination point to a postoperative peritonitis this is the diagnosis irrespective of the presence or absence of bowel sounds.

c. Tachycardia.

Facial flushing.

Tachypnoea.

Signs of early sepsis (bounding pulse, normotensive, brisk capillary return) or late sepsis (weak pulse, hypotension, poor capillary return).

Any three of these responses would score marks. These are all signs of systemic sepsis. They indicate the need for aggressive treatment of the underlying condition.

d. Blood cultures and broad-spectrum intravenous antibiotic therapy (including anaerobic cover).

Parenteral analgesia.

Intravenous fluid resuscitation.

Up-to-date haematology and biochemistry and blood cross-match, in case the patient requires urgent surgery.

These steps will cover all the key management issues for this patient.

Systemic antibiotics will help combat sepsis and must be delivered intravenously. The intravenous route will ensure that therapeutic levels are quickly achieved. Oral antibiotics will not be absorbed in this patient, who has compromised intestinal function. Similarly, oral or intra-muscular routes of delivery are inappropriate routes of delivery for analgesia as absorption will be haphazard.

Major intra-abdominal sepsis is always associated with increased fluid losses. These can usually be replaced by crystalloid (normal saline) and most patients will require a variable amount of fluid resuscitation. As it is likely this patient will require a surgical intervention to deal with the postoperative intra-abdominal sepsis, up-to-date haema-tology and biochemistry will provide a guide to any trans-fusion or biochemical correction that might be required prior to or during surgery.

e. Water soluble contrast enema.

This is the key investigation. The primary cause for post-operative peritonitis in patients who have undergone intestinal resection and anastomosis is an anastomotic leak. Anterior resection is particularly prone to this complication because of the relatively poor blood supply to the rectal stump and distal colon that are used to create this anastomosis. A water soluble contrast medium (such as gastrograffin) is used for safety reasons. If the test is positive and an anastomotic leak is confirmed the con-trast medium will leak harmlessly into the peritoneal cavity. If barium had been used it would provoke an intense inflammatory reaction in the peritoneal cavity at the leak site.

CRQ 3

a. This patient is hypoxic and may be developing respiratory complications.

b. Atelectasis.

Pneumonia.

Respiratory failure.

Fat embolus.

Pulmonary embolus.

Any three of these answers will score marks. They are the commonest causes of hypoxia in a patient in the early postoperative period. Fat embolus must be considered in the orthopaedic patient especially after lower limb surgery or trauma. Pulmonary embolus is less common this early after surgery but may occur in patients who have been bedridden for some days prior to operation.

b. Arterial blood gas.

ECG.

Sputum culture.

An arterial blood gas is an essential step in the assessment of any hypoxic patient. It will accurately determine whether the patient is retaining carbon dioxide, the degree of respiratory failure and whether or not there is an acid–base imbalance.

All patients who are being investigated for respiratory complications should have an ECG to rule out a cardiac event (such as a myocardial infarction), which may be the underlying cause.

Sputum culture will help plan an appropriate antibiotic regime. It should be taken before therapy is commenced so that the treatment does not interfere with the culture result.

c. Oxygen therapy.

Pain control.

Physiotherapy.

Antibiotic therapy.

Nasal cannulae or a variety of masks can be used to deliver up to 60–70% oxygen to a patient. Care must be taken in patients with chronic obstructive airways disease as they have chronic CO_2 retention and are dependent upon a hypoxic drive to maintain their respiratory effort. The oxygen delivery only should be slowly increased in these patients usually to a maximum of 35%.

Adequate pain control is essential. It should be suffi-cient to relieve pain but not cause respiratory depression. Epidural analgesia is ideal.

Physiotherapy will help with retained secretions or any major lobar collapse which is compromising ventilation.

Antibiotics should be administered as this patient is febrile. The choice is usually dictated by local protocols and can be modified if necessary when the results of the sputum cultures are available.

OSCE answers

OSCE 1

a. ECG B shows S waves in lead I and Q waves in lead III and inverted T waves in lead III.

b. These changes are in keeping with a right heart strain secondary to a pulmonary embolus.

c. Tachycardia and tachypnoea are common but non-specific signs. Look for a pleural friction rub, evidence of pleuritic chest pain or haemoptysis; examine the calves for evidence of a deep vein thrombosis.

d. The diagnosis would be confirmed by demonstrating a mismatched ventilation/perfusion defect on V/Q scanning or by CT angiogram.

e. Full systematic anticoagulation is required either with intravenous heparin by continuous infusion or by using fractionated heparin using a single daily therapeutic does given by subcutaneous injection. Both should be followed by 3–6 months of oral anticoagulation with warfarin.

OSCE 2

a. This patient drops his blood pressure to 80 mmHg systolic and develops a tachycardia of 130 beats/min. His CVP increases acutely to +11 cmH$_2$O and he becomes hypoxic with an oxygen saturation of 84%.

b. These changes are in keeping with acute heart failure or a major pulmonary embolus.

c. An ECG would be a useful investigation which might show the acute changes in keeping with a right heart strain secondary to a pulmonary embolus (See OSCE 1) or it may show evidence of a myocardial infarction or a rhythm disturbance.

d. A chest radiograph and arterial blood gas analysis would be important baseline investigations in this patient. Measuring the troponin T level would detect a myocardial infarction. The patient needs an urgent V/Q scan or a CT pulmonary angiogram in order to detect a pulmonary embolus.

OSCE 3

a. A diffuse patchy pulmonary infiltrate affecting both lung fields.

b. Adult respiratory distress syndrome

c. This patient would be hypoxic and may have carbon dioxide retention. The patient would be acidotic

d. Severe intra-abdominal sepsis

   Massive blood transfusion

   Fat embolism

e. Any underlying cause should be treated where possible. A search should be made for any underlying surgical sepsis. Otherwise the treatment is supportive aiming to maintain fluid balance, kidney function and tissue perfusion. Intubation and mechanical ventilatory support is the vital step in maintaining adequate tissue oxygenation. These patients are gravely ill.

Best of 5s answers

1. e. Parenteral nutrition delivered via a tunnelled central venous catheter.

This patient has a short gastrointestinal tract because of previous Crohn's surgery. He also has an entero-cutaneous fistula. Together these conditions limit the absorptive capacity of the small intestine. As a result, this patient requires parenteral nutrition which has to be delivered via a central vein. Parenteral nutrition administered via a standard grey cannula would rapidly cause thrombophlebitis.

2. d.

	Pulse rate (beats/min)	Jugular venous pressure (cmH$_2$0)	Skin	Blood pressure (mmHg)	Urine output (ml/h)
d.	>100	0–5 or negative	Warm	Normal or <100	30

These are the classic features of early septic shock. At this stage, the circulation is hyperdynamic with a bounding full pulse, adequate urine output and warm peripheral circulation. These patients may look deceptively well and require aggressive early treatment with antibiotics and specific treatment of the cause of the underlying infection. If these steps are neglected this patient will slip into irreversible septic shock with hypotension and renal failure.

Multiple choice answers

1. a. **False.** Elective surgery should be postponed for at least 6 months after a myocardial infarction. Thereafter, the risk of reinfarction is about 5%.

   b. **True.** The normal serum potassium ranges from 3.5–5.5 mmol/l. This patient is hypokalaemic (2.6 mmol/l) and is at risk of cardiac arrhythmia if anaesthesia is induced. The hypokalaemia should be corrected by slow intravenous potassium infusion over 24–48 h before proceeding to surgery.

   c. **False.** Patients with previous valvular heart surgery are usually fit enough to undergo surgery. They do require antibiotic prophylaxis to prevent endocarditis, and careful fluid balance to prevent fluid overload, together with close monitoring and a temporary reduction of any anticoagulant therapy.

   d. **True.** Patients with evidence of an upper respiratory infection preoperatively who undergo surgery are at risk of developing major respiratory postoperative complications. Elective surgery should be deferred until any infection is completely resolved.

   e. **True.** This may be the first indication of diabetes in an asymptomatic patient. Surgery tends to promote insulin resistance and may precipitate a diabetic coma in a previously undiagnosed diabetic. If unsuspected glycosuria is detected surgery should be deferred until the diagnosis of diabetes has been confirmed or excluded.

2. a. **False.** Nasogastric aspirates contain large amounts of sodium, potassium and chloride ions in addition to other elements. Nasogastric losses should be replaced volume for volume by 0.9% saline solution with added potassium or by a balanced salt solution (Hartmann's or Ringer's solution).

   b. **False.** Daily potassium requirements average 40 mmol/l.

   c. **False.** Patients with long-standing fluid losses may be deficient of 5 or more litres of extracellular fluid. This should be replaced slowly over the first 48 h to prevent overexpansion of the circulating plasma volume. It is important to remember while calculating the daily fluid balance that these patients will also need fluid to replace any ongoing losses (nasogastric aspirates, etc.) as well as their baseline daily requirements.

   d. **False.** Insensible losses are increased by fever through sweating and exhalation of warm humidified air. Water is lost in excess of sodium and should be replaced by 5% dextrose solution.

   e. **False.** The daily intravenous fluid requirement is 2500 ml (500 ml 0.9% of normal saline, 2000 ml of 5% dextrose).

3. a. **False.** Enteral nutrition is delivered via the gastrointestinal tract and is not associated with any thrombogenic risk. Parenteral nutrition is highly thrombogenic, hence the need for central venous access where high rates of blood flow reduce the risk of thrombosis.

   b. **False.** Patients with a short gut have limited absorptive capacity. They are best fed via the parenteral route.

   c. **True.** Enteral nutrition is hyperosmolar and can stimulate gastrointestinal motility producing diarrhoea and cramps.

   d. **False.** Parenteral nutrition requires strict asepsis to prevent catheter sepsis, thrombosis and septicaemia. Enteral nutrition using the gut is less prone to septic complication.

   e. **False.** Provided these patients have an intact gag and cough reflex they can be fed enterally without a significant risk of aspiration.

4. a. **False.** Opiate overdosage causes respiratory depression.

   b. **False.** Opiates cause pupillary constriction rather than dilatation.

   c. **True.**

   d. **False.** Opiate overdosage causes circulatory collapse producing hypotension and a bradycardia.

   e. **True.** Hypoxaemia is a secondary effect of respiratory depression.

5. a. **True.** The risk of thrombosis is increased even in a relatively short operation in a patient using oral contraception.

   b. **True.** Patients of any age group undergoing surgery that involves a pelvic dissection are at increased risk of thromboembolism.

   c. **True.** Hip surgery is one of the operations with the highest incidence of thromboembolism, up to 50% of patients being affected.

   d. **True.** Patients with malignancy are at increased risk. Prophylaxis should be given even for a short palliative operative procedure.

   e. **False.** Short operations in young patients that are followed by early ambulation do not require prophylaxis.

6. a. **True.** CVP measurements are usually elevated in patients with cardiogenic shock because of right heart failure or fluid overload. CVP measurements are reduced in hypovolaemic shock as a result of diminished venous return.

   b. **False.** Both types of shock are associated with systemic hypotension.

   c. **False.** Hypovolaemic shock will respond to a fluid challenge. Cardiogenic shock may be aggravated by a fluid challenge, which will expand the circulating volume, increase the venous return and aggravate any cardiac failure.

d. **True.** Inotropic support will improve myocardial efficiency and cardiac output.

e. **True.** Cardiogenic shock will lead to renal hypoperfusion and oliguria.

7. a. **False.** The defect following a pulmonary embolus is usually mismatched, i.e. there is a defect on the perfusion scan in an area of normal ventilation.

b. **True.** These features are often the hallmark of a major pulmonary embolus.

c. **False.** A major pulmonary embolus will cause arterial hypoxaemia. Cyanosis will be central and peripheral.

d. **True.** Shallow, fast respiration is a frequent finding.

e. **False.** A major pulmonary embolus causes right ventricular strain caused by a sudden increase in pulmonary artery resistance.

8. a. **False.** Dehiscence usually presents around 7–10 days after surgery.

b. **False.** Recurrence is uncommon.

c. **False.** Most patients make an uneventful recovery after abdominal resuture.

d. **True.** Wound healing is impaired in patients with jaundice.

e. **True.** Steroid therapy impairs wound healing.

9. a. **False.** The right lung is most often affected because the right main bronchus is wider and has a more vertical course. The middle and lower lobe segments are most frequently affected.

b. **True.** These patients are frequently obstructed or require urgent surgery with limited opportunity

for preoperative fasting. The risks of aspiration are increased.

c. **True.** Cricoid pressure during induction of anaesthesia is an essential manoeuvre which protects the airway immediately prior to endotracheal intubation.

d. **True.** Gastric acid can cause an intense chemical pneumonitis that after secondary bacterial infection leads to a severe aspiration pneumonia.

e. **False.** Patients with severe gastro-oesophageal reflux are more likely to regurgitate gastric contents once consciousness is depressed during anaesthesia.

10. a. **True.** Smoking impairs the ciliary clearance mechanism and makes bronchial mucus more viscid.

b. **False.** Upper abdominal incisions inhibit abdominal respiration more than lower abdominal incisions and thus contribute to shallow breathing, a factor linked to postoperative atelectasis and pneumonia.

c. **True.** Bowel obstruction and abdominal distension can lead to diaphragmatic splinting and basal atelectasis.

d. **False.** Atelectasis begins early often within the first 24 postoperative hours.

e. **True.** Oversedation can cause respiratory depression and hypoventilation, which predispose to collapse of the small airways and absorption of alveolar air causing atelectasis. Major airway obstruction may develop because of suppression of the cough reflex.

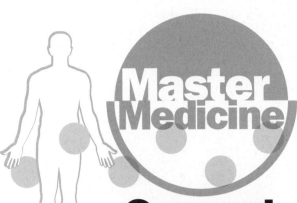

General surgery

Emergency surgery

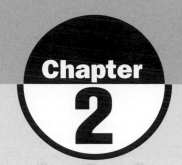

Chapter overview

Trauma, the acute abdomen and major gastrointestinal haemorrhage all require prompt aggressive management to save life and to minimise morbidity. Each is characterised by its own management plan or algorithm. By following strict guidelines vital steps in the diagnosis and treatment of these patients will not be overlooked. This chapter outlines the principles of management that are common to all surgical emergencies.

2.1 Trauma

Learning objectives

You should:

- recognise the vital importance of the 'golden hour' in improving the outcome of trauma
- understand the principles of ATLS in early trauma care
- know the key steps in management of head and neck, thoracic, abdominal and vascular injury.

Trauma is the leading cause of death in people under 40 years of age. Many survivors of injury are left with permanent disabilities. The human and economic cost remains enormous despite efforts at accident prevention through education, engineering and enforcement.

Injury patterns and severity

The greater the amount of energy transferred to the injured party, the more extensive and severe the injury. Road traffic accidents and falls from a height are most likely to cause severe and multiple injuries. Knowing the mechanism of the injury makes it easier to predict the pattern of injuries a patient is likely to have. Therefore, a detailed history is as important in trauma patients as elsewhere. The 'dose' of injury a patient has sustained can be quantified by scoring systems: anatomically, using the Injury Severity Score, or physiologically, using the Trauma Score.

Improving the outcome: the 'golden hour'

Some trauma victims die immediately after injury and are probably unsalvageable because of the severity of their injuries (e.g. brainstem tear or a ruptured aorta). Others die later and there is evidence that better early management – especially airway care, control and correction of blood loss, and an early assessment by experienced clinicians – would save many victims and reduce disability among survivors.

The patient's fate is decided by what is done (or not done) during the 'golden hour' of opportunity after injury. Major trauma is best managed by a team of experts drawn from all the relevant fields (especially accident and emergency medicine, anaesthesia and the various surgical specialities) who work together in an appropriate setting such as an accident and emergency department and keep their skills up to date.

Education and training: ATLS

There has been an explosion of interest in how to develop and to maintain the knowledge and skills of those who treat the seriously injured. Advanced trauma life support (ATLS) courses have spread worldwide from the USA because they offer a safe way to assess and resuscitate the seriously injured.

The ATLS principles of early trauma care are:

- do no further harm to the patient
- assess and resuscitate the patient simultaneously and systematically
- develop a rigid order of priority dealing first with the greatest threats to life (the 'primary survey')
- conduct a thorough search for all other injuries ('secondary survey')
- stabilise the patient before transfer to a definitive trauma care facility.

A systematic approach to trauma care

Many patients die because major injuries or their complications are missed or underestimated, often in the 'golden hour'. Having a systematic approach to assessment makes this less likely to happen. The ATLS system offers an easy-to-remember mnemonic:

A – airway (with cervical spine control)
B – breathing
C – circulation (with control of haemorrhage)
D – dysfunction (of the nervous system)
E – exposure and the environment.

The alphabetical order is also that in which complications threaten life. For example, there is no point in operating on a head-injured patient to remove an intracranial haematoma while the patient dies from a blocked airway or hypovolaemic shock from uncontrolled haemorrhage. Instead, the management of the patient's head injury should begin by clearing the airway (taking great care to protect the potentially injured cervical spine), ensuring he/she is breathing and then correcting the blood loss causing the hypovolaemic shock.

The following sections systematically outline the core points in trauma management once the 'primary survey' has been completed. Further detailed information is provided in the relevant chapters in this book. In a trauma patient, the injuries, which are often multiple, are best categorised by site:

- head and neck
- thorax
- abdomen
- vascular
- urogenital system
- orthopaedic.

Head and neck injuries

The key points in trauma management are:

1. Provide cervical stabilisation with a collar until cervical radiographs rule out a fracture.
2. Prevent airway obstruction with either an airway or an endotracheal tube.
3. Regularly record neurological status (Glasgow Coma Scale: see Ch. 15); consider CT scan if status deteriorates; skull radiograph if there has been a loss of consciousness (see p. 309).
4. Remember that vascular, tracheal and oesophageal injuries can occur from blunt or penetrating cervical trauma.

Thoracic injuries

The key points are:

1. Ensure the patient is breathing with unrestricted symmetrical chest movement.
2. Remember the most frequent serious major chest injuries are:
   - haemothorax/haemopneumothorax
   - flail chest
   - tension pneumothorax
   - cardiac tamponade.
3. Although the diagnosis will be obvious on a chest radiograph, in a critically injured patient there may not be time and a life will be saved after insertion of a chest drain or pericardiocentesis *after an accurate clinical diagnosis*.
4. Occasionally a life will be saved by urgent thoracotomy in the emergency room to arrest haemorrhage from the heart or lung root.

Abdominal injuries

Parenchymal organs or hollow viscera can be damaged by blunt or penetrating abdominal trauma. A blunt injury may be overlooked in a comatose patient with a head and/or chest injury.

The key points are:

1. Major intra-abdominal blood loss usually follows injury to the liver or spleen (either blunt or penetrating) or a penetrating injury that damages the great vessels or mesentery. In a haemodynamically unstable patient, if doubt exists, a diagnostic peritoneal lavage will identify any intra-abdominal bleeding. In a stable patient a CT scan will identify any injury to liver, spleen or kidney. Not all patients with a haemoperitoneum require laparotomy. For example a patient with a fractured pelvis, or a retroperitoneal haematoma with no major vascular injury, may settle without surgical intervention.
2. Rupture of a hollow viscus can be difficult to detect and may be missed on simple radiological studies. A CT scan is the most sensitive test for visceral perforation and can detect minute amounts of free gas in the peritoneal cavity. It should be suspected in a patient who becomes septic for no apparent cause or in any patient who develops progressive abdominal signs.
3. The most frequently injured organs are:
   - Liver: Some patients with a liver injury who are haemodynamically stable can be treated conservatively. For others, bleeding is the major problem; usually this will stop with tamponade or simple suture. Debridement of formal liver resection is rarely required.
   - Spleen: usually requires splenectomy or occasionally splenorrhaphy (surgical repair of the spleen) to control bleeding.
   - Small bowel and stomach: rupture of any part of the intestine causes peritonitis. Usually a small bowel tear or mesenteric injury can be treated by simple oversew or resection.
   - Colon injury: a fresh colonic injury can usually be repaired by primary suture. If the diagnosis has been delayed and there is gross faecal peritonitis and contamination, most surgeons would exteriorise the injured colon to form a colostomy.

Vascular injuries

Worldwide, penetrating injuries caused by gunshot or stab wounds are the most common cause of major arterial injury. Crush injury to the limbs may contuse an artery producing an intimal tear that will impede distal blood flow even though the blood vessel may appear structurally intact. This type of injury frequently accompanies a long bone fracture or dislocation.

Clinical features

Patients may present with an obvious external haemorrhage from a bleeding wound, or the blood loss may be concealed as in a retroperitoneal or thoracic injury, the only clinical evidence being hypovolaemic shock. Alternatively, the patient may present with an ischaemic pulseless limb (pain, pallor, paralysis, paraesthesia, no pulses).

A high index of suspicion is the key to diagnosis, especially in a shocked patient or one with an injury close to a blood vessel or following a fracture/dislocation. Even if distal pulses are present, the proximal vessel can still be injured and if there is any doubt an arteriogram should be performed.

Treatment

Direct compression of a bleeding wound will save a life while emergency resuscitation takes place. Whenever possible, a tourniquet should *not* be used as they can cause further damage to the circulation. Operative treatment involves obtaining control above and below the bleeding vessel, followed by careful exploration of the bleeding point. Sometimes, once the damaged section of vessel has been excised, a primary end-to-end repair can be undertaken. Alternatively, a vein or prosthetic graft can be interposed if the defect is too wide. A careful search should be made for any associated vein or nerve injury.

Urogenital system

Major injury to the renal tract must be suspected in any patient with a loin injury or gross haematuria. An intravenous pyelogram (IVP) is essential.

The kidney should be explored if there are signs of extravasation of urine or continuing haemorrhage. Nephrectomy or partial nephrectomy may be required.

Bladder or urethral injuries may not be so obvious but should be suspected in any patient with a major pelvic injury. Blood dripping from the external urethral meatus or a 'floating' prostate gland on rectal examination is a cardinal sign. Operative repair of the bladder together with suprapubic catheterisation and urinary diversion is the best initial treatment option. Operative reconstruction of a damaged urethra is carried out at a later date.

Orthopaedic injuries

Most orthopaedic injuries can be managed immediately by external splints or external fixation devices which will buy time until other coexisting life-threatening injuries have been dealt with or stabilised. Orthopaedic trauma is dealt with in detail in Chapter 7.

2.2 The acute abdomen

Learning objectives

You should:
- know the common causes of an acute abdomen
- be able to use a case history, physical examination and simple investigations to reach the most likely diagnosis in a patient with an acute abdomen
- be able to outline the principles of management in a patient with an acute abdomen.

An acute abdomen can be defined as a non-traumatic, catastrophic event that affects any of the intra-abdominal organs. Acute severe abdominal pain is usually the hall-

Table 5 Causes of an acute abdomen

Common causes

Acute appendicitis

Acute cholecystitis, biliary colic

Acute pancreatitis

Acute diverticulitis

Acute gynaecological problems: salpingitis, ectopic pregnancy, torted ovarian cyst

Perforated peptic ulcer

Large or small bowel obstruction

Ureteric or renal colic

Less common causes

Leaking aortic aneurysm

Mesenteric ischaemia

Acute colitis or Crohn's disease

mark. Patients with an acute abdomen require urgent investigation, diagnosis and treatment.

There are numerous causes of an acute abdomen. The most important are listed in Table 5.

Clinical features

Most will present with abdominal pain. Although patients will be distressed, time taken to obtain an accurate history is well spent and will frequently point to the diagnosis.

There are five key points in relation to pain and the acute abdomen, namely:

- location
- onset
- progression
- character
- radiation.

Location

There are usually two components to abdominal pain: visceral and parietal.

Visceral pain This type of pain is caused by inflammation or distension of a viscus and is often poorly localised:

- Pain from organs of the foregut (stomach/liver/gallbladder/duodenum) is usually perceived in the epigastrium.
- Pain derived from midgut organs (pancreas/small bowel/appendix/ascending colon) is perceived in the centre of the abdomen (periumbilical).
- Hindgut pain (transverse/descending and sigmoid colon) is perceived in the hypogastrium/suprapubic areas.

Parietal pain Eventually the parietal peritoneum becomes inflamed by pus or bile or an adjacent acutely inflamed viscus and pain will localise to that particular part of the abdomen.

Onset

Sudden/explosive pain This usually heralds an intra-abdominal catastrophe such as a ruptured viscus (e.g. perforated peptic ulcer) or a leaking abdominal aortic aneurysm.

Gradual onset pain This often implies progressive inflammation of a viscus, as in acute cholecystitis or pancreatitis.

Progression

Acute appendicitis is a classic example of the progression of pain from a visceral to a parietal component and underlines the importance of taking an accurate history. Many patients with acute appendicitis will describe pain originating in the centre of the abdomen (the appendix is a midgut organ) before the pain eventually settles in the right iliac fossa when the parietal peritoneum adjacent to the appendix becomes inflamed. A careful history will lead to the diagnosis, which can be simply confirmed on abdominal examination.

Character

The most important features to determine are:

- Is the pain colicky or constant?
- What is the effect of movement?

Colic implies obstruction of a viscus, as in small or large bowel obstruction. Constant pain is in keeping with inflammation of an organ or vascular compromise (e.g. strangulation or ischaemia).

Movement exacerbates pain caused by parietal peritoneal inflammation. A patient with generalised peritonitis caused by a perforated peptic ulcer will lie completely still. In contrast, patients with ureteric or renal colic cannot find a comfortable position and will frequently writhe in agony until they receive adequate analgesia or until the colic subsides.

Radiation

This can often provide an important diagnostic clue. For example, pain from the retroperitoneal organs, such as the pancreas or the aorta, will radiate to the back, whereas pain of biliary origin may radiate to the shoulder tip because of irritation or inflammation of the adjacent diaphragm.

Physical findings

Avoid the temptation to rush to examine the abdomen. The entire patient must be evaluated. Is the patient shocked? Do not forget to examine the chest and cardiovascular system. Resuscitation (see p. 30) may be required while physical evaluation and urgent investigation of the patient continues.

The abdomen

The most important question to answer is: is there an obstruction or peritonitis, or are both present?

In examining the patient, certain key features must be sought.

Inspection Is the abdomen flat or distended? Does the abdomen move with respiration? A distended abdomen suggests obstruction or the accumulation of ascitic fluid.

Palpation Is there any tenderness? Is it localised or generalised? Are there any masses? Generalised tenderness with rebound or guarding is in keeping with a generalised peritonitis; occasionally rectus muscle spasm will be induced, causing 'board-like' abdominal rigidity, for example after a perforated ulcer. If the inflammatory process is localised as in appendicitis or acute diverticulitis, careful palpation to elicit the area of maximum tenderness will point towards the most likely underlying cause. A pulsatile abdominal mass is an abdominal aortic aneurysm until proven otherwise.

Percussion Is the abdomen hyper-resonant or not? A resonant distended abdomen, suggests an obstruction, a dull abdomen, ascites or a mass.

Auscultation Are there bowel sounds present? Are the bowel sounds obstructive? A silent abdomen is usually a grave sign indicating an intra-abdominal catastrophe, for example generalised peritonitis or severe mesenteric ischaemia. Normal bowel sounds may be reassuring, but in the presence of other significant abdominal findings 'normal' bowel sounds should not lead you into a false sense of security. High-pitched 'tinkling' bowel sounds are indicative of a bowel obstruction.

Rectal and vaginal examination

No abdominal evaluation is complete if a rectal examination is omitted. The pelvic organs, a pelvic mass or abscess, or a pelvic appendicitis are protected by the bony pelvic ring and are inaccessible to abdominal palpation. A rectal examination allows access to the pelvis by *palpation* and will reveal areas of tenderness or a mass that would otherwise be missed. If there is any suspicion that the acute pathology is of gynaecological origin then a vaginal examination is mandatory.

Investigations

Often, simple blood tests and radiological investigations will provide diagnostic evidence and will confirm or refute the clinical findings and diagnosis.

Blood tests Patients with an acute abdomen should have blood drawn for:

- full blood count
- urea and electrolytes
- serum amylase
- blood grouping (save serum for cross-match).

These tests will detect anaemia, a leucocytosis, electrolyte imbalance or dehydration and will influence the patient's resuscitation. A massively elevated serum amylase will confirm a diagnosis of acute pancreatitis.

Radiological investigations

Erect chest radiograph The most important feature to look for is subdiaphragmatic gas. Its presence indicates a perforated viscus. Occasionally, a chest radiograph will demonstrate an unexpected cause of a patient's abdominal pain, such as a right-sided basal pneumonia, which clinically had been mistaken for an attack of acute cholecystitis.

Plain abdominal radiology A single supine abdominal film will identify a small or a large bowel obstruction. Critical features such as caecal dilatation with impending perforation or a toxic colonic dilatation will also be identified. Occasionally abnormal calcification in the gallbladder (gallstones), pancreas (pancreatitis), renal tract (ureteric or renal colic) or outlining the wall of a dilated aorta (aneurysm) will point to the underlying diagnosis.

ECG Many patients with an acute abdomen will require surgical intervention. An ECG may be required in view of a forthcoming anaesthetic. Equally important, an underlying cardiac cause for an acute epigastric pain (e.g. an atypical myocardial infarction) may be discovered.

A treatment plan

Much will depend on the diagnosis. Sometimes, despite careful clinical evaluation and investigation, no firm conclusion is reached. Those patients who do not respond to resuscitation or conservative measures will require a diagnostic laparoscopy or laparotomy to establish and treat an elusive diagnosis.

The key management points are:

- resuscitation
- antibiotics
- analgesia
- monitoring the response.

Resuscitation Several immediate steps are necessary: establish an intravenous fluid infusion and replace volume deficits with crystalloid, colloid or blood as appropriate; administer supplemental oxygen therapy.

Antibiotics Many patients will have intra-abdominal sepsis. Until culture and sensitivity reports are to hand (often only as a result of specimens obtained during urgent surgery), antibiotics will have to be chosen based on the likelihood of the infecting organisms. Usually broad-spectrum cover is required to include gram-negative and gram-positive aerobes plus anaerobic organism cover. Take blood cultures first.

Analgesia Adequate parenteral analgesia is essential and should not be withheld once a preliminary assessment has been completed. A carefully titrated analgesic dose will not mask significant abdominal findings but instead will often facilitate abdominal examination by relaxing the patient.

Monitoring the response Fluid resuscitation, antibiotic therapy and adequate analgesia form the cornerstone of conservative management. The patient's vital signs and urine output are a sensitive indicator of the response to treatment.

Getting better?

Some causes of an acute abdomen will respond well to conservative measures, e.g. acute cholecystitis or acute pancreatitis. For others (e.g. a perforated duodenal ulcer), an initial response to conservative treatment simply indicates that resuscitation has been adequate and that the patient is now optimised and ready for surgical treatment. Any untoward delay and the benefits of resuscitation will be lost as sepsis supervenes and compromises the outcome of surgery.

No improvement or a worsening clinical condition?

A falling blood pressure, rising pulse rate and dwindling urine output all indicate a failure to respond to conservative measures. In these patients, the initial diagnosis may have been incorrect or a complication may have supervened (e.g. rupture of a diverticular abscess causing generalised peritonitis). Patients in this category usually require aggressive resuscitation prior to surgical intervention.

Surgery inevitable?

In a third group of patients, the need for surgical intervention is obvious from the outset once a diagnosis has been reached (e.g. perforated peptic ulcer, leaking aortic aneurysm). In this group of patients, conservative management is limited to providing the necessary resuscitation to optimise the patient's condition prior to operation.

2.3 Major gastrointestinal haemorrhage

Haemorrhagic shock is the most common form of shock encountered by surgeons. The clinical picture depends on the extent of blood loss (see Table 6). Patients with a massive, exsanguinating haemorrhage will need a rapid overall evaluation with resuscitation taking priority over a full history and physical examination.

Resuscitation

The initial resuscitation is the same, regardless of the site of blood loss. The key steps are:

Table 6 Clinical features of haemorrhagic shock

Blood loss	Physical findings
Mild shock vasoconstriction (<20% loss of blood volume)	Periphery pale, cold
Moderate shock (loss of 20–40% blood volume)	As above plus oliguria, postural hypotension
Severe shock (loss of >40% blood volume)	As above plus restlessness, supine hypotension

1. Ensure adequate ventilation and oxygenation.
2. Establish venous access using multiple wide-bore peripheral venous cannulae.
3. Pass a nasogastric tube.
4. Obtain blood for cross-match, baseline haemoglobin and coagulation profile.
5. Resuscitate with colloid plasma expanders (e.g. Haemaccel) or crystalloid solutions until matched whole blood is available. In an exsanguinating patient, it may be necessary to use group O negative blood.
6. Monitor response by vital signs; catheterise patient to observe urine output.
7. Consider urgent surgical intervention in any patient who does not respond to 2–3 l fluid resuscitation.
8. Invasive monitoring using central venous access and pressure monitoring is best left until resuscitation is established and the circulating volume restored.

Overall, bleeding stops spontaneously in 80% of patients and these steps will effectively resuscitate most patients and allow time for diagnostic evaluation.

Causes

The main causes of massive upper gastrointestinal haemorrhage are:

- common
  - peptic duodenal or gastric ulceration
  - oesophageal varices
  - acute gastritis
  - Mallory–Weiss tear (a mucosal laceration at the gastro-oesophageal junction caused by repeated retching or vomiting)
- uncommon
  - gastric or oesophageal cancer.

The main causes of massive lower gastrointestinal haemorrhage are:

- common
  - diverticular disease
  - angiodysplasia
  - acute colitis of any cause
- uncommon
  - colon carcinoma
  - haemorrhoids.

On the rare occasions that the small intestine is the site of major gastrointestinal blood loss, angiodysplastic lesions or a Meckel's diverticulum will usually be responsible.

Clinical features

Haematemesis implies a brisk upper gastrointestinal bleed either from oesophagus, stomach or duodenum. Melena, the passage of black tarry stools, indicates blood loss from any point of the gastrointestinal tract as far as the caecum. Haemorrhage from the colon, rectum and anus is characterised by fresh rectal bleeding or passage of dark altered blood per rectum.

Several points in the case history are particularly important:

- drug history
  - anti-inflammatory agents
  - anticoagulants
  - aspirin
- alcohol intake.

Diagnostic difficulties arise because:

- Not all upper gastrointestinal bleeds are associated with haematemesis; some present with melena alone.
- Rapid upper gastrointestinal bleeding may present as rectal haemorrhage rather than melena because of rapid transit through the intestines. These patients are usually profoundly shocked.

The essential diagnostic steps are:

- urgent gastroscopy for all suspected upper gastrointestinal bleeds plus those patients with shock and rectal haemorrhage
- colonoscopy for all patients with suspected lower gastrointestinal bleeds
- selective mesenteric angiography in patients who continue to bleed despite negative endoscopic evaluation.

Treatment

This will depend upon the underlying cause and is covered in detail in Chapter 3. The most frequent urgent procedures are:

- band ligation or sclerotherapy for bleeding oesophageal varices
- eudoscopic treatment or surgery for bleeding peptic ulcers
- angiography and embolization of a bleeding gastric, duodenal or colonic vessel
- colonic resection for angiodysplasia or diverticular disease
- subtotal or total colectomy for acute colitis.

Outcome

Approximately 80% of acute bleeds of whatever cause will stop and these patients will survive provided resuscitation is adequate. For the remainder, the outcome will depend on the cause of the bleed. Those at greatest risk are the elderly or those patients who bleed for a second time (rebleeding) after the initial haemorrhage has stopped.

Self-assessment: questions

Extended matching items questions (EMIs)

EMI 1

Theme: Trauma

A. diagnostic peritoneal lavage

B. immediate laparotomy

C. CT scan abdomen

D. abdominal ultrasound

E. observation alone

F. CT brain

G. mesenteric angiogram

H. skull radiograph

Select the most useful management option with regard to the following trauma patients.

1. A 55-year-old woman is admitted after a road traffic accident. She was a front-seat passenger in a car and sustained a seatbelt injury with bruising across her central abdomen. She is fully conscious and orientated and a primary survey shows no other injury. On admission her blood pressure was 95/60 mmHg and her pulse 120 beats/min. She has stabilised after resuscitation with a litre of crystalloid and a 2-unit colloid transfusion.

2. A 23-year-old man is admitted following an assault. He has three stab wounds in the left side of his abdomen. On examination he is haemodynamically stable and his abdomen is generally tender with guarding away from the stab wound entry sites. A plain abdominal film is normal but an erect chest radiograph shows a large amount of gas under the left hemidiaphragm.

3. A 40-year-old cyclist is knocked off his bicycle. He sustains a head injury and has an obvious fracture of his left femur. No other injuries are apparent on the primary survey and he is haemodynamically stable with normal bowel sounds. The paramedical team who brought him to the casualty department have recorded a deterioration in his neurological status using the Glasgow Coma Scale.

EMI 2

Theme: Gastrointestinal haemorrhage

A. Mallory–Weiss tear

B. caecal angiodysplasia

C. oesophageal varices

D. acute ulcerative colitis

E. anterior duodenal ulcer

F. posterior duodenal ulcer

G. acute mesenteric ischaemia

H. acute diverticulitis

Select from the above options the most likely diagnosis in the following patients.

1. A 79-year-old woman who has recently changed to a new non-steroidal inflammatory medication is admitted with rectal bleeding. She has a normal gastroscopy. Her colonoscopy was technically unsuccessful. She continues to bleed and undergoes a mesenteric angiogram. This shows evidence of blood loss in the right side of her colon.

2. A 17-year-old man is admitted with a haematemesis. The previous night he attended a stag party and drank excessively. He was violently sick before the haematemesis and has not required resuscitation.

3. A 59-year-old man presents with a bright red rectal haemorrhage. He is not shocked. A gastroscopy is normal and an attempt at colonoscopy was of limited success. The mucosa that was seen looked entirely normal.

EMI 3

Theme: Causes of an acute abdomen

A. acute cholecystitis

B. acute pancreatitis

C. leaking abdominal aortic aneurysm

D. acute diverticulitis

E. mesenteric ischaemia

F. acute appendicitis

G. acute colitis

H. renal colic

Read the following case descriptions and match each to one of the above diagnoses.

1. A 70-year-old man is admitted with severe pain. It is difficult to get a clear history. The pain appears predominantly left sided and mainly in his back. He has a soft abdomen and cannot lie still. His vital signs are: blood pressure 155/90mmHg; pulse 120 beats/min.

2. A 66-year-old woman presents with a short history of lower abdominal pain which is made worse when she moves or coughs. She has no backache. When you examine her she is febrile and you think you can feel a non-pulsatile mass in her left iliac fossa.

3. A 58-year-old woman who is diabetic and a lifelong smoker is admitted urgently with abdominal pain. She has previously had a limb amputation and has angina. She complains of a central abdominal pain which is worse after a meal.

Constructed response questions (CRQs)

CRQ 1

A 40-year-old man who has been on a drinking binge is admitted collapsed after a haematemesis. He has a pulse rate of 120 and a systolic blood pressure of 80 mmHg. He is barely conscious.

a. List five of the key steps to his resuscitation

The patient responds to your resuscitation

b. Consider the differential diagnosis in this patient. Name three of the most likely causes for his bleed.

His conscious state improves after several hours.

c. What questions would you ask this patient that might provide clues to the cause of his gastrointestinal bleed? List three.

The patient has a further haematemesis on the day of admission. He remains haemodynamically stable.

d. What should you do?

CRQ 2

An 82-year-old woman who has previously had a coronary artery bypass graft and has a long history of intermittent claudication affecting both legs is admitted with severe abdominal pain. The discomfort she describes is poorly localised, constant not colicky, but was of sudden onset. She describes it as the worst pain she has ever had. On examination she has a diffusely tender abdomen. You also note that she does not have an aortic aneurysm and that her bowel sounds are scanty.

a. What do you think is the likely differential diagnosis? List three important causes.

She was mildy hypotensive on admission but responds initially to fluid resuscitation.

b. List four urgent diagnostic tests that you would arrange in this difficult case.

Two hours after admission, the patient's condition deteriorates further. Her abdominal pain increases and she develops rebound tenderness and guarding. The bowel sounds are now absent.

c. What do these clinical signs indicate.

The patient's family are concerned about her progress and you discuss with them what is likely to happen next while you are waiting for a senior colleague to review the patient.

d. What do you think is the most appropriate management option?

CRQ 3

A 24-year-old man is brought into a casualty department after falling off a motorbike. He was not wearing a crash helmet. He has an obvious fracture of his right humerus and marked bruising over his lower abdomen and pelvis. His blood pressure is 110/60 mmHg with a pulse rate of 96 beats/min.

a. In order of priority list the five key points in the initial assessment of this patient on arrival in the casualty department.

The paramedic tells you he was conscious for a time after the injury but then became unrouseable.

b. How would you evaluate his cerebral injury?

The patient appears stable from your initial assessment.

c. What blood tests would you arrange?

While you are waiting for a senior to review the patient you are asked to complete the patient's radiography request form.

d. What radiological tests would you order to assess the extent of his skeletal injuries?

CRQ 4

A 62-year-old woman is admitted urgently with a short history of cramp-like lower abdominal pains and constipation. There is no history of vomiting, nor has she had any previous surgery. On examination she has a tympanitic, grossly distended abdomen and appears mildly tender in the right iliac fossa. She has high-pitched tinkling bowel sounds.

a. What do you think is the most likely diagnosis?

The patient looks in pain and is dehydrated. You administer analgesia and set up an i.v. infusion.

b. Taking into account the above history, what important step is necessary to complete the examination of this patient's abdomen?

She responds to your resuscitation and you are able to take a full case history.

c. What key points in her history would you seek in order to establish a diagnosis?

The patient's family ask to see you and ask what is to happen next.

d. Name two diagnostic tests this patient is likely to require.

The patient again draws your attention to her lower abdominal discomfort. You re-examine her. She remains mildy tender in the right fossa, there is no guarding and she is afebrile.

e. What do you think is the significance of this patient's right iliac fossa tenderness?

CRQ 5

A 70-year old man is referred to the casualty department with a 24-h history of severe epigastric and back pain. His GP had recently organised an abdominal ultrasound scan which showed he had gallstones. The patient was waiting for an outpatient appointment.

a. Name three possible causes for this patient's emergency presentation.

The casualty officer has undertaken some routine blood tests. These are the most important results:

White cell count 17,000	(3–6,000) normal
Serum amylase 1,850 IU/l	(0–100 U/l) normal
C-reactive protein 220	up to 5 normal

b. What do you think is the diagnosis?

You decide that the patient requires admission to the acute surgical acute receiving unit.

c. List five important steps in the initial management of this patient.

The next day this patient's clinical condition has deteriorated. His oxygen saturation P_aO_2 is 84% on 60% inspired oxygen.

d. What is the most likely reason for this patient's deterioration?

Best of 5s questions

1. A 35-year-old man sustains an isolated head injury when he is hit by a piece of scaffolding on his left temple at work. His Glasgow Coma Scale has changed from 15 to 12 points since the accident 2 h ago. His most appropriate management would be:

   a. admit for neurosurgical observation
   b. provide cervical stabilisation with a collar until cerical radiographs rule out a fracture
   c. arrange a skull radiograph
   d. organise a CT brain scan
   e. immediate intubation and ventilation

2. A 49-year-old woman is a back seat passenger in a car. Despite wearing a seatbelt she sustains an injury to her chest. She becomes acutely breathless and anxious within a few minutes of arrival in the accident and emergency department. Her trachea is deviated to the right and the left side of her chest is hyper resonant. Her correct management is:

   a. cricothyroidotomy
   b. chest radiograph
   c. insert a right-sided chest drain
   d. immediate pericardicentesis
   e. insert a left-sided chest drain

3. A 50-year-old man is a front seat passenger in a road traffic accident. He has a head, chest and pelvic injury and requires intubation and transfer to an intensive care unit. Two days later he becomes septic from no apparent cause. He has a normal chest radiograph. Which of the following investigations will be of most use?

   a. CT abdominal scan
   b. V/Q scan
   c. CT brain scan
   d. peritoneal lavage
   e. CT pulmonary angiogram

4. There are many causes of acute abdominal pain, some of which are treated by conservative means initially. Which of the following always requires urgent surgical intervention upon diagnosis?

   a. acute pancreatitis
   b. acute mesenteric ischaemia
   c. acute diverticulitis
   d. acute cholecystitis
   e. acute Crohn's disease

5. A 66-year-old woman is admitted with acute abdominal pain. You suspect she might have peritonitis. Which one of the following investigations will be of most use?

   a. erect abdominal film
   b. supine chest radiograph
   c. mesenteric duplex scan
   d. erect chest radiograph
   e. supine abdominal film

Multiple choice questions

1. The following points relate to the early management of trauma:

   a. the first priority in a critically injured patient is to establish intravenous access
   b. cervical fractures are usually obvious
   c. supine hypotension usually indicates a greater than 40% loss of blood volume
   d. mediastinal injury is likely in patients with bilateral rib fractures
   e. diagnostic peritoneal lavage will reliably detect visceral rupture in the comatose patient

2. Major peripheral arterial injuries:

   a. inevitably cause loss of peripheral pulses distal to the injury
   b. are reliably diagnosed by arteriography
   c. are rarely accompanied by vein or nerve injury
   d. frequently accompany fracture/dislocations of the long bones

e. should have a tourniquet applied to them to obtain initial control of the blood loss

3. The following points relate to abdominal pain:

   a. The visceral component of duodenal pain is perceived in the periumbilical area.
   b. Patients with renal colic can often alleviate their symptoms by lying very still.
   c. Shoulder tip pain is a characteristic of a perforated peptic ulcer.
   d. Mesenteric thrombosis is rarely associated with colicky abdominal pain.
   e. Parietal pain is often preceded by visceral pain.

4. A supine plain abdominal radiograph can provide useful diagnostic information in the following conditions:

   a. abdominal aortic aneurysm
   b. perforated peptic ulcer
   c. acute appendicitis

   d. acute cholecystitis
   e. large bowel obstruction

5. In patients with upper gastrointestinal bleeding:

   a. the bleeding point is frequently beyond the ligament of Treitz
   b. angiodysplastic lesions are a common cause
   c. the patients always present with haematemesis
   d. diagnostic endoscopy is best deferred for at least 24 h
   e. selective mesenteric angiography is the key diagnostic step

6. Patients with a major rectal haemorrhage:

   a. should have a gastroscopy
   b. almost always require surgery
   c. frequently harbour a colorectal cancer
   d. have angiodysplastic lesions most frequently found in the caecum
   e. should have an emergency barium enema as the key investigation

Self-assessment: answers

EMI answers

EMI 1

Theme: Trauma

1. C. CT abdomen.

This patient's injuries appear localised to the abdomen and have been sufficient to cause hypovolaemic shock which responded well to a limited amount of fluid resuscitation. A CT scan would demonstrate the presence of any blood within the peritoneal cavity and would also provide vital information regarding any parenchymal injury to the liver, spleen and kidneys. This information together with the patient's subsequent clinical progress would help determine whether or not a laparotomy is required.

2. B. Immediate laparotomy.

This patient, who has had a penetrating abdominal injury, requires a laparotomy because he has signs of peritonitis on examination (tenderness and guarding) together with evidence of visceral perforation (large amounts of free intraperitoneal air) on his erect chest radiograph.

3. F. CT brain.

A deterioration in neurological status since the time of injury is the key feature in this patient's clinical progress. As there is no evidence of abdominal injury on the primary survey assessment of the neurological injury by CT scan would be the first priority as soon as the patient was stabilised.

EMI 2

Theme: Gastrointestinal haemorrhage

1. D. Caecal angiodysplasia.

An upper gastrointestinal cause for blood loss has been eliminated in this patient as she has a normal gastroscopy. This would be particularly relevant in a patient who has just received new NSAID medication. As she has rebled and had a failed colonoscopy a mesenteric angiogram is the next logical step. Caecal angiodysplasia will cause blood loss from the right side of the colon.

2. A. Mallory–Weiss tear.

This is a classic history for a patient with a Mallory–Weiss tear. The bleeding inevitably follows a bout of prolonged wretching or vomiting precipitated by a heavy alcohol intake.

3. H. Acute diverticulitis.

This diagnosis is sometimes reached by a process of elimination. The blood loss in this patient was bright red in colour and the patient did not become shocked. This is most in keeping with blood loss from the rectum or left side of the colon. The colonoscopy eliminated an acute colitis from the differential diagnosis as the mucosa appeared normal.

EMI 3

Theme: Causes of an acute abdomen

1. H. Renal colic.

Often it is difficult to obtain a full history when a patient is acutely unwell. The site of the pain and the inability of the patient to keep still point to the agonising discomfort of renal or ureteric colic. An abdominal aortic aneurysm is an important differential diagnosis in any patient who presents with left-sided back pain.

2. D. Acute diverticulitis.

This patient has a febrile illness with left iliac fossa peritonism. She may also have an abdominal mass. These features are the hallmark of acute diverticulitis and may not be associated with any disturbance in bowel function.

3. E. Mesenteric ischaemia.

This patient has several risk factors for mesenteric ischaemia. She is an arteriopath, and she is diabetic. In addition she has postprandial pain, which is the classic pattern of discomfort in patients with chronic mesenteric ischaemia.

CRQ answers

CRQ 1

a. Establish intravenous access; use multiple sites if necessary.

  Draw blood for urgent cross-match, baseline haematology, biochemistry and coagulation screen.

  Give supplemental oxygen.

  Restore circulating blood volume.

  Catheterise the patient.

  Monitor the response.

Any of these responses will score marks. These are the key steps in resuscitation. Use multiple sites for venous access if required. Restore the circulating volume by infusion of colloid (plasma protein substitute) or a plasma expander (such as Haemaccel) together with normal saline while waiting for cross-match blood to arrive.

  Most patients will respond to this initial regimen once 1–2 l crystalloid/colloid have been infused. A failure to respond suggests ongoing haemorrhage. These patients require:

- urgent transfusion of uncross-matched blood (O negative)
- central venous pressure monitoring
- consideration for urgent diagnostic investigation and possible surgical treatment.

b. Oesophageal varices.

  Peptic ulcer.

  Acute gastritis.

  Mallory–Weiss tear.

Any of these responses will score marks. As there is no history of vomiting it is unlikely the bleed has been caused by a Mallory–Weiss tear.

c. Previous dyspeptic symptoms.

Drug history.

Alcohol intake.

The patient should be asked if he has a history of dyspeptic symptoms (epigastric pain, nausea indigestion) or if he takes anti-inflammatory drugs, aspirin or anticoagulants, all of which predispose to gastrointestinal haemorrhage. It is most important that his alcohol intake is recorded.

d. Arrange an upper gastrointestinal endoscopy.

This is the key investigation. It should be performed within the first 24 h of admission or earlier if the patient continues to bleed and is unstable. The oesophagus, stomach and duodenum should be carefully evaluated. Active bleeding from ulcers or varices can be treated by injection or banding during endoscopy. If this fails, surgical intervention will be required, the procedure depending on the cause and the site of the bleeding.

CRQ 2

a. Acute mesenteric vascular occlusion.

Acute pancreatitis.

Intestinal strangulation.

Peritonitis.

Any of these responses will score marks. The history and findings suggest there has been an intra-abdominal catastrophe. This patient is an arteriopath, having previously undergone a coronary artery bypass graft, and presently has symptoms of intermittent claudication. She may have atheromatous disease affecting her mesenteric vessels.

b. Serum amylase.

White cell count.

Baseline biochemistry (and haematology).

Plain abdominal film.

Erect chest radiograph.

Any of these responses would score marks. A massive elevation in the serum amylase would be in keeping with a diagnosis of acute pancreatitis (minor elevations favour mesenteric ischaemia). Although non-specific, a leucocytosis would also support a diagnosis of serious intra-abdominal pathology. Baseline biochemistry and haematology would be important aids to planning resuscitation.

An erect chest radiograph and plain abdominal film are two vital investigations which should detect a perforation or an unexpected bowel obstruction.

c. Generalised peritonitis.

Rebound tenderness, guarding and absent bowel sounds are the key physical signs in peritonitis.

d. Laparotomy.

The condition of this patient has clearly deteriorated. There is nothing to be gained from further non-invasive investigation. The patient should be resuscitated and prepared for an exploratory laparotomy.

CRQ 3

a. Airway.

Breathing.

Circulation.

Dysfunction.

Exposure.

This is the advanced trauma life support (ATLS) systematic approach used to assess this patient and to perform a 'primary survey' in order to deal first with the greatest threats to the patient's life. You would score extra marks for listing the assessment in the correct order.

Airway The airway should be clear with no blood, saliva, vomit or broken teeth likely to cause an obstruction. Before moving the head and clearing the airway, ensure the cervical spine is stabilised with an external collar in case the patient has fractured his cervical spine. It may be necessary to provide the patient with an artificial airway.

Breathing Check there is respiratory movement and symmetrical chest expansion with air entry in both lungs. If not the patient will require intubation and ventilation.

Circulation Check the patient has a cardiac output (carotid pulsation) *and* start regular monitoring of pulse and blood pressure. If there is no cardiac output, cardiopulmonary resuscitation will need to be started. Set up an intravenous infusion. Carefully examine the abdomen, catheterise the patient and decide whether or not the patient requires a diagnostic peritoneal lavage or an abdominal CT scan. These steps will detect any major intra-abdominal bleeding.

Dysfunction A quick neurological examination should be made, concentrating on conscious level, papillary response, peripheral reflexes and limb movements. These will form the baseline for the patient's Glasgow Coma Scale observations.

Exposure The patient should be totally undressed and a complete physical examination carried out to check for other injuries.

b. Neurological examination.

Glasgow Coma Scale.

Cerebral CT scan.

Clinical examination coupled with the Glasgow Coma Scale observations will provide a sensitive index of the patient's progress. In this case we have evidence of a deterioration in the conscious level. This is an indication (in a haemodynamically stable patient) for an urgent cerebral CT scan to detect any haematoma, contusion or brain swelling.

c. Group and cross-match.

Full blood count.

Biochemistry.

These tests will provide a baseline for management and operative intervention if required.

d. Obtain radiographs of:

Cervical spine.

Skull.

Chest.

Plain abdomen.

Pelvis.

Right arm.

This patient has signs of major trauma with a head injury, pelvic injury and limb fracture. He is mildly hypotensive and from the distribution of his bruising may have a fractured pelvis in addition to his fractured right humerus. There has also been a deterioration in his conscious level since the time of injury suggesting he might have a progressive intracerebral injury.

He needs an urgent radiograph of his cervical spine (to exclude a cervical fracture/dislocation), skull (to identify a skull fracture), chest (to exclude a mediastinal injury/haemothorax/rib fractures), plain abdominal film and pelvis (to exclude a pelvic fracture) and a radiograph of his fractured right arm.

CRQ 4

a. Large bowel obstruction.

Gross abdominal distension, low abdominal colicky pain and a relative absence of upper gastrointestinal symptoms are highly suspicious of a large bowel obstruction.

b. A rectal examination.

Examination of the hernia orifices.

A rectal examination is critical and might detect a mass or faecal impaction. A dilated empy rectal ampulla indicates a more proximal colonic obstruction (rectal cancers rarely obstruct).

c. Any change in bowel habit.

Presence or absence of flatus.

Timing of last bowel movement.

It would be important to know of any recent alteration in bowel habit, passage of blood or mucus per rectum. It would also be vital to know when the patient's bowels last moved or if there had been a stoppage to the passage of flatus.

d. Plain abdominal radiograph.

Sigmoidoscopy.

Gastrograffin enema.

Any of these responses will gain marks. A plain abdominal radiograph should be diagnostic. The absence of complete haustral folds and picture frame distribution of the distended intestinal loops would help distinguish a large bowel obstruction from a small bowel obstruction. The characteristic features of a sigmoid colon volvulus would also be detected. A sigmoidoscopy should also be performed in order to identify an obstructing rectosigmoid cancer.

Before any surgery is undertaken it is important that the level and cause of the obstruction is identified in order that the most appropriate operation can be planned. Whenever possible these patients should have a preoperative contrast enema study, preferably using a water-soluble contrast medium such as gastrograffin.

e. A tender caecum.

Right iliac fossa tenderness in a patient with large bowel obstruction is an important physical sign. It usually relates to a tender, distended caecum. This is most common in a closed loop large bowel obstruction where a competent ileocaecal valve prevents reflux of the obstructed colonic contents into the small bowel. Untreated, these patients are at a grave risk of spontaneous caecal perforation which can lead to a fatal faecal peritonitis. The plain abdominal films in all patients with large bowel obstruction must be inspected for evidence of caecal dilatation.

CRQ 5

a. Acute cholecystitis.

Acute pancreatitis.

Perforated peptic ulcer.

Acute mesenteric ischaemia.

Abdominal aortic aneurysm.

Acute gastritis.

Any of the above diagnoses would score marks. The differential diagnosis is wide and these symptoms can be caused by disease in any of the foregut organs. The initial screening tests in any patient with this presentation will help to identify the most likely diagnosis.

b. Acute pancreatitis.

The massively elevated serum amylase level is diagnostic of acute pancreatitis. Small increases in the serum amylase are sometimes seen in patients with mesenteric ischaemiaor a perforated peptic ulcer. The raised white cell count is a marker of infection or an inflammatory response, both may be present in a patient with acute pancreatitis. The CRP level exceeds 150 mg/dl and is in keeping with a severe attack of pancreatitis.

c. Withdraw oral intake.

Establish IV fluids.

Catheterise the patient.

Give supplemental oxygen.

Provide adequate parenteral analgesia.

Obtain a baseline chest radiograph.

Monitor the response.

Any of the above responses will score marks. They are listed in order of priority. Most patients will respond to this 'supportive' treatment regime. Some patients (such as this one) with a severe attack may deteriorate despite apparently adequate treatment and may require care in a high dependency/intensive care setting to optimize function of their vital organs (heart/kidney/lungs).

d. Respiratory failure.

Some patients with severe acute pancreatitis will go on to develop the respiratory complications of the disease.

Pancreatitis stimulates a systemic inflammatory response, which leads to an increased permeability of the pulmonary microcirculation, which interferes with gas exchange between the lung capillaries and the alveoli. Some of these patients will go on to develop adult respiratory distress syndrome (ARDS, Ch. 1, p. 7). A fall in oxygen saturation (P_aO_2) is often the first indication of this condition. It is important also not to overlook other causes of respiratory deterioration, for example pneumonia, fluid overload or an underlying cardiac cause for the symptoms.

Best of 5s answers

1. d. Organise a CT brain scan.

This patient's conscious state, measured by the Glasgow Coma Scale, has deteriorated in the interval between admission and injury. It is vital to exclude intracerebral cause, for example an extradral haematoma, which must be treated by urgent surgical intervention. In this list of options, only a CT scan will provide the relevant information.

2. e. Insert a left-sided drain.

Acute dyspnoea plus a deviation in the trachea with an increase in resonance in the contralateral side of the chest and/or diminished air entry on that side are the hallmark of a tension pneumothorax. In this patient, the trachea has deviated to the right and the left side of the chest has increased resonance to percussion. This patient has a *left*-sided tension pneumothorax. Left untreated, the build-up of pressure in the left pleural cavity will reduce venous return to the heart and death may follow from acute heart failure.

This patient requires urgent insertion of a left-sided chest drain or, if that is not immediately available, a wide-bore intravenous cannula inserted into an intercostal space on the left chest wall will save a life.

3. a. CT abdominal scan.

This patient's radiograph is clear, which makes a respiratory cause for his deterioration unlikely. The most common cause of late sepsis after blunt trauma is a missed intra-abdominal injury. The diagnosis is always difficult to elicit in patients who may have a bruised abdominal wall from superficial trauma or those whose neurological status is depressed after a head injury. A 'burst' injury to the small intestine can occur when the abdomen is suddenly compressed by a seat belt (seat belt injury) during deacceleration at the time of impact. This injury may be silent at the time of primary survey and only become apparent when the patient becomes septic from peritonitis which develops later. A CT scan will detect small amounts of intraperitoneal gas, which are the hallmark of this injury and will not be identified by other less sensitive tests.

4. b. Acute mesenteric ischaemia.

Without urgent revascularisation or surgical resection of the gangrenous segments of intestine, these patients will die of overwhelming intra-abdominal sepsis. The greatest difficulty is establishing this elusive diagnosis. Too often these patients present with established disease which is beyond salvage. It is vital to consider acute mesenteric

ischaemia in every patient with an acute abdomen, especially if they have co-existing peripheral vascular disease or if they are diabetic. Sometimes they have a small elevation in their serum amylase. If there is time, the diagnosis will be clinched by a duplex ultrasound study of the mesenteric vessels which will show impaired or absent flow.

5. d. Erect chest radiograph.

Free intra-abdominal gas is the hallmark of a perforated viscus – the most common cause of generalised peritonitis. Of the tests listed, an erect chest radiograph will be the most helpful. Look beneath the diaphragms on this radiograph in order to detect traces of sub-diaphragmatic gas which will seal the diagnosis.

Multiple choice answers

1. a. **False.** The first priority is to secure the patient's airway. A patient will die of asphyxia before he exsanguinates.

   b. **False.** Cervical spine radiographs are essential to detect a fracture or dislocation. All major trauma victims should be considered to have a cervical fracture until proven otherwise by radiology. For this reason all these patients should have their cervical spine stabilised immediately with a cervical collar.

   c. **True.** Supine hypotension indicates a major loss in the circulating blood volume, usually in excess of 40%.

   d. **True.** Bilateral rib fractures indicate a severe injury to the chest. This group of patients are at a high risk of mediastinal injury.

   e. **False.** Peritoneal lavage is most effective at determining intraperitoneal bleeding: the lavage returns pink or bloodstained.

2. a. **False.** There may still be partial blood flow despite the injury or there may be a transmitted pulsation along the vessel wall.

   b. **True.** This is the key diagnostic step where major arterial injury is suspected. There is no substitute.

   c. **False.** Veins and nerves frequently accompany arteries in a neurovascular bundle. Injury to these structures should always be sought in any major arterial injury.

   d. **True.** This is one of the most common mechanisms that lead to vascular trauma in association with a blunt soft tissue injury. For example, the popliteal artery can be stretched and damaged during a posterior dislocation of the knee.

   e. **False.** A tourniquet is the last resort. It may further damage the blood supply to the distal tissues and will enhance any venous bleeding by obstructing the venous return. Direct pressure over the bleeding point is the best method of providing control.

3. a. **False.** The duodenum is a foregut structure. The visceral component of foregut pain (caused by

distension, inflammation, etc.) is perceived in the epigastrium. Midgut pain is perceived in the periumbilical area.

b. **False.** Renal or ureteric colic is characterised by pain in which *no* position is comfortable. Patients frequently 'writhe in agony'.

c. **True.** This is caused by diaphragmatic irritation from released gastric contents, which track up to lie beneath the diaphragm.

d. **True.** The pain of mesenteric ischaemia is characteristically severe, constant and diffuse.

e. **True.** Parietal pain develops as a consequence of inflammation of the parietal peritoneum by an inflamed viscus, intestinal contents or pus. It may be preceded by a visceral type pain, e.g. in acute appendicitis [periumbilical pain (visceral); right iliac fossa pain (parietal)].

4. a. **True.** The wall of the aneurysm may be calcified and this will be detected on a plain abdominal radiograph.

b. **False.** A plain abdominal radiograph may be normal. The most useful non-invasive test in a suspected perforated ulcer is an erect chest radiograph; this will detect subdiaphragmatic gas in 8 out of 10 patients.

c. **False.** This is essentially a clinical diagnosis. A plain abdominal film will not add to the diagnosis.

d. **True.** Radiopaque gallstones will be detected in 10% of cases.

e. **True.** This is a key diagnostic step in these patients and will confirm or refute the diagnosis.

5. a. **False.** The ligament of Treitz is sited at the duodenal–jejunal flexure. Gastrointestinal bleeding beyond this point presents as melena or rectal haemorrhage (depending on the rate of blood loss).

b. **False.** Angiodysplastic lesions are extremely uncommon in the stomach and duodenum.

Peptic ulcers, gastric and duodenal erosions and oesophageal varices are the main causes of upper gastrointestinal haemorrhage.

c. **False.** Some patients will present with melena alone. The combination of haematemesis and melena usually implies a more major bleed.

d. **False.** The detection rate of the underlying cause of an upper gastrointestinal bleed declines markedly after 24 h. All these patients should undergo a gastroscopy within the first 24 h.

e. **False.** Gastroscopy is the key step. Selective mesenteric angiography is reserved for those patients who continue to bleed but from no obvious source.

6. a. **True.** This is an important part of their work-up. Occasionally a major acute bleed from an upper gastrointestinal source will present as a rectal haemorrhage. The large volumes of blood released are an irritant to the gastrointestinal tract and stimulate a rapid transit through the small and large bowel.

b. **False.** Overall 80% of patients with rectal haemorrhage will settle on conservative treatment.

c. **False.** A major bleed is rarely caused by colorectal cancer. Occult bleeding or small amounts of blood loss with stools would be more likely. Angiodysplasia and diverticular disease are the most common causes of a major rectal haemorrhage.

d. **True.** They can be detected during colonoscopy or by mesenteric angiography.

e. **False.** A barium enema will provide the least information in a patient with an acute bleed. It will not detect any angiodysplastic lesions and may even mislead: diverticular disease is a common finding on any barium enema study and is not necessarily the cause of bleeding.

Surgical gastroenterology

Chapter

3

Chapter overview

Surgical gastroenterology encompasses a heterogeneous group of diseases which can affect the alimentary tract at any point from the mouth to the anus. This chapter outlines the key clinical features of the most important gastrointestinal diseases which are likely to present to a surgeon. As you will see there is a considerable overlap between medical and surgical gastrointestinal problems, and many of the conditions covered will be managed without the need for surgical intervention. In clinical practice some of these diseases are best managed by the close cooperation between surgeons and their medical gastroenterological colleagues.

Others require elective surgical intervention while some need emergency surgery and form the backbone of urgent surgical practice seen on any acute receiving ward. These patients will often require prompt resuscitation, investigation and surgery. The essential steps in the management and operative treatment are outlined in this chapter.

3.1 Diseases of the oesophagus

Learning objectives

You should:
- know the key clinical features of the main oesophageal diseases
- know how to investigate a patient with symptoms of oesophageal disease
- understand the principles of treatment in patients with diseases of the oesophagus.

The oesophagus is a muscular tube that extends from the pharynx to the gastric cardia. Its prime function is to act as a conduit for the passage of food. Muscular sphincters control entry and exit of food into the oesophagus. In health, the lower 2 inches (5 cm) of the oesophagus and the gastro-oesophageal junction lie below the oesophageal hiatus of the diaphragm.

The most important oesophageal diseases are:

H • hiatus hernia with or without reflux oesophagitis
C • carcinoma of the oesophagus
A • achalasia
S • oesophageal strictures and perforation.

CASH

Hiatus hernia with or without reflux oesophagitis

These are separate but related conditions and together are the most common oesophageal disorder. There are two types of hernia: a sliding hernia (Figure 5A) and a paraoesophageal or rolling hernia (Figure 5B). Reflux oesophagitis is caused by acid or bile regurgitation into the oesophagus and is more common in patients with a sliding hiatus hernia. Reflux oesophagitis can occur in patients without a hiatus hernia.

Sliding hiatus hernia
Aetiology
Ageing and obesity slacken the oesophageal hiatus and allow the gastro-oesophageal junction to slide upwards between the crura of the diaphragm into the chest (Figure 5A). In this position, the lower oesophageal sphincter is less effective and allows reflux of gastric contents. Acid, bile and pepsin all contribute to the erosive oesophagitis and oesophageal ulceration.

Clinical features
Heartburn, regurgitation and waterbrash are the primary symptoms. They are worse at night when the patient is recumbent. Chronic aspiration of gastric contents into the lungs can cause recurrent chest infections.

Complications
There are two main complications:

- reflux-induced oesophageal 'peptic' stricture which may require dilatation
- Barrett's oesophagitis.

Chronic irritation of the lower oesophagus by reflux can promote replacement of the normal squamous epithelium with columnar (Barrett's) epithelium. Untreated, long-standing Barrett's oesophagitis is unstable. Mucosal

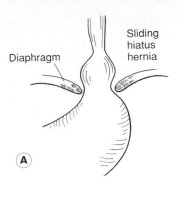

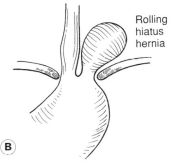

Figure 5 (A) Sliding hiatus hernia. (B) Rolling, paraoesophageal hiatus hernia.

changes will progress from low- to high-grade dysplasia and eventually an adenocarcinoma will develop.

Diagnosis

A sliding hiatus hernia can be detected on a barium swallow and meal examination or, more often, at endoscopy. Biopsy is necessary to assess the severity of any associated oesophagitis or replacement by Barrett's epithelium.

Specialised oesophageal function studies, which include manometry, 24-h ambulatory pH monitoring and radioisotope transit tests, are mandatory prior to surgical treatment and in addition to confirming reflux disease will identify any associated motility disorder.

Treatment

Antacids regimens using a combination of acid suppression therapy (see p. 43) and a mucosal protective agent together with weight reduction form the cornerstone of medical treatment. Elevation of the bed head may relieve night-time symptoms. Patients should also be encouraged to cut down alcohol intake and stop smoking. These measures are effective in 90% of patients; the remainder require surgery either for symptom control or because complications develop. The aim of surgery is to *prevent* gastro-oesophageal reflux by restoring the gastro-oesophageal junction and lower oesophagus to their normal position below the oesophageal hiatus and to strengthen the lower oesophageal sphincter by wrapping the fundus either partly (Toupet procedure) or completely (Nissen procedure) around the oesophagus. The partial wraps are reputed to cause less postoperative dysphagia. The oesophageal hiatus is tightened by suturing together the diaphragmatic crura. Most antireflux procedures are undertaken using a laparoscope. Occasionally the operation is performed through the chest (Belsey repair). 'Gas-bloat' syndrome is the most important side effect after antireflux surgery and leaves 10% of patients unable to belch or vomit.

Paraoesophageal or rolling hiatus hernia

All or part of the stomach herniates through the oesophageal hiatus adjacent to the gastro-oesophageal junction, which remains in its normal anatomical position (Figure 5B).

Clinical features

Usually asymptomatic, the rolling hiatus hernia only presents when complications develop. Incarceration of the hernia causes:

- gastric outlet obstruction
- strangulation
- gastric stasis and ulceration.

Diagnosis

A rolling hiatus hernia is detected by a chest radiograph, barium swallow and meal examination or gastroscopy.

Treatment

Because the complications are dangerous, early surgery is required. The herniated stomach is reduced through an abdominal incision or by laparoscopic surgery and the defect in the oesophageal hiatus repaired.

Carcinoma of the oesophagus

True primary oesophageal cancers are of squamous cell origin. Adenocarcinomas in the lower third of the oesophagus are usually gastric in origin or have developed in a Barrett's oesophagus. Both types of tumour spread by direct invasion of local structures, via the bloodstream to liver, lungs and bone, and by lymphatics to the regional lymph glands. The incidence of oesophageal cancer is increasing.

Aetiology

The causes of carcinoma of the oesophagus are:

- high alcohol and tobacco consumption
- malnutrition
- certain chemicals, e.g. nitrosamines
- stasis of food caused by an oesophageal web, achalasia or stricture.

Clinical features

Progressive dysphagia of solids then liquids with severe weight loss are the hallmark of oesophageal cancer. Chest pain and hoarseness are grave symptoms and indicate local spread within the chest to involve the recurrent laryngeal nerve. Some patients will present with recurrent chest infections or an aspiration pneumonia caused by regurgitation of food from the obstructed oesophagus.

Three

Complications

These include:

- aspiration pneumonia
- inability to swallow saliva
- tracheo-oesophageal fistula.

Diagnosis

A barium swallow will demonstrate an irregular stricture. The diagnosis must be confirmed by endoscopy and biopsy. A computed tomography (CT) scan or a magnetic resonance imaging (MRI) scan of the chest is vital in order to 'stage' the disease and assess resectability.

Treatment

As in all patients with cancer the choice of treatment lies between aggressive surgery/radiotherapy/chemotherapy, in an attempt to cure the patient, and a lesser procedure aimed at relieving (palliating) the patient's symptoms. The decision taken will be based on many factors including the stage or extent of the disease, the age and fitness of the patient and also the patient's wishes.

Surgical resection should be attempted whenever possible as this provides the best symptom palliation. The surgery is complex and the choice of operation depends on the site of the cancer (Table 7). However, many patients are unfit or have advanced disease and only 10% will undergo a successful resection. Many surgeons will undertake a laparoscopy before embarking on resection to identify those patients with metastatic disease (usually liver or peritoneal seedlings) which have not been identified during preoperative screening. This will save these patients with incurable disease an unnecessary laparotomy/thoracotomy. The choice of operation, when resection is possible, depends on the site of the cancer (see Table 7). You do not need to know the precise technical details.

Most *squamous* cell cancers and some adenocarcinomas are sensitive to radiotherapy, which can be used as an alternative to surgery either as primary treatment in an attempt to 'cure' the disease or simply in a palliative dose to relieve dysphagia. Swallowing can also be restored by intubation using an expandable metal stent. This is inserted over a guide wire under fluoroscopic control after dilating the malignant stricture using an endoscope and bougie or balloon dilator and provides better palliation than a pulsion tube (e.g. the Nottingham tube), which is pushed through the tumour from above (through the mouth). Traction tubes (e.g. the Celestin tube), which are pulled into place through a gastrotomy at open operation, are

Table 7 Surgery in oesophageal cancer

Site of cancer	Operation
Cervical oesophagus	Pharyngo-oesophagectomy
Upper third oesophagus	Subtotal oesophagectomy
Middle third oesophagus	Subtotal oesophagectomy
Lower third oesophagus	Oesophagogastrectomy
Oesophago-gastric junction	

used if the cancer cannot be safely dilated using an endoscopic technique.

Prognosis

Survival is poor. Overall, around 10% of all patients with oesophageal cancer will survive 5 years. Surgeons aim to keep operative mortality rates less than 5%. After a successful resection 5-year survival rates increase to 30%.

Achalasia

Achalasia is a functional not a mechanical obstruction of the oesophagus. It is the most important of all the oesophageal motility disorders.

Aetiology

Achalasia is caused by an idiopathic degeneration of the ganglion cells of Auerbach's myenteric plexus, which lie in the muscular wall of the oesophagus. As a result, primary peristalsis is absent and the lower oesophageal sphincter fails to relax on swallowing.

Clinical features

Dysphagia without weight loss is the cardinal symptom. Pain is uncommon.

Complications

These include:

- night-time regurgitation – aspiration pneumonia
- oesophageal stasis – ulceration
- carcinoma of the oesophagus.

Diagnosis

A barium swallow is the primary investigation. The proximal oesophagus is dilated and tortuous and merges into a smooth cone-shaped narrowed segment above the gastro-oesophageal junction.

Oesophageal manometry (pressure studies) will confirm absent primary peristalsis and failure of the lower oesophageal sphincter to relax on swallowing.

During endoscopy, the narrow lower oesophageal sphincter offers no mechanical resistance to the passage of the gastroscope. A mucosal biopsy should be taken to exclude a cancer.

Differential diagnosis It is important to differentiate achalasia from other major causes of dysphagia, e.g. benign strictures, oesophageal carcinoma.

Treatment

Achalasia can be relieved by forceful disruption of the lower oesophageal sphincter using endoscopically guided balloon dilatation or by laparoscopic or open surgical division of the sphincter (Heller's cardiomyotomy). The risks of oesophageal perforation and recurrent achalasia are higher with balloon dilatation, which is usually reserved for patients unfit for surgery.

Oesophageal strictures and perforation

Strictures

Most oesophageal strictures present with dysphagia. The diagnosis is confirmed by barium swallow and endoscopy.

Usually they are the result of long-standing oesophageal reflux. Other important causes are:

- oesophageal cancer
- corrosive ingestion
- collagen diseases, e.g. scleroderma.

The majority of benign strictures can be managed by endoscopic dilatation and treatment of the underlying condition.

Perforation

Perforation of the oesophagus is a recognised complication of forceful dilatation of an oesophageal stricture or during palliative intubation of an oesophageal cancer. It can also complicate diagnostic endoscopy as a result of either a technical error or tearing of the oesophagus by the endoscope against the cervical spine.

Spontaneous oesophageal perforation (Boerhaave syndrome) is the sequel to a violent bout of vomiting or retching, often precipitated by a bout of heavy eating or drinking. The tear usually occurs just above the gastro-oesophageal junction on the left side.

Clinical features
These include:

- agonising pain in the chest, neck or upper abdomen
- cervical crepitus and subcutaneous emphysema
- hydropneumothorax on a chest radiograph caused by air leaking from the oesophageal lumen into the pleural cavity.

Diagnosis
A water-soluble contrast swallow or a CT scan with water-soluble contrast will demonstrate the site of the leak.

Treatment
Most instrumental cervical perforations and some minor intrathoracic perforations can be treated conservatively with systemic antibiotics and oral fluid restriction. All others require thoracotomy, closure of the perforation and chest drainage. If surgery is delayed beyond 24 h in these cases, the survival rate will be less than 50%.

3.2 Diseases of the stomach and duodenum

· ·

Learning objectives

You should:
- know the clinical features of peptic ulcer disease and gastric cancer
- know how to investigate a patient with 'dyspeptic' symptoms
- have a treatment plan for patients with peptic ulcer disease
- understand the role and principles of surgery in patients with peptic ulcer disease or gastric cancer.

The two most important conditions that affect the stomach and duodenum are:

- peptic ulcer disease
- carcinoma of the stomach.

Peptic ulcer disease

This is the most common disorder of the stomach and duodenum. Peptic ulceration occurs at any site where gastrointestinal mucosa is subject to the corrosive action of acid gastric juices. The most frequent sites are:

- duodenum, causing a duodenal ulcer
- oesophagus, causing a peptic stricture
- stomach, causing a gastric ulcer.

It also occurs following gastroenterostomy, causing a stomal ulcer.

Aetiology
The causes of the disease are:

- high gastric acid output
- alcohol and tobacco consumption
- salicylates, steroids, non-steroidal anti-inflammatory drugs
- antral helicobacter infection.

Clinical features
Cyclical epigastric pain relieved by food, milk or antacids characterises uncomplicated peptic ulcer disease but many patients will present with non-specific dyspeptic symptoms. Epigastric tenderness is usual.

Diagnosis
Gastroscopy is the most valuable investigation. It will detect small superficial ulcers and any inflammation, which may be overlooked on a barium meal.

Treatment
Most uncomplicated peptic ulcers respond to medical therapy. Surgery is only occasionally needed.

Medical treatment Histamine H_2 receptor antagonists, such as ranitidine, which reduce gastric acid secretion, are the mainstay of treatment. Peptic ulcers are characterised by a rapid symptomatic response to these drugs and to the withdrawal of any causative agents. Resistant ulcers usually respond to proton pump inhibitors such as omeprazole, which is a more potent inhibitor of acid secretion. Some ulcers respond to chealating agents such as bismuth compounds or sucralfate.

Helicobacter infection In patients with a biopsy-proven gastric helicobacter infection and a duodenal ulcer, eradicating the infection using a combination of antibiotics (clarithromycin, amoxycillin) together with a histamine H_2 receptor antagonist or proton pump inhibitor is the most effective method, inducing permanent healing in more than 90% of patients.

Elective surgery for peptic ulcer disease
Very few patients with peptic ulcer disease will have a persistent ulcer that will require surgery.

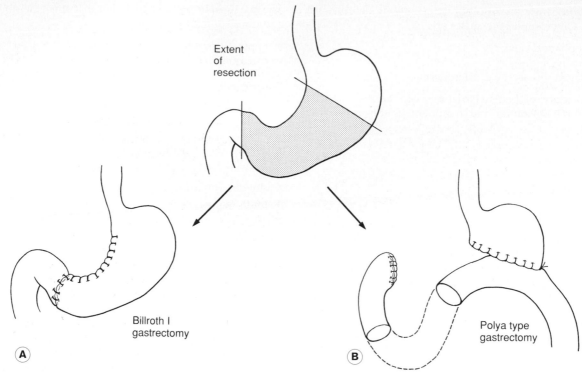

Extent
of
resection

Billroth I
gastrectomy

(A)

Polya type
gastrectomy

(B)

Figure 6 Billroth I (A) and Polya type (B) gastrectomies for peptic ulcers (A or B) or gastric cancer (B).

Operations such as truncal vagotomy and a gastric drainage procedure (either a pyloroplasty or gastroenterostomy) or highly selective vagotomy, both designed to cut gastric acid secretion, have fallen into disuse since the advent of effective medical treatment to suppress gastric acid output. Most surgeons would now opt for a partial gastrectomy (Figure 6) to treat an ulcer which is resistant to medical treatment. It is important that a pathological cause for acid hypersecretion such as Zollinger–Ellison syndrome (a pancreatic islet cell tumour which secretes gastrin) is excluded in these patients.

Despite this change in surgical practice there are still a number of patients who present with the complications of gastric surgery carried out many years ago.

Complications of gastric surgery

The complications seen are:

- recurrent ulceration
- postgastrectomy syndromes
- nutritional deficiencies.

Recurrent ulceration Ulcers that recur after surgery usually develop because the original operation was inadequate or incomplete. They present with ulcer pain or bleeding or both. Reoperation can be complex and difficult. Wherever possible proton pump inhibitors or histamine H_2 receptor antagonists should be tried first to promote healing.

Post gastric surgery syndromes Division of the main vagal nerve trunks inhibits gastric acid output production but it also impairs gastric emptying. These patients would always have a gastric drainage procedure (either a pylo-roplasty or a gastroenterostomy) to prevent gastric stasis. Patients who have undergone partial gastrectomy will also have had a vagotomy. The mechanisms causing post gastric surgery syndromes are poorly understood but seem to relate to the denervation of the gut after vagotomy and precipitous gastric emptying. Two main categories are recognised:

Postvagotomy diarrhoea After truncal vagotomy, 1% of patients develop incapacitating explosive diarrhoea. The mechanism is poorly understood but may be caused by rapid gastric emptying and fast small bowel transit.

Dumping syndrome There are two types:

- Early dumping syndrome (vasomotor dumping). This occurs shortly after eating; patients experience sweating, palpitations, lightheadedness and abdominal cramps and feel compelled to lie down. The cause is uncertain but appears related to the uncontrolled entry of hypertonic food boluses from the stomach into the small bowel. Treatment is difficult. Some patients relieve their symptoms by taking small frequent dry meals.
- Late dumping syndrome or reactive hypoglycaemia. In these patients, rapid absorption of a large glucose load from the small bowel is followed by a 'rebound' hypoglycaemia caused by prolonged insulin action.

Nutritional deficiencies Iron deficient anaemia is common and is caused by a failure to absorb dietary iron. A macrocytic anaemia can also develop because of vitamin B_{12} malabsorption. This can be prevented by 3-monthly vitamin B_{12} injections.

Complications of peptic ulcer disease

There are three major complications:

- haemorrhage
- perforation
- pyloric stenosis.

Haemorrhage

Bleeding is the most frequent and most lethal complication of peptic ulcer disease. Sudden, massive haemorrhage presents with haematemesis, melena and shock. Less often, chronic blood loss can cause anaemia with or without melena. The principles of management of a bleeding peptic ulcer are fully outlined in section 2.3. The most important points are:

- resuscitate with blood products
- confirm diagnosis by endoscopy within 24 h in a stable patient, immediately in an unstable patient
- perform urgent endoscopic treatment or surgical intervention if no response to resuscitation.

Endoscopic treatment Bleeding can be arrested by injecting sclerosing agents, by applying a clip to a bleeding vessel, or by using heater probes or laser coagulation. These procedures are performed at the same time as the diagnostic gastroscopy.

Surgical treatment Three-quarters of all patients will stop bleeding after resuscitation alone or following endoscopic treatment. Continuing haemorrhage (requiring more than a 4-unit blood transfusion) or rebleeding is an indication for emergency surgery. Simple oversew of the bleeding ulcer is effective in combination with histamine H_2 receptor antagonists or proton pump inhibitors to reduce gastric acid output. Major surgery such as a gastrectomy should be avoided if possible because the surgical mortality is increased.

Prognosis Up to 10% of patients with bleeding ulcers will die. Elderly patients or those who have rebled are at greatest risk.

Perforation

Most ulcers that perforate are sited on the anterior wall of the duodenum or stomach. The release of food and digestive enzymes into the peritoneal cavity initially causes a chemical peritonitis. Secondary bacterial peritonitis evolves later.

Clinical features:

- agonising central epigastric pain, shoulder tip radiation
- rigid, silent abdomen
- subdiaphragmatic gas on an *erect* chest radiograph.

Treatment Nasogastric decompression is essential to minimise further intraperitoneal contamination. After intravenous fluid resuscitation, urgent laparotomy and simple oversew of the perforation with an omental 'patch' are required. Thorough peritoneal lavage will minimise the risks of postoperative abscess formation.

Prognosis As with haemorrhage, 10% of these patients will die. At special risk are the elderly and patients in whom a late diagnosis is made.

Pyloric stenosis

This is the result of fibrotic scarring from a long-standing duodenal or pyloric channel ulcer. It can also result from spasm or oedema caused by an acute ulcer. Pyloric stenosis is the least common complication of peptic ulcer disease.

Clinical features:

- a long history of peptic ulcer symptoms
- vomiting unaltered foodstuffs
- weight loss and dehydration
- a succussion splash on examination.

Diagnosis Barium meal and gastroscopy are complementary in the evaluation of gastric outlet obstruction. Barium meal will demonstrate delayed gastric emptying while gastroscopy will help distinguish spasm from fibrosis and exclude a gastric outlet cancer. Before either investigation is attempted, the stomach should be decompressed by nasogastric suction and lavaged to remove food debris.

Treatment Some patients with an acute ulcer and spasm will respond to intravenous histamine H_2 receptor blockade and a period of nasogastric decompression. Most require a gastric drainage procedure (either pyloroplasty or gastroenterostomy) combined with long-term acid suppression using proton pump inhibitors or H_2 receptor blockade, to cut down acid secretion. A few patients will respond to endoscopic balloon dilatation of the pylorus.

Prognosis In contrast to haemorrhage and perforation, the outlook for patients with pyloric stenosis is excellent.

Benign gastric ulcers

These are less common than duodenal ulcers and occur in an older age group. It is *essential* to differentiate them from an ulcerating gastric cancer.

Aetiology:

The causes are:

- high acid output
- non-steroidal anti-inflammatory drugs
- *Helicobacter pylori* infection
- duodenogastric bile reflux.

Clinical features

Epigastric pain, vomiting, weight loss and anaemia are the chief symptoms. They are common to patients with a gastric ulcer or a *gastric cancer.*

Diagnosis

Gastroscopy and biopsy are essential in order to confirm the diagnosis, exclude gastric cancer and to detect helicobacter infection. Classically a punched out ulcer crater is in keeping with a benign gastric ulcer whereas a rolled everted ulcer edge is suspicious of malignancy. Repeated biopsy may be necessary to rule out a gastric cancer.

Treatment

Histamine H_2 receptor antagonists or proton pump inhibitors form the mainstay of treatment. Some ulcers, especially those associated with helicobacter infection, will respond to combinations of antibiotic therapy plus

Three

45

histamine H$_2$ receptor antagonists. Repeat endoscopy after 6–8 weeks of treatment is mandatory to ensure the ulcer heals. Non-response or relapse after treatment is more common in gastric than in duodenal ulceration. It may also indicate that the ulcer is malignant.

A recurring or non-healing gastric ulcer in the body of the stomach is best treated by partial gastrectomy (Figure 6). Local excision plus acid suppression therapy is sometimes effective in elderly patients. Ulcers in the gastric antrum are treated like duodenal ulcers.

Carcinoma of the stomach

Nearly all gastric cancers are adenocarcinomatous in origin. The disease is twice as common in men as in women and has a peak incidence in the sixth decade. Overall, the incidence of gastric cancer is decreasing. Spread occurs by direct invasion of local structures, e.g. the pancreas; via the bloodstream to the liver; by lymphatics to regional lymph glands; and across the peritoneal cavity (transcoelomic) to form peritoneal deposits or metastases in the ovaries (Krukenberg tumours).

Aetiology

Gastric cancer is more common in patients with:

- pernicious anaemia and achlorhydria
- type A blood group
- previous partial gastrectomy
- positive family history
- smoking and spicy foods
- a history of gastric adenomatous polyps.

There are four main pathological types:

- ulcerative
- polypoid
- linitis plastica ('leather bottle stomach'): a diffuse infiltrating cancer affecting all layers of the stomach wall
- superficial spreading cancer: an uncommon variant restricted to the mucosa and submucosa and associated with a better prognosis.

Clinical features

Gastric cancer often presents late. Patients may present with symptoms and signs of the *primary tumour* (dyspeptic symptoms, vomiting, epigastric mass), signs of *secondary disease* (left supraclavicular lymphadenopathy spread via the thoracic duct) or *systemic symptoms* such as weight loss, poor appetite, anaemia. Usually patients have a long history often of initially rather vague symptoms. Tumours that block the cardia and cause dysphagia or those that obstruct the pylorus and cause vomiting present earlier.

Patients with unremitting, gnawing epigastric pain and a palpable epigastric mass or a hard liver edge usually have advanced, inoperable disease.

Diagnosis

Gastroscopy and biopsy is the key investigation. It provides a tissue diagnosis and detects those cancers that because of size or site may be missed on a barium meal examination.

Abdominal ultrasound and CT scanning (or MRI scanning) can be used independently or in combination to look for liver metastases.

Treatment

Once the diagnosis is confirmed, a barium meal is a useful aid in planning the surgical treatment. The surgical management is complex and depends on the site of the cancer. Radical surgical resection provides the only hope of cure. It is also the best way to palliate the patient's symptoms. Cancer of the body of the stomach requires a total abdominal gastrectomy. The entire stomach is removed en bloc with the attached omentum, adjacent lymph nodes and spleen. Continuity of the gastrointestinal tract is restored using the jejunum (Figure 7A). For cancers involving the gastric fundus or cardia the distal stomach can be preserved and used to restore continuity to the oesophagus – a procedure known as proximal gastrectomy (Figure 7B). Alternatively the proximal stomach and distal oesophagus can be removed en bloc. This operation, an oesophagogastrectomy, also uses the distal stomach to restore continuity to the remaining oesophagus. The choice of operation is determined by the site of the cancer in relation to the gastro-oesophageal junction. For a cancer of the antrum or pylorus, the spleen and proximal stomach are preserved and gastrointestinal continuity restored with a Polya type gastrectomy (Figure 6B).

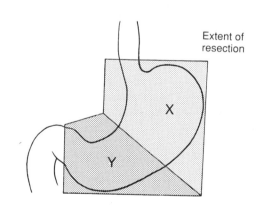

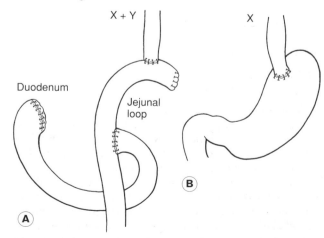

Figure 7 (A) Total abdominal gastrectomy for gastric cancer (resection of X and Y). (B) Proximal gastrectomy for cancer of the gastric cardia (removal of X only).

Radical gastric resection is contraindicated if liver metastases are present. These patients cannot be cured. A lesser gastric resection may be chosen to simply remove the bulk of the tumour. A palliative bypass (gastroenterostomy) may help relieve symptoms caused by an obstructing cancer that cannot be removed.

Prognosis

Because this disease presents late, is locally invasive and disseminates widely, only 10% of patients will survive 5 years. A few patients with superficial spreading cancers that are diagnosed early are the only exception. They can expect a 90% 5-year survival.

3.3 Biliary and pancreatic disease

Learning objectives

You should:

- know the key clinical features of the main biliary and pancreatic diseases
- have a management plan for a patient presenting with jaundice
- know how to treat a patient with acute cholecystitis or pancreatitis
- understand the principles of management in patients with pancreatic cancer.

There are four important biliary disorders:

- common
  - gallstone disease
  - obstructive jaundice
- uncommon
  - cholangiocarcinoma
  - carcinoma of the gallbladder.

The three most important diseases affecting the pancreas are:

- acute pancreatitis
- carcinoma of the pancreas
- chronic pancreatitis.

Biliary disease

Gallstone disease: biliary colic and acute cholecystitis

Gallstones are common. Up to 20% of all individuals over the age of 60 have gallstones. Although the vast majority of gallstones are asymptomatic, cholecystectomy for gallstone disease is the most frequent major elective operation carried out in Britain and the USA today.

There is a considerable overlap between biliary colic and acute cholecystitis. Biliary colic is caused by the transient impaction of a gallstone in the neck of the gallbladder (Hartmann's pouch). Acute cholecystitis implies the development of bacterial infection in the gallbladder wall, which may or may not be preceded by biliary colic.

Clinical features

Biliary colic has the following characteristics:

- sudden onset of right subcostal pain which subsides gradually *over a few hours*
- radiation around costal margin and shoulder tip
- nausea and vomiting
- symptoms that may not be severe enough for the patient to urgently attend hospital
- fever (uncommon).

Acute cholecystitis is the sequel to secondary bacterial infection caused by gut-derived gram-negative bacteria (e.g. *Escherichia coli*), which spread to the gallbladder via the bile or bloodstream.

Additional clinical features are:

- signs of systemic sepsis
- subcostal tenderness (Murphy's sign)
- jaundice
- fever (common).

Acute cholecystitis can also occur without gallstones (acalculous cholecystitis). This condition, which is rare, occurs in debilitated, septic patients, burn victims or intensive care patients on long-term parenteral nutrition.

Diagnosis

This diagnosis is established primarily by history and physical examination. It is confirmed by:

- Ultrasound scan: this will detect 95% of all gallstones.
- Radionuclide biliary excretion scan (HIDA): used when ultrasound scanning is unsuccessful. If diseased, the gall bladder will fail to 'take up' the radionuclide and will not be visible on the scan.
- Oral cholecystogram: *this is of no value* in acute cholecystitis as it requires a functioning gallbladder to produce a result. Today, this test is rarely used.

Medical treatment

The key steps in the initial management of acute cholecystitis are:

1. establish i.v. fluid regimen, restrict oral intake
2. broad-spectrum intravenous antibiotic cover
3. parenteral opioid analgesia.

About 90% of all attacks will resolve using this conservative regimen. Those that do not respond within 24–48 h have usually developed a septic complication of gallstone disease that will require urgent surgery.

Surgical treatment

For the majority of cases that settle with conservative treatment, there are two choices:

- early cholecystectomy: performed during the same hospital admission within 5–7 days of the acute attack
- elective cholecystectomy: 4–6 weeks after the acute attack following convalescence at home.

Three

Early cholecystectomy is preferred as it will prevent further attacks and the patient will not require readmission for surgery at a later date.

Currently, most patients with gallstones will have their gallbladder removed using laparoscopic surgical techniques. Open cholecystectomy is reserved for those patients in whom technical difficulties are encountered or for patients undergoing urgent surgery for the complications of biliary disease. Some surgeons routinely perform an operative cholangiography during cholecystectomy to check the biliary anatomy and to look for common bile duct stones (see below for management of common bile duct stones).

Urgent surgery and the complications of acute cholecystitis

Urgent surgery is required for those patients with acute cholecystitis who do not respond quickly to medical treatment, usually because of the onset of complications. These can be classified according to the site of the gallstones in the biliary tree (see Figure 8).

Stones remaining in the gallbladder (Figure 8A, B):

- common complications
  - pericholecystic abscess
  - empyema
  - mucocele
- uncommon complications
  - gangrene
  - free perforation
  - gallstone ileus.

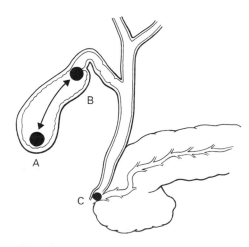

{ A – Acute cholecystitis
{ B – Biliary colic
    – Empyema
    – Pericholecystic abscess
    – Perforation
    – Gangrene
  C – Ascending cholangitis
    – Obstructive jaundice
    – Gallstone pancreatitis

Figure 8 Complications of gallstones.

Stones that migrate to the common bile duct (Figure 8C):

- obstructive jaundice
- ascending cholangitis
- gallstone pancreatitis.

Surgery for gallstones remaining in the gallbladder

There are two surgical options for complicated gallstone disease when the gallstones have remained in the gallbladder.

Emergency cholecystectomy Removing the diseased gallbladder and stones plus draining the associated sepsis.

Emergency cholecystostomy Using a tube to drain the gallbladder after removing the stones. This is a safer option in frail, septic patients or when technical difficulties are encountered. The gallbladder can be removed at a later date when the patient's condition allows.

In a critically ill unfit patient, ultrasound-guided percutaneous cholecystostomy can be performed, draining the gallbladder of pus and bile but leaving the stones in situ.

Surgery for gallstones in the common bile duct

Gallstones are found in the common bile duct (choledocholithiasis) in 5% of all patients with gallstone disease. Most migrate from the gallbladder. Occasionally stones form primarily in the common bile duct. In addition to the three main clinical presentations outlined above, common duct stones can also be silent and present unexpectedly during routine elective or emergency cholecystectomy.

Obstructive jaundice This is caused by common duct stones and may be painless or associated with biliary colic or cholecystitis. The diagnosis is supported by obstructed pattern liver function tests (see below) and a dilated biliary tree on ultrasound scan caused by the mechanical obstruction to the bile duct. Although gallstones are easily seen in the gallbladder with ultrasound they are rarely identified in the common bile duct. There are two options for treatment:

- endoscopic retrograde cholangiopancreatography (ERCP), sphincterotomy and stone removal
- open or laparoscopic common bile duct exploration.

ERCP, sphincterotomy and stone removal The diagnosis of bile duct stones can be absolutely confirmed with this procedure and other causes (e.g. carcinoma of the pancreas) eliminated. ERCP is also used to extract the stones. A special side viewing endoscope is used to advance a catheter into the bile duct via the ampulla of Vater. Once the stones are identified diathermy is used to cut open the ampulla and sphincter of Oddi with a sphincterotome. Stones can then be retrieved from the bile duct using baskets or balloons. The technique has the advantage of avoiding a laparotomy. It is probably the first choice in treatment for all patients with suspected common bile duct stones. It is especially suitable for frail elderly patients whose main symptoms relate to the common bile duct stones and who do not have acute cholecystitis, and also for those patients with common bile duct stones who have previously had a cholecystectomy. Pancreatitis, bleeding and duodenal perforation are occasional complications of this procedure.

Open or laparoscopic common bile duct exploration In this procedure the bile duct is opened and any stones are removed also using baskets or balloons. The bile duct is usually closed over a T tube which decompresses the biliary system after surgical exploration. A T tube cholangiogram is performed before the tube is removed to make sure that no stones have been left behind.

Ascending cholangitis Rigors, jaundice and fever are the hallmark of ascending cholangitis; these are caused by a combination of obstruction and infection in the biliary tree. Untreated, this lethal combination will lead to death from septicaemia and liver abscess. Treatment involves urgent decompression of the biliary tree under antibiotic cover, by either ERCP or open exploration; this is a life-saving measure.

Gallstone pancreatitis (see acute pancreatitis, p. 50).

Prognosis

Elective biliary surgery is characterised by a low morbidity and mortality. Patients at highest risk are those undergoing urgent or emergency surgery for the complications of gallstone disease.

Obstructive jaundice

The main *surgical* causes of jaundice are:

- common causes
  - common bile duct stones
  - pancreatic cancer
- less common causes
  - cholangiocarcinoma
  - extrinsic compression by malignant hilar lymph glands
  - metastatic liver disease.

These conditions have to be differentiated from the many medical causes, the most common being:

- hepatitis A, B and C
- drug-induced jaundice
- primary biliary cirrhosis
- alcoholic liver disease.

Clinical features

Most patients will be obviously jaundiced. Some will have hepatomegaly, which may be smooth or irregular. A palpable gallbladder is suspicious of malignant biliary obstruction with passive massive distension of an obstructed gallbladder. There may be stigmata of cirrhotic liver disease (see section 3.4). Diagnostic tests will be essential to determine the cause.

Diagnosis

The key tests are:

- liver function tests
  - serum bilirubin
  - alkaline phosphatase
  - liver transaminases.

Massive elevation in the liver transaminases is in keeping with a hepatocellular cause for jaundice. Major elevations in serum alkaline phosphatase with normal liver transaminase levels suggest an obstructive jaundice. These tests are not infallible and patients often present with a 'mixed' pattern with elevations in alkaline phosphatase and liver transaminases. Further investigation is always required:

- hepatitis screen, A, B and C
- biliary ultrasound scan
- CT or MRI scan
- ERCP examination.

A hepatitis screen will eliminate any infectious cause. The identification of a dilated biliary tree using ultrasound will confirm the diagnosis of an obstructive jaundice; liver metastases may also be detected. CT or MR scan of the liver, gall bladder and pancreas will detect a cancer or gallstones causing obstruction. ERCP is frequently an essential diagnostic and therapeutic step once biliary tree dilatation is detected; the cause of the obstruction can be identified and endoscopic treatment may be possible.

Treatment

This depends on the underlying cause. Treatment of the various surgical causes of obstructive jaundice is discussed in detail in the relevant sections of this chapter. Any jaundiced patient faced with surgery has three additional problems to surmount:

- coagulopathy
- hepatorenal failure
- increased risk of infection.

Coagulopathy must be corrected before surgery by vitamin K injection plus fresh frozen plasma infusion (contains a high concentration of clotting factors). The risk of hepatorenal failure is minimised by keeping jaundiced patients well hydrated before, during and after surgery. All these patients require antibiotic prophylaxis.

Cholangiocarcinoma

Cholangiocarcinoma is relatively uncommon and can affect any part of the biliary tree.

Seventy per cent of all cholangiocarcinomas arise at the junction of the left and right hepatic ducts in the hilum of the liver (a klatskin tumour). They usually present with jaundice caused by obstruction of the biliary tree.

Treatment

Cure is infrequent; most patients present with advanced disease. The jaundice and intense pruritis that accompany the disease are usually relieved with a biliary stent, which is placed across the tumour to decompress the biliary tree using either endoscopy (ERCP) or percutaneous transhepatic cholangiography (PTC) techniques. Surgical resection of the tumour is possible in about 20% of patients. The operation is complex and, depending on the site of the cancer, it may be necessary to resect part of the liver (a left or right hemihepatectomy).

Carcinoma of the gallbladder

Gallbladder cancer is rare. Most often it is identified as an unexpected finding on histopathological examination in a gallbladder removed for gallstones. Sometimes the disease will present with a painful biliary mass or jaundice, or the diagnosis will be made unexpectedly at operation for 'gallstone disease'. Usually these cancers cannot be removed and the survival is poor.

Diseases of the pancreas

Acute pancreatitis

Aetiology

Gallstone disease or alcohol excess account for 70% of all episodes of acute pancreatitis. A transient obstruction of the ampulla of Vater during passage of a common duct stone is the most likely mechanism in biliary pancreatitis. Alcohol may act as a pancreatic toxin or may damage the pancreas by simultaneously inducing pancreatic hypersecretion and spasm of the sphincter of Oddi. Less common causes of acute pancreatitis include:

Pancreas divisum This is a congenital abnormality in which the body of the pancreas drains into the duodenum via the accessory and not the main pancreatic duct.

Metabolic abnormalities These include hyperlipidaemia and hypercalcaemia.

Trauma This can occur either after a blunt abdominal injury or following a peroperative injury, or after ERCP.

Mumps

Despite thorough evaluation, 10–20% of all cases of pancreatitis will prove to be idiopathic.

The clinical course and outcome depend on the severity of the attack. In a mild attack, the pancreas becomes oedematous. If the injury continues, oedema will progress to haemorrhage and ultimately pancreatic necrosis. All attacks of pancreatitis are aseptic initially. Secondary infection develops in areas of pancreatic necrosis and can cause a pancreatic abscess. Fluid and blood loss into the pancreas and retroperitoneum are caused by an increase in capillary permeability and produce shock. Fluid and pancreatic enzymes may become sequestered in the lesser sac and produce a pseudocyst.

Clinical features

Acute pancreatitis is characterised by a rapid onset of agonising epigastric pain that spreads to the back and flanks. Patients are usually nauseated and will vomit. Early in the attack, abdominal tenderness is maximal in the epigastrium and later becomes more generalised. Some but not all patients will be shocked. The degree of shock will depend on the severity of the attack.

Diagnosis

Almost invariably the diagnosis is confirmed by an elevated serum amylase level. Plain abdominal radiographs may be normal or may show an isolated dilated loop of bowel (a sentinel loop) caused by a local ileus. A swollen oedematous pancreas can be demonstrated on ultrasound or CT examination, which may also detect any gallstones.

Differential diagnosis The two most important conditions that mimic acute pancreatitis and can be associated with an elevated serum amylase are:

- perforated peptic ulcer
- mesenteric vascular ischaemia.

Treatment

Surgery has no role to play in the early management of acute pancreatitis. Aggressive supportive medical therapy forms the cornerstone of treatment. The key features are:

1. Withdraw all oral intake, institute nasogastric suction.
2. Establish intravenous fluid support and resuscitation.
3. Monitor response:
   - catheterise, measure hourly urine volumes
   - record vital signs
   - record central venous pressure.
4. Draw blood for:
   - serum amylase
   - calcium
   - blood glucose
   - arterial blood gases
   - liver and serum biochemistry
   - C-reactive protein.
5. Obtain a baseline chest radiograph.
6. Provide adequate parenteral opioid analgesia.

Most patients respond rapidly to this regimen. A few will progressively deteriorate and develop respiratory and renal failure. Failure to respond indicates a severe (necrotising) attack, development of a complication or an incorrect diagnosis.

Necrotising pancreatitis can be detected on a CT scan; radical surgical debridement of the dead tissue is sometimes the only option.

Complications

The two most important complications of acute pancreatitis are:

- pancreatic pseudocyst
- pancreatic abscess.

Two less common complications of pancreatitis are:

- pancreatic ascites
- pancreatic pleural effusion.

Pancreatic pseudocyst A pseudocyst consists of a fluid collection rich in pancreatic secretions that usually develops in the lesser sac. Pseudocysts present as an epigastric mass about 1 week after the onset of pancreatitis. The diagnosis is confirmed on ultrasound or CT scan. Most resolve spontaneously. Large cysts that persist or cause pain or jaundice can be drained either percutaneously under ultrasound/CT-guided control or internally at laparotomy into the back wall of the stomach (an operation known as a marsupialisation). Occasionally pseudocysts can become infected and form an abscess or may erode a major blood vessel causing haemorrhage and collapse. Both complications need emergency surgical intervention.

Pancreatic abscess This is the sequel to secondary bacterial infection in an area of pancreatic necrosis, usually with a mixed growth of aerobic and anaerobic organisms. This diagnosis should be suspected in patients with pancreatitis who become severely septic with a tender abdominal mass. The diagnosis is confirmed on ultrasound/CT scanning and urgent surgical drainage is mandatory.

Pancreatic ascites and pleural effusion This develops as a result of disruption of the main pancreatic duct by the acute inflamatory process. Leakage of pancreatic secretion into the peritoneal cavity may lead to a pseudocyst (localised leak) or pancreatic ascites (generalised leak) or a pleural effusion if fluid leaks via the diaphragm and mediastinum into the chest. Surgical treatment is complex and the overall outcome is poor.

Prognosis

Of all patients with acute pancreatitis 10–15% will die of their disease. Death is more likely in the elderly with a fulminant, severe attack or in patients with septic complications and multisystem organ failure. The severity of an attack can be predicted from a combination of factors recorded at the time of admission and 48 h later (see Table 8). or by interpretation of the C-reactive protein level (see Table 9) on admission.

Chronic pancreatitis

Chronic pancreatitis is usually the sequel to repeated attacks of alcohol-induced acute pancreatitis. Rarely, it follows an injury to the pancreas caused by surgery or external trauma.

Clinical features

Chronic pancreatitis is characterised by recurrent severe abdominal pain, or signs of pancreatic insufficiency (malabsorption and diabetes mellitus). Most patients give a history of alcohol abuse. Occasionally patients will present with a complication of chronic pancreatitis, e.g. abscess or pseudocyst.

Diagnosis

Plain abdominal film shows pancreatic calcification and endoscopic retrograde cholangiopancreatography (ERCP) or MRCP shows pancreatic duct strictures and dilatation. It is extremely important to exclude pancreatic cancer as the presentation is similar.

Medical treatment

Malabsorption and steatorrhoea can be reduced by oral pancreatic enzyme supplements, which may also reduce narcotic analgesic requirements. Diabetic patients require insulin therapy. Chronic pain is a major clinical problem and is the most frequent cause of urgent surgical admission in these patients. Narcotic addiction is commonplace.

Surgical treatment

The main indication for surgical intervention is relief of pain. Operative treatment is complex and should be reserved for the few well-motivated patients who have a clear structural abnormality in the pancreas detected on CT scan or ERCP. Unreformed alcoholics who are addicted to narcotics are unlikely to benefit from surgery.

There are two main options:

- pancreatic ductal drainage
- major pancreatic resection.

Drainage of a dilated ductal system either by an ampullary sphincteroplasty (Figure 9) or by anastomosing the pancreatic duct to a loop of jejunum using various techniques (Figure 10) will relieve pain. If the pancreatic duct is not dilated, resection of the diseased gland is the only other option. Resection should be tailored to the extent of the disease. Unlike pancreatic resection for cancer, the pylorus and duodenum are preserved whenever possible to minimise the disturbance in gastrointestinal function.

Table 8 Prognostic factors in acute pancreatitis

On admission	
Age	>60 years
Blood glucose	>200 mg/dl
White cell count	>16 000/µl
Serum LDH	>350 IU/l
Serum SGOT	>250 IU/l
During initial 48 h	
Change in haematocrit	>10% fall
Serum calcium	Falls to less than 8 mg/dl
Blood urea	>8 mg/dl
Arterial oxygen tension (pO$_2$)	<60 mmHg
Fluid sequestration estimate	>500 ml

Patients with three or more of these prognostic factors have severe pancreatitis

Table 9 C-reactive protein level in acute pancreatitis

Mild	Severe
<150 mg/l	>150 mg/l

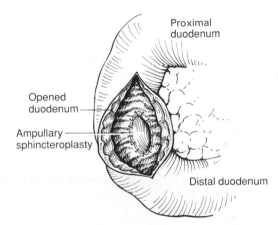

Figure 9 Ampullary sphincteroplasty for chronic pancreatitis.

Proximal duodenum

Opened duodenum

Ampullary sphincteroplasty

Distal duodenum

Three

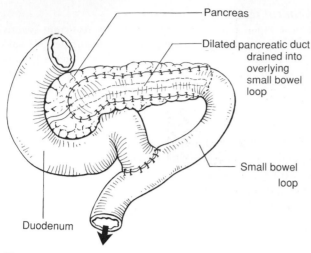

Figure 10 Pancreatic ductal drainage procedure for chronic pancreatitis.

Carcinoma of the pancreas

Pancreatic ductal adenocarcinoma accounts for 90% of all cancers arising from the pancreas. The remainder, which are derived from the ampulla of Vater or the adjacent duodenal mucosa, are termed periampullary cancers. These cancers present earlier with obstructive jaundice, are biologically less aggressive and are associated with a better prognosis. Most pancreatic ductal adenocarcinomas arise in the head of the gland.

Pancreatic cancer is becoming increasingly common in both men and women. Many have advanced disease at presentation and symptom palliation is often all that can be offered.

Clinical features

Weight loss, abdominal pain, back pain and jaundice are the cardinal features of pancreatic cancer. Jaundice is most common in cancers of the pancreatic head (caused by early obstruction of the common bile duct) and is less frequent in a cancer of the body and tail of the gland, where malignant obstruction of the common bile duct occurs later. A mass may be palpable in the epigastrium together with an enlarged liver. In patients with jaundice and pancreatic cancer, the gallbladder may be painlessly distended (Courvoisier's law).

Diagnosis

It is essential to 'stage' these patients accurately. Surgical resection is a major undertaking and it is vital for a surgeon not to embark on this operation only to find that the disease is too extensive to remove.

Abdominal ultrasound and CT/MR scan These are the key investigations. A dilated common bile duct plus a soft tissue mass in the pancreas is virtually diagnostic of pancreatic cancer. Liver metastases may also be detected.

Endoscopic retrograde cholangiopancreatography ERCP can distinguish pancreatic ductal carcinoma from the various periampullary cancers. ERCP techniques are used to insert a stent through a malignant biliary stricture caused by cancer of the pancreas or ampulla and will

relieve obstructive jaundice. This will provide definitive treatment for an elderly/frail patient or in a younger patient with metastatic disease.

Surgical treatment

Cancers of the body and tail of the pancreas are almost inevitably inoperable. Only one in ten patients with cancer of the pancreatic head is resectable and of these very few will be long-term survivors. Resection is prevented either by direct invasion of vital local structures (e.g. portal vein, hepatic or mesenteric vessels) or because of coexistent hepatic metastases.

There are two surgical options for the few patients with early resectable cancer of the pancreatic head. They are:

Pancreaticoduodenectomy (Whipple's operation) En-bloc resection of the pancreatic head bearing the tumour, duodenum, pylorus and distal bile duct (see Figure 11A).

Total pancreatectomy Complete removal of pancreas, duodenum, pylorus and distal common bile duct (see Figure 11B). This operation removes all the pancreatic islet cell tissue and these patients develop insulin-dependent diabetes.

There has been considerable debate as to the relative merits of these two operations. Periampullary cancers are usually treated by Whipple's operation.

Symptom palliation

The three predominant symptoms are:

- Obstructive jaundice: this can be relieved by ERCP and stenting. Sometimes attempts to pass endoscopic stents will fail. In these patients a stent can be passed through the abdominal wall and liver and positioned across the stricture under radiologic control (percutaneous transhepatic stent). Open surgical bypass (cholecyst-jejunostomy) is sometimes used.
- Pain: high doses of oral or subcutaneously infused opioids may be required.
- Pruritus: this requires endoscopic or operative relief of obstructive jaundice.

Prognosis

There are few long-term survivors even after apparently successful pancreatic resection for pancreatic ductal adenocarcinoma. The 5-year survival rate after surgery is less than 5%. Most die of local recurrence. In contrast one in three patients with periampullary cancer can expect to live 5 years after resection.

3.4 Diseases of the liver and spleen

Learning objectives

You should:

- understand the management principles in primary and secondary liver cancer
- recognise how the detection of a liver secondary can affect the management of the associated primary cancer
- know the treatment options in patients with variceal haemorrhage
- know the indications and effects of splenectomy.

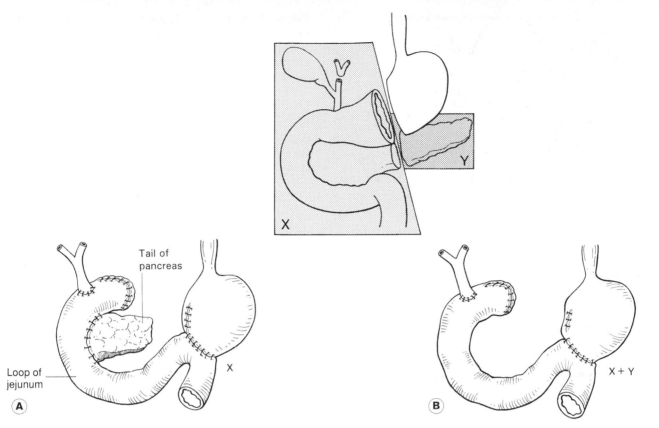

Figure 11 (A) Pancreaticoduodenectomy. (B) Total pancreatectomy.

Surgery has a role to play in two important groups of liver diseases:

- primary and secondary liver cancer
- portal hypertension and cirrhosis.

Primary and secondary liver cancer

Worldwide, primary liver cancer is common. It is only in Europe, North America and Australasia that secondary metastatic liver cancer is seen more often.

Primary hepatocellular carcinoma

Aetiology

Chronic *hepatitis B infection* is the primary aetiological factor. In Africa, for example, 80% of all patients with hepatocellular carcinoma are seropositive. In the USA, *alcoholic cirrhosis* is the major predisposing factor, whereas in the Orient infestation with *liver flukes* is linked to the increased incidence of the disease. Elsewhere, a high dietary intake of *aflatoxins* (products of the mould aspergillus found in wheat and soyabean) coincides with an increased incidence of primary hepatocellular cancer.

Pathology

Usually, the cancer develops as a single mass and later develops satellite nodules. In a fibrous cirrhotic liver, the cancer may be nodular and surrounded by a pseudocapsule. Less often a young adult (usually without any aetiological risk factors) will develop a fibrolamellar carcinoma characterised by multiple nodules separated by fibrous septae. This variant of the disease has a better prognosis. Primary hepatocellular carcinoma spreads to the coeliac and hilar lymph glands and can invade the portal and hepatic veins giving rise to pulmonary metastases.

Clinical features

Patients frequently present late with weight loss, abdominal pain and an upper abdominal mass. Fewer than half will be jaundiced. Some will have stigmata of underlying liver disease. A few will present with spontaneous rupture causing a major intra-abdominal bleed.

Diagnosis

Most patients will have an elevated oncofetoprotein and α-fetoprotein (AFP) level. Ultrasound or CT evaluation of the liver is the key diagnostic test. Tissue diagnosis is confirmed either by ultrasound or CT-guided percutaneous biopsy or by laparoscopy and biopsy.

Treatment

Liver resection offers the only hope of long-term survival. Only one in five patients are suitable. Extensive disease or poor residual liver function resulting from coexisting cirrhosis precludes resection in most patients. Attempts to devascularise the tumour by hepatic artery ligation or to destroy the tumour by direct infusion of cytotoxic agents via the hepatic artery have had limited success. Non-resectable tumours can also be destroyed without resection (in-situ ablation) by freezing techniques (cryotherapy) or by heat (thermal ablation) using specially designed instruments that are inserted into the tumour and cause necrosis.

Prognosis

Long-term survival is poor; most patients are dead within 1 year of diagnosis. Fewer than 20% of the few patients undergoing resection will survive 5 years. The best results are achieved in patients with small tumours who have little background liver disease.

Secondary liver cancer

Almost all primary cancers can metastasise to the liver. The most common primary sites in order of frequency are:

- colorectum
- lung
- pancreas
- breast
- stomach
- unknown primary site.

The deposits, which may be single or multiple, are caused by the spread of primary tumour cells to the liver via the portal or systemic circulation and less often via the lymphatics.

Clinical features

Metastatic liver disease may be detected during the pre-operative work-up of a patient with cancer or is discovered unexpectedly during elective or urgent surgery for cancer. Less often, patients will present primarily with pain, ascites, jaundice or hepatomegaly caused by metastatic disease with a 'silent' underlying primary cancer.

Diagnosis

Diagnosis is by ultrasound, CT or MRI scanning. Any of these tests will confirm the presence of hepatic metastases. Ultrasound or CT can be combined with percutaneous needle biopsy to provide a tissue diagnosis. An alternative is a laparoscopically guided biopsy, which provides the opportunity to inspect the rest of the peritoneal cavity in cases where no primary site is obvious.

Treatment

The detection of liver metastases often alters the surgical management of patients with cancer. Since most of these patients will have incurable disease, the primary goal of surgical intervention is to palliate distressing symptoms rather than undertake radical surgical resection.

The management of colorectal and renal cell cancer metastases is an exception to this rule. Hepatic lobectomy in patients with metastases from colorectal cancer can give a 25% 5-year survival, whereas some renal secondaries will regress after resection of the primary tumour. Up to one-third of patients with colorectal cancer will have liver metastases at presentation.

Some gastrointestinal metastases will respond to chemotherapy using 5-fluorouracil, by either systemic or direct intrahepatic arterial perfusion. Ablation techniques using heater probes or cryotherapy can also be used to palliate metastatic disease.

Prognosis

Overall, less than 10% of patients will survive more than 1 year after diagnosis. The outlook is better for patients with hepatic colorectal metastases; up to one-half will survive 5 years.

Portal hypertension and cirrhosis

Increased resistance to intrahepatic blood flow or extrahepatic portal vein obstruction causes portal hypertension. This leads to the diversion of portal venous blood to the systemic circulation through collateral blood vessels, which exist between the portal and systemic circulations. The most important plexus of these veins lies around the gastro-oesophageal junction. These veins become progressively dilated and varicose, forming oesophageal varices which lie just beneath the oesophageal mucosa. These fragile veins can rupture causing an exsanguinating haemorrhage and death. Surgical treatment is aimed either at mechanically obliterating the varices or at creating a venous shunt between the portal and systemic circulations, which decompresses the portal circulation and thus reduces the pressure and risk of bleeding from the oesophageal varices.

Aetiology

Most cases of portal hypertension are caused by cirrhosis, which is usually the sequel to alcohol abuse or viral hepatitis. Infrequently, portal hypertension can result from isolated thrombosis of the portal or splenic vein (prehepatic causes) or by restriction of blood flow through the hepatic veins (posthepatic causes).

Clinical features

Cirrhotic patients may present with the classic triad of ascites, hepatomegaly and spider naevi. Palmar erythema, gynaecomastia and testicular atrophy are other key physical signs. Some patients will present with a catastrophic haematemesis following oesophageal variceal rupture.

Diagnosis

Gastroscopy is the key investigation that will detect any oesophageal or varices which sit in the fundus of the stomach – 'gastric fundal varices': suspect this diagnosis in every cirrhotic patient who has a haematemesis.

Treatment of the acutely bleeding patient

All patients require immediate resuscitation as outlined on p. 29. Many patients will have a coagulopathy because of their underlying liver disease coupled with the massive blood losses. This requires correction with fresh frozen plasma, clotting factors and vitamin K.

The following steps should be taken to arrest the haemorrhage:

Variceal banding injection sclerotherapy This is performed at the same time as the diagnostic gastroscopy. The bleeding varix can be occluded using rubber band ligation or by injection of a sclerosant (e.g. ethanolamine oleate) into or around the bleeding site.

Splanchnic vasoconstriction Vasopressin, somatostatin or propranolol may reduce splanchnic blood flow and portal venous pressure and hence stop bleeding.

Balloon tamponade A Sengestaken–Blakemore tube (Figure 12) can be used to control bleeding by applying direct pressure to the varices. It can be particularly useful in controlling gastric fundal varices, which, because of their position, may be difficult to control with bands or sclerotherapy. Occasionally, in patients who are exsanguinating, immediate placement of a Sengestaken–Blakemore tube will be a lifesaving manoeuvre carried out in advance of sclerotherapy or endoscopy.

Emergency surgery Patients who do not respond to these measures or who rebleed require one of the following procedures.

Transhepatic intravascular porto-systemic shunt (TIPS) This is a relatively new technique which reduces the portal venous pressure by creating a fistula between a branch of the portal vein (high pressure) and one of the hepatic veins (low pressure) within the liver. This complex technique is usually performed by an interventional radiologist and can avoid the need for a major operation.

Oesophageal transection Direct obliteration of the bleeding varices using a staple gun to completely transect and reanastomose the oesophagus.

A porto-systemic shunt procedure See below.

Treatment of patients who are not bleeding acutely

Patients with varices who have bled but are no longer acutely bleeding can be treated by two main options:

- variceal banding injection sclerotherapy
- elective surgery.

Varices can be obliterated by a programme of repeated band applications or sclerosant injections, which produces fibrosis and thrombosis. This reduces the death rate from bleeding, but these patients will still die from their underlying cirrhotic liver disease.

Operative diversion of blood from the portal to the systemic circulation (porto-systemic shunt) will decompress the varices and prevent further bleeding. Its use is restricted to a selected group of patients who have previously bled, are at a high risk of rebleeding and are fit enough to undergo the procedure. Overall, the operative death rate is 10%. Diversion of blood away from the liver by the procedure can lead to an increased risk of liver failure and hepatic encephalopathy. Patient selection is difficult and is aided by Child's criteria, which use hepatic function and patient nutritional status to identify those patients suitable for surgery.

There are many types of shunt operation, but the three most commonly used are:

- end-to-side portacaval (Figure 13)
- side-to-side portacaval (Figure 14)
- distal splenorenal shunt (Figure 15).

Both portacaval shunts decompress high-pressure portal venous blood into the low-pressure inferior vena cava. A

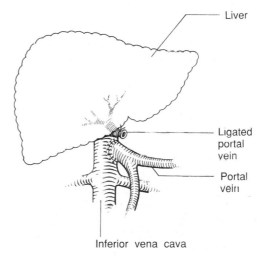

Figure 13 End-to-side portacaval shunt.

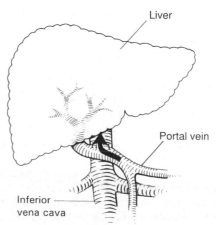

Figure 14 Side-to-side portacaval shunt.

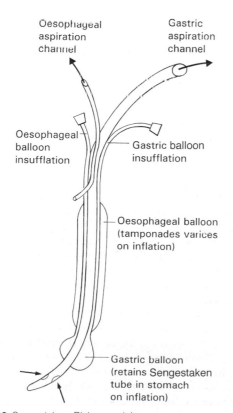

Figure 12 Sengestaken–Blakemore tube.

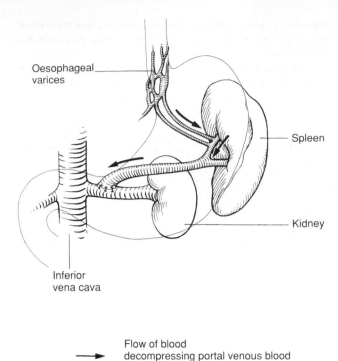

Figure 15 Distal splenorenal shunt.

major advantage of the distal splenorenal shunt is that it selectively decompresses the oesophageal varices and preserves the liver perfusion. It is a more difficult operation.

Surgery and the spleen

In the adult, the spleen produces plasma cells, monocytes and lymphocytes and functions as a filter to remove defunct circulating red blood cells. It also functions as a store for platelets and has a pivotal role in antibody production. Despite its protected position behind the left costal margin, the spleen remains vulnerable to trauma, particularly after a violent acceleration or deceleration injury.

There are three main indications for splenectomy:

- trauma
- incidental splenectomy during elective intra-abdominal surgery
- symptomatic splenomegaly or hypersplenism.

Trauma

Splenic rupture should be considered in any blunt or penetrating injury to the upper abdomen or lower chest. Patients may show signs of hypovolaemic shock, although this may be absent in the early stages after injury. Rib fractures or a complaint of left shoulder tip pain caused by the subdiaphragmatic collection of blood should also raise suspicion of injury. In patients with multiple trauma, the diagnosis may be overlooked unless a CT abdominal scan or a diagnostic peritoneal lavage is performed.

Occasionally a delayed splenic rupture may occur several weeks following the initial injury after late rupture of a slowly expanding subcapsular haematoma.

Diagnosis

In a shocked patient following major trauma with no other overt sign of blood loss, it may be necessary to proceed immediately to a lifesaving diagnostic laparotomy. Here, the diagnosis may be made at operation.

In less urgent circumstances, the diagnosis may be suspected by a positive diagnostic peritoneal lavage and confirmed by CT or ultrasound abdominal scan.

Treatment

Total splenectomy is often the only operative option. Occasionally it may be possible to conserve the spleen by repair of any isolated tears (splenorrhaphy) or by tamponade (wrapping the organ in an absorbable woven mesh).

Splenectomy during intra-abdominal surgery

The spleen may be removed as part of a radical surgical procedure for cancer of the oesophagus or stomach in an attempt to ensure complete removal of the lymphatic drainage bed. Splenectomy may also be necessary as a result of inadvertent injury during surgery of the stomach and gastro-oesophageal junction or during mobilisation of the splenic flexure during colonic surgery.

Symptomatic splenomegaly or hypersplenism

Congenital haemolytic anaemias Splenectomy will prevent haemolysis in congenital haemolytic anaemias (e.g. hereditary spherocytosis, thalassaemia) or in auto-immune haemolytic anaemia.

Idiopathic thrombocytopenic purpura This condition, characterised by a shortened platelet lifespan causing a bruising and bleeding tendency, can be effectively treated by splenectomy if patients fail to respond to steroid therapy. In this disease, the spleen may function as a source of circulating antiplatelet antibodies as well as the site of platelet extraction from the circulation.

Hodgkin's disease Splenectomy is now rarely performed in staging Hodgkin's disease.

Chronic lymphatic leukaemia The spleen may need to be removed in these patients because of hypersplenism leading to thrombcytopaenia or anaemia requiring repeated blood transfusion.

The consequences of splenectomy

After splenectomy, there is often a massive rise in the circulating platelet level (up to 0.5–1.0 million platelets/μl). This can persist for up to 12 months, but the risks of thrombosis are slight and patients do not need anticoagulation.

All patients after splenectomy are at risk of a severe postsplenectomy infection. The infection starts as a flu-like illness and rapidly progresses to septicaemia causing multiple organ failure and death. The increased risk is greatest in the first 2 years after surgery but persists throughout life. The most common pathogen is *Streptococcus pneumoniae*. All patients undergoing splenectomy should be immunised preoperatively, when possible, with a pneumococcal vaccine, followed by lifelong antibiotic prophylaxis with a low-dose penicillin.

3.5 Diseases of the small bowel and appendix

Learning objectives

You should:

- know how to diagnose and treat a patient with acute appendicitis
- know the key clinical features of the main small bowel diseases
- have a management plan for small bowel obstruction
- understand the place of medical and surgical treatment in Crohn's disease.

Small bowel disease falls into three major categories:

- small bowel obstruction
- inflammatory disease of the small bowel
- mesenteric ischaemia.

Acute appendicitis is the most important surgical condition that affects the appendix.

Small bowel obstruction

Aetiology

The two main causes of small bowel obstruction are:

- postoperative adhesions
- irreducible external hernias, e.g. inguinal, femoral or umbilical.

Less frequent but important causes are:

- caecal carcinoma obstructing the ileocaecal valve
- Crohn's disease
- ischaemic stricture from radiation enteritis or mesenteric ischaemia
- food bolus or foreign body
- congenital adhesions
- intussusception
- small bowel volvulus
- gallstone ileus.

Clinical features

Colicky abdominal pain is the most constant feature of small bowel obstruction. Other symptoms and signs depend upon the level of obstruction.

Distal small bowel obstruction is associated with progressive abdominal distension and dehydration.

Mid small bowel obstruction is characterised by severe colic.

High small bowel obstruction can be deceptively pain-free with profuse vomiting and rapid dehydration. Abdominal distension may be absent.

Physical examination classically reveals a tympanitic distended abdomen with tinkling bowel sounds together with clues as to the likely underlying cause of the obstruction, e.g. an irreducible hernia or a previous laparotomy scar.

Diagnosis

This is usually established on clinical grounds and confirmed by plain abdominal radiograph. Distended small bowel loops on a supine film and multiple fluid levels on an erect film are the hallmark of small bowel obstruction (Figure 16).

Strangulation This is a life-threatening complication and implies obstruction of the blood supply to the affected segment of small bowel by either venous congestion or arterial occlusion. It is more common in:

- a closed loop obstruction (where a single loop of bowel becomes obstructed between two fixed points and rapidly distends)
- small bowel volvulus (where loops of bowel twist along the long axis of their mesentery and compromise their own blood supply)
- irreducible incarcerated external hernias.

Differential diagnosis Clinical and biochemical indices differentiate poorly between strangulating and 'simple' small bowel obstruction, but strangulation should be suspected in patients with:

- localised abdominal tenderness
- fever, leucocytosis, tachycardia
- constant rather than colicky pain.

Treatment

Urgent surgery is indicated only if there is a suspicion of strangulation. At least half of episodes of simple adhesive obstruction will settle with conservative treatment and will not need surgery. Those patients who do not settle after 1–2 days or who have an obvious underlying cause, e.g. an external hernia, all require surgery after appropriate preoperative preparation.

The key steps to conservative management and preoperative preparation are:

- stop oral intake
- apply nasogastric suction
- provide intravenous fluid replacement and resuscitation
- correct any fluid and electrolyte imbalance.

Surgery

Most cases of small bowel obstruction needing operation are the result of adhesions. The surgery involves meticulously unravelling the entire small intestine by careful division of all adhesive bands. Any non-viable segments of bowel (as a result of strangulation) should be resected. Any associated disease (e.g. hernia or colon cancer) should be dealt with at the same time.

Prognosis

Surgery for simple small bowel obstruction is a low-risk procedure. If strangulation supervenes, death rates may reach 10%, especially in the elderly. This emphasises the need for careful appraisal and prompt management of patients in whom strangulation is suspected.

Inflammatory diseases of the small bowel

Crohn's disease is the most important condition in this category. In addition, there are many infective causes of small bowel inflammation:

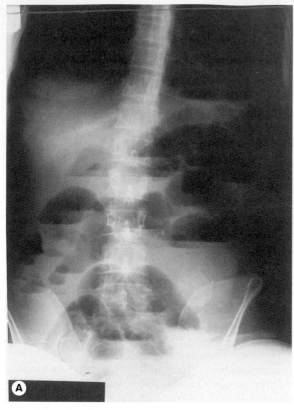
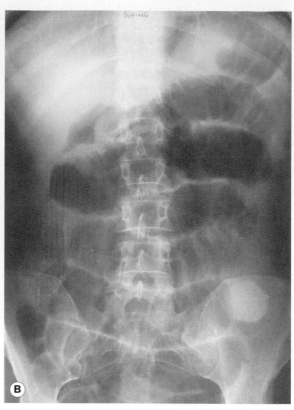

Figure 16 Radiograph appearances of a small bowel obstruction – erect abdominal film (A); supine abdominal film (B).

- *Campylobacter coli*
- *Yersinia enterocolitica*
- *Salmonella typhi*
- Tuberculous enteritis.

Crohn's disease

Aetiology and pathology

Crohn's disease is an idiopathic transmural inflammatory disease of the intestinal wall. It can affect any part of the gastrointestinal tract from the mouth to the anus. The disease is characterised by focal areas of lymphocytic infiltration and the presence of non-caseating epithelioid granulomas. Mucosal ulceration, skip lesions (segments of normal bowel interspersed between grossly diseased bowel) and deep fissures, which sometimes connect with adjacent viscera causing fistulation or abscess formation, are the hallmark of Crohn's disease.

The most frequent distribution of the disease is:

- terminal ileum and caecum
- perineum
- colon.

Clinical features

Most patients will present with one or a combination of the following symptoms:

- gastrointestinal
  - colicky abdominal pains
  - diarrhoea
  - perianal sepsis, abscesses and fistulae

- chronic systemic disease
  - weight loss, malnutrition, anaemia
  - failure to thrive.

Occasionally the disease presents acutely and mimics appendicitis.

Although some patients will exhibit no gross abnormal physical signs in the early stages of the disease, others will exhibit a range of physical findings:

- evidence of recent weight loss
- small bowel obstruction
- abdominal mass caused by matted intestinal loops
- entero-cutaneous fistula
- chronic perianal sepsis.

Diagnosis

Depending on the symptom pattern, confirmation of Crohn's disease can be obtained by two main methods.

Barium studies A barium follow-through is the single most useful examination for small bowel Crohn's disease. Cobblestone mucosa, rose thorn fissures, multiple small bowel strictures, interloop fistulae and 'skip lesions', appearing in any combination, are classic features of small bowel Crohn's disease (Figure 17).

CT/MRI scan These tests can be used to detect an associated intra-abdominal abscess.

Sigmoidoscopy/colonoscopy This provides direct visualisation of Crohn's ulceration and biopsy evidence

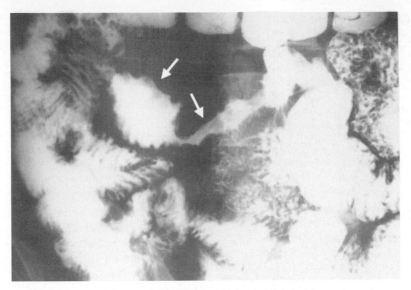

Figure 17 Radiograph appearances of small bowel Crohn's disease showing strictured and dilated segments.

of pathognomonic granulomata if the large intestine is involved.

Differential diagnosis The differential diagnosis of Crohn's disease is extremely wide, encompassing almost all intra-abdominal pathologies. Two important conditions in the differential diagnosis of small bowel Crohn's disease which should not be overlooked are:

- tuberculous enteritis
- small bowel lymphoma.

Both these conditions may present with weight loss and a right iliac fossa mass, with similar radiological findings on a small bowel follow-through. Often the diagnosis is only realised after surgical resection and histopathology examination.

In a young patient if is easy to confuse an acute Crohn's presentation with a late appendicitis presenting with an appendix mass or abscess.

Complications The two most important groups of complications are:

- fistula and abscess formation
  - entero-cutaneous
  - entero-enteric
  - entero-vesical
  - interloop abscess
- small bowel obstruction.

Treatment

The natural history of Crohn's disease is of spontaneous relapses and remissions. This makes evaluation of any therapy difficult. Generally, the first-line management is medical, with surgery reserved for the management of complications.

Medical therapy Steroids and/or immunosuppressive therapy combined with nutritional support form the cornerstone of medical treatment.

Steroids Intermittent high-dose courses are used alone or in combination with low-dose steroid maintenance therapy.

Azathioprine, methotrexate or cyclosporin These immunosuppressive agents suppress the chronic inflammatory reaction associated with Crohn's disease.

Metronidazole or sulphasalazine These agents are most effective in colonic Crohn's disease (see p. 67).

Nutritional support Total parenteral or enteral nutrition can effectively treat malnutrition caused by Crohn's induced malabsorption, although it is unlikely to influence the course of the disease.

Surgery in Crohn's disease Conservative surgery is the keynote of operative management in Crohn's disease. Abscesses and fistulae are the main indications for surgery in small bowel Crohn's disease. Wherever possible, the affected segments of bowel should be resected and gastrointestinal continuity restored rather than performing a bypass operation that short-circuits but leaves behind the affected Crohn's disease segment. Surgery is sometimes required for chronic small bowel obstruction caused by a strictured segment of Crohn's disease. The same surgical principles apply. Provided at least 150 cm of small intestine remain after surgery these patients can survive without needing parenteral nutrition support.

Prognosis

Management of patients with Crohn's disease is a lifelong task best provided by a dedicated team of gastroenterologists and surgeons with a special interest in the disease. Surgery does not cure the disease and some patients will require repeated surgical procedures. Overall, the death rate of Crohn's disease patients is two to three times higher than that of the general population.

Mesenteric ischaemia

Lack of blood supply to the small intestine can be acute or chronic. Whereas the blood supply to the foregut (from the coeliac axis) or to the hindgut (from the inferior mesenteric artery) can be sustained by collateral blood flow immediately after an acute occlusion, the blood supply to the midgut cannot, hence the catastrophic consequences of an acute occlusion of the superior mesenteric artery.

The three most important types of occlusion are:

- acute superior mesenteric artery occlusion
- acute mesenteric venous occlusion
- chronic superior mesenteric artery occlusion.

Acute superior mesenteric artery occlusion

Acute occlusion is caused by arterial embolisation, usually from a mural thrombus in the heart or great vessels or by thrombosis of an atherosclerotic superior mesenteric artery.

Clinical features

Agonising abdominal pain, vomiting and diarrhoea, and gastrointestinal blood loss are the hallmarks of an acute occlusion. Typically, the patient is elderly, has atrial fibrillation and may have a previous history of peripheral vascular disease.

Generalised tenderness is evident on abdominal examination. Without treatment, sepsis and irreversible shock rapidly supervene.

Diagnosis

Making the diagnosis can be suprisingly difficult as there are few specific signs. The following features suggest a diagnosis of acute mesenteric ischaemia:

- massive leucocytosis
- a mild hyperamylasaemia, which can cause diagnostic confusion with acute pancreatitis
- lack of intestinal gas on plain abdominal radiograph.

Treatment

There is rarely time for sophisticated investigation and in many cases a suspected diagnosis will be confirmed only at an urgent laparotomy after resuscitation.

In elderly patients with total small bowel infarction, surgery has no role to play. Laparotomy merely confirms the diagnosis and inevitably there is a fatal outcome. Less extensive infarction is amenable to resection. In other patients, revascularisation by either embolectomy or bypass grafting may revive an ischaemic but not an infarcted bowel.

Mesenteric venous thrombosis

Venous infarction is much less common than arterial occlusion. It is usually idiopathic but may be the result of sepsis, liver disease or other hypercoagulable states. The presentation and management are essentially the same as for an acute mesenteric arterial occlusion.

Chronic superior mesenteric artery vascular occlusion

Incomplete occlusion of the superior mesenteric artery causes chronic small bowel ischaemia. This manifests as postprandial pain coupled with weight loss and diarrhoea caused by malabsorption. The clinical picture may mimic advanced malignancy and requires either a mesenteric duplex ultrasound scan or a superior mesenteric angiogram to clinch the diagnosis.

Endarterectomy or the use of a vein graft to bypass the occlusion can produce a dramatic resolution of the symptoms.

Prognosis The overall prognosis for patients with mesenteric ischaemia is poor. Over 50% of patients will die of the acute event.

Acute appendicitis

Appendicectomy for acute appendicitis is one of the most common surgical emergencies. The disease can occur at any age and overall mortality rates are less than 1%. Those at greatest risk of dying of the disease are the very young and the very old.

Aetiology

There is no single satisfactory explanation for the cause of appendicitis. A combination of luminal obstruction by faecoliths or lymphoid follicular hyperplasia with secondary bacterial invasion of the appendicular wall by enteric organisms have been implicated.

Clinical features

The initial symptoms are vague. Patients complain of nausea, anorexia and a poorly localised abdominal discomfort. Later, as serosal inflammation of the appendix develops, pain localises in the right iliac fossa and becomes aggravated by movement. A low-grade fever with tenderness and guarding over McBurney's point (one-third of the way along a line drawn from the anterior superior iliac spine to the umbilicus) are classic physical signs. Rectal examination is essential to detect pelvic appendicitis.

The history and physical signs will differ depending on the site of the appendix (Figure 18) and in patients at the extremes of life.

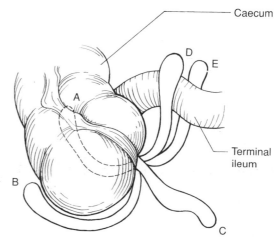

Figure 18 Anatomical positions of the appendix in relation to the caecum and ileum. (A) Retrocaecal. (B) Paracaecal. (C) Pelvic. (D) Preileal. (E) Postileal.

Retrocaecal appendicitis Pain remains poorly localised as the appendix is not in contact with the parietal peritoneum. It can mimic renal colic or pyelonephritis.

Pelvic appendicitis There are no abdominal signs; patients may have diarrhoea or urinary frequency because of irritation of the rectum or bladder by the inflamed appendix. It can mimic gastroenteritis, cystitis or acute salpingitis.

Appendicitis and an abnormally sited caecum In patients with a high caecum or those with a malrotation, appendicitis may mimic cholecystitis or diverticulitis.

Diagnosis

In the majority of cases, the diagnosis of acute appendicitis is based on the case history and physical examination. Special investigations have little role to play except in young women, in whom the diagnosis may be difficult to distinguish from gynaecological disease. In these patients pelvic ultrasound examination and/or diagnostic laparoscopy are essential steps.

Diagnosing appendicitis in children can be difficult as the history may not be clear. Appendicitis may also be overlooked in the elderly patient with a lax abdominal wall where guarding cannot be elicited.

Differential diagnosis The differential diagnosis in acute appendicitis is wide and is summarised in Table 10.

Complications

Perforation This is more common in the young and the elderly or where there is a delay in diagnosis.

Appendix mass The acutely inflamed appendix, which may have perforated, becomes 'walled off' from the peritoneal cavity by adjacent loops of intestine and omentum that prevent a generalised peritonitis. A tender mass is palpable in the right iliac fossa.

Treatment

Appendicectomy either by open or laparoscopic surgery is mandatory once the diagnosis has been made and the patient made fit for surgery; the only exception is an appendix mass that can be treated conservatively with

Table 10 Differential diagnosis of acute appendicitis

Common
Mesenteric lymphadenitis
Gastroenteritis
Salpingitis
Ruptured ovarian follicle
Pyelonephritis/ureteric colic

Uncommon
Ectopic pregnancy
Torted ovarian cyst
Acute Crohn's disease
Cholecystitis

antibiotics, intravenous fluids and bed rest until the mass resolves. In these cases, appendicectomy is undertaken at a later date unless an appendix abscess develops that requires drainage.

Tumours of the appendix

These are rare and of two types:

- benign and malignant carcinoid tumours
- adenocarcinoma of the appendix.

Benign and malignant carcinoid tumours

The appendix is the most common primary site for these tumours. They develop from specialised cells, namely the argentaffin cells, which have an endocrine function. These tumours are usually found by chance at the tip of the appendix during appendicectomy and they have a characteristic yellow-brown colour. Although microscopically they have many of the features of an invasive carcinoma, their biological behaviour is benign and only a few will metastasise.

A carcinoid tumour of the tip of the appendix can be treated by appendicectomy. Carcinoid tumours of the base of the appendix are more likely to invade adjacent structures and are best treated by right hemicolectomy. Appendicular carcinoids are usually incidental findings during laparotomy or appendicectomy. Occasionally they present late when metastatic liver deposits give rise to the carcinoid syndrome (flushing, diarrhoea, borborygmi) caused by the release of vasoactive amines, C_5 hydroxytryptamine, into the systemic circulation.

Adenocarcinoma of the appendix

This diagnosis is rarely made preoperatively and may be difficult to distinguish from a caecal carcinoma. A right hemicolectomy is the treatment of choice.

Uncommon small bowel diseases

Radiation enteritis and small bowel lymphoma are two uncommon but important small bowel diseases.

Radiation enteritis

Irradiation injury to the small bowel is usually the sequel to pelvic radiotherapy for gynaecological cancer. The early mucosal injury presents with bloody diarrhoea and abdominal cramps. Injury to the blood vessels can present up to 20 years later with chronic ischaemia causing formation of fibrotic strictures and symptoms of chronic small bowel obstruction or malabsorption.

Treatment

Early symptoms resulting from the mucosal injury are treated conservatively and usually settle spontaneously. Major small bowel resection is required to relieve the late obstructive symptoms.

Small bowel lymphoma (non Hodgkin's and T-cell lymphoma)

The presenting symptoms are similar to small bowel Crohn's disease. Sometimes the diagnosis is confirmed

Three

only after resection of the affected segment of small intestine. Radiotherapy and chemotherapy are usually used in conjunction with surgery.

3.6 Diseases of the large intestine

Learning objectives

You should:
- recognise the key features of the main colorectal diseases
- know how to investigate a patient with altered bowel habit or rectal bleeding
- know how to treat a patient with diverticular disease
- understand the role of medical therapy and the indications for surgery in patients with ulcerative colitis and Crohn's colitis
- have a management plan for a patient with large bowel obstruction.

The most important surgical diseases affecting the large bowel are:

- carcinoma of the colon
- colonic polyps
- Crohn's colitis and ulcerative colitis
- diverticular disease.

All of these conditions usually present with an alteration in bowel habit often associated with the passage of blood, mucus and slime. The principles of investigation are common to all; namely, a careful contrast radiological evaluation of the colon coupled with endoscopy and biopsy using sigmoidoscopy or colonoscopy as appropriate. Some affected patients will present acutely with a large bowel obstruction.

Carcinoma of the colon (and rectum)

Carcinoma of the colon and rectum are closely related and are considered together. Colorectal cancer is a common malignancy and is second only to lung cancer in incidence. It develops slowly and has usually been present for several years before becoming clinically apparent. The distribution of colorectal cancer is shown in Figure 19. Primary cancers in the caecum and ascending colon develop into a large fungating mass that rarely obstructs the intestinal lumen. Elsewhere, colonic cancer slowly encircles the bowel and will eventually produce obstruction. The disease spreads via the lymphatics to regional and distant lymph node groups and by haematogenous routes to liver and lungs. Spread also occurs across the peritoneal cavity to form multiple metastatic serosal seedlings.

Survival is closely linked to the pathological stage (Dukes staging or TNM staging) at the time of resection (Table 11). Up to 5% of patients will have more than one bowel cancer (synchronous tumours) when they present or will develop a further bowel cancer (metachronous tumour) later in life.

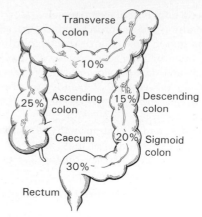

Figure 19 Distribution of colorectal cancer.

Table 11 Dukes staging for colorectal cancer

Stage	Extent	5-year survival (%)
A	Limited to bowel wall	80
B	Extends through bowel wall; no lymph node metastases	60
C	Lymph node metastases	30
D	Distant metastases	10

Aetiology

The most important aetiological factors predisposing to carcinoma of the large intestine are:

- diet: a high ratio of animal protein to fat, low-fibre diet
- strong family history of colon cancer
- adenomatous colonic polyps
- familial polyposis coli
- hereditary non-polyposis colorectal cancer
- chronic ulcerative colitis.

Clinical features

The presentation depends on the site of the cancer:

Right hemicolon: anaemia, tiredness, abdominal mass and vague abdominal pain.

Left hemicolon: altered bowel habit, blood mixed with stools and large bowel obstruction.

Rectum: altered bowel habit, rectal bleeding and a mucous rectal discharge, tenesmus. The cancer may be palpable on rectal examination.

Carcinoma of the rectum and right-sided large bowel cancer rarely present with obstruction.

Diagnosis

Investigations must visualise the entire colon, using a combination of three tests.

Rigid or flexible sigmoidoscopy Up to 50% of all colonic cancers can be reached by these simple endoscopic tests and a diagnostic biopsy obtained.

Double-contrast barium enema This will outline the entire colon and detect the majority of cancers and colonic polyps.

Colonoscopy With an experienced endoscopist, the entire colon can be directly visualised. It has the advantage that diagnostic biopsy can be obtained and that any dysplastic polyps, the precursors to bowel cancer, can be removed. The main disadvantage is that the caecum may not always be reached. In the UK, it is reserved for those patients for whom a barium enema raises suspicion of cancer but is not diagnostic, or patients with iron deficient anaemia where an upper gastrointestinal source of blood loss has been ruled out.

Screening for colorectal cancer using a faecal occult blood (FOB) test is currently being evaluated and is offered to patients over 50 years of age. Those who test positive are offered colorectal investigation. Early indications show an increase in detection of pre-malignant polyps, malignant polyps and early stage cancers.

Once the diagnosis of a bowel cancer has been confirmed the liver should be carefully examined for metastases by CT/MR scan. The pelvis is scanned in patients with rectal cancer to assess resectability and to decide whether preoperative radiotherapy is required to shrink the cancer prior to removal.

Surgical treatment: colonic carcinoma

The goal of surgery is to remove the tumour-bearing areas of the colon together with a wide margin of normal bowel and the adjacent regional lymphatic drainage. Gastrointestinal continuity is restored usually by an end-to-end anastomosis. Liver metastases are not a contraindication to resection. Solitary and sometimes multiple metastases can be res-ected; the decision requires close collaboration between the colorectal and hepatobiliary surgeon.

The precise colonic operation depends on the site of the tumour.

Cancer in the right colon requires a right hemicolectomy (Figure 20).

Cancer in the transverse colon requires either an extended right hemicolectomy or an extended left hemicolectomy depending upon the position of the cancer in the transverse colon (Figures 21, 22A).

Cancer in the left colon requires a left hemicolectomy (Figure 22A).

Cancer in the sigmoid colon requires a sigmoid colectomy (Figure 22B).

Surgical treatment: rectal carcinoma

Treatment of rectal carcinoma is more complex. The surgical options depend upon the size and site of the tumour, together with the build of the patient. Of great importance is the pelvic rectal dissection which must incorporate the entire mesorectum to ensure adequate tumour clearance (total mesorectal excision, TME).

Carcinoma of the upper rectum can be dealt with by an extended sigmoid resection and reanastomosis (anterior resection, Figure 23A). Cancers of the lower rectum, usually those that can be felt on rectal examination, require excision of the entire rectum and anal canal with the formation of a permanent end colostomy in the left iliac fossa (abdomino-perineal resection, Figure 23B). Cancers in the mid rectum are the most difficult to manage. A large tumour in a small male pelvis may require an abdomino-

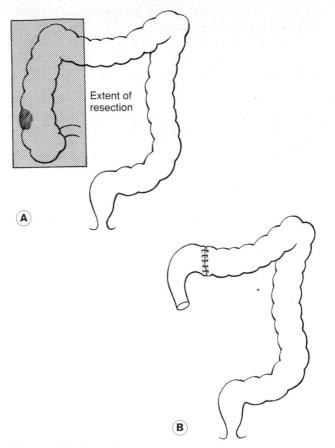

Figure 20 Right hemicolectomy.

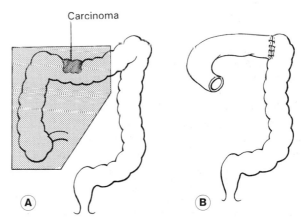

Figure 21 Surgery for cancer of the transverse colon: extended right hemicolectomy.

perineal resection, whereas a small tumour in a wide female pelvis may be manageable by a low anterior resection.

Complications of surgery

A leak from the bowel anastomosis is the most serious complication after bowel surgery. Untreated it will cause a lethal peritonitis. The risk is minimised by meticulous surgical technique ensuring a good blood supply and tension-free anastomosis. Leaks are more common after 'low' anterior resection or emergency colonic surgery for

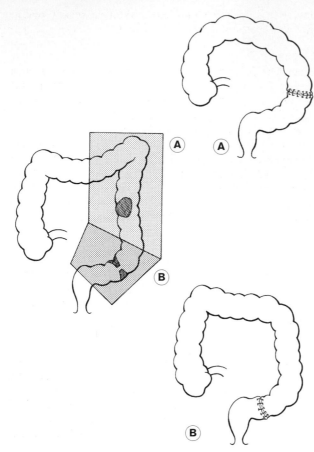

Figure 22 (A) Left hemicolectomy. (B) Sigmoid colectomy.

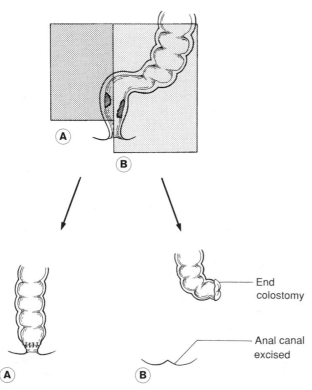

End colostomy

Anal canal excised

Figure 23 (A) Anterior resection. (B) Abdomino-perineal resection.

obstruction. A defunctioning 'loop' ileostomy is often used to rest a difficult bowel anastomosis to optimise the conditions for healing and to allow any small leaks to heal without the risks of faecal peritonitis.

Radiotherapy and chemotherapy in colon and rectal cancer

Adjuvant radiotherapy can be used pre- or postoperatively to reduce the risk of local recurrence in rectal cancer. It has no role in the treatment of colon cancer. It may also be administered preoperatively to 'downstage' a large rectal cancer and increase the likelihood of a successful surgical resection.

5-Fluorouracil-based chemotherapy regimens confer a survival advantage in lymph gland positive (Dukes stage C) colon and rectal cancers and may help certain 'at-risk' patients with Dukes stage B cancer where, for example, there may be evidence of vascular invasion but no sign of any lymph gland involvement. Chemotherapy can be used in combination with radiotherapy in patients with rectal cancer.

Prognosis

Outcome is closely linked to the pathological staging at the time of resection (see Table 11). It is worse for patients who undergo urgent surgery for obstructed or perforated cancers. After successful resection all patients with colorectal cancer should undergo regular follow-up colonoscopy to check for local recurrence, to remove any new polyps or to detect metachronous cancers.

Colonic polyps

Colonic polyps are of great importance because they are the precursor to colon cancer. They have the following characteristics:

- up to 50% of polyps 2 cm or greater in size are malignant
- one-third of patients with colon cancer also have colonic polyps
- colonic polyps can recur or develop at new sites
- malignant potential is also related to the histological type of the polyp (villous > tubulo-villous > tubular adenoma).

Clinical features

Most polyps will be asymptomatic and may not present until the patient develops symptoms of colonic cancer. Some asymptomatic polyps will be detected by screening programmes. Rectal bleeding is the most frequent symptom.

Diagnosis

Colonoscopy is the most sensitive test and can be used for diagnosis and treatment (see below). The detection of a polyp or polyps during sigmoidoscopy is an indication for total colonoscopic inspection of the colon as other polyps or cancers may be present in the remaining colon. A double contrast barium enema is the least sensitive test and will always need to be followed by colonoscopy when polyps are detected and need to be removed.

Treatment

Single polyps Most polyps are on a stalk and can be snared and removed during sigmoidoscopy or colonoscopy. Sessile polyps, which cannot be safely snared, may require colonic resection. All polyps must be subject to a careful histological examination. Pedunculated polyps bearing a focus of malignancy but no evidence of any invasion of the stalk require no further treatment. Other polyps with malignant invasion of the stalk require resection of the segment of colon bearing the polyp.

Multiple polyps Colonic polyps are often multiple and the detection of a single polyp demands evaluation of the entire colon and complete clearance of any additional polyps.

Familial polyposis coli Occasionally, this rare autosomal dominant condition will be encountered. It is characterised by the development of hundreds of polyps throughout the colon after the age of puberty and the development of cancer in at least one of these polyps by the age of 40. There are two treatment options.

Panproctocolectomy Total removal of the colon, rectum and anus with formation of a permanent ileostomy (see Figure 24C).

Near total colectomy As above, with preservation of the anal canal to allow either an ileo-anal anastomosis or construction of an ileal pouch or reservoir (see Figure 24).

Prognosis

Regular colonoscopy follow-up is essential in patients who have had colonic polyps. In this way, recurrent or new polyps can be removed before malignancy supervenes.

Diverticular disease

Multiple colonic diverticulae (mucosal herniation through the large bowel circular muscle layers) are a common finding. Although they can develop in any part of the colon, they are most frequent in the sigmoid colon. Diverticular disease is a condition of Western society and is linked to a low dietary intake of fibre.

Clinical features

Diverticular disease may be an incidental finding on a barium enema or sigmoidoscopy. Colonic symptoms should not be attributed to it until full colonic investigations have ruled out any coexisting pathology.

Acute diverticulitis is caused by infection of one or more diverticulae and inflammation of the adjacent colon. Patients present with left iliac fossa pain of variable severity, systemic signs of sepsis and an altered bowel habit (either diarrhoea or constipation). On examination, there may be tenderness in the left iliac fossa or signs of local peritonitis or an abdominal mass.

Diagnosis

Acute diverticulitis is a clinical diagnosis and the immediate treatment is based on the history and physical findings. Once the patient's condition has responded to treatment, the diagnosis is confirmed by flexible sigmoidoscopy or barium enema examination.

Treatment

Intravenous antibiotic therapy, bowel rest and analgesia are the cornerstone of medical management. Most patients will settle on this regimen. Those who do not or who develop complications require resection of the diseased segment of bowel. Because of the surrounding inflammation and infection, it is often necessary to perform a Hartmann's procedure (Figure 25).

Complications

There are five major complications:

- pericolic abscess
- perforation
- major haemorrhage
- diverticular stricture
- fistula formation, usually to the bladder or vagina, causing a vesico-colic or a vagino-colic fistula. The patient will complain of pneumaturia and cystitis or the passage of flatus and faeces per vagina. Less

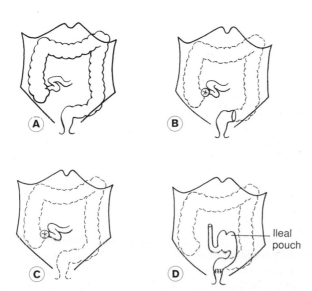

Figure 24 Surgery of the large bowel and rectum. (A) Normal anatomy. (B) Subtotal colectomy. (C) Panproctocolectomy. (D) Total colectomy, ileo-anal anastomosis with ileal pouch.

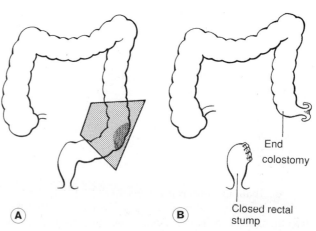

Figure 25 Hartmann's operation.

frequently Crohn's disease and colorectal cancer can also cause this complication.

Some patients will present primarily with these complications, which usually require urgent surgery after resuscitation. Again, a Hartmann's procedure is the most useful operation. Occasionally a primary resection and reanastomosis is possible.

Large bowel inflammatory disease

Ulcerative colitis and Crohn's colitis are the two most common causes of large bowel inflammatory disease. The clinical picture may vary from a chronic low-grade colitis that may persist for many years to an acute fulminant attack of colitis. Infective colitis and ischaemic colitis are two other important causes of acute colitis.

Clinical features

Bloody diarrhoea is the key presenting symptom in acute colitis. In a severe attack, patients may be septic with abdominal pain and tenderness. Patients may also present with chronic colitis causing loose stools, weight loss, anaemia and malaise.

Diagnosis

A plain abdominal film is essential in all patients presenting acutely with colitis in order to detect toxic dilatation or colonic perforation (see p. 67).

The three most important elective investigations are:

- stool cultures: to detect any infective causes of colitis
- sigmoidoscopy, colonoscopy and biopsy: to obtain a tissue diagnosis
- barium enema: to assess the extent and severity of the disease.

Treatment

The key steps in managing an acute severe attack of colitis are:

- intravenous fluid resuscitation
- restrict oral intake
- intravenous steroid therapy once infective or ischaemic colitis ruled out
- consider subtotal colectomy if no remission after 5 days of intensive medical therapy or if complications supervene.

Ulcerative colitis

This idiopathic condition is characterised by mucosal and submucosal inflammation. In contrast to Crohn's disease, the muscular and serosal layers are spared. During active phases of the disease, the mucosa is densely infiltrated with leucocytes and plasma cells, and crypt abscesses form at the base of the villae. Mucosal ulceration develops as the disease progresses. The disease only affects the colon and rectum.

Exacerbations and remissions of the disease, which causes diarrhoea and rectal bleeding, are typical. In addition there are a variety of extracolonic disorders that affect some but not all patients (Table 12).

Table 12 Extracolonic manifestations of ulcerative colitis

Eye disorders	Iritis
	Conjunctivitis
Joint disorders	Arthralgia
	Ankylosing spondylitis
	Sacroiliitis
Skin disorders	Erythema nodosum
	Pyoderma gangrenosum
Liver disorders	Sclerosing cholangitis

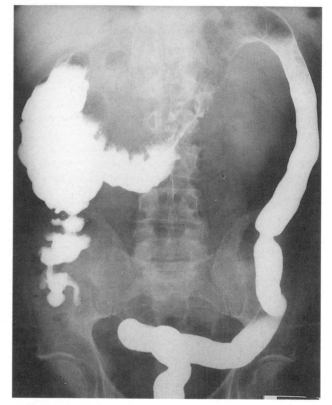

Figure 26 Radiological appearance of ulcerative colitis.

Diagnosis

Diagnosis is by barium enema, where the classical features are a shortened colon (lead pipe appearance) in chronic ulcerative colitis with mucosal ulceration (Figure 26) and pseudopolyps in acute colitis. Flexible sigmoidoscopy/colonoscopy will provide a tissue diagnosis and show confluent mucosal inflammation.

Medical treatment

Most mild attacks will respond to treatment with:

- oral or topical (enema or suppository) steroids
- oral or rectal administration of sulphasalazine compounds.

Low doses of these agents either alone or in combination are used to maintain disease remission. Severe attacks require treatment with intravenous steroids.

Surgical treatment

There are four main indications for surgical intervention:

- failure of medical therapy
- acute, fulminant disease
- onset of complications
- malignant change.

Excision of the colon, rectum and anus (panproctocolectomy) will cure the disease (Figure 24C) but has the disadvantage of leaving the patient with a permanent ileostomy. This operation is a major undertaking in an ill, toxic patient with complications of the disease. A subtotal colectomy [excision of the colon with preservation of the rectum and anus (Figure 24B)] is less extensive and better tolerated by these patients and leaves options for further surgery at a later date – either removal of the rectal stump and ileal pouch–anal anastomosis (a restorative proctectomy) or complete excision of the rectal stump and anal canal leaving the patient with a permanent ileostomy.

A single stage total colectomy, proctectomy and ileoanal anastomosis with an ileal pouch [a restorative proctocolectomy (Figure 24D)] is an alternative to these procedures. It is a complex operation which has the advantage of avoiding the need for a permanent ileostomy and is usually reserved for fit patients undergoing elective surgery. Usually this surgery will be protected by a temporary defunctioning loop ileostomy which will be closed at a later date.

Complications

There are four major complications of ulcerative colitis:

Toxic dilatation Gross dilatation of the transverse colon in a severely ill patient. This is an indication for urgent colectomy before perforation occurs.

Massive haemorrhage

Perforation This may occur without dilatation in acute fulminant colitis.

Urgent sub-total colectomy is the procedure of choice for these three groups of patients.

Malignant change Dysplasia and eventually malignancy will develop in 10–20% of patients who have poorly controlled *total* colitis of 10 or more years in duration. They require either a restorative proctocolectomy or a panproctocolectomy.

Crohn's colitis

Unlike ulcerative colitis, acute colitis caused by Crohn's disease is a transmural inflammation with classic microscopic Crohn's features (see p. 58). Macroscopically, the inflammation may be patchy with areas of normal colon interspersed between areas of disease. Sometimes the rectum is spared. There is often severe perianal disease with multiple fistulae and abscesses.

Treatment

Medical treatment is with steroids (systemic or topical) and rectal metronidazole.

When medical treatment fails colectomy is the only option. Sometimes if only a segment of colon is diseased a limited resection can be undertaken, e.g. a right hemicolectomy. If the entire colon is involved the patient will

Table 13 Infective causes of acute colitis

Shigella sonnei

Salmonella typhimurium

Escherichia coli

Staphylococcus aureus

Clostridium welchii

Entamoeba histolytica (amoebic dysentery)

Schistosoma mansoni (schistosomiasis)

require a panproctocolectomy or, if the rectum is spared, a subtotal colectomy with an ileorectal anastomosis. Ileal pouches are avoided because of the risk of developing Crohn's disease in the pouch itself.

Infective colitis

Acute colitis may also be caused by various infections (Table 13). Usually these infections are self-limiting or respond to an appropriate course of antibiotics. Surgical intervention is rarely required.

Antibiotic-associated colitis

Overgrowth of *Clostridium difficile*, a normal component of the intestinal flora, can follow ampicillin, clindamycin or cephalosporin therapy. Endoscopic examination of the colon will reveal a pseudomembrane made up of necrotic epithelium and leucocytes. The diagnosis is confirmed by stool culture. The causative antibiotic should be withdrawn and oral vancomycin therapy instituted. Occasionally colectomy is required.

Ischaemic colitis

This condition usually affects elderly arteriopaths. It is caused by acute or chronic occlusion of the inferior mesenteric artery. The left side of the colon is mainly affected. Clinically, the condition can be difficult to differentiate from other causes of colitis. The diagnosis is usually made on the barium enema appearances: either oedematous mucosa and 'thumb-printing' or a diseased strictured segment of colon in the region of the splenic flexure at the 'watershed' between the colonic blood supply from the superior and inferior mesenteric arteries. Most patients settle on conservative management; otherwise resection is necessary.

Large bowel obstruction

The obstructed colon distends progressively as the small bowel continues to pour its contents through the ileocaecal valve. As the distended colon contracts and attempts to overcome the obstruction, the peristaltic waves are perceived as colic. If the ileocaecal valve is competent (Figure 27B) and prevents reflux of the intestinal contents back into the small intestine, a closed-loop obstruction develops with massive and rapid distension of the colon. Left untreated, the thin-walled highly distensible caecum will perforate. If the ileocaecal valve is incompetent

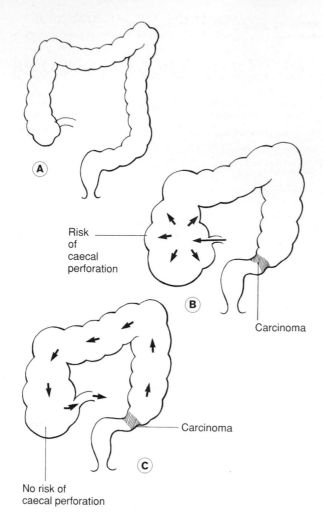

Risk
of
caecal
perforation

Carcinoma

Carcinoma

No risk of
caecal perforation

Figure 27 Large bowel obstruction. (A) Normal anatomy. (B) Closed-loop large bowel obstruction. (C) 'Open' loop obstruction with retrograde decompression of the colon into the small bowel.

(Figure 27C), intestinal contents will flow back into the small bowel, which will in turn distend and eventually cause vomiting.

Aetiology

Cancer of the colon is by far the most common cause of large bowel obstruction (see p. 62).

Less frequent causes are sigmoid or caecal volvulus, 'pseudo-obstruction', chronic constipation and faecal impaction, and finally a diverticular stricture or acute diverticulitis.

Clinical features

Large bowel obstruction is characterised by colicky lower abdominal pains, abdominal distension and an alteration in bowel habit. As the obstruction progresses, constipation becomes absolute and the passage of flatus ceases. Unlike small bowel obstruction, vomiting is a late feature.

Physical examination often reveals a tense tympanitic distended abdomen in a dehydrated patient. The bowel sounds are high-pitched and tinkling. Localised tenderness, particularly over the caecum, suggests imminent caecal perforation.

Diagnosis

Large bowel obstruction is investigated by a combination of the following tests.

Plain abdominal radiograph Gross colonic dilatation in a picture-frame distribution around the margins of the abdomen are evident on a supine abdominal film. Large bowel fluid levels are the classical features on an erect film. The extent of any caecal dilatation in a closed-loop obstruction will also be evident.

Sigmoidoscopy and/or gentle contrast enema examination

CT abdomen Wherever possible, the level of the obstruction must be assessed prior to surgery. These tests are essential in order to help plan the most appropriate operation and to rule out a pseudo-obstruction or faecal impaction, which can be treated without operation.

Treatment

Once the patient has been adequately resuscitated, rapid surgical relief of the mechanical obstruction is the primary aim of treatment in order to prevent colonic perforation and a potentially lethal faecal peritonitis. Treatment depends on the cause of the obstruction.

Carcinoma of the colon An obstructing cancer of the caecum or ascending colon can usually be treated by right hemicolectomy with an immediate reanastomosis (Figure 20, p. 63). Left-sided cancers that obstruct are more difficult to manage. Primary reanastomosis after resection can be achieved after an 'on-table' lavage is used to decompress and empty the colon of faecal matter. In frail, ill patients, a defunctioning transverse colon loop colostomy may be lifesaving. Primary resection without reanastomosis (Hartmann's operation, Figure 25, p. 65) is a good alternative in a fitter patient. The choice of operation calls for a skilled judgement by an experienced surgeon.

In patients with an obstructed colonic cancer it is important to determine whether or not they have any metastatic liver disease and these patients need a CT scan. If extensive metastatic disease is identified, which is unlikely to be treated surgically, other treatment options should be considered that might avoid a laparotomy. A left-sided cancer can be treated with an endoluminal stent, which can be positioned radiologically. This may save giving a colostomy to a patient who has just a few months to live. Alternatively, it may be used to relieve an acute obstruction allowing an easier bowel resection at a later date once the obstruction has settled.

Sigmoid or caecal volvulus Decompression of a sigmoid volvulus (Figure 28) using a flatus tube introduced per rectum can be a lifesaving manoeuvre. The volvulus is likely to recur and wherever possible resection either with or without primary reanastomosis should be attempted. A caecal volvulus is less common. Here the caecum is abnormally mobile and may twist, compromising its own blood supply and causing an intestinal obstruction. A right hemicolectomy is the operation of choice.

Pseudo-obstruction This condition mimics a true mechanical bowel obstruction. It is caused by abnormal gut motility and the diagnosis is confirmed by a contrast enema examination, which will fail to show any evidence

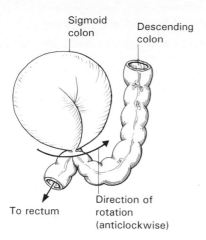

Sigmoid colon

Descending colon

To rectum

Direction of rotation (anticlockwise)

Figure 28 Sigmoid volvulus.

of a mechanical obstruction despite the plain abdominal radiograph findings. A pseudo-obstruction often responds to correction of any electrolyte imbalance, rehydration and supplemental oxygen. Occasionally, massive caecal distension will occur and it will be necessary to decompress the colon either by colonoscopy or caecostomy.

Faecal impaction Faecal impaction, often in elderly bedridden patients, can present as a large bowel obstruction that can be relieved by either manual disimpaction or a series of enemas. These patients should be investigated by sigmoidoscopy and barium enema to exclude an underlying cause for their impaction.

In neglected cases with gross constipation the colon sometimes perforates (a stercoral perforation) and can cause a lethal peritonitis.

Prognosis

This depends on the cause. The mortality rates after laparotomy for large bowel obstruction are about 15% and are doubled in patients with faecal peritonitis from an associated perforation.

Colonic angiodysplasia

This is the most common cause of an obscure gastrointestinal haemorrhage (i.e. when routine investigation has failed to find an obvious cause). The caecum and ascending colon are the most frequent sites for these submucosal capillary blood lakes to develop. They can cause a chronic anaemia or a torrential haemorrhage.

Diagnosis

Diagnosis is by angiography during active haemorrhage or by colonoscopy, which allows direct visualisation of the angiomata. Sometimes the bleeding vessels can be embolised during angiography.

Barium enema examination will not detect these vascular lesions.

Treatment

Frequently the bleeding will cease spontaneously and often the precise site of blood loss is never determined. A right hemicolectomy is the operation of choice for patients who continue to bleed when angiography has failed.

3.7 Diseases of the rectum and anus

Anorectal problems are a frequent presenting complaint for patients with surgical diseases. They can be conveniently grouped:

The principle minor anorectal diseases are:

- anorectal sepsis
- haemorrhoids
- anal fissures
- pilonidal sinus.

The two important cancers are:

- carcinoma of the rectum (see p. 63)
- carcinoma of the anal canal.

The most important functional disorders of the rectum and anus are:

- rectal prolapse
- faecal incontinence
- faecal impaction
- chronic constipation.

Anorectal sepsis

Most episodes of acute anorectal sepsis start with an infection in the intersphincteric space, usually in an anal gland. A primary infection of the anal gland will produce an intersphincteric abscess. Infection from here will spread in several directions (Figure 29) and lead to:

- perianal abscess
- ischio-rectal abscess
- supralevator abscess or pelvic abscess.

Spontaneous or surgical external drainage will produce a fistula if the connection between the underlying anal gland and the anal canal remains patent. Occasionally, a deep abscess will rupture and drain into the rectum to produce a high fistula (Figure 29).

Chronic anorectal sepsis results from:

- incomplete treatment of the acute infection
- a persisting fistula-in-ano
- underlying chronic inflammation, e.g. Crohn's disease, tuberculosis
- carcinoma of the rectum or anus.

Clinical features

Perianal pain, swelling and erythema are the hallmarks of anorectal sepsis. Pain is maximal in those lesions

Three

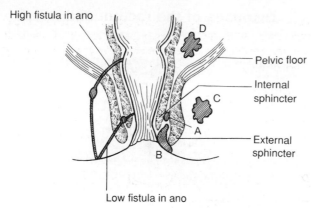

High fistula in ano

D — Pelvic floor

— Internal sphincter

C

A

B — External sphincter

Low fistula in ano

Figure 29 Perianal sepsis and fistulae. (A) Intersphincteric abscess. (B) Perianal abscess. (C) Ischio-rectal abscess. (D) Pelvic abscess.

nearest the anal verge. Swelling and tenderness may be less apparent in deep-seated ischio-rectal or supralevator abscesses and may be only detected on rectal examination. These patients will show signs of systemic sepsis.

Treatment

An acute abscess needs prompt incision and drainage under general anaesthetic. A deep ischio-rectal abscess may contain multiple loculi and may extend behind the anal canal into the opposite ischio-rectal fossa (a horseshoe abscess). A careful sigmoidoscopic examination plus biopsy of the abscess wall is important to rule out any associated serious pathology.

A fistula-in-ano may present as an abscess or as a spontaneously discharging opening on the perineum (Figure 29). The principle of surgery is to lay open the fistula between its internal and external openings and to allow healing by secondary intention. A careful examination under anaesthetic is essential in order to assess the relationship of the fistula to the underlying sphincters, division of which would lead to incontinence. Immediate control of the fistula is obtained by external surgical drainage coupled with the use of a seton, a non-absorbable ligature, which is threaded along the fistula tract and through the internal opening of the fistula. Both ends are then tied loosely outside the anal canal. Remarkably this allows the sepsis to resolve and allows the surgeon time to carefully assess the relationship of the fistula to the sphincter muscle complex using MRI scans, endoanal ultrasound or both techniques.

Some low fistulas can be laid open at a later date, especially in those male patients who have a more robust sphincter complex. The management of intermediate or high fistulas is difficult and technically demanding. Some patients benefit from leaving the seton in situ long term.

Multiple fistulas, recurrent perianal abesesses and anal fissures are the hallmark of perianal Crohn's disease. Whenever possible, surgery is conservative (because healing is poor) and concentrates on draining any pockets of infection. Many of these patients will respond to a course of rectal metronidazole.

Haemorrhoids and anal fissures

More than 50% of the population have symptoms caused by haemorrhoids at some stage of their lives. The condition should be considered a variant of normal.

Haemorrhoids develop when the normal prolapse of the anal mucosa and its underlying venous plexus becomes exaggerated and leads to symptoms.

Clinical features

Rectal bleeding with or without pain is the hallmark of haemorrhoids. Because these symptoms can also be caused by many other colorectal diseases, in particular *colorectal cancer*, all patients should be carefully evaluated to exclude other more serious causes for their rectal bleeding.

Haemorrhoids are classified according to their severity:

First degree: rectal bleeding
Second degree: prolapse with spontaneous reduction
Third degree: prolapse requiring manual reduction
Fourth degree: permanent prolapse with or without thrombosis.

Diagnosis

Diagnosis is by proctoscopy and flexible sigmoidoscopy. Coexisting colorectal pathology should be excluded using a barium enema in all patients over 45 years of age.

Treatment

Dietary measures Promoting increased stool softness and bulk by increasing intake of fibre will 'cure' most first- and second-degree haemorrhoids.

Band ligation or injection sclerotherapy These simple measures are effective for persistent bleeding and mild prolapse.

Haemorrhoidectomy This is reserved for major prolapse (third and fourth degree) or where other measures fail to control the symptoms.

Acutely prolapsed thrombosed piles

This painful condition can be treated by urgent surgery to excise the thrombosed pile. Alternatively the acute thrombosis can be resolved with bed rest, icepacks, analgesia and laxatives. Some patients will require an elective haemorrhoidectomy at a later date.

Anal fissure

An anal fissure is an ulcer at the mucocutaneous junction between the anal canal and the rectum. It usually lies in the posterior or anterior midline. Often, the underlying cause is unknown. Sometimes it is associated with underlying inflammatory bowel disease.

Clinical features

Patients present with fissures that cause excruciating anal pain during defecation. The discomfort, which lasts for several hours after each bowel movement, is prolonged by a reflex spasm of the anal sphincters. Patients with fissures frequently defer defecation in order to avoid pain. The constipation that results aggravates the symptoms. Bleeding is usually slight but bright red in colour.

Inspection of the perineum sometimes reveals a sentinel pile at the site of the fissure caused by oedema and inflammation of the adjacent perianal skin. Rectal examination and proctoscopy is usually impossible because of pain and intense spasm of the anal sphincters.

Differential diagnosis:

- carcinoma of the anal canal
- perianal Crohn's disease.

Treatment

Healing of the fissure occurs rapidly once spasm of the anal sphincters is reduced. This can be induced by topical application of glyceryl trinitrate (GTN) ointment or diltiazem paste, which acts locally to relax muscle spasm. If this fails there is a surgical option:

Lateral sphincterotomy Surgical division of the lower part of the internal anal sphincter under general anaesthetic.

The aim is to relax the anal canal enough to allow healing of the fissure. Anal dilatation, an uncontrolled forceful manual partial disruption of the anal sphincters under general anaesthetic, is not recommended.

Prognosis

Most fissures rapidly resolve after surgery. Incontinence as a result of treatment is uncommon.

Pilonidal sinus

Aetiology

A pilonidal sinus is the result of an ingrowth of dead hairs through small pits usually in the midline of the natal cleft between the buttocks. It occurs in hirsute men and women and usually only presents when infection supervenes, often around puberty when hair growth and sebaceous gland activity peak.

Clinical features

Most patients present with pain, swelling and discharge or with an acute abscess between the buttocks that sometimes ruptures spontaneously before treatment to produce a chronically discharging sinus. Inspection usually reveals the sinus opening, often stuffed with protruding hairs some distance from the abscess itself, although both are connected by a subcutaneous tunnel.

Treatment

As with any abscess, incision and drainage is the key treatment. All underlying granulation tissue and ingrown hairs should be removed and the underlying cavity deroofed. Postoperative care is particularly important if recurrence is to be avoided. The area must be kept clean and shaved and allowed to heal by *secondary intention*.

Prognosis

Despite meticulous attention, up to 20% of patients will develop a recurrence.

Carcinoma of the anal canal

This disease is rare in comparison with carcinoma of the rectum. In the early stages, it may present as a small nodule that eventually will ulcerate and become fixed to the underlying sphincters. As well as local invasion, the cancer will spread to the pelvic lymph glands and to the *inguinal* lymph glands. The disease is confirmed by proctoscopy and biopsy.

Treatment

Radiotherapy and chemotherapy are the first-line treatment. Surgical excision by abdomino-perineal resection (Figure 23B, p. 64) is reserved for patients who do not respond or have recurrent disease.

Rectal prolapse and faecal incontinence

Rectal prolapse

Rectal prolapse is most common at the extremes of life. In a complete rectal prolapse, the entire rectal wall including its coverings turns inside out and slides out of the anus. Thus it is anatomically different from a simple rectal mucosal prolapse, which is associated with haemorrhoids.

Adult rectal prolapse predominates in the elderly and is more common in women. The underlying problem does not appear to be muscular damage caused by previous childbirth but instead is a reduction in tone of the anal sphincters.

Clinical features

The rectum prolapses as a conical mass outside the anal canal. Initially this follows defecation and spontaneous reduction occurs. Eventually with progressive muscular laxity, a permanent prolapse develops which causes soiling and excoriation and may eventually ulcerate.

Treatment

Most prolapses can be easily reduced manually only to recur as soon as the patient strains or becomes ambulant. The most effective surgical procedure is a transabdominal rectopexy, hitching the rectum to the sacrum either with sutures or with a non-absorbable mesh. This operation is often combined with a sigmoid colectomy (a resection rectopexy), which reduces the incidence of constipation after the procedure.

Alternatively, the redundant mucosa can be prolapsed through the anal canal and excised. In a frail, unfit patient another option is to encircle the anal canal with a non-absorbable submucosal suture (Thiersch wire technique) which constricts the anus and prevents prolapse. Faecal impaction is quite common after this procedure, which has become unpopular.

Faecal incontinence

This implies the loss of voluntary control of defecation. It often accompanies rectal prolapse but may occur independently. Incontinence may be secondary to birth trauma or surgical injury or organic disease of the anorectum, such as Crohn's disease or cancer. Many cases are idiopathic and these patients have a combination of defects of the anal sphincters, pelvic floor and their innervation.

Treatment

Some mild cases respond to pelvic floor exercises. Iatrogenic sphincter damage (e.g. during haemorrhoidectomy)

Three

71

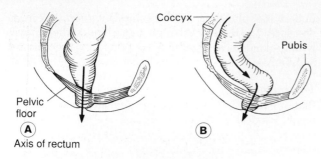

Pelvic floor

Axis of rectum

Coccyx

Pubis

(A)   (B)

Figure 30 Postanal repair for faecal incontinence.

is amenable to surgical repair or sphincteroplasty. A general tightening of the pelvic floor muscles and anal sphincters *behind* the anal canal [postanal repair (Figure 30)] is the most frequently used operation for idiopathic faecal incontinence. Surgical intervention in these patients should only take place after careful preoperative evalua-

tion of the rectal and anal physiology using manometry and ultrasound techniques.

Faecal impaction

Faecal impaction can occur at any age. It is especially frequent in the elderly bedridden patient who may be recovering from an operation. Opiates or other constipation-inducing analgesic agents, which contain codeine, may cause constipation that progresses to faecal impaction. Paradoxically, the initial presentation may be a spurious diarrhoea caused by overflow of liquid faeces and mucus from the proximal colon around the impacted faecal bolus. The diagnosis is confirmed by rectal examination.

Treatment

Sometimes the faecal bolus can be broken up by enemas and stool softeners. More often, digital breakdown followed by a manual evacuation is required. Oral laxatives are important to prevent recurrence, and a sigmoidoscopy should be undertaken to make sure an underlying carcinoma has not precipitated the impaction.

Self-assessment: questions

Extended matching items questions (EMIs)

EMI 1

Theme: The jaundiced patient

A. viral hepatitis

B. carcinoma of the pancreas

C. liver metastases

D. carcinoma of the gallbladder

E. ascending cholangitis

F. common bile duct stones

G. acute pancreatitis

For each patient described below select the most likely diagnosis from the list above.

1. A 72-year-old man who had a right hemicolectomy for a Dukes stage C carcinoma of the caecum 2 years ago presents with weight loss and a poor appetite. He has not noticed any change in the colour of his stools or urine but when you examine him you note he is jaundiced and feel a fullness in the upper abdomen.

2. A 52-year-old woman presents with a 3-month history of weight loss. Over the last month her appetite has been poor and this week she noticed her urine had become dark and her stools pale. There has been no pain. Last year she was diagnosed as a maturity-onset diabetic. On examination you can feel a smooth painless mass in the right upper quadrant.

3. A 30-year-old man is admitted with abdominal pain and a fever. A week previously he had an episode of right upper quadrant pain which had settled spontaneously. When you examine him he is tender in the upper abdomen and is shivering. You note that he is jaundiced and has a temperature of 39°C. His pulse rate is 130 beats/min and he has a systolic blood pressure of 95 mmHg.

EMI 2

Theme: Upper gastrointestinal tract investigation

A. gastrograffin swallow

B. biliary HIDA scan

C. endoscopic retrograde cholangiopancreatogram (ERCP)

D. barium follow-through

E. barium meal

F. oesophageal function tests

G. ultrasound scan

H. barium swallow

I. gastroscopy and biopsy

Select from the above list of options the most appropriate investigation for the following patients with upper gastrointestinal symptoms.

1. A 32-year-old man presents with symptoms of progressive dysphagia. He has not lost any weight. The symptoms have been present for 12 months. His GP had arranged a barium swallow, which shows a mild dilatation of the distal oesophagus, and asks for a gastroscopy. This is reported as a normal examination.

2. A 57-year-old man has a 1-month history of painless jaundice. He has the following liver profile: alanine transaminase (ALT) 75 U/l (normal range 0–40 U/l); alkaline phosphatase 420 U/l (normal range 70–230 U/l); serum bilirubin 91 µmol/l (normal range 2–20 µmol/l).

3. A 39-year-old woman is admitted with fever and severe upper abdominal pain. Her serum amylase is normal. She was tender in the center and right side of her upper abdomen. An ultrasound examination was unsuccessful because of her build. No abnormalities were detected on gastroscopy.

EMI 3

Theme: Treatment of oesophageal disease

A. cardiomyotomy

B. oesophageal stent

C. palliative oesophagogastrectomy

D. Nissen fundoplication

E. oesophageal balloon dilatation

F. two-stage oesophagectomy

G. treatment with prokinetic drugs

H. acid suppression treatment

Select from the list above the most appropriate treatment option for the following patients.

1. A 74-year-old man with achalasia of the cardia. He has severe angina and has had recurrent chest infections over the past 6 months.

2. A 53-year-old man with biopsy-proven adenocarcinoma of the gastro-oesophageal junction. He has solid dysphagia and ultrasound evidence of liver metastases.

3. A 55-year-old woman with reflux oesophagitis. Despite medical therapy she has developed a peptic oesophageal stricture and required two oesophageal dilatations in the last 18 months.

EMI 4

Theme: Acute abdominal pain

A. acute appendicitis

B. acute cholecystitis

C. mesenteric ischaemia

D. distal small bowel obstruction

E. perforated peptic ulcer

F. acute diverticulitis

G. leaking abdominal aortic aneurysm

H. sigmoid colon cancer

I. large bowel obstruction

For each of the following patients select the most appropriate diagnosis from the list above.

1. A 63-year-old man is admitted with a 4-day history of lower abdominal pain. He has been anorexic but has had no alteration in bowel habit. On examination he is febrile and generally tender in the lower abdomen. There is evidence of peritonism in the left iliac fossa.

2. A 70-year-old woman presents with a 2-day history of vomiting and colicky abdominal pain. She has not moved her bowels for 72 h. The key features on abdominal examination were dehydration, abdominal distension and tenderness in the right iliac fossa. A plain abdominal radiograph shows distended loops of intestine with incomplete haustral markings in a 'picture-frame' distribution.

3. A 49-year-old man with a long history of rheumatoid arthritis is admitted with collapse associated with severe upper abdominal pain. Two weeks ago his arthritic symptoms had worsened and he increased his non-steroidal medication. On examination he was hypotensive and distressed with a rigid, silent abdomen. A chest radiograph revealed an abnormal gas shadow under the right hemidiaphragm.

EMI 5

Theme: Surgical management of colonic disease

A. left hemicolectomy

B. right hemicolectomy

C. extended right hemicolectomy

D. panproctocolectomy

E. anterior resection

F. Hartmann's procedure

G. restorative proctocolectomy

H. abdomino-perineal resection

I. subtotal colectomy

Choose the correct treatment option from the list above for the following patients.

1. A 42-year-old man is admitted with severe diarrhoea and rectal bleeding and dehydration. He is known to have ulcerative colitis. His symptoms do not respond to a 5-day course of intensive steroid therapy.

2. A 75-year-old woman is admitted with severe lower abdominal pain and peritonism. A plain abdominal radiograph is unremarkable. She is resuscitated and because of her ongoing symptoms an abdominal CT

scan is arranged. This shows severe diverticular disease with a free perforation into the peritoneal cavity.

3. A 69-year-old woman is admitted with large bowel obstruction. An urgent gastrograffin enema shows a malignant stricture in the transverse colon.

EMI 6

Theme: Perianal diseases

A. examination under anaesthesia and rectal biopsy

B. lateral internal sphincterotomy

C. band ligation or sclerotherapy

D. insertion of a seton

E. incision and drainage

F. a 5-day course of broad-spectrum intravenous antibiotics

G. rectal metronidazole

H. a 4-week course of steroid enemas

I. lay open fistula

For the following patients select the most appropriate treatment from the list of options above.

1. A 42-year-old man who complains of severe pain after defecation which lasts several hours. He finds your rectal examination too painful to tolerate. You note that he has a sentinel pile.

2. A 60-year-old man presents with a history of swelling and pain in his bottom. On the morning of his admission he discharges some pus per rectum. When he is examined under anaesthetic your consultant identifies an opening adjacent to the anal canal which appears to communicate with a separate opening in the rectum above the pelvic floor.

3. A 55-year-old woman who is known to have terminal ileal Crohn's disease presents with 'a rectal discharge'. You attend theatre with your registrar. A sigmoidoscopy shows some inflammation in the lower rectum which is biopsied. You notice the patient has several anal fissures and two sinuses on the left side of the perineum which discharge mucoid material.

EMI 7

Theme: Upper gastrointestinal haemorrhage

A. underrun bleeding ulcer, truncal vagotomy and gastroenterostomy

B. total abdominal gastrectomy

C. gastroscopy and injection therapy

D. insertion of Sengestaken tube

E. 4-unit blood transfusion

F. nasogastric suction, intravenous fluid therapy

G. oesophageal transection

H. urgent gastroscopy and 4-unit blood transfusion

I. simple underrun bleeding ulcer

Select the most appropriate surgical management from this list for the following patients.

1. A 66-year-old man is admitted with haematemesis. He requires a 4-unit blood transfusion. An emergency gastroscopy is performed once he is resuscitated. This reveals an actively bleeding prepyloric ulcer which is controlled by saline and adrenaline (epinephrine) injection. The next morning he drops his blood pressure and has another haematemesis.

2. A 44-year-old man with cirrhosis is admitted with haematemesis. He is resuscitated and undergoes sclerotherapy for bleeding varices. Six hours later he rebleeds and cannot be controlled by further sclerotherapy.

3. A 29-year-old man is admitted with a haematemesis. He is shocked on arrival but quickly resuscitated. Prior to admission he had been passing black tarry stools for 24 h. His admission haemoglobin was 12.2 g/dl.

Constructed response questions (CRQs)

CRQ 1

A 59-year-old man presents with a 6-week history of jaundice and pruritis. He had a cholecystectomy for acute cholecystitis 12 years ago.

a. Name three of the most likely causes for this patient's jaundice.

You arrange a liver profile for this patient. These are the results:

Serum bilirubin 142 μmol/l	(2–20 μmol/l) normal range
Alkaline phosphatase 530 U/l	(70–230 U/l) normal range
Transaminase 66 U/L	(0–40 U/l) normal range

b. What other investigations would you arrange to determine the cause of the jaundice?

These investigations suggest there is an abnormality at the lower end of the bile duct. Your consultant asks you to arrange an ERCP.

c. What complications do you know of the procedure? List two.

This patient is deeply jaundiced and has abnormal liver function.

d. List three additional risks that any jaundiced patient may encounter during any surgical intervention.

CRQ 2

A 70-year-old woman presents with a 2-week history of cystitis and pneumaturia.

a. What is the clinical diagnosis?

You examine her abdomen and discover a mass in the left iliac fossa.

b. Name three diseases which can cause this condition.

Within a few hours of admission she develops a fever.

c. What steps would you take?

The following day her clinical condition has improved.

d. Name two diagnostic tests you could use to confirm the diagnosis.

The decision is made to treat this patient by surgery.

e. What operation do you know that would help this patient?

CRQ 3

A 70-year-old woman who had a laparotomy for perforated appendicitis 20 years ago is admitted with a 3-day history of colicky abdominal pain and vomiting. Her bowels have not moved and she has not passed flatus for 24 h.

a. What is the most likely diagnosis?

You undertake a full history and examination.

b. What features on abdominal examination would support this diagnosis?

You decide to arrange a plain abdominal radiograph.

c. What features would you expect to find on this radiograph?

When you examined the patient you decided there was no sign of any peritonism or peritonitis.

d. Outline five key steps in the conservative management of this patient.

Two days later the condition of the patient has not changed.

e. What are the options?

Sometimes these patients require urgent surgery.

f. List three clinical signs that would make you abandon conservative management and seek advice regarding urgent surgery.

CRQ 4

A 55-year old man presents with lower abdominal discomfort and tiredness. He has recently felt short of breath.

a. What other important points would you elicit from the history? List four.

When you examine him you think he is anaemic and you discover a mass in his right iliac fossa which seems tender on palpation.

b. List three important possible diagnoses.

You are concerned the patient might have an intra-abdominal abscess.

c. What investigation would be most helpful?

There is no sign of any abscess but the test shows a solid mass in the right iliac fossa. Your investigation reveals an apple-core shaped lesion in the ascending colon.

d. What is the most likely cause and what operation do you think the patient will require?

CRQ 5

A 69-year-old man is referred by his GP with a history of rectal bleeding. There has been no alteration in bowel habit. His haemoglobin was checked in the surgery and measured 8.6 g/dl. You confirm the history and can find nothing abnormal on abdominal or rectal investigation.

a. How would you investigate this patient and what dictates your choice of test?

The patient had a sessile sigmoid colon polyp which was simply removed.

b. When might a sigmoid colectomy be necessary in some patients with this condition?

Later, the decision is made to perform a sigmoid colectomy in this patient. He is anxious about his surgery and asks about the risks.

c. What complications do you know that are specific to this type of surgery?

The patient makes an uneventful recovery from his operation despite his fears.

d. What specific follow-up would you arrange for this patient?

CRQ 6

A 60-year-old woman presents with a 4-week history of progressive dysphagia. She has had a long previous history of heartburn and reflux oesophagitis.

a. What investigations would you arrange for this patient?

The examinations confirm that this patient has a carcinoma in the lower third of the oesophagus

b. What is the most likely histological type?

The patient is keen to be considered for surgical treatment, having previously been fit and well.

c. What investigation would you choose to assess whether or not the cancer could be resected?

Unfortunately your investigations show that cancer is inoperable.

d. What features would indicate that this cancer should not be resected?

This patient is keen to pursue other treatment options.

e. How else could you treat this patient's cancer?

Finally, this patient asks you about her life expectancy.

f. How long do patients who have inoperable oesophageal cancer live?

CRQ 7

A 44-year-old woman presents with a short history of jaundice and right upper quadrant pain. She is shivering uncontrollably on admission. Her stools have been pale and her urine dark.

a. What is the clinical diagnosis and what is the most likely cause?

You arrange some liver function tests which show the following profile:

Serum bilirubin 230 μmol/l	(2–20 μmol/l) normal range
Alkaline phosphatase 380 μmol/l	(70–230 μmol/l) normal range
AST 22 μmol/l	(0–40 μmol/l) normal range

You decide to arrange a biliary tract ultrasound examination as a result.

b. What abnormalities would you look for on this test?

Your consultant decides to organise an ERCP examination for this patient based on the interpretation of the ultrasound scan.

c. Why is this test useful in patients with this clinical presentation?

You are asked to prepare this patient for the procedure.

d. What would you do?

Unfortunately, the ERCP examination was technically unsuccessful.

e. Are there any other treatment options for this patient?

CRQ 8

A 78-year-old man visits his GP because he has lost 2 stone in weight and has daily upper abdominal pain. He has become increasingly concerned because he is vomiting especially towards the end of the day. He has noticed what appears to be undigested food in the vomit. His GP is concerned he has a gastric cancer.

a. What clinical signs might you find on clinical examination? List four of them.

You decide the patient is dehydrated and arrange his admission for rehydration.

b. What investigation would you arrange to confirm the diagnosis?

The examination confirms there is a cancer in the outlet of the stomach.

c. What specific tests would you arrange to determine whether this cancer was operable; what would you look for?

The investigations show that this patient is a suitable candidate for surgery.

d. What would be the most appropriate operation?

Objective structured clinical examination questions (OSCEs)

OSCE 1

Examine this barium swallow (Figure 31). Read the accompanying case history, then answer the following questions

A previously healthy 47-year-old man presents with an 18-month history of dysphagia for solids. Recently he has had several prolonged chest infections. A barium swallow has been arranged by his general practitioner.

a. What is the most likely diagnosis?
b. How would you confirm the diagnosis?
c. What is the cause of the recurrent chest infections?
d. What treatment would you advise?

OSCE 2

Look at the accompanying radiographs (Figure 32A, B), then answer the questions below.
a. What is this radiograph examination?
b. What abnormality can you see (Figure 32A)?
c. What are the treatment options?
d. List three complications of this procedure.

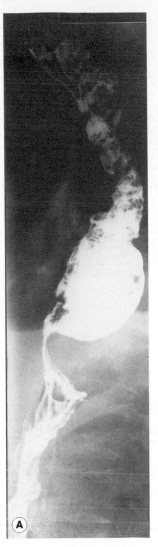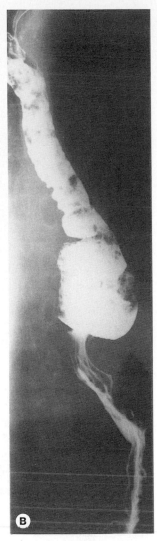

Figure 31 Barium swallow.

OSCE 3

A 35-year-old woman has a 2-month history of diarrhoea. She has lost 10 kg in weight. On examination she looks rather pale; the abdominal examination is unremarkable. She has a barium enema examination. This radiograph (Figure 33) is taken from her barium enema series. Examine the film and then answer the questions.

a. What abnormal features are shown on this radiograph?
b. What is the diagnosis?
c. What complications can develop?

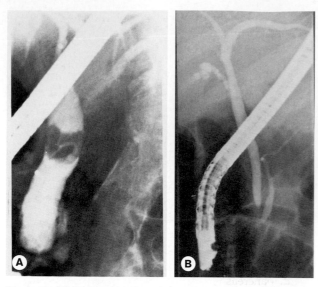

Figure 32 (A) (B) Normal radiograph for comparison.

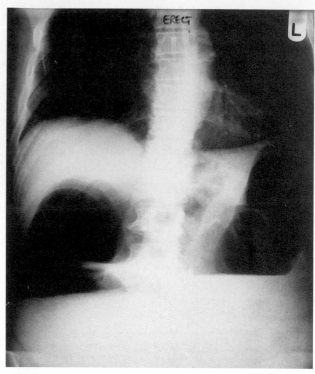

Figure 34 Erect abdominal radiograph.

OSCE 4

A 75-year-old man is admitted to hospital with abdominal distension and intermittent abdominal pains. He is dehydrated and has a tympanitic abdomen. You order a plain abdominal radiograph (Figure 34).

a. What is the diagnosis?
b. How would you confirm the cause?
c. What is the risk if treatment is delayed?

OSCE 5

A 36-year-old woman presents with a third episode of abdominal pain. On this occasion, as previously, she describes a band-like discomfort across the upper abdomen which is associated with nausea and lasts several hours before it spontaneously subsides. Look at the accompanying investigation (Figure 35).

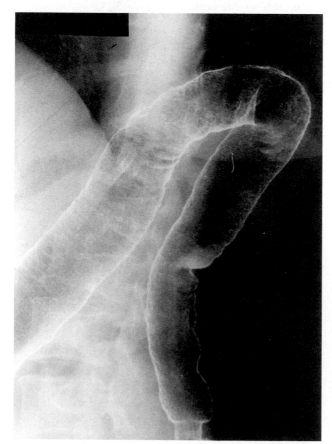

Figure 33 Barium enema.

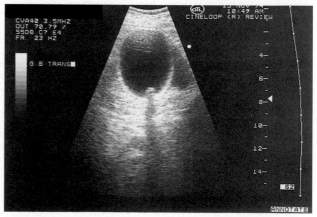

Figure 35

a. What examination is this an example of?

b. What abnormality is shown?

c. How else can this diagnosis be confirmed?

Best of 5s questions

1. A 58-year-old woman has noticed an alteration in her bowel habit. She has a barium enema examination and later a colonoscopy. These tests show she has a carcinoma in the descending colon. Which operation should she undergo?

   a. transverse colectomy

   b. right hemicolectomy

   c. panproctocolectomy

   d. left hemicolectomy

   e. extended right hemicolectomy

2. A 35-year-old woman is admitted with profuse diarrhoea and lower abdominal pain. The previous week she had completed a course of clindamycin for a cutaneous infection. A flexible sigmoidoscopy showed a pseudomembrane. Which organism is responsible for her infection?

   a. *Campylobacter coli*

   b. *Salmonella typhi*

   c. *Clostridium difficile*

   d. *Mycobacterium tuberculi*

   e. *Yersinia enterolytica*

3. A 21-year-old man is admitted with weight loss, abdominal colic and diarrhoea. He has a tender mass in his right iliac fossa. He undergoes a CT scan which shows some abnormal loops of small intestine in his lower abdomen. There is no abscess. A small bowel follow-through confirms that he has Crohn's disease of the terminal ileum. The correct initial treatment is:

   a. immunosuppression with methotrexate

   b. resection of his terminal ileum

   c. oral metronidazole

   d. high-dose oral steroids

   e. oral sulphasalazine

4. A 74-year-old man has a biopsy-proven carcinoma of the rectosigmoid junction. His disease is staged with a CT abdominal scan. Unfortunately this shows widespread metastases affecting both lobes of the liver. He develops signs of a colonic obstruction. What is the most appropriate treatment for this patient?

   a. defunctioning transverse colostomy

   b. endoluminal stenting

   c. palliative anterior resection

   d. sigmoid colectomy

   e. palliative abdomino-perineal resection

5. A 25-year-old man with familial polyposis coli has multiple polyps identified on his most recent surveillance colonoscopy. Which of the following options is the most appropriate treatment?

   a. subtotal colectomy

   b. repeat colonoscopy and polyp clearance

   c. abdomino-perineal resection

   d. annual colonoscopic surveillence

   e. restorative proctocolectomy, pouch anal anastomosis

6. A 64-year-old patient presents with lassitude, weight loss and an abdominal mass. An ultrasound examination of his liver shows that he has multiple liver metastases. Of the following list which is the most common primary site?

   a. colorectum

   b. breast

   c. lung

   d. pancreas

   e. stomach

7. A 35-year-old alcoholic patient presents with a major haematemesis. Attempts to control the bleeding endoscopically are not successful. What should the next treatment step be?

   a. TIPS procedure

   b. balloon tamponade

   c. oesophageal transaction

   d. distal splenorenal shunt

   e. side-to-side portacaval shunt

8. A 45-year-old woman is admitted with severe upper abdominal pain and mild jaundice. She has an ultrasound scan which confirms the presence of gall stones and a serum amylase of 720 IU/l. A diagnosis of gallstone pancreatitis is made. Which one of the following criteria is not in keeping with a severe attack?

   a. arterial oxygen tension (pO$_2$) <60 mmHg

   b. blood urea >8 mg/dl

   c. C-reactive protein 50 mg/l

   d. serum calcium <8 mg/dl

   e. serum SGOT >250 IU/l

9. A 55-year-old man presents with epigastric pain and weight loss. He has a barium meal and a gastroscopy which show he has a cancer halfway along the greater curvature of the stomach. His CT scan does not show any metastatic disease. Which is the most appropriate operation for this patient?

   a. distal gastrectomy

   b. oesophagogastrectomy

   c. gastroenterostomy

   d. total abdominal gastrectomy

   e. proximal gastrectomy

10. Which of the following is an unlikely presentation in a patient with common bile duct stones?

    a. gallstone ileus

    b. ascending cholangitis

    c. gallstone pancreatitis

    d. obstructive jaundice

    e. an unexpected finding on a routine intraoperative cholangiogram during cholelystectomy

Multiple choice questions

1. Barrett's oesophagus is:

   a. unrelated to gastro-oesophageal reflux

   b. best diagnosed using contrast radiology

   c. best treated by surgical resection

   d. a premalignant condition

   e. associated with stricture formation

2. A paraoesophageal hiatus hernia:

   a. is a common cause of gastro-oesophageal reflux

   b. is less common than a sliding hiatus hernia

   c. is usually repaired through the chest

   d. is lined by Barrett's epithelium

   e. can cause gastric outlet obstruction

3. The following statements are true regarding instrumental oesophageal perforation:

   a. it may cause a pneumothorax

   b. a mediastinal crunch can be detected on auscultation

   c. it always requires operative intervention

   d. it follows a prolonged bout of vomiting

   e. it is infrequently detected using contrast radiology

4. The following statements relate to peptic ulcer disease:

   a. ulcers are most reliably detected by a barium meal

   b. pyloric stenosis is the least frequent complication

   c. elective surgery is rarely required

   d. a drainage procedure is always required after truncal vagotomy

   e. radiological evidence of subdiaphragmatic gas is always present after peptic ulcer perforation

5. Malignant gastric ulcers:

   a. can be reliably diagnosed on barium meal examination

   b. can be differentiated from benign peptic ulcers on history alone

   c. respond to histamine H_2 receptor antagonists

   d. can cause pyloric stenosis

   e. are usually cured by partial gastrectomy

6. The following are classical features of a perforated peptic ulcer:

   a. succussion splash on examination

   b. a long antecedent history

   c. shoulder tip pain

   d. rebound tenderness

   e. absent bowel sounds

7. The following statements are true concerning gastric carcinoma:

   a. it is twice as common in females as in males

   b. it is linked to patients with type O blood group

   c. it often presents with a major gastrointestinal haemorrhage

   d. it is sited mainly on the lesser curvature of the stomach

   e. it can metastasise to the ovaries

8. Ascending cholangitis:

   a. can cause collapse in the elderly

   b. is caused by stone impaction in Hartmann's pouch

   c. can be treated endoscopically

   d. is cured by cholecystectomy

   e. is usually caused by gram-positive organisms

9. In patients with acute cholecystitis:

   a. gallstones are always present

   b. diagnosis is usually confirmed by an oral cholecystogram

   c. a pericholecystic abscess is the most common complication

   d. the presence of icterus invariably implies a coexisting common bile duct stone

   e. complications are more likely if the patient is a diabetic

10. The following statements relate to common bile duct stones:

    a. most are formed primarily in the common bile duct

    b. most are associated with an elevated serum alkaline phosphatase

    c. about 50% are asymptomatic

    d. they are often associated with a palpable gallbladder

    e. they cause at least one-third of all episodes of pancreatitis

11. An elevated serum amylase is seen in:

    a. mesenteric ischaemia

    b. acute cholecystitis

    c. idiopathic pancreatitis

    d. perforated peptic ulcer

    e. acute hepatitis

12. Necrotising pancreatitis:

    a. complicates half of all episodes of acute pancreatitis

    b. is associated with a poor outcome

    c. can be diagnosed on ultrasound scanning

d. responds to radical surgical debridement

e. is usually sterile

13. In patients with pancreatic cancer:

   a. cancer of the tail of the gland can often be treated by distal pancreatectomy

   b. maturity-onset diabetes is not uncommon *T several years*

   c. obstructive jaundice is infrequent *F*

   d. periampullary cancers have a better prognosis *T - early jaundice less aggress*

   e. they can present with a deep vein thrombosis *T - unknown*

14. Injection sclerotherapy:

   a. is particularly useful in controlling gastric fundal varices

   b. can cause an oesophageal stricture

   c. reduces blood flow through the varices through vasopressin release

   d. can be used in conjunction with balloon tamponade

   e. causes variceal thrombosis

15. The following statements relate to surgery and the spleen:

   a. after splenectomy the circulating platelet count falls *F*

   b. it is the first-line management for patients with idiopathic thrombocytopenic purpura

   c. isolated tears in the spleen can be repaired *T*

   d. a delayed splenic rupture usually occurs within 48 h *F 1-2 weeks*

   e. postsplenectomy pneumococcal infection is more common in young patients

16. Strangulating small bowel obstruction is more common in:

   a. small bowel volvulus *T*

   b. high small bowel obstruction *F*

   c. an incarcerated external hernia *T*

   d. obstructed patients with constant not colicky abdominal pain *T*

   e. a closed-loop obstruction *T*

17. Crohn's disease:

   a. rarely fistulates *F*

   b. may present as a recurrent perianal abscess *T v. common*

   c. can involve the mouth *T*

   d. is characterised by caseating epithelioid granulomas

   e. is a frequent cause of fulminant colitis *F - UC*

18. In small bowel mesenteric ischaemia:

   a. an absence of intestinal gas is a common finding

   b. a history of atrial fibrillation is common *T*

   c. the coeliac axis is usually occluded *F Sup Mes*

   d. venous infarction is more common than arterial occlusion *F*

   e. about 50% of patients die of the acute event *T*

19. The following statements relate to large bowel obstruction:

   a. caecal perforation is more likely if the ileocaecal valve is incompetent *F*

   b. it is usually caused by carcinoma of the colon *T*

   c. vomiting is an early feature *F - 2nd to S Bowel*

   d. distension is usually marked *T*

   e. the rectum is usually dilated and empty *T*

20. In colorectal cancer:

   a. at least 50% of all cancers are in the rectum and sigmoid colon *T*

   b. low anterior resection is easier in males than in females *F vide pelvis*

   c. 60% of patients with lymph gland involvement will survive 5 years *F 30%*

   d. most 1-cm polyps contain a focus of cancer *F*

   e. alteration in bowel habit is uncommon in right-sided cancers *F*

21. With regard to diverticular disease:

   a. this is the most common cause of a colovesical fistula

   b. it can present with massive rectal haemorrhage

   c. colonic resection and primary reanastomosis is the treatment of choice for severe acute perforated diverticulitis

   d. diverticulae are a common incidental finding on a barium enema examination

   e. colorectal cancer is rare in patients with diverticular disease

22. Ulcerative colitis is characterised by:

   a. mucosal skip lesions *F*

   b. rectal sparing *F*

   c. crypt abscesses *T*

   d. transmural inflammation *F*

   e. a lead pipe appearance on barium enema examination *T*

23. Carcinoma of the anal canal:

   a. is usually treated by abdomino-perineal resection

   b. can present with an inguinal lymphadenopathy

   c. is less common than rectal cancer

   d. is usually painless

   e. is radiosensitive

24. The following are characteristic of ischio-rectal abscesses:

a. they are usually situated above levator ani
b. they can be multilocular
c. they cause severe perianal tenderness
d. they are common in patients with ulcerative colitis
e. recurrence is often related to an underlying fistula

25. A pilonidal sinus:
    a. is usually congenital F – e hair + poo
    b. is best treated by primary excision and closure F
    c. affects men more than women T
    d. rarely recurs F
    e. frequently presents at puberty T

Self-assessment: answers

EMI answers

EMI 1

Theme: The jaundiced patient

1. C. Liver metastases.

This is a sinister history in a patient who has previously undergone surgery for cancer. The original histopathological staging (a Dukes stage C carcinoma) indicates that the tumour had spread to the lymph glands by the time of the original surgery. Patients like this are at high risk of developing liver metastases at a later date. A liver ultrasound scan would confirm the diagnosis.

2. B. Carcinoma of the pancreas.

Pale stools and dark urine are the hallmark of an obstructive jaundice. The lack of pain and a palpable enlarged gallbladder make gallstone disease unlikely. Two additional clues comes from the history. The patient has lost weight and has recently developed diabetes – both features are associated with a diagnosis of pancreatic cancer.

3. E. Ascending cholangitis.

This patient's presentation includes all the features of ascending cholangitis, a combination of jaundice, fever and rigors caused by obstruction and ascending infection in the common bile duct. These patients are much more ill in comparison with patients who have cholecystitis plus common bile duct stones. His vital signs show evidence of systemic sepsis. From the history this episode appears to have been preceded by an episode of biliary colic.

EMI 2

Theme: Investigation of upper gastrointestinal symptoms

1. F. Oesophageal function tests.

The only abnormality detected on barium swallow and gastroscopy was a mild dilatation of the lower oesophagus. These tests have not identified a stricture or evidence of reflux disease to explain his symptoms. Because of this a motility disorder must be considered. The dilatation of the lower oesophagus would be in keeping with an early achalasia.

2. G. Ultrasound scan.

This patient's liver function tests show a mixed picture with evidence of obstructive jaundice and hepatocellular dysfunction. Always start with simple non-invasive (and often less expensive) investigations. In this patient a liver ultrasound scan should be used to look for evidence of bile duct dilatation (to differentiate obstructive from hepatocellular jaundice) as well as identifying any possible cause, e.g. gallstones, liver metastases or pancreatic cancer.

3. B. Biliary HIDA scan.

This patient's history is in keeping with acute cholecystitis. Obesity and gas-filled loops of bowel are the main causes of failure of ultrasound examination. A HIDA scan which shows non-function of the gallbladder is diagnostic of cholecystitis when ultrasound fails.

EMI 3

Theme: Treatment of oesophageal disease

1. E. Oesophageal balloon dilatation.

Balloon dilatation and cardiomyotomy are the main treatment options for achalasia. This patient had recurrent chest infections which are probably caused by night-time aspiration of oesophageal contents. He needs treatment to improve swallowing and to prevent pneumonia. In view of his cardiac history balloon dilatation is the best option.

2. B. Oesophageal stent.

This patient has metastatic disease and is incurable. Treatment must be aimed at palliating his symptoms. An oesophageal stent will relieve his dysphagia and obviates the need for open surgery.

3. D. Nissen fundoplication.

This patient has developed a serious complication of reflux disease despite medical treatment. Failure of medical therapy is an indication for surgery in reflux disease. A Nissen fundoplication is one of the surgical options in the treatment of reflux disease.

EMI 4

Theme: Acute abdominal pain

1. F. Acute diverticulitis.

The history and clinical findings are characteristic of acute diverticulitis. A gastrograffin enema or an abdominal CT scan would confirm your clinical diagnosis and would demonstrate whether or not there was a colonic perforation associated with this episode.

2. I. Large bowel obstruction.

This patient's presentation has all the hallmarks of an acute intestinal obstruction. The abdominal distension and acute change in bowel habit point toward a colonic obstruction. This is confirmed on the plain abdominal radiograph which demonstrates the key features of a large bowel obstruction – distended loops of bowel with incomplete haustral folds together with a picture-frame rather than a central distribution of the bowel loops which would be in keeping with small bowel obstruction.

3. E. Perforated peptic ulcer.

Sudden-onset agonising abdominal pain and collapse are the hallmark of intra-abdominal catastrophe. A rigid silent abdomen supports the diagnosis of generalised peritonitis.

In addition, the original distribution of the pain in the upper abdomen together with the use of NSAIDs raise suspicion of a peptic perforation. Sub-diaphragmatic gas clinches the diagnosis.

EMI 5

Theme: Surgical management of colonic disease

1. I.   Subtotal colectomy.

This is the operation of choice for any patient with acute colitis irrespective of cause which does not respond to intensive medical treatment. The majority of the colon is removed and the rectal stump is preserved. This step avoids the need for complex surgery in the pelvis (to remove the rectal stump), which can be hazardous in a sick patient with severe colitis. In addition, when the patient has recovered, it allows for other surgical options which may avoid the patient having a permanent ileostomy.

2. F.   Hartmann's procedure.

Demonstration of a free perforation into the peritoneal cavity by the gastrograffin enema indicates that this patient is at risk of an uncontrolled faecal peritonitis. Resecting the sigmoid colon containing the diverticular disease, creating an end colostomy and a blind rectal stump (Hartmann's operation), will prevent further contamination of the peritoneal cavity. This operation avoids a bowel anastomosis in unfavourable conditions where healing may be compromised by infection.

3. C.   Extended right hemicolectomy.

This procedure has the advantage of removing the cancer along with its lymphatic and vascular drainage and also removes all of the proximal obstructed colon which will be loaded with faeces. This enables a safe reanastomosis of the colon and will avoid the need for a defunctioning stoma.

EMI 6

Theme: Perianal diseases

1. B.   Lateral internal sphincterotomy.

This patient's presentation is characteristic of an anal fissure. Urgent sphincterotomy under general anaesthesia will relieve the muscle spasm and allow the fissure to heal. In some patients with less severe symptoms the fissure may heal with topical application of glyceryl trinitrate (GTN) ointment.

2. D.   Insertion of a seton.

The clinical findings are of a high fistula-in-ano where the internal opening lies above the anal sphincters which control continence. Any attempt to lay open the track from the internal to the external opening of the fistula may render this patient incontinent. A seton (a drain which is inserted along the track of the fistula and then has both ends tied together outside the anal canal) is a safe method of controlling the fistula while healing takes place.

3. G.   Rectal metronidazole.

Multiple fissures and perineal sinuses are the hallmark of perianal Crohn's disease. Treatment should be conserva-

tive and surgery avoided whenever possible. The symptoms often respond dramatically to a topical course of metronidazole.

EMI 7

Theme: Upper gastrointestinal bleeding

1. I.   Simple underrun bleeding ulcer.

Rebleeding after endoscopic therapy is an indication for surgery. As the patient has already had a 4-unit blood transfusion it is important that surgical intervention is prompt. In these critically ill patients surgery should be kept simple, concentrating on arrest of the haemorrhage.

2. D.   Insertion of a Sengestaken tube.

This is the next step once sclerotherapy fails. It almost always controls the bleeding and allows time to resuscitate and stabilise the patient while definitive treatment is planned.

3. C.   Gastroscopy and injection therapy.

Urgent endoscopy is the key diagnostic step in any patient with a brisk upper gastrointestinal haemorrhage. In addition to confirming the diagnosis the technique allows control of any ongoing bleeding using sclerotherapy.

CRQ answers

CRQ 1

a. common bile duct stone

   carcinoma of the pancreas

   cholangiocarcinoma

   acute hepatitis

   hepatic metastases

Any of the above diagnoses would score marks.

b. ultrasound of liver, biliary tract and pancreas

   CT scan liver, bile duct and pancreas

   liver serology for hepatitis

   An ultrasound scan would be the most important non-invasive test.

   This might show:

- biliary tree dilatation
- evidence of a pancreatic mass
- liver metastases.

If a pancreatic cancer is suspected, a CT scan would be useful in determining the extent of disease if surgical resection is to be considered. Liver serology is important to exclude hepatitis A, B and C.

c. pancreatitis

   bleeding

   duodenal perforation

Any two of these answers would score marks. Pancreatitis is the most common complication. Bleeding usually only occurs after a sphincterotomy and can often be treated conservatively by transfusion.

d. coagulopathy

   hepatorenal failure

   infection

These are the commonest causes of major morbidity in patients with jaundice who undergo surgery. The patient's coagulation profile should be checked preoperatively and prophylactic vitamin K administered. Fresh frozen plasma may also be required in the perioperative period.

Postoperative renal failure is a major problem in patients with jaundice. It can be prevented by ensuring the patient is well hydrated before the procedure using intravenous fluids. Mannitol or dopamine can be used to maintain the diuresis perioperatively.

Jaundiced patients are at special risk of infection. Appropriate broad-spectrum antibiotic prophylaxis should be used.

CRQ 2

a. Colovesical fistula.

The presence of pneumaturia indicates this patient has an enterovesical fistula, a connection between the bowel and the bladder. The cystitic symptoms are secondary to infection of the bladder by enteric organisms. Most fistulae to the bladder are colonic in origin.

b. Diverticular disease.

Crohn's disease.

Carcinoma of the sigmoid colon.

These are the most likely causes of a colovesical fistula.

c. Undertake a clinical reassessment.

Take blood cultures.

Start antibiotic therapy.

It is important to rule out a significant deterioration in the patient's overall condition. Provided she is stable it would be appropriate to begin broad-spectrum antibiotics to cover aerobic and anaerobic organisms *after* taking blood cultures. A combination of a cephalosporin and metronidazole would be suitable.

d. Barium enema.

CT abdominal and pelvic scan.

Cystoscopy.

Sigmoidoscopy.

Any of these responses would score marks. Often a combination of these tests will be required. A CT scan is often a useful starting point as it is non-invasive and will give detailed information regarding the relationship of the intestines and the bladder. The diagnosis is confirmed by demonstrating air in the bladder on CT or the passage of contrast into the bladder during a CT or barium study. Cystoscopy will reveal a 'telltale' patch of cystitis at the fistula site which is usually on the dome of the bladder. A sigmoidoscopy will enable a tissue diagnosis to be obtained if the underlying cause is cancer or Crohn's disease.

e. Surgical resection of the diseased section of bowel.

A colovesical fistula is unlikely to heal spontaneously. The patient will require a laparotomy and resection of the affected segment of bowel together with oversew of the bladder fistula. There are two main surgical options:

- resection and primary anastomosis
- resection and exteriorisation (Hartmann's procedure).

The choice will depend on the degree of inflammation and infection present at the time of operation. A primary anastomosis is unsafe in the presence of severe infection and localised peritonitis.

CRQ 3

a. Adhesive small bowel obstruction.

With a history of a previous laparotomy for a septic intra-abdominal condition plus colicky pains and a cessation of bowel function, a bowel obstruction secondary to adhesions would be the most likely diagnosis.

b. Abdominal distension.

A tympanitic abdomen.

Obstructed, tinkling bowel sounds.

An empty rectum.

These are the key features you should look for in a patient with intestinal obstruction. Look also in the groin to check for a strangulated hernia.

c. Distended loops of small intestine.

In an established small bowel obstruction (the most usual finding in adhesive obstruction) it is usual to find a ladder pattern of distended small bowel loops sited centrally in the abdomen. The plain radiograph would also help to distinguish a large bowel obstruction, unrelated to the previous surgery – although this diagnosis would be unlikely from the presenting history.

d. Establish i.v. access for fluid resuscitation and maintenance.

Obtain baseline blood for biochemistry and haematology.

Restrict oral intake.

Use a nasogastric tube to decompress the stomach.

Catheterise the patient.

Fluid resuscitate the patient.

Maintain careful fluid balance.

These are the key steps in conservative management of an intestinal obstruction. Any of these responses will gain marks.

e. Surgical intervention.

Non-response to 24–48 h conservative management is an indication for surgery. Progress should be assessed on clinical grounds (decreasing distension, passage of flatus, etc. all indicate an improvement) and by repeated radiology, looking for resolution of the small bowel distension and/or the presence of gas in the large intestine.

f. Abdominal tenderness.

Continuous not colicky pain.

Fever.

These are all features of strangulation, which is a complication of adhesive small bowel obstruction, and are an indication for urgent surgery.

CRQ 4

a. Nature of the abdominal pain.

Any alteration in bowel habit.

Any rectal bleeding.

Loss of weight.

Change in exercise tolerance.

Cardiac symptoms.

Ankle swelling.

Any of these answers would score marks. It is critical to determine the characteristics of his abdominal pain (is it colicky, signifying an obstructive component?). The distribution of his pain is in keeping with hindgut disease and it is vital to check for any colorectal symptoms. Tiredness and dyspnoea are symptoms associated with anaemia and it is important to look for any other related symptoms (e.g. cardiac).

b. Carcinoma of the caecum.

Crohn's disease.

Appendix mass.

These are the three most likely causes for a right iliac fossa mass in a male patient. In a woman, gynaecological pathology such as an ovarian cyst should also be considered in the differential diagnosis.

c. Abdominal ultrasound scan.

CT abdominal scan.

These are the key investigations. Of the two, a CT scan would yield the most information and usually would identify any underlying pathology in the colon or small bowel. These tests would also show whether there is any associated liver disease, for example, hepatic metastases.

d. Carcinoma of the ascending colon.

Right hemicolectomy.

An apple-core lesion on a barium enema examination is the cardinal feature of a colon cancer. The most appropriate treatment is a right hemicolectomy. This operation will remove the terminal ileum, caecum, ascending colon and hepatic flexure together with the blood supply (ileocolic and right colic arteries) to the tumour and the draining lymph glands. Continuity of the intestine is restored by joining together the small intestine and the transverse colon.

CRQ 5

a. Colonoscopy.

Barium enema and flexible sigmoidoscopy.

A colonoscopy is the preferred test in a patient with anaemia and rectal bleeding. It provides the opportunity to directly inspect the lining of the large intestine, to obtain biopsies and to undertake a therapeutic procedure such as removal of a polyp (polypectomy). A barium enema will also evaluate the entire colon but offers no opportunity for biopsy or treatment such as polypectomy. A flexible sigmoidoscopy will evaluate at least the rectum and sigmoid colon, which contains at least 70% of the colonic pathology.

Biopsy and polypectomy can also be undertaken. This test is frequently combined with a barium enema examination and is used when resources for colonoscopy are limited.

b. If the polyp is malignant.

If removal is incomplete.

Under either of these circumstances it may be necessary to proceed to a sigmoid colectomy. If the polyp is malignant, removal of the sigmoid colon is the only way to be certain that the sessile polyp has been completely removed along with an adequate margin of surrounding healthy colon. Also, it allows the draining lymph glands, which may also contain cancer, to be removed. Even if the polyp is benign it is sometimes necessary to remove the sigmoid colon completely in order to completely remove a sessile polyp which has a broad base.

c. Anastomotic leakage.

Ureteric injury.

An anastomotic leak is the most serious complication after a sigmoid colectomy. The usual cause is an inadequate blood supply or excessive tension at the anastomosis site. Both are usually a result of poor surgical technique and prevent healing at the site where the two ends of the bowel are joined together (the anastomosis). The sigmoid colon and its blood supply lie close to the left ureter and this vital structure can be damaged or divided during this operation.

d. Regular colonoscopy.

CT liver scan.

This patient should have follow-up colonoscopy at least every 5 years to detect any further polyps or cancers. He should have at least one liver CT scan probably 2 years after surgery to check for any liver metastases.

CRQ 6

a. Gastroscopy.

Barium swallow.

Both tests have their uses. A barium swallow will detect and outline the cause of this patient's dysphagia. Gastroscopy has the added advantage of providing a biopsy for tissue diagnosis and also the opportunity to undertake dilatation in those patients who have a benign oesophageal stricture.

a. Adenocarcinoma.

Carcinoma in the lower third of the oesophagus is usually adenocarcinoma in origin and often arises in a segment of Barrett's oesophagus (see p. 40). The majority of squamous cancers arise in the upper third of the oesophagus. This patient has a long history of reflux disease, which is also associated with Barrett's oesophagus.

b. Chest radiograph.

CT mediastinum, liver.

These investigations will demonstrate whether or not the patient has metastatic disease (lung or liver) and will also help determine the size of the cancer itself.

c. Lung or liver metastases.

Involvement of adjacent vital structures, e.g. heart, trachea, bronchus.

All of the above rule out surgical resection of the tumour. Even if the cancer could be removed itself, it is inappropriate if the patient has liver or lung metastases and cannot be cured. Alternatively a large tumour which invades vital local structures such as the heart or trachea cannot be removed irrespective of the presence or absence of metastases.

d. Oesophageal stent.

Radiotherapy.

As the cancer cannot be removed, the patient's treatment must be aimed at palliating any symptoms such as dysphagia. An endoluminal stent placed either under radiologic or endoscopic control is the best option. Sometimes stenting is combined with radiotherapy.

d. Less than 5% 5-year survival.

Unfortunately, the prognosis in this group of patients is poor.

CRQ 7

a. Ascending cholangitis.

Common bile duct stones.

Rigors, jaundice and right upper quadrant pain are the hallmark of ascending cholangitis and indicate a severe biliary infection coupled with obstruction in the extrahepatic biliary tree (usually the common bile duct). Gallstones are the most common cause of this clinical presentation with one or more stones obstructing the flow of bile in the bile ducts.

b. Evidence of gallstones.

Dilatation of the biliary tree.

The liver function test profile is in keeping with an obstructive jaundice, the alkaline phosphatase level is markedly elevated and the liver transaminases are almost normal. A biliary tract ultrasound scan will detect any dilatation of the biliary tree reflecting the obstruction and will detect any gallstones in the gallbladder. Common bile duct stones are not always detected on this examination.

c. It will confirm the diagnosis.

The obstructing stone can be removed.

ERCP has the advantage of directly outlining the biliary tree with a radiopaque contrast, which is introduced once the ampulla of Vater is cannulated. Bile duct stones or any other pathology causing obstruction will be directly identified. Because it is an invasive test with some serious complications (e.g. pancreatitis, bleeding, perforation of the duodenum) it is not used until there is clear evidence from a non-invasive test, for example ultrasound or CT, that the bile duct is obstructed.

d. Establish intravenous access.

Check the patient's coagulation profile.

Prescribe antibiotic cover for the procedure.

These are the most important steps and are common to many invasive procedures. Intravenous access is important should any drugs need to be administered during the procedure, and provides a route of access should the patient develop a complication and require urgent resuscitation. If bile duct stones are present the sphincter of Oddi is cut open using a special diathermy blade called a sphincterotome. The coagulation profile is checked because of the risk of bleeding. Any coagulopathy must be corrected before the patient undergoes the procedure. Finally, ERCP itself can introduce infection into the biliary tree, and prophylactic antibiotic cover, usually cefuroxime, must be prescribed.

e. Surgical exploration of the common bile duct.

Percutaneous drainage of the obstructed biliary tree.

These are the main two options. In a critically ill patient a percutaneous drainage of the biliary tree may be a lifesaving manoeuvre decompressing the obstructed biliary system and allowing control of the infection before proceeding to a definitive surgical procedure such as exploration of the common bile duct and retrieval of the gallstones causing the blockage.

CRQ 8

a. An epigastric mass.

Supraclavicular lymphadenopathy.

Succussion splash.

Jaundice.

This is a sinister history. The epigastric pain, major weight loss and postprandial vomiting of undigested food point to a gastric outlet obstruction usually caused by a cancer in this age group. Seek evidence of an epigastric mass caused by the cancer, look for supraclavicular lymphadenopathy indicating widespread lymphatic metastases, and check for jaundice caused either by metastatic disease or extrinsic compression of the bile duct by a lymph gland mass. A succussion splash is sometimes heard when the patient's abdomen is rocked from side to side, and is caused by retained foodstuff within the stomach.

b. Gastroscopy.

This is the definitive test; it will directly visualise the cancer and also provides the opportunity for biopsy and a tissue diagnosis. Sometimes the retained foodstuffs will hamper this test and it may be necessary to wash out the stomach with a nasogastric tube before proceeding with the examination.

c. Chest radiograph.

CT abdomen and liver.

Assess general fitness of patient.

A chest radiograph plus an abdominal scan will help detect any metastatic disease in the lungs and liver. A palliative gastric drainage procedure such as a gastroenterostomy may still be appropriate in a patient with metastatic cancer in order to relieve the disabling symptoms of gastric outlet obstruction in a patient with metastatic gastric cancer. Surgery for gastric cancer is quite a major procedure and it is important that the overall fitness of the patient is assessed prior to making the decision to proceed with a major operation in an elderly patient.

d. Distal gastrectomy.

This operation will remove the cancer, its blood supply and the draining lymph glands. The surgical reconstruction after this procedure is illustrated in Figure 6B.

OSCE answers

OSCE 1

a. Achalasia. The proximal oesophagus is dilated and contains food debris. There is a smooth cone-shaped area of narrowing in the distal oesophagus.

b. A gastroscopy would rule out other causes of dysphagia such as carcinoma or a peptic stricture. The diagnosis could be confirmed using oesophageal manometry to demonstrate absent primary peristalsis and a failure of the lower oesophageal sphincter to relax on swallowing.

c. Aspiration pneumonia caused by night-time regurgitation of food debris retained in the oesophagus.

d. In a young, fit patient, a Heller's cardiomyotomy would be the procedure of choice rather than a balloon dilatation.

OSCE 2

a. An endoscopic retrograde cholangiopancreatogram.

b. A stone in the common bile duct.

c. Endoscopic sphincterotomy and balloon or basket extraction of the stone.

d. Complications:
- acute pancreatitis
- bleeding
- duodenal perforation.

OSCE 3

a. This is a featureless 'lead pipe' colon.

b. Ulcerative colitis.

c. Complications:
- toxic dilatation
- perforation
- haemorrhage
- malignant change.

OSCE 4

a. Large bowel obstruction.

b. Sigmoidoscopy (rigid or flexible) plus a gastrograffin enema.

c. Perforation leading to faecal peritonitis.

OSCE 5

a. An ultrasound scan of the gallbladder.

b. A gallstone in the gallbladder.

c. A CT abdominal scan.

Best of 5s answers

1. d. Left hemicolectomy.

This is the operation of choice for any cancer in the left (descending) side of the colon. The extent of the resection ensures that the cancer with an adequate surrounding margin of normal tissue is removed along with its blood supply (arising from the inferior mesenteric artery) and its associated lymph gland drainage.

2. c. *Clostridium difficile.*

Clostridium difficile causes a severe form of antibiotic associated diarrhoea. Clindamycin is a frequent culprit. The characteristic appearances on sigmoidoscopy of a pseudomembrane are caused by a layer of necrotic tissue which lies over the mucosa. In its most severe form the infection may precipitate a toxic dilatation of the colon. Oral metronidazole or vanomycin are the first line of treatment in these patients.

3. d. High-dose oral steroids.

Steroids will usually induce a remission in an acute Crohn's ileitis. However, many patients run a remitting and relapsing course requiring frequent courses of steroids or other immunosuppression (such as azathioprine, methotrexate) which are used when steroids are not well tolerated or are no longer effective. Surgery is often required when patients no longer respond or require a prohibitively high dose of steroids to maintain remission.

4. b. Endoluminal stenting.

It is inappropriate to proceed with a major colonic resection in this patient because he has widespread metastatic liver disease involving both lobes of his liver. An endoluminal stent will relieve his obstruction without the need for a defunctioning stoma and is the best way to palliate his symptoms.

5. e. Restorative proctocolectomy, pouch anal anastomosis.

Any patient with familial polyposis coli has the ability to form polyps and eventually cancers at any point in the colon or rectum. The surgery must be designed to remove all the at-risk areas (i.e. the entire colon and rectum). All the procedures listed apart from the restorative proctocolectomy leave some part of the colon behind and are inadequate. The restorative proctocolectomy is so named because it enables preservation and function of the anus. As a final step in the procedure a pouch is constructed from the small intestine to form a reservoir for the stools. This is connected to the anal canal once the colon and rectum are removed. The operation saves the patient having to live with an ileostomy.

6. a. Colorectum.

Colorectal cancer is the commonest primary site for liver metastases. A search for the primary site is often futile as little can be offered to the majority of these patients who have a primary gastrointestinal cancer but present with symptomatic multiple metastases. Patients with metastatic breast cancer are perhaps an exception. The disease may respond to endocrine manipulation or chemotherapy.

7. b. Balloon tamponade.

These patients can die from exsanguinating haemorrhage. Balloon tamponade is the most effective way to control bleeding when endoscopic therapy fails and will allow resuscitation to catch up with blood loss and coagulopathy. Tamponade alone may be enough to arrest haemorrhage especially when coupled with a further attempt at endosopic therapy. Not infrequently, however, these patients will require more invasive therapy, usually a transhepatic intravascular porto-systemic shunt (TIPS) procedure.

8. c. C-reactive protein 50 mg/l.

This patient's CRP level is less than 150 mg/l. Values which exceed 150 mg/l are in keeping with a severe attack.

9. d. Total abdominal gastrectomy.

This is the procedure of choice and is the only operation listed which will enable removal of the cancer, its blood supply and associated lymph gland drainage. A proximal or distal gastrectomy would not provide adequate tumour clearance. An oesophagogastrectomy would be inappropriate as the oesophagus is not diseased in this patient.

10. a. Gallstone ileus.

Gallstone ileus is usually caused by a gallstone eroding its way through the wall of the gallbladder either into the duodenum or colon. If the stone is large enough it will cause intermittent obstruction as it passes through the small intestine. Some will eventually impact in the terminal ileum and cause a permanent obstruction which requires surgical treatment. A clue to the diagnosis can be obtained from a plain abdominal radiograph. Because there is a false connection between the intestine and the biliary tree the biliary system is often outlined by air in these patients.

Multiple choice answers

1. a. **False.** Barrett's oesophagus is caused by gastro-oesophageal reflux.
   b. **False.** It is a tissue diagnosis usually confirmed by endoscopic biopsy – there may be no evidence on a barium swallow.
   c. **False.** Barrett's oesophagus usually responds to standard antireflux treatment. Surgery is restricted to patients with the complications of Barrett's oesophagus such as a stricture or malignant change.
   d. **True.** Severe dysplasia or in situ carcinoma may develop in an area of Barrett's oesophagitis that does not respond to medical therapy.
   e. **True.** Stricture formation is a complication of long-standing Barrett's oesophagitis.

2. a. **False.** The gastro-oesophageal junction lies in its anatomically correct position; the lower oesophageal sphincter continues to function normally; reflux does not occur.
   b. **True.** This type of hiatus hernia is relatively uncommon.
   c. **False.** This type of hiatus hernia is most easily repaired through the abdomen. The hernia usually contains stomach lined by normal gastric mucosa.
   d. **False.** Barrett's epithelium is an abnormal columnar epithelium lining the lower oesophagus in association with a sliding hiatus hernia.
   e. **True.** Large portions of the stomach can slip into the chest causing acute angulation of the gastric outlet and obstruction.

3. a. **True.** Rupture of the intrathoracic part of the oesophagus may cause a pneumothorax; air enters the pleural space through the oesophageal perforation.
   b. **True.** A mediastinal crunch is caused by the heart beating against air-filled tissues.
   c. **False.** Cervical perforations are usually treated conservatively with antibiotics and fluid restriction, as are many minor perforations of the thoracic oesophagus.
   d. **False.** Perforation following instrumentation is usually a direct result of damage during diagnostic endoscopy or forceful dilatation of an oesophageal stricture.
   e. **False.** Water soluble contrast studies are the best way of identifying the site of perforation.

4. a. **False.** Ulcers are best detected by gastroscopy. Small ulcers and erosions can be missed by barium studies.
   b. **True.** The complications of peptic ulcer disease in order of decreasing frequency are: haemorrhage, perforation and pyloric stenosis.
   c. **True.** Most ulcers will heal by medical means using histamine H_2 receptor blocking drugs or proton pump inhibitors.
   d. **True.** Truncal vagotomy denervates the pylorus and the antral mill. Either a pyloroplasty or a gastroenterostomy is needed to prevent gastric stasis.
   e. **False.** Subdiaphragmatic gas will be absent in at least 10% of patients; if the rest of the history and examination fits, the diagnosis must still be considered.

5. a. **False.** Gastroscopy is the key investigation as it allows direct visualisation of the ulcer plus a biopsy for tissue diagnosis.
   b. **False.** Peptic ulcer and gastric cancer symptoms have a considerable overlap. The diagnosis must be confirmed by gastroscopy and biopsy.
   c. **True.** Histamine H_2 blocking drugs can partly heal malignant ulcers and provide symptomatic relief. This underlines the importance of establishing a firm diagnosis in gastric ulceration before starting treatment.
   d. **True.** A malignant ulcer in the gastric antrum or pyloric ring can cause gastric outlet obstruction.
   e. **False.** Most gastrectomies for gastric cancer are palliative. Overall 5-year survival is around 20%.

6. a. **False**. A succussion splash is pathognomonic of gastric outlet obstruction usually caused by pyloric stenosis.

   b. **False**. Perforation is usually unexpected, with no antecedent history.

   c. **True**. Shoulder tip pain is caused by diaphragmatic irritation from gastric contents released into the peritoneal cavity, which track upwards between the liver and diaphragm.

   d. **False**. Rebound tenderness is unusual. Most patients exhibit a board-like abdominal rigidity caused by spasm of the rectii muscles.

   e. **True**. The severe peritonitis after perforation induces a generalised ileus.

7. a. **False**. Gastric cancer is twice as likely in males as in females.

   b. **False**. Gastric cancer is more common in patients with blood group A. Peptic ulceration has been linked to blood group O patients.

   c. **False**. Blood loss from a gastric ulcer is usually occult. Patients may present with an undiagnosed anaemia.

   d. **True**. Approximately one-half are found in this location.

   e. **True**. These are known as Krukenberg deposits.

8. a. **True**. Although rigors, jaundice and fever are the classical triad of symptoms, septicaemia caused by cholangitis can cause collapse in the elderly and must be considered in the differential diagnosis.

   b. **False**. This is more likely to cause empyema or acute cholecystitis. Cholangitis is caused by a combination of infection and obstruction in the common bile duct.

   c. **True**. Cholangitis caused by common bile duct stones or a stricture can be relieved by ERCP coupled with sphincterotomy and stone extraction or endoscopic stenting techniques.

   d. **False**. The bile duct obstruction must be relieved. Cholecystectomy will cure cholecystitis or other gallbladder-related complications of gallstones.

   e. **False**. Most cases of cholangitis are caused by Gram-negative organisms such as *Escherichia coli* or *Klebsiella* spp.

9. a. **False**. Acalculous cholecystitis can occur in immunocompromised patients or critically ill patients in an intensive care setting. It can also affect patients who have been on prolonged parenteral nutrition.

   b. **False**. Oral cholecystography is completely unreliable in acute cholecystitis as it requires a functioning gallbladder to concentrate and reveal the contrast medium. The diagnosis is confirmed by ultrasound or biliary scintiscanning.

   c. **True**. A pericholecystic abscess is the most common cause of a palpable gallbladder mass.

   d. **False**. The presence of an acutely inflamed gallbladder lying adjacent to the common bile duct is enough to cause cholestasis and jaundice in some patients.

   e. **True**. Diabetic patients are at special risk. They are more likely to develop the complications of acute cholecystitis.

10. a. **False**. Most common duct stones are formed in the gallbladder and migrate to the common bile duct.

    b. **True**. Major elevations in the serum alkaline phosphatase with lesser elevations in the liver transaminases are the hallmark of obstructive jaundice.

    c. **True**. At least 50% of common duct stones are silent.

    d. **False**. A palpable gallbladder is associated with malignant biliary obstruction caused by pancreatic cancer or a primary cholangiocarcinoma. In patients with gallstone disease, the gallbladder is usually shrunken from chronic inflammation.

    e. **True**. 'Gallstone' pancreatitis is one of the most common causes of acute pancreatitis. The other is alcohol abuse.

11. a. **True**. Mesenteric ischaemia causes severe abdominal pain. It can often only be differentiated from acute pancreatitis by laparotomy.

    b. **False**. Acute cholecystitis alone rarely elevates the serum amylase. Gallstone pancreatitis is associated with the passage of a gallstone through the ampulla of Vater.

    c. **True**. Idiopathic pancreatitis accounting for 10% of all episodes is associated with hyperamylasaemia.

    d. **True**. The elevation in amylase is usually small.

    e. **False**. The amylase level is normal. Liver transaminases are massively raised.

12. a. **False**. Necrotising pancreatitis complicates fewer than 10% of all episodes of pancreatitis.

    b. **True**. Mortality rates exceed 30%.

    c. **False**. CT scanning with intravenous contrast enhancement will delineate the necrotic (non-enhancing) from the viable (enhancing) pancreatic tissue.

    d. **True**. Pancreatic debridement (necrosectomy) is sometimes the only treatment option for pancreatic necrosis that becomes secondarily infected.

    e. **False**. Secondary bacterial infection with a mixture of aerobic and anaerobic organisms is common.

13. a. **False**. Cancer of the pancreatic tail is usually inoperable by the time it presents.

    b. **True**. Diabetes often pre-dates pancreatic cancer by several months or years.

    c. **False**. Obstructive jaundice is the most common presenting symptom in pancreatic cancer.

d. **True.** They present early with jaundice and biologically are less aggressive.

e. **True.** Pancreatic and gastric cancer can present with a DVT. The reason is unknown.

14. a. **False.** Gastric fundal varices are difficult to treat endoscopically. Often they can be controlled only by tamponade (using a Sengestaken–Blakemore balloon) or by surgery.

b. **True.** Repeated sclerotherapy induces fibrosis, which can cause an oesophageal stricture.

c. **False.** Vasopressin has to be exogenously infused. It reduces variceal blood flow by decreasing the splanchnic blood flow.

d. **True.** A combination of sclerotherapy followed by tamponade is often effective in stopping variceal bleeding.

e. **True.** Sclerotherapy obliterates varices by thrombosis and fibrosis.

15. a. **False.** The platelet count rises following splenectomy.

b. **False.** Splenectomy is reserved for patients who do not respond to steroid therapy.

c. **True.** The spleen can be conserved following minor injuries.

d. **False.** Delayed rupture of a subcapsular haematoma usually follows 1–2 weeks after the initial injury.

e. **True.** Children and young adults are especially at risk. Pneumococcal vaccine should be given prior to splenectomy followed by a lifelong course of low-dose penicillin V.

16. a. **True.** A small bowel volvulus rotates around the axis of its mesentery, rapidly occluding the mesenteric blood supply and causing strangulation.

b. **False.** Strangulating obstruction can occur at any level of small bowel obstruction. It is perhaps less common in high obstruction.

c. **True.** An incarcerated hernia often has a tight neck that interferes with the blood supply to the trapped small bowel loops.

d. **True.** Constant severe pain is one of the hall-marks of strangulation.

e. **True.** A closed-loop small bowel obstruction rapidly distends. This increase in internal pressure within the loop compromises the blood supply and predisposes to strangulation.

17. a. **False.** Fistulae are common in Crohn's disease and reflect the transmural inflammatory process.

b. **True.** Recurrent perianal sepsis is one of the commonest presentations of Crohn's disease.

c. **True.** Crohn's disease can affect the entire gastrointestinal tract from the mouth to the anus.

d. **False.** Crohn's granulomas are non-caseating. Caseating granulomas are usually tuberculous.

e. **False.** Crohn's disease is an infrequent cause of fulminant colitis, which is usually caused by ulcerative colitis.

18. a. **True.** The radiological features are often non-specific: absent gas shadows or, alternatively, gaseous small bowel distension.

b. **True.** Most patients are arteriopaths. A recent myocardial infarction or a history of atrial fibrillation is common.

c. **False.** The superior mesenteric artery is occluded.

d. **False.** Arterial occlusion is more common than venous infarction.

e. **True.** Many patients are elderly with extensive or total small bowel infarction.

19. a. **False.** An incompetent ileocaecal valve will allow reflux of colonic contents back into the small bowel preventing overdistension of the colon and reducing the risk of perforation.

b. **True.** Pseudo-obstruction, volvulus and constipation are infrequent causes.

c. **False.** Vomiting occurs late, once small bowel obstruction develops secondary to the large bowel obstruction.

d. **True.** The abdomen is usually massively distended and tympanitic with tinkling bowel sounds.

e. **True.** Unless the obstruction is caused by constipation, the rectum is often dilated and empty.

20. a. **True.** The caecum is the second most common site for a colorectal cancer.

b. **False.** The wide female pelvis often facilitates this operation.

c. **False.** Patients with a Dukes grade C tumour have a 30% 5-year survival rate.

d. **False.** Polyps of 1 cm are rarely malignant. Cancer is associated with polyps greater than 2 cm in size.

e. **False.** Right-sided cancers present with anaemia, malaise or a right iliac fossa mass

21. a. **True.** Crohn's disease and colorectal cancer are less frequent causes of a colovesical fistula.

b. **True.** Haemorrhage can be life-threatening and an indication for urgent colectomy.

c. **False.** This operation carries a risk of anastomotic dehiscence especially if there is faecal peritonitis. A Hartmann's resection is the procedure of choice.

d. **True.** However, they should not be assumed to be the source of a patient's symptoms.

e. **False.** Patients with diverticular disease are as likely as any to have a bowel cancer. The two conditions frequently coexist.

22. a. **False.** Skip lesions are a characteristic of Crohn's disease.

b. **False.** Rectal sparing is a feature of Crohn's disease. In ulcerative colitis the rectum is frequently the most diseased segment of the colon.

c. **True.** Crypt abscesses on biopsy are a hallmark of ulcerative colitis.

d. **False.** Inflammatory changes in ulcerative colitis are confined to the mucosa and submucosa. Transmural inflammation typifies Crohn's disease.

e. **True.** This is caused by chronic inflammation and a generalised shortening of the bowel.

23. a. **False.** Radiotherapy is the first-line treatment for anal cancer.

b. **True.** Anal cancers drain to the inguinal lymph glands.

c. **True.** Anal cancer is comparatively rare.

d. **False.** A painful ulcer is a common presentation.

e. **True.** Anal cancers are highly sensitive to irradiation.

24. a. **False.** They are centred in the ischio-rectal fossae below levator ani.

b. **True.** An ischio-rectal abscess is usually multilocular. All loculi must be broken down to provide satisfactory surgical drainage.

c. **False.** Severe perianal tenderness is characteristic of a perianal abscess. An ischio-rectal abscess is deep seated and may only be detected on rectal examination.

d. **False.** Underlying Crohn's disease is more likely.

e. **True.** An undetected fistula at the primary operation is the most common cause of recurrence.

25. a. **False.** Most are acquired by the ingress of hair and faecal matter into the natal cleft caused by movement and friction.

b. **False.** Most pilonidal sinuses are infected. After excision the wounds are best left open to heal by secondary intention.

c. **True.** The condition is particularly common in hirsute men.

d. **False.** Recurrence is not uncommon.

e. **True.** During this period hair growth and sebaceous gland activity increases.

Peripheral vascular surgery

Chapter overview

Arterial disease is common: up to 1 in 10 of all adults have evidence of atherosclerotic peripheral vascular disease. Many of these patients will present with chronic or acute symptoms of arterial insufficiency either to the lower limbs (claudication or critical limb ischaemia) or to the brain (transient ischaemic attack or stroke). Not all will benefit from surgery; careful evaluation of symptoms and the underlying extent of atheromatous disease is essential to provide accurate patient selection. Recent advances have led to alternatives to major vascular reconstruction – thrombolysis, angioplasty and intravascular stent insertion all have a role to play. Some patients will continue to be best served by conservative treatment and others, unfortunately, by amputation.

Venous disease is even more common, and it has been estimated that up to 50% of the population have varicose veins and account for a large number of outpatient referrals to a vascular surgeon. Only a few of these patients require surgery and again careful assessment is essential in order to identify those patients who will benefit from an operation.

This chapter will describe all the common types of arterial and venous disease which present to a vascular surgeon and outlines the principles behind their investigation and treatment.

4.1 Arterial disease

Learning objectives

You should:
- know the risk factors in atherosclerotic disease
- understand how atherosclerosis leads to the symptoms and signs of arterial disease.

Atherosclerosis

Atherosclerotic occlusive disease is common; it affects at least 40% of men over 50 years of age. Currently, 50% of all deaths are caused by circulatory diseases, principally myocardial infarction and stroke. Up to 10% of all adults have evidence of *peripheral* atherosclerotic occlusive disease (PAOD).

Atherosclerosis is a diffuse disease process that affects most blood vessels. In many patients with peripheral atherosclerotic disease, it is often the coexisting cardiac component that causes death.

Epidemiology

The main epidemiological factors are:

- diabetes
- smoking
- hypercholesterolaemia
- hypertension
- family history
- geographic considerations
- hyperhomocysteinaemia.

Patients with multiple risk factors from this list are at a greater risk of developing atherosclerosis than those with a single risk factor.

Pathophysiology

Atherosclerosis is an inflammatory response to the deposition of lipids within an arterial wall. It is commonly found in areas of maximum blood flow turbulence, principally at vessel bifurcations. The following is the most likely sequence of disease progression:

1. fatty streaks or patches
2. intimal lipid deposits
3. superficial fibrosis, overlying the lipid deposit
4. atheromatous plaque formation producing:
   - stenosis/occlusion causing distal ischaemia
   - disruption/ulceration causing acute thrombosis with subsequent distal ischaemia or embolisation.

Symptom patterns

These vary depending upon the region of the body most affected by the disease (for example):

- coronary artery disease leads to a cardiac symptomatology
- lower limb disease causes claudication and limb ischaemia.

The reason why one area of the body should be affected more than another is unknown. There are also interesting local geographic variations, even within the UK. One region may have a very high coronary arterial problem (e.g. West of Scotland) whereas other areas have a relatively higher incidence of lower limb disease (e.g. Tayside, Scotland).

The rate of development of atherosclerosis is also extremely important. Slowly developing disease allows compensating mechanisms to develop (e.g. a collateral arterial supply). This can reduce symptoms to an extent that they are barely noticed. In contrast, acute occlusion of an otherwise relatively healthy artery causes severe symptoms.

4.2 Lower limb arterial disease

Learning objectives

You should:
- know how to diagnose and investigate a patient with symptoms of peripheral vascular disease
- understand the role of conservative and interventional treatment (angioplasty or surgery) in these patients
- be able to recognise a patient with a critical limb ischaemia.

Classification

The Fontaine classification is most widely used:

Fontaine I: asymptomatic lower limb arterial disease
Fontaine IIa: claudication >200 metres
Fontaine IIb: claudication <200 metres
Fontaine III: rest pain
Fontaine IV: ulceration and/or gangrene.

Clinical features

A detailed history and examination paying particular attention to the cardiovascular system is essential. The key points are:

- history of stroke, transient ischaemic attack
- diabetes
- angina, myocardial infarction
- shortness of breath/exercise tolerance
- smoking history
- claudication distance, ability to climb stairs, etc.
- chronic obstructive pulmonary disease (COPD)
- hypertension
- hyperlipidaemia
- drug therapy.

It is important to ascertain how much a patient's symptoms interfere with his/her lifestyle and to gauge the quality of life.

Claudication The most common clinical presentation of PAOD is pain during exercise, a symptom known as claudication. Typically, claudication occurs most often in the calf, but may also involve the thigh or buttocks. Frequently, two or even three muscle regions become symptomatic. The pain is cramp-like, only comes on with exercise and is relieved by rest. It is exacerbated by walking quickly, climbing hills, cold weather and some medica-

tions (e.g. beta blockers). Claudication is an extremely common symptom.

The natural history of claudication is difficult to determine. Approximately 25% will deteriorate with time and up to 10% of patients ultimately develop critical limb ischaemia. Of the remainder, some improve, although many suffer repeated cycles of symptom regression/improvement owing to the stepwise progression of the disease.

Differential diagnosis of intermittent claudication

Most patients with claudication are middle-aged or elderly and often have coexisting degenerative musculoskeletal disease which can mimic claudication. Examples include soft tissue sprains and hip or knee osteoarthritis. The lumbar spine is also a source of leg pain which may be sciatic in nature or, alternatively, a dull calf ache on standing or walking. These symptoms are only relieved by sitting or lying down or by taking the weight off the affected leg. The pain can take up to 30 min to ease (in contrast to claudication) and can be distinguished by taking a careful history.

Physical examination

It is important to evaluate the entire cardiovascular system, not only the peripheral circulation. Listen to the heart, check for arrhythmias; look for signs of right or left heart failure. Measure the blood pressure. Examine for an aneurysm and check for vascular bruits particularly in the abdomen and neck.

Clinical examination of the peripheral vascular system includes careful assessment of femoral and distal pulses together with a search for hair loss, temperature differences, ulceration or any other features of chronic ischaemia.

The detection of iliac and/or femoral bruits is also important. Reduced femoral pulses or bruits indicate aorto-iliac disease.

Although palpation of pulses can be unreliable, it is a widely recognised method of assessment. Pulses can be documented as either present or absent, but it is more useful to grade pulses according to the following system:

- +++ aneurysmal pulse
- ++ normal pulse
- + diminished pulse
- 0 absent pulse.

Unfortunately, most patients with significant claudication have absent distal pulses, and it is often impossible to discriminate between a limb that is not in any particular danger and a 'threatened' limb with critical ischaemia solely on the basis of absent pulses. In general, pulses give an idea of the anatomy of the occlusive disease but not of the severity of ischaemia.

Buerger's test

This test can help identify or confirm critical lower limb ischaemia. The patient lies down on a couch and both legs are elevated as high as possible for at least 30 s. If the circulation to one or both legs is critical because of arterial occlusive disease, the lower limb arterial pressure is insufficient to perform the additional work needing to be done against gravity to drive blood to the feet. A critically isch-aemic leg will become pale. At this point, energy require-ments are met by anaerobic metabolism with lactic acid, which causes vasodilatation of the cutaneous microcircu-lation, produced as a waste product. The patient then sits up and the feet are hung over the side of the couch. Blood now flows into the leg with the assistance of gravity and fills the dilated cutaneous microcirculation resulting in the typical rubor of reactive hyperaemia.

None of these sequential changes take place in a patient with no or non-critical limb ischaemia.

Diagnosis

Routine blood tests All patients with peripheral vas-cular disease should have a full blood count, urea and electrolyte, serum glucose and serum cholesterol assay.

ECG and chest radiograph These investigations should be performed in patients who are to undergo arterio-graphy with a view to intervention, as many will have occult cardiac disease. Also, as these patients are usually heavy smokers there is an increased risk of finding coexisting respiratory disease, especially carcinoma of the bronchus.

Doppler-derived arterial pressure measurements These should always be made to confirm the presence of arterial disease. Usually, they will be performed with the pressure cuff on the thigh, calf and ankle (Figure 36). In some patients (e.g. diabetics) arterial calcification of the vessel media renders the vessels incompressible and causes false 'high' readings. In these patients, toe pressure

measurements may be of value. The sensitivity of pressure measurements may be enhanced by exercising the patient for 1 min on a treadmill and assessing the recovery time following exercise.

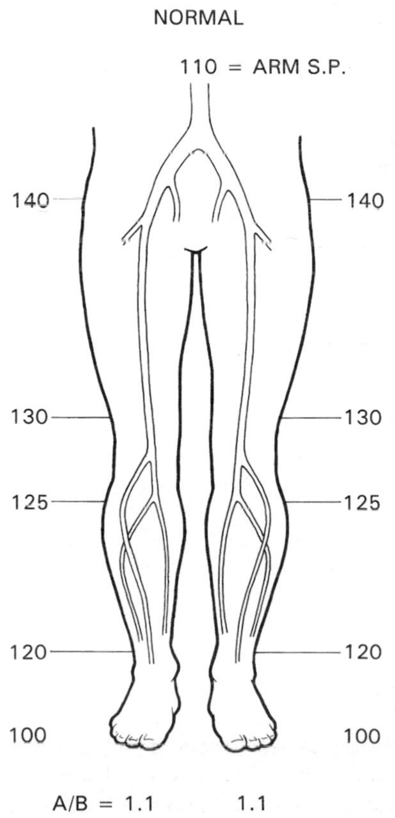

Arteriography This is only used if any form of thera-peutic intervention is being considered. Preliminary colour duplex scans can be used to identify regions of stenosis that might be treated during the initial arteriography. Arte-riography (Figure 37) is usually performed by a retrograde Seldinger technique. This involves passing a catheter per-cutaneously over a guide wire from the common femoral artery up into the aorta. Using this technique, day-case and outpatient angiography is easy to perform and the risk of complications is minimal. Digital subtraction techniques (DSA) are now universal. Intravenous DSA can be used if arterial access is difficult but the images are not as good. Non-invasive duplex scans and magnetic resonance augio-grams (MRA) are useful alternatives/replacements for diagnostic catheter angiography.

Duplex ultrasound scanning

Traditional anatomical ultrasound imaging can be aug-mented by the addition of Doppler information gained from the frequency shift resulting from the reflection of ultrasound off a moving object, in this case the blood-stream. Arterial stenoses can be seen on the anatomical image and the effect of the stenosis on the blood flow is shown by a colour change derived from the Doppler infor-mation. In experienced hands this technique is able to give an accurate description of the distribution of arterial disease, especially in the legs, neck and arms. Although bowel gas makes Duplex ultrasound scanning less useful in the abdomen, the images obtained are often sufficient to plan intervention without the need to resort to invasive imaging.

Magnetic resonance angiography (MRA)

Coils, imaging software and intravenous gadolinium con-trast now combine to produce excellent angiographic images from MR scanners. The technique can allow plan-ning of interventions in all areas of the arterial tree, but care should be taken in the calf in critical ischaemia where the information may not be so accurate. The technique has the advantage of producing images similar to conventional

NORMAL

110 = ARM S.P.

140 — 140

130 — 130

125 — 125

120 — 120

100 — 100

A/B = 1.1   1.1

Figure 36 Doppler-derived arterial pressure measurements in mmHg.

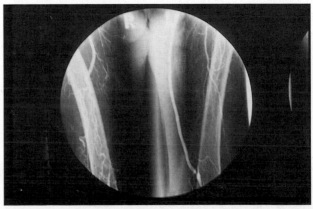

Figure 37 Arteriogram showing right common femoral occlusion.

Four

angiography without the radiation dose, without the need to puncture an artery and with less risk of contrast nephropathy.

Computerised tomographic angiography (CTA)

Newer multislice CT scanners and post-processing allow angiographic style images to be obtained after intravenous contrast. The advantages over conventional angiography are not as great as with MR angiography, however, and the technique is probably most valuable in patients who cannot undergo MR scanning and in whom catheter angiography should be avoided.

Treatment

There are two options:

- conservative management
- intervention by angioplasty or surgery.

Usually the treatment of intermittent claudication is conservative. In every patient the risks of intervention (which, if unsuccessful, may lead to limb loss) must be weighed against the benefits of pursuing a conservative management regime in which the patient learns to live with the symptoms and adapt his or her lifestyle accordingly. Intervention is reserved for critical limb ischaemia or patients whose claudication causes severe lifestyle limitations (e.g. inability to work).

Conservative management. The key points are:

- all patients must be encouraged to stop *smoking*
- optimise medical control of hypertension
- institute cholesterol reduction programmes: a simple modification of dietary intake seems to benefit many patients
- encourage exercise in all patients: a gradual exercise programme will substantially increase a patient's claudication distance over a period of time
- drug treatment using statins, anti-platelet agents, angiotensin-converting enzyme (ACE) inhibitors or folic acid supplements.

Percutaneous transluminal angioplasty Percutaneous transluminal angioplasty (PTA) has revolutionised the management of patients with aorto-iliac disease and some types of superficial femoral artery disease. Localised stenosis or complete occlusion of the common iliac artery or the external iliac artery can be recanalised with excellent immediate results and low risk to the patient. Five-year patency rates exceed 70%. Where disease is limited to the superficial femoral artery, PTA may still be used, although long-term patency rates are not as good as with bypass surgery (see below) and the clinical results may be no better than what can be achieved with a supervised exercise programme.

Technique PTA is usually carried out under local anaesthesia in the radiography suite. An angioplasty catheter is passed percutaneously from the groin over a guide-wire into the narrowed area and a sausage-shaped balloon is placed across the stenosis or occlusion and inflated. In some cases, a metallic stent may be used to maintain luminal integrity after the dilatation. Angioplasty is often performed as a day-case procedure. Afterwards, patients are kept on low-dose aspirin therapy as an anti-platelet agent.

Infra-inguinal bypass surgery This is usually reserved for patients who have critical ischaemia or who have a severely restricted lifestyle. Most infra-inguinal bypasses (Figure 38) are performed under regional anaesthesia. Patency rates at 1 year are between 70% and 80%. There is always a small but finite risk of limb loss if a bypass graft fails, so surgery should not be undertaken lightly. The risks and potential benefits should be carefully explained when informed consent is obtained. Modification of a patient's expectations is often an easier option than surgical intervention.

Aorto-femoral/iliac bypass Where severe aorto-iliac occlusion is present that is not amenable to PTA, aorto-femoral (or iliac) bypass (Figure 39) is an option. Although 5-year graft patency rates of >90% may be obtained, the operative mortality and morbidity with this major surgery are not inconsiderable.

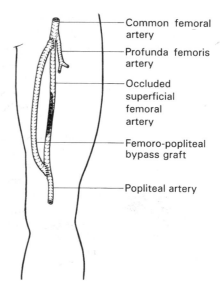

Figure 38 Infra-inguinal bypass.

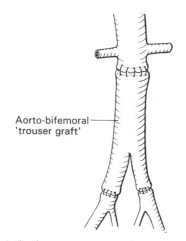

Figure 39 Aorto-iliac bypass.

Prognosis

Up to one-third of all claudicants will die within 5 years of diagnosis, principally from coincidental cardiac disease.

Critical limb ischaemia (CLI)

Critical limb ischaemia (CLI) can be defined as a limb with rest pain of at least 2 weeks' duration or tissue loss caused by arterial disease. The ankle systolic pressure is less than 50 mmHg or the toe pressure is less than 30 mmHg when measured using Doppler techniques. Without intervention these limbs will be lost.

Clinical features

These patients present with:

- rest pain
- gangrene
- ulceration
- a combination of these symptoms.

Rest pain This means pain that affects the toes and/or forefoot and is worse when the patient lies horizontally. In this position, the net perfusion pressure to the foot is significantly decreased. Rest pain is worse at night and, in severe cases, patients will sleep upright to avoid discomfort. Rest pain is relieved by standing up and taking a few steps around the bed. Eventually, secondary orthostatic oedema sets in and perfusion is further compromised. Rest pain may be relieved by cooling the foot to reduce metabolic requirements.

Gangrene Gangrene means tissue necrosis caused by an inadequate blood supply. Usually this is *dry* and affects the most distal extremities (the toes) first. *Wet* gangrene develops if infection supervenes. Wet gangrene spreads rapidly and leads to a severely compromised limb, systemic sepsis and death if there is no intervention. Such a sequence of events is more likely to occur in a diabetic patient.

Ulceration The following factors predispose to ulceration:

- neuropathy (e.g. diabetes)
- poor nutrition
- severe ischaemia
- prolonged bed rest
- infection
- trauma.

Ulceration is most commonly seen over pressure areas such as the heel, tips of the toes and the first metatarsal head. Although the intact foot may withstand markedly reduced skin perfusion, an ulcerated lesion requires a greatly enhanced blood flow to heal; therefore, many ulcers fail to heal where critical ischaemia exists.

Assessment of critical ischaemia

This can be difficult because distal pulses will invariably be absent and it can be hard to tell which limbs are critically ischaemic and warrant urgent investigation and treatment in contrast to those limbs that have chronic *sub*critical ischaemia, which requires less urgent management. The length of history and speed of progression of symptoms are of value in assessing critical ischaemia. A short history with rapid progression indicates limb-threatening disease. Muscle tenderness in acute limb ischaemia (ALI) suggests muscle necrosis and the limb may be non-viable. Fixed mottling of the skin (i.e. mottling which does not blanch on pressure) also suggests non-viability.

Femoral pulses Palpation of the femoral pulses is essential and will indicate whether there is aorto-iliac disease, which in turn often determines subsequent management. Treatment of aorto-iliac disease alone may sufficiently improve the inflow of blood to the limb so that it is no longer critically ischaemic.

Investigations Doppler pressure measurements and urgent angiography are carried out. The foot vessels should be visualised by either DSA or duplex imaging. Non-visualisation of these vessels on angiography does not always mean they are absent, but the outcome after surgery is likely to be much worse.

Treatment

This depends upon the fitness of the patient, surgical expertise and the availability of an autologous vein from the patient that can be used as a bypass graft.

The treatment options for patients with established critical limb ischaemia are:

- conservative (i.e. analgesia and general supportive measures) (10%)
- primary amputation (10%)
- angioplasty (10%)
- surgical revascularisation (65–70%).

All patients require vigorous treatment of any coexisting medical disorders. In many cases, improving the cardiac output alone will produce a sufficient increase in peripheral perfusion to abolish rest pain. However, when ulceration or gangrene is present, it is nearly always necessary to improve the blood supply with either angioplasty or surgery.

Acute limb ischaemia

Acute limb ischaemia may be either acute or 'acute-on-chronic'. More commonly acute ischaemia is caused by thrombosis at the site of underlying disease. Patients with a good collateral blood supply will have a less severe ischaemic insult. The most frequent causes are:

- embolism (look for evidence of atrial fibrillation, recent cardiac infarct, proximal arterial disease, aortic aneurysm)
- acute-on-chronic thrombosis (underlying PAOD), which may have a good collateral circulation
- thrombosis of a peripheral aneurysm (e.g. a popliteal aneurysm)
- thrombosis of a previous bypass graft (e.g. femoro-popliteal bypass)
- trauma (direct or indirect)
- intra-arterial injection (e.g. drug abusers) causing embolisation into healthy vessels.

Clinical features

Classically, an acutely ischaemic limb presents abruptly with severe distal ischaemia characterised by the 'six Ps', although not all will necessarily be present:

Pain: constant and with muscle tenderness.
Pulseless.
Pallor: white limb which eventually mottles suggesting irreversible ischaemia.
Paraesthesia: indicates inadequate circulation for survival. The term 'paraesthesia' encompasses altered/reduced/absent sensation.
Paralysis: a late sign that suggests underlying muscle necrosis; some limbs with foot drop alone can be salvaged if revascularisation is promptly carried out. Paralysis may also arise from severe nerve ischaemia before muscle necrosis occurs.
Perishing cold: the acutely ischaemic limb is extremely cold when compared with the other side.

Acute or chronic ischaemia usually presents with varying degrees of the 'six Ps'; some or all will be present depending on the degree of ischaemia. Survival of the limb at presentation may depend on the existence of good colateral vessels supplying enough blood to preserve the leg.

Treatment

Most of these patients are extremely ill. However, active intervention is usually justified. The first-line *management* is:

- adequate parenteral analgesia
- full anticoagulation with heparin or low molecular weight heparin if immediate treatment is not planned
- optimise cardiovascular status.

If the ischaemia is present for longer than 24 h, consideration should be given to primary amputation.

If revascularisation appears possible, this should be achieved by:

- thrombolysis
- embolectomy/bypass/PTA
- a combination of these methods.

Thrombolysis This technique is ideal as it allows targeted treatment to the underlying lesion and overlying thrombosis by:

- initial visualisation of the disease by angiography
- lysis of the clot
- angioplasty, if necessary.

Lysis is best achieved using recombinant tissue plasminogen activator or streptokinase infused via an intra-arterial catheter directly into the clot and the affected artery. If the artery remains blocked after 12 h of treatment, surgical intervention may be required. Close cooperation between surgeon and radiologist is essential.

Surgery Surgery for limb salvage is a major undertaking. Often an operation that sets out to be a simple 'embolectomy' will fail and only a distal bypass procedure (e.g. a bypass from the femoral artery to the posterior tibial artery) will save the limb. The surgeon must be able and willing to undertake this technically demanding procedure from the outset should embolectomy be unsuccessful. True emboli are less common; many suspected emboli turn out to be an acute or chronic arterial thrombosis.

Anaesthesia Local anaesthesia is rarely suitable for these procedures, which should be undertaken under regional anaesthesia. If revascularisation is successful, the affected limb may swell acutely (the postoperative compartment syndrome). For this reason, decompression fasciotomies may be required at the time of the original operation to prevent this complication, which can endanger a satisfactorily revascularised limb.

Reperfusion syndrome The greatest danger to these patients after successful revascularisation is the 'reperfusion syndrome'. This is caused by the release of toxic metabolites and oxygen free radicals into the systemic circulation from the ischaemic limb. This can cause a profound cardiovascular collapse with renal and sometimes respiratory failure. For this reason revascularisation should not be used in patients with signs of muscle necrosis – primary amputation is better.

Prognosis

The duration of limb ischaemia is crucial to the final outcome. If it is less than 6 to 8 h, a good result can be expected. Any longer and the limb may suffer irreversible damage. Up to 25% of patients with an acutely ischaemic leg will die without leaving hospital. Of the remainder, up to 20% will require a major amputation.

Amputation

Incidence

PAOD and/or diabetes is the cause of >90% of major limb amputations in Western Europe. In the UK, between 5000 and 7000 major limb amputations are performed annually. Up to 40% of amputees die within 2 years of amputation and a further 30% may develop critical ischaemia in the remaining limb that requires either a second amputation or limb salvage surgery.

Indications

Although unsuccessful revascularisation procedures carry a high perioperative morbidity, primary amputation should only be offered when revascularisation is considered inappropriate; for example:

- in bedridden patients
- in a functionally useless limb
- in patients with life-threatening sepsis
- where revascularisation is technically impossible.
- where there is extensive muscle necrosis.

Calf tenderness, a raised CK and a prolonged, profound paralysis or sensory loss may also dictate primary amputation.

Amputation may also have to be considered if revascularisation fails leaving a patient with:

- gangrene/necrosis of part of a limb
- severe ulceration
- rest pain
- a combination of these features.

Investigations

Most patients considered for amputation should have already had an arteriogram and have been seen by a vascular surgeon with consideration given to salvaging the limb.

Major amputations Above knee amputation (AKA) or 'transfemoral amputation' is associated with a much poorer outcome. Although more likely to heal, rehabilitation is less successful. These patients are often more unwell than those needing a below knee amputation (BKA). After a below knee or 'transtibial amputation', up to 80% of patients become independently mobile because the knee joint is preserved and also because a lighter prosthesis is used.

Minor amputations Toe and transmetatarsal resections are rarely possible in the presence of critical ischaemia without first revascularising the limb. Some diabetic patients with little arterial disease develop neuropathies or osteomyelitis. Minor amputation or debridement may be successful.

Treatment

Patients who require amputation are usually elderly, have end-stage peripheral vascular disease and frequently have life-threatening coexistent medical conditions. The key points in their *management* are:

- a careful preoperative cardiovascular renal and pulmonary evaluation
- amputation under regional anaesthesia
- antibiotic prophylaxis
- aggressive treatment of any established infection
- adequate analgesia.

Early fitting of a temporary prosthesis and early mobilisation in an acute rehabilitation unit (with the aid of occupational therapists and physiotherapists) will maximise the chance of a successful independent return to the community.

Prognosis

Emergency amputation carries a mortality of up to 50% because of severe sepsis and the effects of tissue necrosis.

4.3 Cerebrovascular disease

Learning objectives

You should:
- know what can cause a stroke
- understand the role of carotid endarterectomy in cerebrovascular disease.

Epidemiology

Stroke (a cerebrovascular accident or CVA) is the third most common cause of death in Western society and causes an enormous financial and sociological burden to the community. Currently, strokes are becoming less common because of dietary improvements and better control of systemic hypertension.

Up to 25% of patients will die following their first stroke. Of the remainder:

- one-third recover fully
- one-third have a non-disabling deficit
- one-third require permanent support.

Of these survivors, one-third will have a second CVA within 5 years and almost one-half will die from myocardial ischaemia during the same period.

Aetiology

There are three major causes for CVAs:

- small vessel intracerebral disease (arteriosclerosis) usually secondary to hypertension (50%)
- extracranial cerebrovascular cause (30%): of this group, the vast majority have carotid bifurcation disease
- haemorrhage (20%), either subarachnoid or intracerebral.

The major risk factors for CVA are:

- hypertension
- smoking
- hyperlipidaemia
- diabetes.

A combination of these risk factors places an individual at a much greater risk of having a stroke than any single factor.

Pathophysiology

Carotid disease causes CVAs mainly by acting as a source for distal emboli (Figure 40), which occlude the cerebral circulation. The brain can tolerate slowly progressive carotid disease remarkably well and sometimes both the internal carotid and the vertebral arteries can be completely occluded with minimal symptoms! In contrast, acute occlusion or embolisation to an important area (e.g. speech) can be devastating. Major carotid stenoses are associated with compound haemorrhagic plaques and intimal disruption and, hence, an increased risk of embolisation.

Clinical features

Cerebrovascular disease can present in several different ways:

Asymptomatic carotid artery stenosis Usually detected by eliciting a carotid bruit in an otherwise asymptomatic patient. Frequently these bruits are caused by external carotid artery disease.

Amaurosis fugax A transient monocular loss of vision, often described as 'a veil' coming down across the eye. Acute permanent loss of vision in one eye is caused by occlusion of the central retinal artery or a retinal vein thrombosis. Eye signs are a frequent finding in cerebrovascular disease because the ophthalmic artery is the first branch of the internal carotid artery.

Transient ischaemic attacks (TIAs) These are defined as focal neurological symptoms in which the motor and/or sensory deficit lasts less than 24 h. Although there are other causes of TIAs, embolisation from the carotid

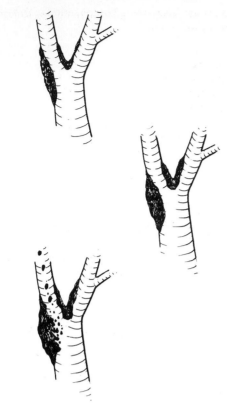

Figure 40 Carotid plaque causing stenosis and giving rise to distal emboli.

bifurcation is of the greatest importance because it can be effectively treated.

Stroke This is the first symptom for many patients with cerebrovascular disease, although close questioning will often elicit preceding symptoms.

Dizziness, vertigo and fainting These are very poor indicators of cerebrovascular disease and only a few patients with these non-localising symptoms will have significant carotid artery disease.

Diagnosis

A careful case history and physical examination is the key step in evaluating patients who have had symptoms or signs of a cerebral insult. Only patients who appear to have carotid disease should be subject to further carotid investigation.

All patients with suspected carotid disease should have their blood pressure and cardiac status evaluated fully and treated.

Duplex scanning is the key diagnostic test. The technique combines B-mode ultrasound with pulsed Doppler wave-form analysis and has almost replaced the need for carotid angiography even when surgery is contemplated. Duplex scanning enables an accurate evaluation of the degree of stenosis and plaque morphology. The method is cheap, non-invasive and easily repeatable.

Treatment

The form of treatment depends on the results of these investigations. The aim of surgery is prophylaxis, i.e. to prevent a stroke. Unless contraindicated, all patients should receive aspirin.

1. Patients with a symptomatic stenotic lesion of over 70% should undergo carotid endarterectomy if their life expectancy is more than 1 year.
2. Surgery should not be undertaken for stenoses of less than 70%.
3. Carotid enarterectomy is of less benefit in patients with asymptomatic disease and is only appropriate in a few carefully selected cases.

Prognosis

The major causes of death in these patients are a catastrophic cardiac event and a perioperative stroke. Patients at highest risk are those with previous CVAs or severe contralateral carotid disease. However, it is this group of patients who are most likely to benefit from surgery.

4.4 Aneurysms

> **Learning objectives**
>
> You should:
> - be able to recognise a patient with an abdominal aortic aneurysm
> - understand the principles of treatment in a patient with an abdominal aortic aneurysm.

An aneurysm is a localised or a diffuse dilatation of an artery. There are two types of aneurysm:

- true aneurysm, in which the wall is made up of diseased arterial tissue
- false (or pseudo-) aneurysm, in which the wall is made up partly of artery and partly of compressed surrounding tissue. These are usually the result of arterial trauma, angiography or surgery.

Aneurysmal disease is associated with peripheral vascular disease, hypertension, advancing age and smoking. It is not clear why some patients develop occlusive vascular disease while others develop aneurysmal disease.

Abdominal aneurysms

Abdominal aortic aneurysms (AAAs) (Figure 41) are frequent and invariably fatal if untreated after rupture. Aneurysms account for 1–2% of male deaths in Western Europe and are five times more common in men than in women. Up to 10% of all patients with peripheral vascular disease will have a detectable AAA. Some will also have a peripheral aneurysm.

The natural history is unpredictable: some gradually increase in size over a number of years; some expand in a stepwise fashion; others remain static.

Clinical features

Most AAAs present either as an asymptomatic finding on routine examination (a pulsatile abdominal mass) or as an acute rupture causing collapse and hypotension. In a thin

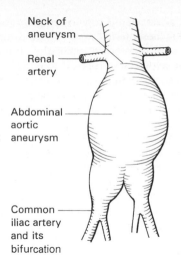

Neck of
aneurysm

Renal
artery

Abdominal
aortic
aneurysm

Common
iliac artery
and its
bifurcation

Figure 41 Aortic aneurysm.

patient a normal-sized aorta may be felt and an ultrasound (see below) may be necessary to differentiate this from an aneurysm. Other symptoms include distal embolisation by clot originating from the aortic sac and non-specific abdominal and/or loin pain and backache.

The majority of patients with AAAs >5 cm will have a palpable abdominal mass in the epigastrium that is pulsatile; in some obese patients, even very large AAAs may be impossible to detect.

Over 95% of AAAs arise from below the renal arteries. Aneurysms that extend above the renal arteries are more difficult to repair and there is an increased morbidity.

Diagnosis

Ultrasound is the simplest definitive test. It allows accurate sizing of the aneurysm although the proximal extent is usually poorly visualised. A CT scan may provide important preoperative information about the neck of the aneurysm in relation to the renal arteries. Also, in stable patients with backache a CT scan may confirm if a leak has taken place.

Treatment

Symptomatic aneurysms of any size require urgent or emergency surgery. Rupture is much more common if the antero-posterior diameter of the AAA is greater than 5.5 cm. Surgery should be offered for all *asymptomatic* patients with an AAA of more than 5.5 cm who are fit enough to withstand major surgery. Aneurysms less than 5.5 cm should be kept under surveillance using ultrasound scanning.

The operation involves replacing the aneurysmal segment of the aorta with a straight tube prosthetic graft or a bifurcated ('trouser') graft if the iliac vessels are involved in the aneurysm. Endovascular aneurysm repair (EVAR), using percutaneous techniques, is less invasive and is currently under evaluation. In a fit patient, EVAR appears to be as good as open repair in the medium term with a lower operative mortality. If a patient is unfit for open repair then EVAR does not prolong life and efforts should be directed, where possible, to make the patient fitter for surgery.

Complications The main complications after aneurysm surgery are:

- early
  - haemorrhage
  - myocardial infarction
  - renal failure
  - distal embolisation
- late
  - colonic ischaemia
  - graft infection
  - chest infection
  - limb ischaemia.

Prognosis

The mortality rate from elective surgery varies from 2% to 10%, depending upon the selection criteria: older patients with larger aneurysms are at higher risk of perioperative death, especially if they have coexistent cardiac disease. The mortality rate increases dramatically after rupture to 30–80%.

After successful AAA surgery, most patients return to a normal lifestyle and a near normal life expectancy.

Peripheral aneurysms

These are often multiple. The more common sites for peripheral aneurysms are:

- popliteal: often bilateral, sometimes associated with an aortic aneurysm
- femoral: often a pseudo-aneurysm
- iliac: isolated iliac aneurysms are uncommon, they are often associated with an aortic aneurysm
- carotid: rare
- splenic: associated with pregnancy; best treated by therapeutic embolisation
- renal: relatively benign.

If any single aneurysm is identified, a careful search should be undertaken to ensure that another potentially more serious aneurysm does not coexist.

Popliteal aneurysms These are the most frequent type of peripheral aneurysm and most should be repaired if greater than 2 cm in size. Untreated they may thrombose or embolise causing acute limb ischaemia. Occasionally they will rupture. Simple ligation and bypass is all that is required.

Femoral aneurysms True femoral aneurysms are uncommon and most are secondary to previous vascular surgery. Repair can be difficult as an underlying graft infection may be the cause.

4.5 Other peripheral arterial diseases

Learning objectives

You should:
- always remember mesenteric vascular disease as a cause of abdominal pain.

Four

Visceral artery vascular disease

Renal artery atherosclerosis

This is usually asymptomatic. Occasionally it causes hypertension or renal failure. These patients are usually high-risk surgical candidates and are frequently unsuitable for surgery. The diagnosis is often made as part of a work-up for other vascular disease.

The treatment options are:

- angioplasty
- bypass grafting
- endarterectomy.

Although the renal failure often responds to treatment, the hypertension frequently persists.

Mesenteric arterial vascular disease

Although quite common, this diagnosis is often made too late, either at laparotomy or at postmortem examination. Acute mesenteric ischaemia may result from:

- embolus
- acute-on-chronic arterial thrombosis.

Clinical features

In an acute case, the abdominal findings are often minimal but pain is severe. The presence of significant arterial disease elsewhere (e.g. the legs) is a clue. Weight loss may be marked in acute-on-chronic cases and is often erroneously attributed to malignancy. *Chronic* mesenteric ischaemia (abdominal angina) is much less common. It is characterised by:

- weight loss
- postprandial pain
- evidence of generalised peripheral vascular disease
- obvious abdominal bruits on auscultation.

Many of these patients will have had long-standing undiagnosed abdominal pain and have been investigated extensively without a diagnosis.

Diagnosis

The definitive diagnosis is made by:

- mesenteric angiography
- laparoscopy
- laparotomy.

In acute mesenteric ischaemia, a high degree of clinical suspicion is required in order to clinch the diagnosis in time to save the patient. Any delay in reaching the diagnosis may mean that bowel necrosis will supervene and the patient will become inoperable. In acute cases with an embolus, the opportunity for intervention is only a few hours.

In chronic disease, there is sufficient time for mesenteric angiography to be performed. In these cases usually at least two of the three main visceral arteries (coeliac, superior and inferior mesenteric arteries) are occluded.

Treatment

Management must be aimed at revascularisation with or without resection of any non-viable small bowel. In most cases this is achieved by constructing an aortocoeliac or aorto-superior mesenteric artery bypass using either vein or a synthetic graft. Very occasionally, an embolectomy will be possible. Often, a 'second look' laparotomy after 24 h will be necessary to ensure the bowel remains viable. A small bowel resection alone is rarely enough to ensure a patient's survival.

Uncommon causes of mesenteric ischaemia

Non-occlusive mesenteric infarction This can develop in patients who have cardiac low output syndrome (e.g. hypovolaemia, cardiogenic shock, sepsis). There is usually extensive patchy necrosis of the entire gut and no evidence of mesenteric insufficiency on an arteriogram. Treatment is directed toward correcting the underlying problem.

Mesenteric venous thrombosis This condition presents in a similar way and in the same group of patients. Full heparinisation is the cornerstone of treatment. Outcome depends upon the extent of the venous thrombosis and the amount of secondary arterial infarction.

Thoracic outlet syndrome

This is a group of symptoms linked together because of a common aetiology: compression at the thoracic outlet.

Most present with neurological signs and symptoms of the upper arm while 1 in 10 have symptoms secondary to compression of the subclavian artery or vein. A cervical rib is the most common cause of these symptoms although, in some patients without a cervical rib, adhesions resulting from fibrous scalene muscle bands may be responsible.

Clinical features

Symptoms reflect the principal nerve root(s) involved from C8 to T1. Complaints include:

- pain in the shoulder or arm
- tingling down a dermatome
- weakness in a muscle group
- loss of fine movement in a hand.

Occasionally, where the artery is compressed, upper arm claudication may occur or, very rarely, a stenosed segment may give rise to distal emboli.

Diagnosis

History and examination are crucial steps to the diagnosis, as there is no definitive test to confirm that where a cervical rib exists *it is responsible* for the symptoms. Exclusion of local nerve compression problems such as carpal tunnel syndrome or ulnar nerve compression is important. The presence of cervical spondylosis would suggest that this may be the most likely cause for symptoms. Nerve conduction studies may help clinch the diagnosis of a neurological thoracic outlet syndrome.

Treatment

Conservative treatment Conservative measures should be tried first. A supervised exercise programme is used to improve posture and shoulder girdle movements. Where a neurological deficit is already present, treatment is urgent and is aimed at avoiding further deterioration.

Surgical treatment Where pain is excessive or every-day activity limited, surgical correction may be required. The cervical rib is excised, often together with a first rib resection, by either a transaxillary or a supraclavicular approach. The results of surgical decompression can dramatically benefit this group of patients. Overall, some patients derive less benefit than others from thoracic outlet decompression. Careful case selection is the key to getting good results.

Arteriovenous malformations

These are a spectrum of disorders in which there are abnormal connections between the venous and arterial systems. The classification is complex and depends upon their histopathology and the nature of their development. Almost all are congenital, although many lie dormant for long periods. Some are soft with predominantly venous elements. Others, comprising mainly arterial elements, are almost aneurysmal. Invariably they are all far more extensive than apparent clinically and their management and treatment is highly specialised.

Clinical features
The lesions are usually:

- warm
- pulsatile
- compressible
- painless.

Some are slow growing and never become a significant problem to the patient: these can be safely left alone. Others will have spurts of growth (typically at adolescence and during pregnancy) but may otherwise be dormant. Others have an aggressive course with gross enlargement and involvement of a major part of the body.

Complications These include:

- development of high output cardiac failure
- limb hypertrophy and distortion
- skin necrosis
- major bleeding.

Diagnosis
These malformations are usually confirmed by arteriography and MRI.

Treatment
The treatment has changed dramatically over the last 10 years as our understanding of these lesions has improved. Excision should rarely be performed unless for a limb-threatening or life-threatening complication. Likewise, ligation of a 'feeder' artery not only is of little value but also destroys a route of access for therapeutic embolisation, which has become the mainstay of treatment. Embolisation is carried out usually in stages and can be repeated if regrowth occurs.

Raynaud's disease and Raynaud's phenomenon

Raynaud's 'disease' was originally described as signs and symptoms caused by an oversensitivity to the sympathetic nervous drive. The exact pathophysiology of the disorder is still uncertain.

The term 'Raynaud's disease' has been superseded by the classification of this syndrome into primary and secondary Raynaud's phenomenon.

Primary Raynaud's phenomenon
This is an episodic, vasospastic disorder of the extremities causing hypersensitivity of the hands and feet to cold and stressful stimuli. Attacks are irregular and unpredictable and are characterised by digital blanching followed by cyanosis and reactive hyperaemia as the vasospasm abates. This rewarming is accompanied by quite severe pain in the affected digits. The whole attack generally lasts less than 30 min. The symptoms are usually bilateral and patterns of digital involvement are symmetrical. Primary Raynaud's phenomenon is extremely common and affects up to 5% of young women. It is a self-limiting benign condition and probably never leads to digital necrosis or ulceration. A few of these patients will, in time, be shown to have secondary Raynaud's phenomenon.

Treatment
Management for primary Raynaud's phenomenon is supportive, such as heated gloves and socks. Nifedipine (a calcium channel blocker that relaxes vascular smooth muscle) is used to provide maintenance therapy, with increased doses for acute exacerbations.

Secondary Raynaud's phenomenon
This is more serious and implies an underlying pathology, usually a collagen vascular disease (vasculitis). Common causes are:

- scleroderma
- rheumatoid arthritis
- systemic lupus
- vibration white finger (prolonged use of vibrating tools, e.g. road drills)
- atherosclerosis
- malignancy.

Treatment
The management of secondary Raynaud's phenomenon is directed at treating the underlying pathology, when known. Severe exacerbations require hospitalisation, especially during the winter months, in order to treat digital ulceration and/or necrosis. Intravenous prostacycline relieves the symptoms in some of these patients, who sustain a benefit of up to several months with just one infusion course.

Acrocyanosis
This is one form of the spectrum of vasospastic disorders in which there is a more constant cyanotic element to the extremity. This is quite common in young patients. Treatment is as for Raynaud's.

Erythromyalgia
This is another sympathetic nerve disorder, in which the prevailing symptom is a burning (painful) extremity that is hyperaemic.

Vibration white finger syndrome

This is caused by protracted exposure and sensitivity to many types of vibration tool, as used in industry. Establishing this diagnosis is important because morphological changes in the arterioles and nerves will eventually supervene, with long-standing symptoms. It is recognised as an occupational disease and attracts many claims for compensation.

4.6 Venous disease

Learning objectives

You should:
- know how to assess a patient with varicose veins
- understand the role of conservative and operative management in these patients
- be able to recognise a patient with deep venous insufficiency.

Varicose veins

Primary varicose veins and deep venous insufficiency are the main venous diseases that present to the surgeon. Varicose veins are common and affect up to half the population at some time during their life. Curiously, varicose veins are almost non-existent in many non-Western countries.

Varicose veins can be classified as primary (idiopathic) or secondary.

Secondary varicose veins are a consequence of deep venous insufficiency. In order to understand the management of venous disease, it is important to have a working knowledge of the anatomy, physiology and pathophysiology of the venous system.

Anatomy and pathophysiology

There are two venous systems in the leg:

- superficial veins that drain the skin and subcutaneous tissue; the long and short saphenous veins are the major vessels
- deep veins that drain the muscles of the leg.

Both systems are connected by numerous perforating veins, which normally have competent valves that allow blood to flow from the superficial to the deep systems only. Normally, the superficial system drains into the deep system at the sapheno-femoral junction (long saphenous vein) and at the sapheno-popliteal junction (short saphenous vein).

Sustained high venous pressure in the superficial veins is prevented by:

- the muscle pump effect (when walking), which squeezes blood from the distal venous system proximally
- deep vein valves and perforator vein valves, which prevent retrograde flow into the superficial venous system.

Together, these mechanisms facilitate flow from the superficial venous system into the deep venous system. Failure of either the perforator valves or the deep venous valves allows blood to flow back into the superficial system and will cause a high superficial venous pressure.

Deep venous insufficiency develops when the deep valves are incompetent. This creates a constant high deep venous pressure, known as ambulatory venous hypertension.

Clinical features

Cosmetic problems, aching, discomfort and a sensation of heaviness of the legs on standing are the main complaints. Severe pain is not usually a symptom unless there is evidence of superficial phlebitis. Four out of five of all patients are women.

Careful assessment of all patients with 'primary' varicose veins is extremely important. Any history suggestive of a previous deep venous thrombosis (DVT) should be elicited. Evidence of possible underlying deep venous insufficiency should be sought, e.g. leg swelling (especially if it is unilateral), haemosiderin staining of the skin and a history of previous or current leg ulceration. If there is any doubt, a more detailed investigation with a duplex ultrasound scan, photoplethysmography and/or venography may also be needed.

Physical examination should identify sapheno-femoral reflux either using a finger to palpate a thrill or using a hand-held Doppler probe to detect reflux in the groin and popliteal regions.

Investigations

Trendelenburg test Finger tip or tourniquet control of the sapheno-femoral junction can be used to demonstrate sapheno-femoral incompetence.

Photoplethysmography This can be used to assess venous refilling time after mild exercise. This non-invasive technique correlates well with direct venous pressure measurements. Application of superficial tourniquets and repetition of this test may identify whether the deep or superficial system is contributing most to the venous refilling.

Treatment

There are four treatment options for primary varicose veins:

- reassurance
- compression stockings
- injection sclerotherapy
- surgery.

Reassurance Conservative management with or without support stockings is often possible once patients with minor varicosities realise there is no absolute need for treatment.

Compression stockings These are specially manufactured stockings that provide graduated compression from the foot to the thigh and should be worn during periods of prolonged standing; because they lose their elasticity, they should be renewed at least every 6 months.

Sclerotherapy The original concept was to inject sclerosant at sites of perforator incompetence. However, accurate identification of these sites is often difficult. The benefit of treatment mainly relates to the obliteration of superficial varicosities. Sclerotherapy is performed on an outpatient basis and may require multiple courses of injections. The technique is useful for minor below knee varicosities and residual varicosities after surgery but not for major varicosities. There is a risk of damage to the deep veins by the highly irritant sclerosant, which may cause permanent deep venous insufficiency, skin staining and ulceration.

Surgical treatment Surgery for primary varicose veins involves three steps:

1. sapheno-femoral ligation
2. above knee saphenous stripping
3. multiple avulsion of varicosities.

With meticulous surgery, the results are excellent (less than 5% recurrence rates). If the primary treatment is inadequate, recurrence rates may be over 20%. Surgery is best performed under regional anaesthesia and can be performed on a day-case basis. After surgery, patients are advised to wear support stockings for 3 to 6 weeks to minimise bruising and maximise comfort.

Newer treatment modalities for varicose veins

Less invasive treatments for varicose veins than conventional surgery are now being evaluated. These essentially involve percutaneous ablation of the lumen of the long saphenous vein from the groin to the knee. This can be achieved by inserting a suitable catheter into the vein at the knee and passing it up to the groin. Heat is then produced at the catheter tip either by a radiofrequency generator or by a laser, and the catheter is slowly withdrawn along the length of the long saphenous vein in the thigh. The heat ablates the lumen, so mimicking a sapheno-femoral ligation and stripping. As a result, the calf varicose veins get smaller as they are not subject to such a high pressure.

An alternative technique involves the injection of sclerosant liquid in the form of a foam into the saphenous vein. The foam is prevented from entering the deep system in the groin by ultrasound-guided direct pressure on the sapheno-femoral junction. An advantage of this technique is that individual varicosities can also be ablated by separate injections of sclerosant.

All these techniques are currently being compared to conventional surgery in terms of their efficacy, longevity of results and side effects.

Complications

These are uncommon. Leg ulceration is rarely the sequel to primary varicose veins. Superficial thrombophlebitis is more common with severe varicosities and may be mistaken for a deep venous thrombosis. It is treated with anti-inflammatory drugs and support bandages. Only if thrombophlebitis extends to the sapheno-femoral junction is there any danger of pulmonary embolisation. Urgent sapheno-femoral ligation may be required.

Deep venous insufficiency

Deep venous insufficiency exists when the deep valves have been previously damaged, usually by a DVT. It is particularly common after limb fractures, major surgery, pregnancy and prolonged bed rest. In many cases, the previous DVT will have been asymptomatic and the clinical features of deep venous insufficiency can take 10–20 years to manifest.

Patients may present with various symptoms:

- common
  - leg swelling
  - secondary varicose veins
  - eczema
  - thickened sclerotic skin (lipodermatosclerosis)
- less common
  - ulceration
  - venous claudication (very rare).

Diagnosis

The key investigations are: photoplethysmography, duplex scanning of veins and venography.

Treatment

The management of deep venous insufficiency depends upon the symptoms. In fit patients, surgery to coexisting superficial varicose veins combined with long-term compression stockings is the optimum treatment.

Venous ulceration

Ulceration is most likely in patients who have constant ambulatory venous hypertension. Where ulceration is present, Doppler arterial pressures should be checked to ensure there is no coexisting arterial component. The mainstay of treatment to *pure* venous ulceration is the application of sustained compression therapy to improve deep venous flow and reduce superficial venous stasis. The most consistent and reliable compression pressures will be obtained with support stockings placed over appropriate dressings.

Venous ulceration accounts for 80–90% of all leg ulcers and accounts for a considerable amount of time lost from work. The exact pathophysiology of ulceration secondary to venous disease is uncertain but it is probably caused by a combination of factors leading to hypoxia in the skin itself. The medial aspect of the calf is most frequently affected.

Other causes of lower limb ulcers are:

- arterial
- neuropathic
- malignant.

Arterial ulcers are usually sited on the toes or lateral aspect of the calf above the malleolus. It is important to differentiate them as compression treatment will make them worse. Neuropathic ulcers occur in weight- or pressure-bearing areas (e.g. sole of the foot); they are aggravated by impaired sensation (e.g. in diabetes). In any ulcer which refuses to heal, the possibility of malignant change should be considered and a biopsy will be necessary.

Treatment
Healing can be extremely slow, but is improved by:

- foot elevation
- compression
- local treatment of infection.

Occasionally, skin grafting (especially pinch skin grafting) may speed up healing. Antibiotics are only used if there is evidence of systemic sepsis or severe cellulitis in the limb.

Once an ulcer is healed, the patient will need to wear support stockings for life to prevent recurrence.

Self-assessment: questions

Extended matching items questions (EMIs)

EMI 1

Theme: Differential diagnosis of leg pain

A. groin pain on walking

B. pain in the legs on standing with rapid relief on elevation

C. pain in the calf on walking relieved rapidly by rest

D. leg weakness on walking relieved by standing still

E. pain on standing or walking relieved after sitting for 30 min

F. knee pain, worse in the mornings

G. leg pain on walking relieved after standing still for 5 min

H. acute posterior thigh pain radiating to the calf

I. pain in the buttock, thigh and calf on walking relieved rapidly by rest

Which of the above symptoms are most likely to be found in the following diagnoses?

1. spinal canal stenosis

2. intermittent claudication

3. intermittent claudication in patients with diabetic neuropathy

4. intermittent claudication with femoro-popliteal occlusive disease

5. varicose veins

EMI 2

Theme: Investigations in peripheral vascular disease

A. colour duplex ultrasound scan

B. CT scan

C. B-mode ultrasound scan

D. resting ankle brachial pressure indices

E. pre- and post-exercise ankle brachial pressure indices

F. photoplethysmography

G. MR angiogram

H. intra-arterial digital subtraction angiogram

I. intravenous digital subtraction angiogram

Which of the above investigations are most suitable in the following conditions?

1. diagnosis of a possible ruptured aortic aneurysm in a stable patient

2. detailed arterial imaging immediately prior to angioplasty

3. investigation of possible carotid artery disease

4. investigation of claudicants with possible iliac disease

5. confirmation of a clinical diagnosis of claudication

6. surveillance of small aortic aneurysms

EMI 3

Theme: Drugs in peripheral vascular disease

A. statins

B. non cardio-selective beta blockers

C. aspirin

D. clopidogrel

E. ACE inhibitors

F. loop diuretics

G. folic acid

H. metformin

I. thiazide diuretics

Which of the above drugs best fits the following descriptions?

1. used to treat hyperhomocysteinaemia

2. may cause metabolic acidosis after contrast enhanced radiology

3. side effects include muscle pains

4. worsen symptoms of claudication

5. may worsen renal function in the presence of renal artery stenosis

6. an anti-platelet agent acting as an ADP receptor antagonist

EMI 4

Theme: Cerebrovascular disease with recent symptoms

A. episodic dizziness with a left ICA stenosis of 70% and a right ICA stenosis of 50%

B. amuarosis fugax in the right eye with a right ICA stenosis of 80% and a left ICA stenosis of 30%

C. right homonomous hemianopia

D. disabling left hemiplegia

E. a right upper limb monoparesis with good recovery and an 85% left internal carotid stenosis

F. dizziness on using the left arm with a proximal left subclavian stenosis

G. acute stroke with a left hemiparesis and a 90% right internal carotid stenosis

H. TIAs affecting left arm with recurrent right internal carotid stenosis of 80% following previous right carotid endarterectomy and neck radiotherapy for lymphoma

For which of the above clinical scenarios are the following treatments best suited?

1. medical therapy with risk factor modification and anti-platelet treatment
2. left carotid endarterectomy
3. right carotid endarterectomy
4. left subclavian artery angioplasty or left carotid-subclavian bypass
5. right internal carotid artery stenting

EMI 5

Theme: Lower limb ulcers

A. pale thin skin
B. healthy pink granulation tissue
C. occur commonly on the medial side of the ankle
D. deep punched out
E. occur commonly under pressure points
F. overhanging with callus
G. necrotic slough
H. thickened haemosiderin pigmented skin
I. sloping with spreading epithelialisation
J. occur commonly on the lateral side of the ankle

Which of the above descriptions best fits the following ulcer types?

1. the edge of an ischaemic ulcer
2. the edge of a neuropathic ulcer
3. the base of a venous ulcer
4. skin surrounding an ischaemic ulcer
5. the site of a venous ulcer

Constructed response questions (CRQs)

CRQ 1

A 65-year-old man presents with paralysis of his right arm and leg and with expressive dysphasia. A carotid duplex scan shows a 30% stenosis of the right internal carotid artery with the left internal carotid being occluded.

a. What other investigations would be useful?

His symptoms improve fairly rapidly and after a week his speech and motor function have returned to normal.

b. How should he be treated?

Three years later he re-presents with a TIA affecting his left arm. A carotid duplex scan now shows a 70% stenosis of the right internal carotid artery while the left internal carotid is still occluded.

c. What treatment should now be recommended?

The patient is concerned about the risks of surgery.

d. List three possible serious complications.

CRQ 2

A 55-year-old man presents with left calf intermittent claudication at 200 m. Some features of his pain suggest there may be a musculoskeletal component.

a. How would you confirm a diagnosis of claudication?

Your investigations confirm significant arterial disease.

b. What should be the initial management?

The patient is concerned about his future progress.

c. What is the natural history of claudication?

Eighteen months later this gentleman returns with progressive symptoms and he is now housebound.

d. If his symptoms become disabling, what investigations will guide arterial reconstruction (balloon angioplasty/stenting/arterial bypass)? Name two.

You review the results of his investigations with your consultant.

e. Which arterial segments are generally considered suitable for reconstruction in patients with claudication?

CRQ 3

A 68-year-old man complains of feeling palpitations in his abdomen. He is otherwise asymptomatic. On examination he has a non-tender pulsatile mass in his central abdomen in keeping with an abdominal aortic aneurysm.

a. What investigation is most appropriate to confirm the diagnosis?

The aneurysm is confirmed and measured at 4.2 cm maximum diameter.

b. How should the patient be managed?

Two years later the decision is made to repair the aneurysm.

c. What would be the indications for repair of the aneurysm?

The patient is admitted for an elective (planned) surgical procedure.

d. What investigations might be useful before elective repair?

CRQ 4

An 80-year-old lady has a relatively pain-free chronic ulcer on the medial side of her lower right calf. It has a sloping edge with a pink-looking base formed of granulation tissue.

a. What is the most likely diagnosis?

b. What would you expect the skin to look like around the ulcer?

The patient explains that the ulcer has been long-standing and began after a minor abrasion to the area did not heal.

c. What aetiological factors should you seek in this patient's history?

The patient has poor home circumstances and is admitted for assessment.

d. What investigations should be performed and how will they help in management?

These investigations confirm that the ulcer is not arterial in origin.

e. How should the ulcer be dressed and what are the chances of it healing with this type of dressing?

CRQ 5

A 70-year-old lady presents with a 2-h history of pain in her left foot leg. An acutely ischaemic leg is suspected.

a. What other clinical features would you expect to find in acute ischaemia?

Your physical examination confirms the diagnosis of an acutely ischaemic limb.

b. Which clinical features are used to determine the degree of severity of the ischaemia and which blood test may help confirm the diagnosis?

You take the patient's full case history.

c. What other symptoms of cardiovascular disease should you seek in this patient's history?

You are asked to prepare this patient for theatre.

d. What specific investigations would help the surgeon decide whether or not an operation would help this patient? List two tests.

Objective structured clinical examination questions (OSCEs)

OSCE 1

Figure 42 shows the intravenous digital subtraction angiogram of a 62-year-old woman who was admitted with severe claudication in both legs.

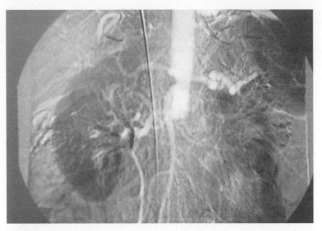

Figure 42

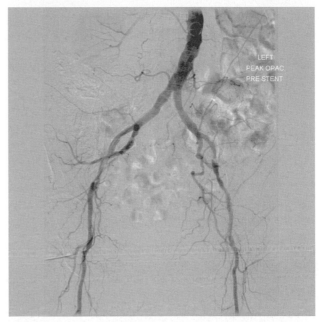

LEFT
PEAK OPAC.
PRE STENT

Figure 43

a. Describe the appearance.

b. What is the diagnosis?

c. What further investigations should be performed?

d. How should she be managed?

OSCE 2

A 66-year-old man presents with left buttock and thigh claudication at 100 m. Study the radiograph (Figure 43) and answer the following questions.

a. Name the type of investigation.

b. Describe the abnormality that is shown.

c. Suggest possible treatment plans.

OSCE 3

Look at the two CT scans (Figure 44A, B) from different patients.

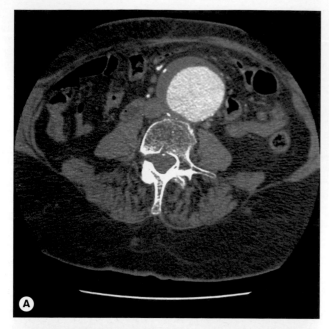

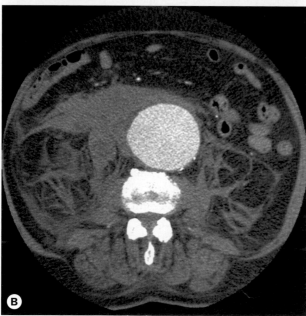

Figure 44 (A), (B)

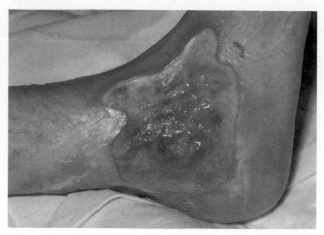

Figure 45

a. Explain what they show.

b. What is the patient likely to complain of?

c. Explain the pathophysiological reason behind the drop in post-exercise pressures on the right.

OSCE 5

Look at the clinical photograph (Figure 45).
a. Describe the appearance of the ulcer.

b. What is the likely aetiology.

c. What further investigations should be done?

OSCE 6

Compare the two pictures (Figure 46A, B).
a. What are the differences?

b. Which requires more urgent treatment and why?

c. What would that treatment be?

d. How can the likelihood of Figure 46A developing into Figure 46B be reduced?

Multiple choice questions

1. Atherosclerosis:
    a. is caused by being overweight
    b. is more common in non-Western countries
    c. is most commonly found in the radial arteries
    d. may be found in the arteries of children
    e. is more common in men

2. In the management of intermittent claudication:
    a. quality of life is more important than absolute walking distance
    b. the absence of femoral pulses suggests inoperability
    c. arteriography should always be performed
    d. most patients should be offered surgery
    e. exercise should always be encouraged

3. In critical ischaemia:
    a. rest pain may be relieved by taking a few steps around the bed

a. What does each show?

b. How may the two patients have presented?

c. What is the appropriate treatment for each?

OSCE 4

Here is a set of ankle–brachial pressure index measurements.

	Right	**Left**
At rest	0.95	1.01
Post exercise	0.65	1.15

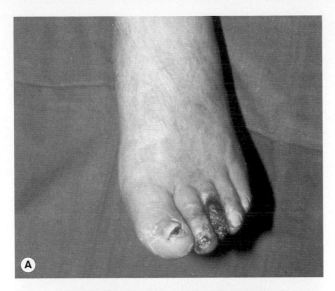

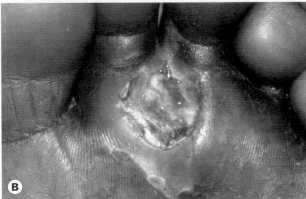

Figure 46 (A), (B)

b. rest pain may be found in the calf muscles

c. the diagnosis is confirmed by the absence of pulses

d. most patients will require revascularisation

e. primary amputation of gangrenous toes is usually successful

4. The following points relate to drugs commonly used in vascular disease:

a. beta blockers can improve muscle blood flow

b. aspirin reduces cardiac mortality

c. tissue plasminogen activator is a major cause of acute thrombosis

d. anticoagulation with warfarin should aim for an INR (international normalised ratio) of >10

e. sensitivity to heparin can cause thrombosis

5. In patients with cerebrovascular disease:

a. most strokes are caused by intracerebral haemorrhage or arterial occlusive disease

b. carotid surgery should always be carried out for stenosis >50%

c. about one in four stroke patients will die from their initial CVA

d. dizziness is a common symptom of carotid disease

e. duplex ultrasound is the investigation of choice for carotid disease

6. Deep venous thrombosis:

a. is best diagnosed clinically

b. is always preventable by subcutaneous heparin

c. is common after pelvic surgery

d. may lead to venous ulceration in later life

e. should usually be treated with a vena cava filter

7. Varicose veins:

a. are a rare cause of pulmonary embolus

b. usually are asymptomatic

c. are best dealt with by surgery

d. are generally secondary to deep venous insufficiency

e. affect 2% of the population

8. The following features are characteristic of venous ulcers:

a. they are never painful

b. they are usually found on the medial aspect of the lower leg

c. they are best treated with high compression (class II) support hose

d. they usually require hospitalisation

e. they are 10 times more common than arterial ulcers

9. The following statements relate to aortic aneurysms:

a. they never rupture if less than 3 cm in diameter

b. they are more common in men

c. repair should be undertaken if they are >5.5 cm in diameter

d. most are found incidentally in patients

e. they are associated with a >10% elective operative mortality

10. Raynaud's phenomenon is:

a. extremely common in young women

b. best treated with cervical sympathectomy

c. usually secondary to an underlying disorder

d. also known as acrocyanosis

e. associated with a benign course in most patients

11. Which of the following statements concerning peripheral vascular disease are true?

a. treatment of hypertension reduces the risk of stroke

b. diabetics are less likely to require amputation for arterial disease

c. atherosclerosis is more common in diabetics than in non-diabetics

d. amputation for critical limb ischaemia is best performed above the knee

e. balloon angioplasty of the iliac arteries is generally unsuccessful

Self-assessment: answers

EMI answers

EMI 1

Theme: Differential diagnosis of leg pain

1. E. Pain on standing relieved after sitting for 30 min.

Spinal canal stenosis is caused by a combination of disc prolapse, osteophyte formation and disc collapse. In the upright position this narrows the spinal canal and causes pressure on the cauda equina resulting in referred pain in the leg. On sitting the space in the spinal canal is opened up. The pressure on the cauda equina is relieved, but nerve compression pain takes some time to wear off.

2. G. Leg pain on walking relieved after standing still for 5 min.

At rest there is sufficient oxygen for aerobic metabolism to provide a muscle's energy requirements. The increased energy requirements of exercise cannot be met by aerobic metabolism as the oxygen supply is limited by the arterial disease and so anaerobic metabolism takes over. The pain of intermittent claudication is caused by a build-up of lactic acid in muscle which has to use anaerobic metabolism to produce energy. After stopping the exercise, anaerobic metabolism and lactic acid production cease and the pain eases off once the residual lactic acid is washed out by the blood supply. This takes only a few minutes and is independent of the position the patient takes up on resting.

3. D. Leg weakness on walking relieved by standing still.

This is the same description as for Question 2, but the peripheral neuropathy of diabetes means that these patients may not feel the pain of claudication. They simply experience muscle weakness instead as anaerobic metabolism produces less energy than aerobic metabolism.

4. C. Pain in the calf on walking relieved rapidly by rest.

The more proximal the arterial disease, the more proximal the patient feels the symptoms of claudication. Generally the claudication is felt one segment lower than the site of arterial narrowing.

5. B. Pain in the legs on standing with rapid relief on elevation.

The pain of varicose veins is caused by the excessive distension of the veins. When elevated the distension disappears and the pain is rapidly relieved.

EMI 2

Theme: Investigations in peripheral vascular disease

1. B. CT scan.

Although not 100% specific or sensitive, a CT scan is the best investigation in this situation to show the rupture haematoma. It should not be performed if there is a risk of the patient destabilising in the scanner. In this situation the diagnosis has to be made clinically.

2. H. Intra-arterial digital subtraction angiogram.

Immediately prior to balloon placement for angioplasty, the stenosis or occlusion has to be accurately identified. This is almost universally done by contrast injection into the artery with digital subtraction imaging. A few centres have tried using ultrasound to guide balloon placement.

3. A. Colour duplex ultrasound scan.

This has become the standard investigation in this situation and gives good images almost always. Catheter angiography of the carotids carries a small stroke risk but is still occasionally required, although the role of CT angiography and MR angiography is being investigated in the small number of cases where duplex fails.

4. G. MR angiogram.

MR angiography is non-invasive and the contrast used (gadolinium) is less toxic than that used for conventional angiography. As techniques and equipment improve it is likely to replace diagnostic catheter angiography.

5. E. Pre- and post-exercise ankle brachial pressure indices.

This test gives a functional assessment of the perfusion of the legs under stressed conditions and is analogous to an exercise ECG. The other tests give information regarding the anatomy of the arterial disease, but cannot indicate whether that anatomy is causing the patient's pain. The patient's history is usually sufficient to make a diagnosis of claudication, but in uncertain cases a functional test is required.

6. C. B-mode ultrasound scan.

Simple ultrasound can see the aorta in 99% of cases and has been shown to measure its size accurately and reproducibly. It is cheap, quick and non-invasive.

EMI 3

Theme: Drugs in peripheral vascular disease

1. G. Folic acid.

Hyperhomocysteinaemia is now a recognised risk factor for arterial disease. Homocysteine can be metabolised to methionine by remethylation. Folic acid is the precursor of the methyl donor in this conversion.

2. H. Metformin.

The combination of diabetic nephropathy, contrast nephropathy and the tendency of metformin to induce lactic acidosis dictates the withdrawal of metformin around the time of contrast-enhanced radiology. This reduces the risk of a renal-induced metabolic acidosis.

3. A. Statins.

Statins can cause muscle pain as a result of myositis or myopathy. The creatine kinase may be elevated in which case the drug should be stopped. A high degree of suspicion is required as the symptoms may mimic the muscle pain of claudication.

4. B. Non cardio-selective beta blockers.

These drugs cause peripheral vasoconstriction and so can worsen the symptoms of claudication.

5. E. ACE inhibitors.

Angiotensin II is important in the maintenance of glomerular filtration pressure (and so glomerular filtration rate) through its selective vasocontriction of the efferent arteriole. If renal perfusion, and so afferent arteriolar pressure, is reduced by renal artery stenosis then loss of the angiotensin II induced efferent arteriolar constriction can cause a rapid and significant fall in glomerular filtration rate.

6. D. Clopidogrel.

ADP binding to platelets induces aggregation directly and by activation of the glycoprotein GPIIb/IIIa receptor. Clopidogrel irreversibly binds to the platelet ADP receptor and so inhibits platelet aggregation for the life of the platelet.

EMI 4

Theme: Cerebrovascular disease with recent symptoms

1. A. Episodic dizziness with a left ICA stenosis of 70% and a right ICA stenosis of 50%.

Episodic dizziness has a wide variety of causes and will not be caused by carotid disease except possibly in the rare circumstance of severe (>95%) bilateral internal carotid stenosis with global cerebral hypoperfusion. Whenever carotid disease is found full risk factor treatment and antiplatelet therapy should be started to reduce the risk of stroke and other vascular events.

2. E. A right upper limb monoparesis with good recovery and an 85% left internal carotid stenosis.

Embolisation from a tight left internal carotid stenosis into the motor cortex of the left cerebral hemisphere will cause right arm or leg symptoms. Carotid endarterectomy in these circumstances has been shown to reduce the risk of subsequent stroke.

3. B. Amaurosis fugax in the right eye with a right ICA stenosis of 80% and a left ICA stenosis of 30%.

Embolisation from the right internal carotid stenosis can cause ipsilateral retinal artery occlusion via the ophthalmic artery – the first branch of the internal carotid. Again, carotid endarterectomy in these circumstances has been shown to reduce the risk of subsequent stroke.

4. F. Dizziness on using the left arm with a proximal left subclavian stenosis.

A stenosis in the left subclavian artery proximal to the origin of the vertebral artery reduces arm blood flow. When the arm is exercised its peripheral vascular resistance may

fall to a lower level than the brain. Under such circumstances the pressure at the origin of the vertebral artery may be lower (because of the proximal subclavian stenosis and because of the reduced vascular resistance in the arm) than at its termination in the circle of Willis (if this provides adequate colaterals). Blood therefore flows retrogradely in the vertebral artery towards the arm. This reduces cerebellar perfusion and causes dizziness. Treatment of the subclavian stenosis can resolve these symptoms.

5. H. TIAs affecting left arm with recurrent right internal carotid stenosis of 80% following previous right carotid endarterectomy and neck radiotherapy for lymphoma.

Treatment of a symptomatic tight restenosis after carotid endarterectomy is appropriate, but redo surgery after cervical radiotherapy would be hazardous and would risk carotid and cranial nerve trauma. Angioplasty and stenting under these circumstances would be safer.

EMI 5

Theme: Lower limb ulcers

1. D. Deep punched out.

Ischaemic ulcers show no attempt at healing because the blood supply is insufficient. The edge of the ulcer is therefore sharply demarcated with no ingrowth of epithelium.

2. F. Overhanging with callus.

Neuropathic ulcers develop when a callus (formed as a result of long-term pressure) breaks down centrally to reveal the cavity under it (caused by tissue having been torn by differential movement between the callus and underlying bone). The cavity is often larger than breakdown in the callus, hence the overhanging edge.

3. B. Healthy pink granulation tissue.

Venous ulcers have a good arterial blood supply and so attempts at healing are made. The base is well vascularised and so healthy granulation tissue forms.

4. A. Pale thin skin

The skin of a chronically ischaemic leg is thin and pale.

5. C. Occur commonly on the medial side of the ankle.

Venous ulcers commonly (but not exclusively) form on the medial side of the ankle, possibly owing to high pressure reflux from incompetent perforating veins at this site.

CRQ answers

CRQ 1

a. CT brain scan – to differentiate between infarct and haemorrhage. The majority of strokes are ischaemic, but it is important to detect haemorrhagic infarcts as the treatment is different. Anticoagulation must not be used in a haemorrhagic infarct – it may promote further bleeding. A search should also be made for an intracranial aneurysm in these patients.

Angiography – depending on the views obtained on duplex scanning, it may be necessary to confirm occlusion of the left internal carotid artery with catheter-based, CT or MR angiography.

ECG – to determine the cardiac rhythm.

Echocardiogram – to look for intra-cardiac thrombus.

A full arterial risk factor screen, with blood pressure, lipid profile, blood glucose.

b. Optimise medical management of all his risk factors including stopping smoking, the use of a statin and possibly an ACE inhibitor. Consider an anti-platelet agent such as aspirin or clopidogrel.

Carotid endarterectomy has no role as the operation is prophylactic and intended to prevent embolisation of particulate matter from a stenosis into the ipsilateral carotid artery territory. It is very unlikely for an occluded artery to be a source of embolisation.

c. A right carotid endarterectomy.

d. Stroke or mortality.

Myocardial infarction.

Postoperative haematoma and stridor from laryngeal oedema.

Cranial nerve injury.

Any of these complications will score marks. For most patients the risk of stroke is less than 3%.

CRQ 2

a. Measure the ankle brachial indices, at rest and after exercise. The post-exercise ratio will be lowered in claudication even if the extent of arterial disease is not sufficient to lower the ratio at rest.

b. Minimise the patient's lifestyle and medical risk factors (stop smoking, use statins to lower cholesterol, control hypertension, control diabetes, look for hyperhomocysteinaemia).

Use anti-platelet treatment.

Encourage regular exercise by walking – may be as part of a supervised exercise programme.

c. The majority of claudicants (up to 80%) do not deteriorate and some may improve with medical therapy. About 20% will deteriorate; the majority of these will do so slowly. The risk of limb loss is very low at about 1% at 5 years

d. Duplex scan.

MR angiography.

Catheter angiography.

Any of these responses will score marks. Usually the least invasive tests are used first (as listed).

e. Aorto-iliac

Femoro-popliteal

These are large vessels and are more suitable for reconstruction because of the relatively large lumen and high blood flow rates. The calf vessels (crural/tibial vessels) are small and have lower flow. This results in a greater risk of bypass failure. Bypass failure risks arterial thrombosis and consequent worsening of symptoms. Reconstruction of these vessels is therefore generally not considered appropriate for claudication.

CRQ 3

a. Ultrasound scan.

b. Keep the aneurysm under surveillence with 6-monthly ultrasound scans in order to detect any enlargement.

c. Increase in size to 5.5 cm.

Increase in size of 1 cm in a year.

The development of pain or tenderness in the aneurysm (repair should be urgent).

Rupture (repair as an emergency).

Any of the above developments (listed in order of increasing danger) is an indication for surgery.

d. Full blood count.

Biochemical profile.

Renal function tests (either simply by urea and creatinine or by formal assessment of glomerular filtration rate).

ECG.

Echocardiography.

Stress testing of myocardial function/perfusion (exercise ECG, stress echocardiogram, tetrofosmin scan, coronary angiography).

Chest radiograph.

Lung function tests.

CT scan – to show the relation of the aneurysm to the renal arteries and give more detail about the iliac arteries.

Angiography – if there is concern about any occlusive disease.

All of these tests have a role to play in the evaluation of a patient before elective aneurysm surgery. These patients often have significant comorbidity affecting the heart, lungs and kidneys, all of which must be taken into account before deciding to operate.

CRQ 4

a. A venous (varicose) ulcer. The position of the ulcer and the lack of pain are all hallmarks of varicose ulceration.

b. Look for evidence of lipodermatosclerosis – thickened, tight skin with patchy or confluent reddish-brown discolouration. This is another feature of venous ulceration.

c. Previous deep vein thrombosis.

Varicose veins.

History of intermittent claudication.

Varicose veins or a history of a previous deep vein thrombosis predispose to venous ulceration. Ask specifically about these points in the history. Also, it is important to check for a history of intermittent claudication. An arterial component to the ulcer will alter the treatment options.

d. Ankle brachial index – to determine if there is an arterial component to the ulcer.

Arterial duplex/angiography – if arterial impairment is a possibility.

Venous duplex scan – to assess the presence of any superficial or deep venous incompetence or deep venous occlusion.

Plethysmography/ambulatory venous pressure – to assess the relative contribution of superficial and deep venous incompetence to the ulcer and to guide whether superficial venous surgery may help.

e. Four-layer compression bandaging results in healing of about 60% of venous ulcers in 12 weeks.

CRQ 5

a. All the **P**'s. As well as **p**ain;

diminished, altered (**p**araesthesia) or absent sensation;

muscle weakness or **p**aralysis;

pallor;

pulselessness;

perishing cold.

b. Fixed mottling is a grave sign – it implies capillary death with extravasation of blood.

Absence of sensation implies total sensory nerve ischaemia.

Paralysis implies no muscle perfusion or absence of motor nerve perfusion.

Calf muscle tenderness implies muscle necrosis.

All of these signs are associated with a poor outcome. These patients may require amputation rather than revascularisation.

An elevated serum creatine kinase level indicates muscle necrosis.

c. Look for a history of cardiac disease, either chronic (previous myocardial infarction or angina) or acute with the current presentation. An ECG is important as some of these patients will have suffered an acute myocardial infarction.

A previous stroke, transient ischaemic attack or history of amaurosis fugax is also important. Seek evidence of intermittent claudication or any previous arterial surgery or angioplasty. Also, these patients often have renal artery disease and may be hypertensive or have impaired renal function.

d. Ankle brachial indices, duplex arterial scan, angiogram.

Collectively, these tests will play a key role in assessing what role surgery may play in this patient's management.

OSCE answers

OSCE 1

a. This is an intravenous digital subtraction angiogram of the aorta and iliac arteries. There is a complete occlusion of the aorta at the level of the renal The left renal artery is occluded but the sple hepatic, right renal and superior mesenteric can be seen.

b. The patient has an aortic occlusion. This is likely to be a chronic occlusive rather than an acute occlusive episode because of the widespread collateral blood supply, which would have gradually developed over a long period of time.

c. Further investigations include a Doppler pressure assessment and a full cardiac and pulmonary assessment.

d. Depending upon the severity of this patient's symptoms and the effect this has on her quality of life, there are several options:

- it may be possible to manage this patient conservatively
- alternatively, an aorto-iliac or aorto-femoral bypass will be required
- because of the extent of the disease, angioplasty or intravascular stenting is unlikely to help.

OSCE 2

a. This is a catheter an angiogram.

b. The examination shows a left external iliac stenosis.

c. First, look for any risk factors in this patient – for example, smoking, diabetes, hypercholesterolaemia, hypertension and hyperhomocysteinaemia. Thereafter, the initial treatment plan is usually conservative.

Medical management of any risk factors should be optimised (stop smoking, control hypertension, institute a dietary cholesterol reducing programme, etc.). Many patients will also require statins, anti-platelet agents (such as aspirin), ACE inhibitors or folic acid supplements (the latter to counter the effects of hyperhomocysteinaemia). Finally, and of great importance, this patient should be encouraged to embark on a graduated exercise programme which will increase his claudication distance over a period of time.

If this regime is unsuccessful or the patient's symptoms become progressively severe a combination of Doppler ultrasound and vascular imaging (usually arteriography or CT/MR angiography) are used to assess the role of angioplasty or arterial surgery in the patient.

OSCE 3

a. Figure 44A shows an abdominal aortic aneurysm with an intact aneurysm sac. Figure 44B shows an aneurysm which has ruptured. There is a large amount of blood clot lying outside the aneurysm sac.

b. In the patient without rupture the aneurysm may be an 'incidental' finding detected by the patient feeling the mass within his abdomen, or, having become aware of its pulsation. The ruptured aneurysm is likely to have led to an acute presentation with crippling abdominal or back pain of sudden onset associated with hypotension and collapse.

c. An intact aneurysm should be repaired if its transverse diameter as measured by ultrasound or CT scan exceeds 5.5 cm or if it has grown by 1 cm in 1 year or if it is tender/painful. In each case, the benefit of repair (prevention of rupture) must be weighed against the risk of surgery and the overall fitness of the patient. If the aneurysm has ruptured emergency surgical repair should be undertaken provided the patient's comorbidity and quality of life suggest a reasonable chance of survival.

OSCE 4

a. The ankle pressures at rest are essentially the same as the brachial pressures. After exercise the ankle pressure on the right has fallen, suggesting there is occlusive arterial disease on the right.

b. The patient is likely to complain of intermittent claudication in the right leg.

c. A relatively minor stenosis may transmit sufficient arterial pressure to prevent a significant pressure drop at the ankle at rest, the ankle pressure being maintained by the vasoconstricted muscle vasculature at rest. During and after exercise, the muscle vasculature vasodilates, lowering the peripheral vascular resistance. The minor stenosis would limit the increase in blood flow during exercise which, coupled with the fall in peripheral vascular resistance, lowers the pressure in the ankle relative to the arm.

OSCE 5

a. An ulcer with thin surrounding skin, a deep punched out edge and a base composed of necrotic slough.

b. This ulcer is likely to be arterial/ischaemic origin.

c. The three most useful investigations are:
   i. ankle:brachial pressure indices to confirm the aeiology
   ii. arterial duplex/angiography to show the anatomy of the occlusive disease
   iii. venous duplex to determine if there is a venous component.

OSCE 6

a. Figure 46A is an illustration of dry gangrene of the forefoot. The boundary between dead and viable is clearly marked and there is little surrounding cellulitis. Figure 46B illustrates wet gangrene. The demarcation between dead and viable tissue is less clear and there is a marked surrounding inflammatory response.

b. Wet gangrene is an indication for urgent surgical intervention as, unchecked, the infection will destroy tissue as it spreads rapidly through the ischaemic limb.

c. Treatment involves amputation of the infected necrotic material, if necessary before any attempt is made to revascularise the limb. Parenteral antibiotics are used to help control infection.

d. By keeping the foot dry and clean and avoiding moist dressings.

Multiple choice answers

1. a. **False.** Excess fat is not a cause of atherosclerosis although it may be a secondary phenomenon.
   b. **False.** It is a disease of Western environments and perhaps genetic make-up.
   c. **False.** It is most commonly seen at bifurcations and in the lower limbs.
   d. **True.** Atheroma has been detected in the arteries of children before their teens.
   e. **True.** Atherosclerosis is more frequently seen in men.

2. a. **True.** The patient's existing quality of life is the most important determinant for intervention in claudication.
   b. **False.** Femoral pulses may often be absent (indicating aorto-femoral disease); these patients are usually operable.
   c. **False.** Arteriography should only be performed if intervention is being considered.
   d. **False.** Most patients are treated conservatively.
   e. **True.** By encouraging exercise with a graduated exercise programme many patients will develop an improvement in their claudication distance and the need for surgery will be obviated.

3. a. **True.** In critical ischaemia, rest pain is paradoxically relieved by standing out of bed and taking a few steps.
   b. **False.** True rest pain occurs in the toes and the foot.
   c. **False.** Absent pulses are a common finding in arterial disease and do not necessarily signify critical ischaemia.
   d. **True.** Revascularisation is usually the only option if the critically ischaemic limb is to be saved.
   e. **False.** Primary toe amputations rarely heal in the absence of pure diabetes; preliminary revascu-larisation of the limb is usually required.

4. a. **False.** Beta blockade reduces muscle blood flow.
   b. **True.** Aspirin has been clearly shown to reduce both the frequency of myocardial infarction and the mortality following infarction.

c. **False.** Tissue plasminogen activator is a naturally occurring thrombolytic agent and may be given by the intra-arterial or intravenous route to achieve thrombolysis.

d. **False.** An INR of >10 is extremely dangerous: doses should aim at a therapeutic range of between 2 and 3.5 depending upon the indication.

e. **True.** Hypersensitivity to heparin can induce thrombocytopenia; this is an uncommon but extremely important cause of intravascular thrombosis as the treatment is cessation of heparin. Watch out for a platelet count of <100 000 during prolonged heparin therapy.

5. a. **True.** Most strokes are caused by intracerebral haemorrhage or infarction; only some are caused by extracranial carotid disease producing thrombosis or embolism.

   b. **False.** Carotid endarterectomy should be carried out for symptomatic stenoses >70% in those who are fit. Most patients with a 50–70% stenosis can be treated conservatively.

   c. **True.** About 25% of stroke patients will die from their initial CVA.

   d. **False.** Non-localising/non-lateralising symptoms such as dizziness are rarely caused by carotid artery disease.

   e. **True.** Duplex ultrasound is the gold standard investigation in carotid disease; it has replaced angiography as the procedure of choice.

6. a. **False.** Clinical evaluation is inaccurate; a DVT is only present in 25–50% of clinically suspicious limbs. A duplex scan is the best diagnostic tool.

   b. **False.** Although subcutaneous heparin administration reduces the incidence of a DVT and may reduce the incidence of a fatal pulmonary embolism, these conditions are not completely prevented.

   c. **True.** DVT is particularly common after pelvic or major orthopaedic surgery.

   d. **True.** A DVT may lead to chronic deep vein insufficiency which may progress to venous ulceration.

   e. **False.** Inferior vena cava filters should only be used if there is a contraindication to anticoagulation or in patients who have suffered pulmonary emboli despite apparently adequate anticoagulation.

7. a. **True.** Varicose veins are an extremely uncommon cause of pulmonary emboli. Very occasionally they are a source if there is thrombophlebitis involving the sapheno-femoral junction.

   b. **True.** Most varicose veins are asymptomatic. Cosmetic problems or an ill-defined ache are the most common reasons for referral for surgery.

   c. **True.** In patients with varicose veins whose symptoms warrant treatment, surgical treatment is the best line of management.

   d. **False.** Most varicose veins are primary or 'idiopathic' and not secondary to underlying deep venous insufficiency.

   e. **False.** At least 10% of the population at any given time have varicose veins.

8. a. **False.** Venous ulcers are rarely painful. Discomfort usually develops when infection supervenes.

   b. **True.** They are usually found on the medial aspect of the ankle and lower calf. Arterial ulcers, in contrast, are often sited on the lateral aspect of the calf or on the foot.

   c. **True.** Extrinsic compression using specially designed support stockings is the best management.

   d. **False.** Patients with venous ulcers rarely require hospitalisation and can be treated on an ambulatory basis.

   e. **True.** Venous disease is the most common cause of lower limb ulceration in Western civilisation. It is about 10 times more common than arterial ulceration.

9. a. **False.** Any aortic aneurysm carries a risk of rupture, although aneurysms of less than 3 cm are very unlikely to rupture.

   b. **True.** They are five times more common in men than in women.

   c. **True.** All aneurysms should be repaired if they are greater than 5.5 cm in diameter provided the patient is fit enough to undertake the operation. The incidence of rupture dramatically increases in aneurysms above this size.

   d. **True.** Most aneurysms are found incidentally on examination. Some present with lower abdominal or back pain and others with acute collapse or death after rupture.

   e. **False.** Although the overall mortality for ruptured aneurysms is approximately 50%, the operative mortality for elective aneurysms is around 2–10%.

10. a. **True.** Raynaud's phenomenon is a very common finding in young women.

    b. **False.** Cervical sympathectomy is no longer recommended even in severe cases. Although a temporary improvement was sometimes obtained after this operation, recurrence was frequent within a year.

    c. **False.** Raynaud's phenomenon is usually primary or 'idiopathic'. Only a small number are secondary to an underlying disorder, usually a collagen vascular disease.

    d. **False.** Acrocyanosis is a distinct entity characterised by a persistent cyanosis of the extremities.

    e. **True.** Primary Raynaud's phenomenon has a benign course.

11. a. **True.** Careful treatment of hypertension substantially reduces the risk of stroke in later

years. This has been one of the main reasons for the reduction in incidence of cerebrovascular accidents.

b. **False.** Diabetes is one of the major causes of lower limb amputation.

c. **True.** Atherosclerosis is much more common in diabetics. Many diabetics who require amputation have a combination of diabetic microangiopathy and atherosclerosis.

d. **False.** When amputation is necessary for critical limb ischaemia, it should be carried out below the knee (transtibial) if at all possible. Successful rehabilitation is much more likely after a below knee amputation compared with an above knee amputation.

e. **False.** Transluminal angioplasty of the iliac arteries is very successful. Eight out of 10 vessels so treated will remain patent 5 years after the procedure.

Breast and endocrine surgery

Chapter overview

Most patients with *breast disease* present with a lump in the breast or a painful breast. This chapter emphasises the importance of careful clinical assessment in all patients with breast symptoms in order to rule out an underlying breast cancer and outlines the principles of care in benign and malignant breast disease.

Patients with *endocrine disorders* usually present for surgery either because an endocrine gland has become enlarged (e.g. a thyroid goitre) or because a gland has become overactive (e.g. a phaeochromocytoma causing a hypertensive crisis). Although endocrine underactivity can cause serious medical disorders (e.g. diabetes mellitus caused by β cell failure in the pancreatic islets) an underactive endocrine gland is infrequently an indication for surgery. When malignancy is encountered the prognosis is often good in comparison to malignancy in non-endocrine organ systems.

5.1 Breast disease

Learning objectives

You should:

- know the main causes of a lump in the breast
- be able to use triple assessment to evaluate a patient presenting with symptoms or signs of breast disease
- understand the principles of treatment in patients with benign breast disease and breast cancer.

Symptoms and signs

Breast problems may present with one or a combination of the following features:

- a lump
- skin changes
- nipple discharge
- breast pain.

Always ask how long the lump or lumps have been present and whether the patient has noticed any changes in the skin or nipple distortion. Check if there has been a nipple discharge. If so, is it from one or both breasts? Is it blood-stained? Finally ask about breast pain – where is it? How does it relate to the menstrual cycle?

Triple assessment

This is the key to breast assessment. It comprises:

- clinical history and examination
- mammography ± ultrasound
- cytology/pathology.

Triple assessment is used to decide whether an abnormality in the breast is malignant or non-malignant. A full clinical history of breast symptoms should be supplemented by an endocrine history (see Table 14). Clinical examination should focus on both breasts, the regional lymph glands in the axillae and neck plus a check for hepatomegaly.

Radiological evaluation (Figure 47)

Two-view mammography is the key investigation in women over 35 years of age supplemented by ultrasound. Because the breasts are dense in women under 35 years of age, mammography becomes difficult to interpret and ultrasound is used as the lead investigation.

Histopathological analysis

A tissue diagnosis can be obtained by:

- fine needle cytology
- large bore needle core biopsy (under local anaesthetic)
- open diagnostic biopsy (under local or general anaesthetic).

Benign breast disease

There are seven important breast conditions that frequently present as surgical problems:

- fibrocystic breast changes
- breast pain
- breast cysts
- fibroadenoma
- gynaecomastia
- breast sepsis
- nipple discharge.

It is very common for women to develop areas of lumpy breast tissue, most often before their menses. Any

Table 14 Hormone history in breast disease

Age at menarche

Age at menopause

Use of exogenous hormones
  Oral contraceptive
  Hormone replacement therapy

Family history of malignancy

Number of pregnancies and live births

Previous breast problems

Hysterectomy or oophorectomy

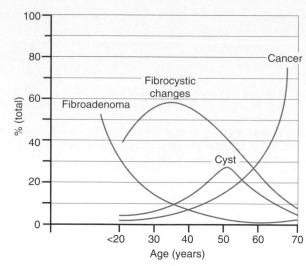

Figure 48 Age and diagnosis in breast disease.

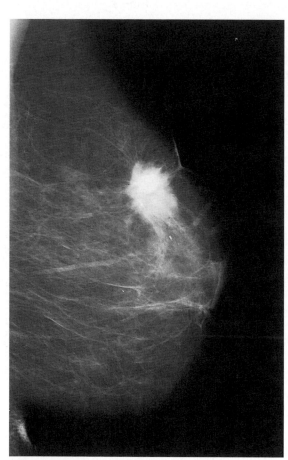

Figure 47 Mammogram – breast cancer.

persistent lump should be properly assessed and triple assessment undertaken if a focal lump is detected. The most likely diagnosis varies with the age of the patient (Figure 48).

Fibrocystic changes

This term encompasses the triad of pain, nodularity and cyst formation in the female breast. Symptoms are often cyclical and worse in the premenstrual period. The peak incidence occurs between 35 and 45 years of age. The

condition is rare after the menopause. The treatment is reassurance once pathology has been excluded by triple assessment.

Breast pain

Pain may affect one or both breasts or even just a small area of a single breast. For some the pain is cyclical, in others there is no relation to the menstrual cycle (acyclical). Reassurance and psychological support are often all that is needed once cancer or an underlying breast infection has been ruled out. The symptoms will often respond to simple measures which include:

- a firm, correctly fitted supportive bra (also worn at night)
- avoiding caffeine (tea, coffee, soft drinks)
- paracetamol

A few patients will have severe pain. Completion of a pain chart over a period of 3–6 months will give an indication of the pattern of symptoms. Severe cyclical mastalgia may respond to the antiestrogen tamoxifen or bromocriptine, which suppresses pituitary gonadotrophin secretion.

Breast cysts

These are often multiple although a single dominant cyst may present. They are most common in women aged 30–50, are probably hormone driven and can be treated by needle aspiration during triple assessment. Recurrent breast cysts or those containing bloodstained fluid should be excised because of the chance of malignancy in the cyst wall.

Fibroadenoma

This is the most common cause of a single breast lump in women under 30 years of age. It is considered to be an abnormality of normal development and involution (ANDI) of the breast tissue. A fibroadenoma is character-ised by a firm, painless, smooth, often highly mobile lump in the breast. Occasionally a giant fibroadenoma develops which grows rapidly.

Diagnosis and treatment

Following triple assessment a fibroadenoma can be treated by excision, or simply monitored if the patient prefers to avoid surgery for cosmetic reasons. If the fibroadenoma remains unchanged over 6–9 months or if it involutes it may be safely left alone. Because the breast tissue is usually very dense in these patients ultrasound is the lead assessment tool.

Gynaecomastia

Gynaecomastia is caused by hypertrophy of the male breast tissue. It can be unilateral or bilateral and is sometimes painful. Gynaecomastia occurs in two age groups:

- in teenage boys/young adults
  - *rarely, testicular tumour*
  - *physiological, at puberty*
- older men
  - *drug induced, e.g. by cimetidine, spironolactone, digoxin*
  - *disease induced, e.g. by cirrhosis, hyperthyroidism, Kleinfelter syndrome, pituitary tumour.*

Treatment

Physiological gynaecomastia usually resolves spontaneously. Surgical excision should be reserved for large symptomatic gynaecomastia.

Breast sepsis

Infection can develop in relation to the nipple (subareolar infection) or in the peripheral glandular mass of the breast. Breast sepsis occurs most often in breastfeeding mothers (usually staphylococcal) or in middle-aged female smokers (anaerobic infection). Usually the infection involves one or more segments of the breast.

The typical features of acute inflammation are present. The breast is painful and tender with erythema and induration. Without treatment, the cellulitis will progress to a breast abscess and it then presents as a fluctulant mass.

A subareolar infection can develop from:

- cuts or abrasions on the nipple caused by breastfeeding
- a blocked lactiferous duct [this can spontaneously discharge through the skin and lead to a mammary duct fistula (Figure 49)].

In older women, dilatation of the nipple duct system associated with a surrounding chronic inflammatory cell infiltrate leads to a condition called mammary duct ectasia or plasma cell mastitis. Chronic inflammation and scarring will lead to indrawing and slit-shaped inversion of the nipple. If secondary infection supervenes, a mammary duct fistula can also develop.

Treatment

During the cellulitic stage, before an abscess forms, infection can often be resolved with an appropriate course of antibiotics (amoxycillin plus clavulanic acid). A breast

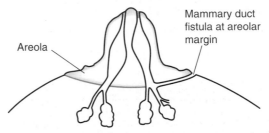

Figure 49 Mammary duct fistula.

abscess can be treated under local or general anaesthesia by:

- aspiration – using a wide bore needle under antibiotic cover
- incision and drainage.

Always culture any pus.

Breastfeeding mothers should be encouraged to continue to feed on the side with sepsis, smokers should be encouraged to stop smoking. Patients with chronically diseased ducts in mammary duct ectasia or a mammary duct fistula require a subareolar excision of the affected ducts.

Nipple discharge

In the non-lactating breast, the four most common causes of nipple discharge are:

- fibrocystic breast changes
- mammary duct ectasia
- intraduct papilloma
- breast cancer.

Clinical features

It is important to determine whether the discharge is:

- unilateral or bilateral
- from a single duct or from multiple ducts
- bloodstained.

The discharge associated with fibrocystic change is usually green/brown in colour, has the associated features of fibrocystic change outlined above and may issue from multiple ducts or from both breasts. Mammary duct ectasia also causes a similar discharge. A serosanguinous discharge from a single duct is more likely to be caused by an intraduct papilloma or a carcinoma. A frankly bloodstained discharge from one or more ducts with an underlying breast mass is usually caused by a breast cancer.

Diagnosis

The nipple discharge can be tested for blood using a urine testing stick. All these patients must also undergo triple assessment.

Treatment

Treatment is only required for persisting discharge or where an underlying pathology is suspected and can involve:

1. exploration and excision of a single lactiferous duct (microdochectomy) to remove an intraduct papilloma
2. subareolar resection of one or more ducts for mammary duct ectasia
3. the appropriate management of any underlying breast disease such as carcinoma.

Breast cancer

Carcinoma of the breast is the most common cancer occurring in women. In the UK it causes more than 10 000 deaths each year and is the leading cause of death in women aged between 40–50 years. Worldwide it afflicts an estimated 1 million women. Currently 1 in 10 women can expect to develop the disease during their lifetime.

Aetiology

The aetiology is uncertain although in 10% there is a familial basis for the disease (women whose mothers and sisters have had breast cancer). Other important factors associated with an increased incidence are:

- nulliparous women or those who have a late first pregnancy, or a late menopause
- lifetime number of menstrual cycles
- family history of ovarian cancer
- use of oral contraceptives or HRT
- smoking, alcohol and obesity.

Despite these risk factors, the disease is unexpected in most women. This has led to the introduction of nation-wide mammography-based screening programmes to detect impalpable cancers. Breast screening is aimed at the 50–70 years age group seeking to detect early cancers which are potentially curable.

Pathology

Most breast cancers grow slowly and may take several years before they are palpable. By local growth, they will eventually invade the underlying pectoral muscles and chest wall and the overlying breast skin. Lymphatic dissemination occurs early to the axillary and internal mammary nodes and later to the supraclavicular nodes. Distant spread by bloodstream occurs to the liver, lungs, pleura and bones. Less often the brain and adrenal glands are involved.

The underlying pathological process is an invasive adenocarcinoma developing from the terminal duct lobular unit within the breast. Some tumours (about 20%) show distinct patterns of growth (see Table 15) and have a better prognosis. The remainder, tumours of no special type, are graded according to the degree of differentiation of the

Table 15 Special pathological types of breast cancer

Lobular
Tubular
Mucoid
Cribriform
Papillary
Medullary

tumour. Pre-invasive cancer (ductal carcinoma in situ; lobular carcinoma in situ) accounts for 10–20% of malignant lesions detected.

Clinical features

Most women will present either with a painless lump detected during self-examination or with radiologically detected evidence of cancer from a breast screening programme. Less frequently, nipple discharge or retraction, nipple crusting or itching, or breast pain will be the presenting symptom. A few patients still present with an advanced cancer breaking through the skin.

Careful inspection and palpation of the breast and axillae provide the key to the clinical diagnosis.

Inspection

The most important features on inspection are:

- breast asymmetry
- skin tethering
- nipple indrawing
- skin oedema or *peau d'orange*.

Palpation

The most important features on palpation are:

- a non-tender lump
- a poorly defined edge between the lump and surrounding breast tissue
- a bloody nipple discharge
- fixity to skin or underlying pectoral muscles
- the presence or absence of axillary or supraclavicular lymphadenopathy.

Diagnosis and staging

The diagnosis of breast cancer is confirmed by triple assessment (clinical/radiological/cytological features). An irregular radiodense breast mass with a spiculated border, which sometimes contains areas of fine 'pepper pot' calcification (microcalcification) is the hallmark of a breast cancer on a mammogram (see Figure 47).

Because survival and treatment options are closely related to the extent of disease at presentation, accurate staging of the disease is essential. The TNM classification (tumour, nodes, metastases) is used most often (Table 16). Other key investigations are:

- full blood count
- liver function tests
- chest radiograph.

Table 16 TNM classification of breast cancer

Tis	Carcinoma in situ
T1	<2 cm
T2	2–5 cm
T3	>5 cm
T4	Involvement of chest wall/skin
N0	No regional node metastases
N1	Palpable, mobile ipsilateral involved axillary nodes
N2	Fixed involved ipsilateral axillary nodes
M0	No evidence of metastases
M1	Distant metastasis

If metastatic disease of the liver or bone is suspected or if the cancer is large or a lymph node mass is present then distant metastases should be sought by:

- liver ultrasound scan
- isotope bone scan.

Differential diagnosis:

- benign breast disease (see p. 119)
- traumatic fat necrosis.

Traumatic fat necrosis may closely mimic a breast cancer in appearance. Despite the name, there may be no obvious history of injury. Although the condition spontaneously resolves, triple assessment may be necessary to exclude a cancer.

Unusual clinical forms of breast cancer

Ductal carcinoma in situ

Ductal carcinoma in situ is a tumour which develops within the glandular ducts and has not yet invaded the surrounding parenchyma. It is usually detected following biopsy of areas of microcalcification identified on mammography. As a result of screening programmes this type of breast cancer is being diagnosed more frequently. Untreated it may progress to invasive breast cancer in some but perhaps not all cases. If the tumour is multifocal total mastectomy is the best treatment. Usually only one breast is affected.

Inflammatory breast cancer

This is a highly aggressive form of breast cancer. Women present with an enlarged, inflamed, erythematous painful breast, which may be mistaken for a breast abscess. These appearances are caused by lymphatic invasion by the cancer. The disease is often widely disseminated and beyond surgical resection by the time of presentation. Survival is poor even after aggressive treatment with a combination of radiotherapy and chemotherapy.

Paget's disease of the breast

Paget's disease occurs in 1 in 50 breast cancers. These patients present with symptoms of nipple disease. They complain of itching, weeping or bleeding of the nipple or areolar, which appears excoriated or covered with a scaly rash on examination. Although an underlying breast mass is rarely present in the early stages of the disease, these patients often have an associated ductal carcinoma in situ and if untreated will go on to develop breast cancer.

The diagnosis is confirmed by nipple biopsy and mammography, with treatment as for carcinoma of the breast.

Breast cancer in pregnancy and lactation

This is uncommon but the outcome is poor. The disease is often detected late because it may be masked by the physiological changes occurring in the breast during pregnancy. The same principles of treatment apply as for breast cancer in non-pregnant or non-lactating women.

Cancer of the male breast

Of all breast cancers, 1 in 200 occur in men. Because the breast is small, spread occurs early to the lymph glands, skin and chest wall. As a result, the disease is often advanced by the time of presentation and the outcome after surgery in men is not as good as in women.

Treatment of breast cancer

There is still controversy regarding the best way to treat breast cancer. Today, radical breast surgery has been replaced by more conservative techniques that provide a better cosmetic result without increased risk of recurrence.

Treatment of localised breast cancer (T1–T3;N0–N1;M0)

Surgery and radiotherapy are used for local disease control on the chest wall and axilla. Since more than one-half of patients with breast cancer who have no evidence of distant disease at the time of diagnosis will ultimately die of distant disease without evidence of local recurrence, various adjuvant therapies are used in an attempt to kill occult metastases that are present at the time of surgery.

Local therapy

Localised breast cancer can be treated by wide local excision plus radiotherapy to the remaining breast or by mastectomy. Survival is identical in either group. Radiotherapy to a conserved breast or chest wall is used to reduce the risk of recurrent local disease. As the bulk of the breast tissue is preserved after a wide local excision there is a considerable cosmetic benefit. Large tumours in a small breast are an exception and are best treated by mastectomy. If a mastectomy is performed breast reconstruction should be considered. These factors and patient preference dictate the choice of operation. In either case the regional (axillary) nodes are sampled or removed for the following reasons:

- to stage the axilla (lymph node positive or negative)
- to provide guidance for chemotherapy and/or radiotherapy
- to achieve local disease control.

Systemic therapy

The following factors are taken into account before deciding on treatment:

- axillary node status
- estrogen receptor status of the tumour
- is the patient pre- or postmenopausal?

The aim of 'adjuvant' therapy is to protect the patient from the development of future metastatic disease. Adjuvant chemotherapy is often given as a combination of a number of drugs (combination chemotherapy) and is used mainly in axillary node positive women whether pre- or postmenopausal. Chemotherapy can be given prior to surgery ('neoadjuvant' chemotherapy) and is used to shrink down the tumour and render an inoperable cancer operable.

Endocrine therapy is particularly effective for estrogen receptor positive tumours. Tamoxifen, an estrogen receptor antagonist, or aromatase inhibitors, which block the production of estrogen in postmenopausal women, will benefit 20% of all patients. Oophorectomy is also very effective in premenopausal women with estrogen receptor positive cancer.

Newer 'biological' therapies targeting specific genes (such as the Her2 gene) can also improve survival.

Treatment of advanced breast cancer (T4;N2;M1)

Patients with locally advanced cancer, metastatic cancer or recurrent disease fall into this category. As treatment is palliative, it must be individualised to provide the maximum benefit with the minimum morbidity for each patient.

Treating the primary cancer
Radiotherapy, hormonal therapy or chemotherapy is used. Sometimes it is necessary to perform a 'toilet' mastectomy in order to control locally advanced but resectable disease.

Treating the metastases
Bone and soft tissue metastases usually respond well to hormonal manipulation. Visceral metastases (e.g. liver) respond better to chemotherapy. Bisphosphonates or radiotherapy are particularly useful in treating painful bone metastases.

In general, the order of choice for treatment of primary or metastatic breast disease is:

1. aromatase inhibitors*
2. antiestrogen therapy: tamoxifen*
3. chemotherapy.

Breast cancer follow-up
Close follow-up of breast cancer patients provides psychological support and aims to detect recurrence and to screen for cancer in the remaining breast.

Prognosis
Survival depends on:

- the number of axillary nodes involved with the tumour (see Figure 50)

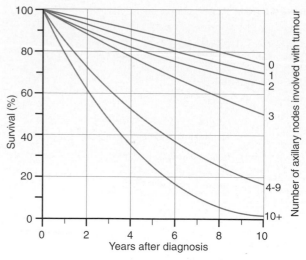

Figure 50 Correlation of survival with the number of axillary nodes involved with tumour.

- the size of the cancer
- the histological grade of the tumour
- the treatment received.

In general there is a 5-year survival of 80% and a 10-year survival of 60% in the UK. Despite appropriate treatment, however, many women will ultimately die of their disease.

5.2 Thyroid disease

Learning objectives
You should:
- know the main clinical features, investigation and treatment of hyperthyroidism
- understand the diagnostic steps in patients with a thyroid nodule
- understand the principles of thyroid surgery and the most common complications.

Patients with thyroid disease present most commonly with one or a combination of the following:

- hypothyroidism
- a lump in the neck which is of thyroid origin (a goitre)
- hyperthyroidism

Hypothyroidism

Hypothyroidism is common, affecting 5% of the female population (female–male ratio 10:1). It is an autoimmune disease caused by antibodies to the thyroid peroxidase enzyme (TPO) enzyme which is essential for thyroid hormone production. Patients can present with cold intolerance, lethargy, weight gain and constipation. They may have a small firm goitre.

* If estrogen receptor positive.

Diagnosis:
- raised thyroid-stimulating hormone (TSH) levels
- low serum-free T_4 and T_3 levels
- elevated TPO antibody levels.

Treatment:
- thyroxine replacement therapy.

Hyperthyroidism

Hyperthyroidism is caused by excess circulating thyroid hormones [usually thyroxine (T_4), occasionally triiodothyronine (T_3)] coupled with a loss of control of the feedback mechanisms regulating hormone secretion (suppressed TSH).

Most cases of hyperthyroidism are autoimmune in origin and produce a diffuse smooth swelling of the thyroid gland (Graves' disease). Less often, hyperthyroidism develops in a multinodular goitre or a solitary toxic adenoma (a single hyperfunctioning nodule).

Clinical features

There is usually a distinctive combination of symptoms and signs:

- irritability, fatigue, palpitations
- weight loss, increased appetite
- menstrual irregularities
- tremor, tachycardia
- goitre with a bruit ⎫ (with Graves'
- eye signs: lid lag, exophthalmos ⎬ disease only).

Diagnosis

The clinical diagnosis is confirmed by radioimmunoassay of the circulating thyroid hormone levels, which reveals:

- elevated serum T_4 or T_3 levels
- suppressed TSH levels
- thyroid antibodies (in Graves' disease TSH receptor antibody, TRAb).

Treatment

There are three treatment options.

- antithyroid drugs
- radioiodine
- thyroidectomy.

Antithyroid drugs Carbimazole and propylthiouracil are the drugs of choice. Both act by interfering with thyroid hormone synthesis. Treatment is continued for 1–2 years in the hope of inducing long-term remission. Recurrent thyrotoxicosis occurs in three out of four patients. Permanent agranulocytosis is an occasional but serious side effect of these drugs.

Radioiodine (^{131}I) therapy Radioiodine is taken up by the thyroid follicles and destroys the acinar cells, thus reducing T_3 and T_4 production. Its use is avoided in children and pregnant women because of the potential irradiation hazard. It is a highly effective treatment but in the long term leads to hypothyroidism and most patients ultimately need thyroid hormone replacement therapy. It is of most value in an older patient or one who is unfit for surgery.

Thyroidectomy Thyroidectomy controls thyrotoxicosis by reducing the functional mass of thyroid gland tissue. It is especially helpful in patients who do not comply or respond to antithyroid drug therapy or in patients who have a significant goitre. Nowadays, surgeons usually remove the entire thyroid gland to avoid possible recurrence of thyrotoxicosis. Postoperatively all these patients will require lifelong thyroid replacement therapy. In patients with severe thyrotoxicosis the conditions for surgery are optimised preoperatively by administering Lugol's iodine (potassium iodide) orally to reduce the vascularity of the gland, and by beta-adrenergic blockade, such as propranolol, to block the cardiovascular and central nervous system symptoms of thyrotoxicosis.

Post-thyroidectomy complications There are three important complications following thyroid (or parathyroid) surgery:

- postoperative haemorrhage, causing respiratory distress by tracheal compression
- hypocalcaemia caused by damage or inadvertent excision of the parathyroid glands
- recurrent laryngeal nerve injury, causing vocal cord paralysis and hoarseness.

Goitres

A goitre is an enlargement of the thyroid gland. Goitres may be toxic or non-toxic depending whether there is any associated hyperthyroidism. There are three main types:

- diffuse
- multinodular
- solitary thyroid nodules.

Diffuse goitre

These are usually physiological, the gland increasing in size during times of increased demand, e.g. during puberty or pregnancy.

Multinodular goitre

If the stimulus causing the goitre is prolonged, some areas of the gland will involute and others will enlarge, leading to a multinodular goitre. In areas where there is a dietary lack of iodine, this may lead to an endemic goitre; this can affect up to 70% of the population of that area.

Solitary thyroid nodules

Solitary thyroid nodules are common – 5% of women will develop a nodule in their lifetime. The vast majority (95%) are benign. There are four main causes of a single thyroid nodule:

- a prominent nodule within a multinodular goitre
- a thyroid cyst
- thyroid adenoma
- thyroid cancer.

Clinical features

A neck swelling is the primary complaint of most patients with a goitre. Other important symptoms are stridor and occasionally dysphagia (caused by local pressure effects on the trachea and oesophagus respectively) or symptoms of hyperthyroidism. Hoarseness or pain are rare and may indicate malignant infiltration from a thyroid cancer.

Goitres are midline in origin and move on swallowing (as the thyroid is invested in the pretracheal fascia). Occasionally, in adolescents, a thyroglossal cyst can also present as a midline swelling. These cysts develop along the line of the thyroglossal tract, an embryological remnant, which connects the back of the tongue to the thyroid gland. This connection means that a thyroglossal cyst will move on tongue protrusion (the thyroid gland does not) as well as on swallowing. It is important to ask a patient to swallow and also to stick out their tongue when examining a midline cervical swelling. The type of goitre can be determined by palpation, either nodular or smooth. A special check should be made for evidence of:

- tracheal deviation
- cervical lymphadenopathy
- signs of thyroid over- or underactivity.

Diagnosis

There are two key steps in the evaluation of a thyroid goitre or nodule:

- thyroid function tests (TSH, T_3 and free T_4)
- fine needle aspiration cytology (FNAC). FNAC will determine whether the follicular cells are benign, suspicious or frankly malignant.

Other useful tests include:

- thyroid ultrasound scan to differentiate cystic or solid areas and to guide the fine needle aspiration
- radiograph thoracic inlet to detect tracheal compression/deviation
- thyroid isotope (technetium) scan – useful if there is a solitary nodule and suppressed TSH, to look for a solitary toxic adenoma.

Treatment

A diffuse physiological goitre rarely requires surgical intervention. These patients are euthyroid and the goitre frequently regresses once the physiological stress (such as puberty or pregnancy) has passed.

In patients with multinodular goitre, surgery (usually total thyroidectomy) may be indicated for:

- pressure symptoms in the neck
- cosmetic reasons
- thyrotoxicosis.

The treatment of a solitary thyroid nodule depends on the FNAC result. If benign, the nodule can be left alone and a repeat FNAC performed in 6–12 months. If the FNAC is suspicious, a thyroid lobectomy is carried out, as a quarter of these nodules are malignant. If the FNAC is frankly malignant, a total thyroidectomy is carried out.

If the FNAC reveals the nodule to be a cyst, the treatment is different. Small cysts (<4 cm) which do not recur can be left alone. Larger cysts (>4 cm), or any cyst which recurs, are best treated by thyroid lobectomy because of the risk of malignancy.

Carcinoma of the thyroid gland

Thyroid cancer is uncommon compared to breast, colon and lung cancer. It accounts for 1% of all cancers in adults. There are four types of thyroid cancer. Although they all have similar clinical features initially, they differ in biological behaviour and response to therapy.

- differentiated thyroid cancer
  - papillary
  - follicular
- undifferentiated cancer
  - medullary cancer
  - thyroid lymphoma.

Papillary carcinoma This is the most common cancer and has the best prognosis. Disease spread is to the lymph nodes and by direct invasion into the neck. Distant metastases are infrequent.

Follicular carcinoma This tumour develops later in life than papillary cancer. Spread is mainly via the bloodstream with distant metastases to the bones, liver and brain.

Medullary carcinoma This uncommon cancer develops from the calcitonin-secreting parafollicular cells in the thyroid gland. It is sometimes associated with tumours in the parathyroid and adrenal glands – MEN (multiple endocrine neoplasia) type 2 syndrome.

Undifferentiated carcinoma This is the most aggressive thyroid malignancy. It is locally invasive to vital structures in the neck and has a poor prognosis.

Thyroid lymphoma This type of thyroid cancer usually presents as a rapidly increasing thyroid mass in an elderly female patient with long-standing hypothyroidism.

Clinical features

Almost all thyroid cancers present as a solitary thyroid nodule in a euthyroid patient. They occasionally develop in a multinodular goitre. There may be a history of irradiation to the head and neck during childhood or a family history of thyroid carcinoma.

Examination will usually reveal a hard mass, which may be fixed, with or without cervical lymphadenopathy. Patients are usually euthyroid.

Diagnosis

The investigations carried out are:

- thyroid function tests
- FNAC
- chest radiograph (to look for pulmonary metastases).

Treatment

Total thyroid lobectomy and total thyroidectomy are the main treatment options. If the FNAC shows definite malignancy most surgeons opt for total thyroidectomy. If the FNAC shows suspicious follicular cells, a thyroid lobectomy is carried out.

Lymph node or distant metastases can be effectively treated with radioiodine. Iodine is taken up by normal and differentiated (papillary or follicular) thyroid cancer cells. Following thyroidectomy any remaining thyroid cancer cells will take up and be destroyed by radioactive iodine. Differentiated thyroid cancers are also sensitive to TSH. In order to suppress the cellular activity of any remaining thyroid tissue, these patients are given sufficient doses of thyroxine to maximally suppress their endogenous TSH production.

Undifferentiated thyroid cancers are usually inoperable, have an extremely poor prognosis, and may be treated by external beam radiotherapy or chemotherapy. After biopsy, thyroid lymphoma is usually treated by chemotherapy alone or in combination with radiotherapy.

Prognosis

Survival ranges from 90% at 10 years for papillary cancer to 15% at 1 year for an undifferentiated cancer.

5.3 Parathyroid gland disease

Learning objectives

You should:
- understand the difference between primary, secondary and tertiary hyperparathyroidism
- know the clinical features of hyperparathyroidism
- be able to interpret the biochemical tests in patients with hyperparathyroidism
- understand the role of surgery in parathyroid disease.

Usually there are four parathyroid glands; occasionally there are three or five. Anatomically, they are arranged in pairs, the superior pair on the posterior surface of the thyroid gland intimately related to the recurrent laryngeal nerves, the inferior pair closer to the lower pole of the thyroid gland. The position of the glands and their number is variable and locating them at operation can be difficult.

The parathyroid glands secrete parathormone (PTH), which plays a vital role in calcium metabolism by mobilising calcium from the bones, reducing renal calcium excretion and promoting renal phosphate excretion. The secretion of PTH is inversely related to the circulating calcium level.

Overproduction of PTH can be classified into three groups depending on the cause:

- primary hyperparathyroidism (most common)
- secondary hyperparathyroidism
- tertiary hyperparathyroidism.

Primary hyperparathyroidism

This is an autonomous production of PTH by the parathyroid glands, which is not inhibited by the prevailing circulating calcium level. It is caused, in order of frequency, by:

1. a single parathyroid adenoma (85%)
2. generalised parathyroid hyperplasia (15%)
3. parathyroid carcinoma (1%).

Clinical features

Today, most patients with hyperparathyroidism are discovered incidentally during routine biochemical screening that includes a serum calcium determination.

Hitherto, many patients presented with a complex of symptoms caused by long-standing hyperparathyroidism, including:

- muscle weakness and arthralgia
- peptic ulcer disease
- abdominal pain and constipation
- renal calculi
- psychiatric disorders
- hypertension.

Diagnosis

The diagnosis is confirmed with biochemical tests:

- a high serum calcium level coupled with a low serum phosphate level is highly suggestive of hyperparathyroidism
- an elevated serum parathormone level coupled with a raised urinary calcium excretion completes the diagnosis.

In long-standing disease there may be several radiological changes:

- subperiosteal bone resorption in the phalanges
- generalised skeletal demineralisation
- renal calculi or nephrocalcinosis.

Differential diagnosis There are many conditions associated with an elevated serum calcium level. The most important are:

- metastatic cancer
- sarcoidosis
- myeloma.

Treatment

In a fit patient, surgery is the treatment of choice even when the disease is asymptomatic. Parathyroid exploration is a demanding operation as the glands may be difficult to locate. A sestamibi isotope scan is useful to localise the adenoma preoperatively.

An attempt should be made to identify all four glands, which usually are red/brown in colour. An adenomatous gland is usually enlarged and the diagnosis may be confirmed by frozen section analysis. Multiple adenomas should be removed and the normal glands left undisturbed. If four gland hyperplasia is present, a 'three and one-half' (subtotal) parathyroidectomy is performed leaving a fragment of one gland to act as functioning parathyroid tissue.

After surgery, a careful check on the serum calcium must be maintained as the circulating calcium levels can drop precipitously and cause symptomatic hypocalcaemia. Oral or intravenous calcium supplements may be needed.

Secondary hyperparathyroidism

This develops as a result of some of the complex metabolic changes associated with chronic renal failure, which tend to produce a low serum calcium level and an elevated serum phosphate level. As patients with chronic renal failure now live longer as a result of dialysis and renal transplantation, secondary hyperparathyroidism is becoming more common.

Unlike primary hyperparathyroidism, the primary treatment is medical, aimed at reducing circulating serum phosphate levels and boosting the dietary intake of calcium. The condition usually resolves after renal transplantation.

Tertiary hyperparathyroidism

In this infrequent condition, the parathyroid glands develop autonomous function in patients who have had long-standing secondary hyperparathyroidism. It is often only detected after a successful renal transplantation, where patients develop a persistent hypercalcaemia and should be treated by subtotal parathyroidectomy.

5.4 Adrenal gland disease

Learning objectives

You should:

* recognise the importance of adrenal disease in patients presenting with hypertension
* understand the complex diagnostic and treatment pathways in patients with phaeochromocytoma or primary hyperaldosteronism
* recognise the difference (and the relationship) between Cushing syndrome and Cushing's disease.

Patients with adrenal disease rarely present for surgery because of an abdominal mass arising from one or other of the adrenal glands. Instead, oversecretion of adrenal medullary or cortical hormones leads to a variety of complex syndromes that can be resolved by surgical removal of the diseased adrenal gland.

There are three surgically treatable disorders:

* phaeochromocytoma
* primary hyperaldosteronism
* Cushing syndrome and Cushing's disease.

Phaeochromocytoma

A phaeochromocytoma is a neuroendocrine tumour that arises from the chromaffin cells in the adrenal medulla. It affects both sexes, usually in early adult life. Phaeochromocytomas produce an excess of catecholamines [noradrenaline (norepinephrine) and adrenaline (epinephrine)] either intermittently or continuously. 10% are bilateral, 10% are malignant and 10% are extra-adrenal in position.

Clinical features

Patients present in two ways:

* dramatically, in a hypertensive crisis with sweating, palpitations, severe headache and occasionally a myocardial infarction or cerebrovascular accident
* insidiously, with diastolic hypertension.

Classically, the hypertensive attacks can be provoked by exercise, straining or abdominal palpation, all of which lead to the release of a pulse of catecholamines.

Diagnosis

As approximately 1 in 1000 of all newly diagnosed hypertensive patients have an underlying phaeochromocytoma, some physicians recommend that all young hypertensive patients should be screened for this disease.

Metabolite levels The key diagnostic test is based on the detection of elevated catecholamine levels (dopamine, noradrenaline and adrenaline) in a 24-h urine collection.

Tumour localisation CT scanning and magnetic resonance imaging (MRI) are the primary means of identifying the tumour. Radioisotope scanning using metaiodobenzylguanidine (MIBG) may be used to confirm the diagnosis. Uptake of the radioisotope by the neuroendocrine tissue creates 'hotspots' on the scan identifying the location of the tumour.

Treatment

Because surgical manipulation of a phaeochromocytoma is likely to provoke massive catecholamine release, these patients require careful preoperative preparation and perioperative care in order to prevent wild and potentially fatal fluctuations in heart rate and blood pressure.

Usually, alpha-adrenergic blockade (phenoxybenzamine) is started some time before surgery, with agents such as nitroprusside and propranolol being used to control the blood pressure and heart rate during the operation.

The site of the phaeochromocytoma is localised preoperatively by the above imaging and most can be removed by laparoscopic surgery.

Prognosis

Surgery is usually curative, although a mild hypertension may persist. Patients should be followed up by annual 24-h catecholamine collections. Untreated, most patients with phaeochromocytoma will ultimately die during a hypertensive crisis.

Primary hyperaldosteronism (Conn syndrome)

The primary function of aldosterone (a mineralocorticoid) is to maintain the circulating intravascular volume. This is achieved by promoting renal sodium reabsorption in exchange for renal potassium loss. In normal individuals, the secretion of aldosterone is closely regulated by the renin–angiotensin mechanism (Figure 51).

Most cases of primary hyperaldosteronism are caused by unilateral adrenal cortical adenomas. Some cases are caused by bilateral adrenal cortical hyperplasia. It is important to differentiate these preoperatively as hypertension caused by adrenal cortical hyperplasia should be treated medically.

Clinical features

These are very non-specific. The diagnosis is usually suspected based on biochemical tests that show an unexplained hypokalaemia in a hypertensive patient. Vague headaches, muscle weakness and fatigue are the most common complaints. Approximately 1% of hypertensive patients have primary hyperaldosteronism.

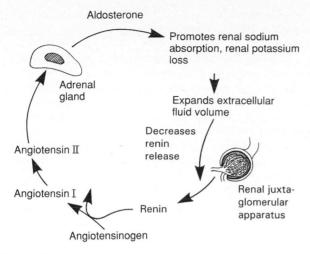

Figure 51 Renin–angiotensin mechanism.

Diagnosis

Establishing the diagnosis can be a complex and time-consuming task. Three blood tests are used in combination to detect inappropriately elevated aldosterone levels in the face of suppressed plasma renin levels:

- urea and electrolytes (↓ serum potassium)
- ↑ plasma aldosterone
- ↓ plasma renin.

This triad of results is diagnostic of primary hyperaldosteronism. If only two criteria are met the tests are repeated after administering a high-sodium diet. Primary hyperaldosteronism is confirmed if the plasma aldosterone levels remain elevated.

Tumour localisation

A CT or MRI scan may identify an adrenal tumour. If no tumour is detected an iodocholesterol (NP-59) isotope scan is used to identify small unilateral tumours from bilateral hyperplasia.

Treatment

Bilateral hyperplasia is best treated medically using large doses of spironolactone, which acts as an aldosterone antagonist. A unilateral laparoscopic adrenalectomy is the treatment of choice for an adrenal adenoma.

Cushing syndrome and Cushing's disease

Cushing syndrome is caused by an excess secretion of glucocorticoids (cortisone and corticosterone) by the adrenal cortex. There are three main causes:

- Secondary to increased adrenocortical stimulation by ACTH (adrenocorticotrophic hormone) produced by a basophil pituitary adenoma. This is Cushing's disease and accounts for 75% of cases of Cushing syndrome. These patients have bilateral adrenocortical hyperplasia.
- Adrenocortical tumours (20% of cases), most of which are benign adenomas; carcinomas are rare.
- Ectopic sites of ACTH production (usually cancers) (5%).

In each case, it is important to be certain of the precise cause, as the management of each group is different.

Clinical features

Cushing syndrome is at least 10 times more common in women than in men. One or more of the following features will be present:

- truncal obesity, moon face, buffalo hump
- abdominal striae, hirsutism
- menstrual disturbance
- psychological disturbance.

Many of these patients will be mildly hypertensive or diabetic.

Diagnosis

The two key questions are:

1. Is there excess glucocorticoid secretion?
2. If so, is it pituitary dependent (Cushing's disease)?

A combination of tests are required to provide the answer. Excess glucocorticoid secretion is proved if:

- the normal diurnal variation of ACTH and cortisol secretion (with plasma levels peaking in the early morning and reaching a nadir in the evening) is lost
- 24-h urinary cortisol excretion levels are elevated
- the administration of dexamethasone, a potent synthetic glucocorticoid, does not suppress endogenous corticosteroid production (dexamethasone suppression test).

These tests collectively will confirm the diagnosis of Cushing syndrome. It remains to determine whether or not this is secondary to excess pituitary ACTH secretion (Cushing's disease). This is confirmed by:

- plasma ACTH measurements using radioimmunoassay; high ACTH levels are diagnostic of pituitary tumours, low levels are diagnostic of adrenal adenomas
- CT or MRI scanning of the adrenal glands and pituitary fossa, which will localise the adenoma in most cases.

Treatment

There are two surgical options:

- pituitary ablation
- adrenalectomy.

Pituitary ablation ACTH-secreting pituitary tumours can be removed by neurosurgeons using microsurgical techniques. Currently, the favoured approach is through the sphenoid bone and the operation is termed a trans-sphenoidal hypophysectomy. In patients who are unfit for surgery, pituitary ablation can be performed by external beam irradiation.

Adrenalectomy Patients with Cushing syndrome are often obese and prone to infection and heal poorly. As a result, transabdominal bilateral adrenalectomy for Cushing's disease is only considered when attempts at pituitary ablation have failed. Adrenalectomy is the only option for those patients with a hypersecreting adrenal adenoma or carcinoma.

Multiple endocrine adenomatosis

Parathyroid hyperplasia is occasionally associated with a familial tendency to develop multiple functioning endocrine adenomas known as multiple endocrine adenomatoses. Occasionally a carcinoma will develop. The two commonest combinations are:

MEN type 1 syndrome. Parathyroid hyperplasia; pituitary chromophobe adenoma; pancreatic islet cell adenoma.

MEN type 2 syndrome. Parathyroid adenoma; medullary thyroid carcinoma; phaeochromocytoma.

Patients present either with clinical features caused by the secretions of these functioning adenomas or with a mass in the abdomen or neck caused by the growing tumour. The individual tumours may grow synchronously or metachronously. Treatment is complex but is usually directed at removing the adenoma if this is technically possible.

Self-assessment: questions

Extended matching items questions (EMIs)

EMI 1

Theme: Breast disease

A. Paget's disease

B. fibroadenoma

C. breast cyst

D. breast carcinoma

E. mammary duct ectasia

F. mammary duct fistula

G. fibrocystic disease of the breast

H. gynaecomastia

What is the most likely diagnosis in the following patients?

1. A 47-year-old woman who has been aware of a painful right nipple for 2 months. For the last 2 weeks she has been aware of a discharge from that nipple. Since then the pain has been less severe. When you examine her you notice that a greenish discharge can be expressed from a single opening at the outer margin of the areola.

2. A 69-year-old woman who complains of an itch affecting the right nipple over the last 4 months. She attends because she has noticed some 'crusting' over the nipple and a discharge which stains her bra.

3. A 25-year-old woman who presents with a 6-month history of a left breast lump. On examination you detect a 3 cm firm, painless lump with a well defined margin which feels quite mobile within the surrounding breast tissue.

4. A 72-year-old man who takes digoxin for atrial fibrillation presents with bilateral tender swollen breasts.

EMI 2

Theme: Thyroid disease

A. subtotal thyroidectomy

B. 6 months' treatment with carbimazole

C. 24 months' treatment with carbimazole

D. thyroid lobectomy

E. near-total thyroidectomy

F. cervical radiotherapy

G. radioactive iodine, followed by lifelong thyroxine supplements

H. 6 weeks' Lugol's iodine therapy

Which of the above treatments is most appropriate in the following patients?

1. A 55-year-old woman who presents with a swelling in the left side of her neck. This appears to be a 5-cm cyst on ultrasound and this is confirmed on needle aspiration. This is the third time this cyst has recurred in the last 6 months.

2. A 34-year-old woman who presents to her GP with 'anxiety attacks'. On examination she has a resting tachycardia and a mild tremor. She has a small goitre and her serum free thyroxine level is 60 pmol/ml (normal range 10–30 pmol/ml).

3. A 65-year-old woman who presents with a neck swelling. On examination she appears euthyroid and has a hard irregular swelling that diffusely involves the entire gland. The swelling appears fixed and on needle aspiration appears to be a poorly differentiated carcinoma.

4. A 55-year-old man who has undergone a near-total thyroidectomy for a follicular carcinoma which had arisen in the left lobe of the gland.

EMI 3

Theme: Thyroid disease

A. Graves' disease

B. autoimmune hypothyroidism

C. thyroid lymphoma

D. thyroglossal cyst

E. multinodular goitre with retrosternal extension and tracheal compression

F. papillary thyroid cancer

For each of the following presentations select the most appropriate diagnosis. Each diagnosis may be used once, more than once or not at all.

1. A 35-year-old female presents with hoarseness and a firm irregular mass on the right side of the neck with ipsilateral cervical lymphadenopathy.

2. A 70-year-old male presents with stridor; a chest radiograph shows a superior mediastinal mass with tracheal deviation.

3. A 30-year-old female presents with tiredness and lethargy and on examination is found to have a small firm goitre.

4. A 25-year-old female presents with increased appetite, weight loss and irritability. On examination she has lower eyelid retraction and a firm smooth goitre with an audible bruit.

5. An elderly female patient with long-standing hypothyroidism presents with a recent onset of a rapidly enlarging thyroid mass.

Constructed response questions (CRQs)

CRQ 1

A 58-year-old woman presents with a 2-cm painless lump in the right breast that she detected during self-examination.

a. What features on clinical examination would make you suspect the lump was malignant?

Examination confirms your clinical suspicion.

b. List three questions you would ask this patient to assess whether she was at an increased risk of developing breast cancer.

c. How would you confirm the diagnosis?

Your tests confirm a diagnosis of breast cancer.

d. Name two tests that would be useful in a search for metastatic disease.

Assessment of this patient's breast cancer confirms the disease is localised to the breast.

e. What surgical options would you recommend?

The pathology after her surgery shows an estrogen receptor positive cancer with metastasis to 2 of 10 axillary lymph nodes.

f. What systemic adjuvant therapy might be offered?

CRQ 2

A 36-year-old woman presents with a swelling in the right side of her neck. In addition she tells you she has lost 8 kg in weight in the last 3 months. When you examine her she appears to have a 5-cm nodule in the right lobe of her thyroid gland. You wonder if she might be thyrotoxic.

a. What physical signs would you look for to support this diagnosis? List three of them.

Physical examination confirms a clinical diagnosis of thyrotoxicosis.

b. What specific blood tests would you ask for to confirm the diagnosis?

c. These tests confirm the diagnosis. What further investigations would you arrange before treatment?

The patient asks you about the diagnosis.

d. What are the treatment options?

e. What would you recommend?

CRQ 3

A 50-year-old man presents with a swelling in his neck. His general practitioner is certain it is a thyroid gland swelling.

a. What are the relevant points in this patient's history? List three.

You agree with the general practitioner's clinical diagnosis.

b. How would you confirm on clinical examination that the lump is thyroid in origin?

You tell the patient the most likely diagnosis and explain that several tests will be required.

c. List three specific diagnostic tests which will be useful in this patient.

The results of these tests confirm that the patient will require a total thyroidectomy. The patient asks about the risks of this operation.

d. List three complications of thyroidectomy.

Objective structured clinical examination questions (OSCEs)

OSCE 1

Examine the accompanying photograph (Figure 52) then answer the following questions.

a. What is the most likely diagnosis?

b. What tests would you use to confirm the diagnosis?

c. What is the underlying disease process?

d. What is the most appropriate treatment?

OSCE 2

Look at this radiograph (Figure 53) then answer the following questions.

a. What is this examination?

b. What abnormal features can you identify?

c. What is the most likely diagnosis?

d. How would you confirm the diagnosis?

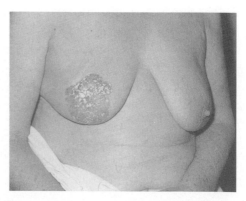

Figure 52

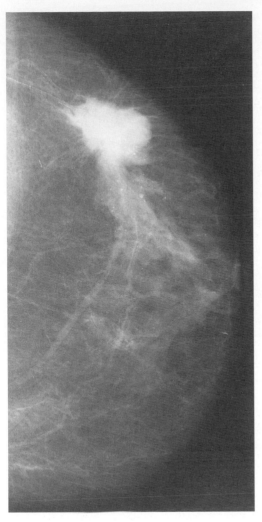

Figure 53

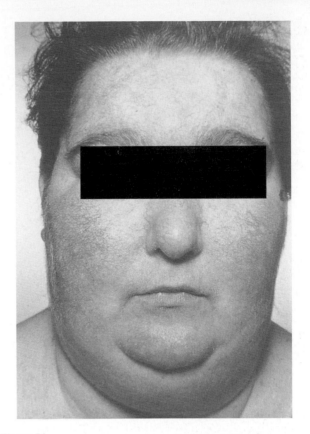

Figure 54

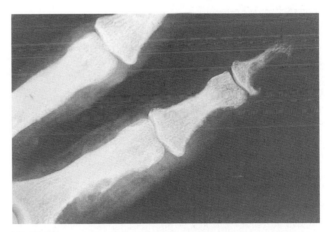

Figure 55

OSCE 3

Look at the accompanying clinical photograph (Figure 54) then answer the following questions.

  a. What abnormal features can you identify?

  b. What can cause this appearance?

  c. Describe three other clinical features you would look for.

  d. A drug history confirms this patient is not taking any medication. How would you confirm the diagnosis?

OSCE 4

Look at this radiograph (Figure 55) then answer the following questions.

  a. What abnormalities are present on this radiograph?

  b. What other radiological abnormalities might you identify in the same patient?

  c. What is the most likely cause?

  d. How would you confirm the diagnosis?

Best of 5s questions

1. A 28-year-old female presents with a 4-month history of a right solitary thyroid nodule. She is otherwise asymptomatic. Investigations show a TSH of 3.5 mU/l (normal range 0.4–4.0 mU/l) and her FNAC is reported as highly suspicious of papillary thyroid cancer.

Her subsequent treatment should consist of:

    a. lifelong thyroxine to suppress her TSH

    b. 2 years' treatment with carbimazole

    c. total thyroidectomy with postoperative diagnostic radioactive iodine

    d. radioactive iodine alone

    e. external beam radiotherapy

2. A 45-year-old man presents with uncontrolled hypertension. A 24-h urinary catecholamine excretion shows a significantly raised adrenaline level. Subsequent CT scanning shows a 3-cm mass in the right adrenal gland.

This patient should be treated by:

    a. immediate adrenalectomy

    b. preparation with beta blockade followed by adrenalectomy

    c. preparation with alpha blockade followed by adrenalectomy

    d. antihypertensive drugs only

    e. therapeutic MIBG scan

Multiple choice questions

1. In patients with fibrocystic breast changes:

    a. axillary lymphadenopathy is common

    b. the incidence peaks between 35 and 45 years of age

    c. symptoms are worse after menstruation

    d. gammalinoleic acid can improve symptoms

    e. the incidence of breast cancer is doubled

2. The following points relate to mammography:

    a. all patients over 35 years of age with a nipple discharge need a mammogram

    b. all patients with fibrocystic breast changes need mammography

    c. stellate lesions on mammography require biopsy

    d. areas of microcalcification on mammography require biopsy

    e. it can detect cancers up to 2 years before they become palpable

3. Gynaecomastia:

    a. is usually drug induced

    b. resolves spontaneously in most cases

    c. is more common in patients over 25 years of age

    d. can be bilateral

    e. is occasionally caused by hypothyroidism

4. A bloodstained nipple discharge is associated with:

    a. mammary duct ectasia

    b. an intraduct papilloma

    c. a fibroadenoma

    d. Paget's disease of the breast

    e. breast carcinoma

5. Breast cancer is more common in women:

    a. with a family history of breast cancer

    b. who have undergone bilateral oophorectomy

    c. who have had endometrial cancer

    d. who smoke

    e. who have had a late first pregnancy

6. In Paget's disease of the breast:

    a. there is usually an underlying intraduct papilloma

    b. itching is an early symptom

    c. an underlying breast mass is a common feature

    d. the diagnosis is made primarily on mammography

    e. radiotherapy is the primary treatment

7. In the treatment of advanced breast cancer:

    a. painful bone metastases respond best to chemotherapy

    b. 60% of patients are expected to live 5 years

    c. mastectomy still has a role to play

    d. estrogen receptor status may influence management

    e. chemotherapy may be useful in the treatment of liver metastases

8. The following points relate to goitres:

    a. they often cause hoarseness

    b. stridor is an indication for thyroidectomy

    c. diffuse goitres are associated with iodine deficiency

    d. hot nodules are rarely malignant

    e. most patients with multinodular goitres are euthyroid

9. In thyroid cancer:

    a. papillary tumours spread mainly to the bones

    b. a preceding multinodular goitre is common

    c. a thyroid isotope scan is likely to show a cold area

    d. radioiodine is the treatment of choice for secondary deposits from follicular cancers

    e. cervical lymphadenopathy is more frequent with papillary cancers

10. The following statements relate to radioiodine therapy:

    a. recurrent thyrotoxicosis is uncommon

    b. agranulocytosis is a significant side effect

    c. post-treatment hypothyroidism is infrequent

    d. it is the treatment of choice for recurrent thyrotoxicosis

    e. it should be avoided in childhood thyrotoxicosis

11. In primary hyperparathyroidism:

    a. a single parathyroid adenoma is the most likely cause

b. renal phosphate excretion is increased

c. most patients have radiological evidence of sub-periosteal bone resorption in the phalanges

d. chronic renal failure is uncommon

e. most patients will complain of polyuria and polydypsia

12. A phaeochromocytoma:

    a. usually presents early in adult life

    b. is diagnosed by an elevated serum catecholamine level

    c. is caused by adrenal cortical hyperplasia

    d. may be a cause of stroke

    e. can be bilateral

13. A patient with Conn syndrome:

    a. is usually hyperkalaemic

    b. may present with hypertension

    c. can be treated medically with spironolactone

    d. has an elevated plasma renin

    e. usually has an underlying adrenal cortical adenoma

14. A patient with Cushing syndrome:

    a. will occasionally have a visual field defect

    b. is more likely to be male

    c. will have a low evening serum cortisol level

    d. may be diabetic

    e. may have an associated thyroid cancer

Self-assessment: answers

EMI answers

EMI 1

Theme: Breast disease

1. F. Mammary duct fistula.

This history is in keeping with an episode of sepsis in the nipple which has resolved when the infected material spontaneously discharged through the skin. Once the pressure was released, the pain subsided. The identification of a discharging sinus at the outer margin of the nipple areola confirms the diagnosis of a mammary duct fistula. This is usually a consequence of a blocked lactiferous duct or mammary duct ectasia.

2. A. Paget's disease.

This history bears the hallmark of Paget's disease – a nipple itch, eczematous changes in the nipple, areola and surrounding skin, together with bleeding or discharge from the nipple. These changes are inevitably associated with an underlying breast cancer.

3. B. Fibroadenoma.

The clinical description of the breast lump and the age of the patient provide the key clues to the diagnosis. A fibroadenoma is characteristically smooth, firm, has a well-defined margin and is highly mobile within the breast (hence the term 'breast mouse'). It is the commonest cause of a breast lump in a woman in her mid-20s. The diagnosis would be confirmed by ultrasound as the breast will be too dense for mammographic interpretation.

4. H. Gynaecomastia.

Breast swelling in men is usually physiological (in young men) or secondary to systemic disease which results in elevated estrogens (e.g. cirrhosis) or secondary to medications (digoxin included). Based on the history and examination, which should demonstrate a tender swelling but normal skin and nipple, reassurance or surgery (if particularly tender or large) may be offered.

EMI 2

Theme: Thyroid disease

1. D. Thyroid lobectomy.

This patient has a large recurrent cyst in the left lobe of her thyroid gland. The size of the cyst and the frequency of recurrence over a short period of time are all indications for surgical treatment. A thyroid lobectomy will remove the cyst-bearing tissue while endocrine function will be preserved by the remaining lobe of the gland.

2. C. 24 months' carbimazole.

Mild disease, a young patient and a small goitre are all good indications for using antithyroid drugs as first option in the management of thyrotoxicosis. A prolonged course of treatment (usually more than 18 months) is required to secure remission.

3. F. Cervical radiotherapy.

Undifferentiated thyroid carcinoma usually invades the structures surrounding the thyroid gland (trachea/carotid sheath etc.) and is rarely resectable. Progress of the tumour is usually rapid and the symptoms (stridor, pain, dysphagia) can only be palliated either with radiotherapy alone or in combination with chemotherapy. These tumours do not respond to treatment with radioiodine therapy.

4. G. Radioactive iodine followed by lifelong thyroxine supplements.

This patient has undergone a near-total thyroidectomy for follicular cancer. This tumour is sensitive to thyroid stimulating hormone which can stimulate regrowth of the cancer. To prevent this, patients are given lifelong thyroxine supplements after surgery, which will suppress their production of thyroid-stimulating hormone.

EMI 3

Theme: Thyroid disease

1. F. Papillary thyroid cancer.

Hoarseness and a firm mass point to a probable thyroid cancer, with direct involvement of the recurrent laryngeal nerve, leading to ipsilateral vocal cord palsy and subsequent hoarseness. The surrounding lymphadenopathy suggest a papillary thyroid carcinoma, as this spreads by invasion of local lymph nodes.

2. E. Multinodular goitre with retrosternal extension and tracheal compression.

Stridor is caused by narrowing of the windpipe (tracheal compression). Long-standing multinodular goitres tend to have a retrosternal component, which can displace the trachea, causing deviation and compression of the trachea.

3. B. Autoimmune hypothyroidism.

Classically, autoimmune hypothyroidism presents with these features of an underactive thyroid. A small firm smooth goitre is also usually present.

4. A. Graves' disease.

The symptoms suggest an overactive thyroid (hyperthyroidism) and the bruit and eye signs point to Graves' disease (autoimmune thyrotoxicosis).

5. C. Thyroid lymphoma.

Be wary of an elderly hypothyroid female patient who presents with a quickly enlarging thyroid mass. These are the typical features of a thyroid lymphoma.

CRQ answers

CRQ 1

a. indrawn nipple

   peau d'orange skin

a non-tender lump

irregular lump with poorly defined edge

bloodstained nipple discharge

skin or chest-wall tethering

axillary or supraclavicular lymphadenopathy

Any of these responses will score marks. In any individual patient a combination of some but not all of these physical signs will be present.

b. a family history of breast cancer

a late first pregnancy or a late menopause

family history of ovarian cancer

use of oral contraceptives or HRT

Any of these responses will score marks. A family history of breast cancer (women whose mothers and sisters have had a breast cancer) is most important and is present in 10% of all cases.

c. clinical history plus examination

mammography ± ultrasound

cytology/pathology

These are the essential steps in the 'triple assessment' of any breast lump. For most women, clinical examination is followed by mammography and FNAC. In the unlikely event that a firm tissue diagnosis is not obtained, the diagnosis could be confirmed either by a large bore needle core biopsy under local anaesthetic or by open diagnostic biopsy under local or general anaesthetic.

d. chest radiograph

liver ultrasound scan

isotope bone scan

Any of these responses will score marks. The lungs, bones and liver are the commonest sites for breast cancer metastases. Most surgeons would only look for metastases in patients with a large primary cancer or an axillary lymph gland mass or in those patients with abnormal liver function tests.

e. wide local excision plus radiotherapy plus axillary gland clearance or axillary sample

mastectomy plus axillary gland clearance or axillary sample

The choice of operation would be determined by the size and site of the tumour relative to the breast (a large tumour in a small breast is better treated by mastectomy) and would also take into account the patient's wishes about conservation of the breast. In either case axillary node clearance (or axillary gland sampling) is essential to 'stage' the axilla (lymph gland positive or negative) and to provide guidance for any adjuvant chemotherapy or endocrine therapy in addition to providing local disease control.

CRQ 2

a. tremor

resting tachycardia

thyroid bruit

eye signs – lid lag, exophthalmos

Any of these responses will score marks. Tremor and tachycardia are common to almost all patients with thyrotoxicosis. 75% will have a thyroid bruit and almost 50% will have eye signs.

b. Serum T_4 or T_3 levels

Thyroid stimulating hormone (TSH) levels.

An elevated serum T_4 (or T_3) level with a suppressed TSH level will clinch the diagnosis.

c. FNAC

isotopic thyroid scan

thyroid ultrasound scan

radiograph thoracic inlet

Any of these responses will score points. A thyroid isotope scan would confirm that the palpable nodule is functional (hot nodule) and an FNAC will identify any cytological abnormalities. An radiograph of the thoracic inlet would check for tracheal deviation or a mediastinal component to the thyroid gland.

d. antithyroid drugs

radioiodine treatment

surgical resection: thyroid lobectomy

Any of these responses will score points.

e. right thyroid lobectomy

Antithyroid drugs are of most use in small diffuse goitres. The presence of a large nodule in the thyroid gland would be a relative contraindication to this treatment. Radioiodine therapy would probably be effective but is better reserved for patients who are over 40 years of age or who are unfit for surgery. A thyroid lobectomy is probably the best option for a young patient with a toxic thyroid nodule.

CRQ 3

a. any history of symptoms suggestive of hyper- or hypothyroidism

family history of thyroid disease

past medical history of neck irradiation

any history of hoarseness

Hoarseness is a *significant* symptom, suggesting vocal cord palsy, caused by tumour infiltrating the recurrent laryngeal nerve. A family history of thyroid cancer or previous neck radiotherapy is a possible pointer to thyroid malignancy.

b. ask the patient to swallow, ask the patient to protrude his tongue

A thyroid lump will move on swallowing, as the thyroid is invested by the pre-tracheal fascia. If the lump also moves up on protrusion of the tongue, then it is a thyroglossal cyst, which is connected by a tract to the back of the tongue.

c. thyroid function tests

FNAC

thyroid isotope scan

ultrasound of the thyroid

The key two tests are to check the thyroid function (by measuring the TSH) and to do a fine needle aspiration of the lump, which will determine whether the lump is benign, suspicious or malignant. Ultrasound will show whether the lump is cystic; an isotope scan will show if the nodule is 'hot' (takes up the isotope) – this is useful in patients whose TSH is suppressed (i.e. hyperthyroid).

d. haematoma

recurrent laryngeal nerve palsy

hypoparathyroidism

hypothyroidism

The main complications to know are damage to the recurrent laryngeal nerve (about 3% of cases) and damage to the parathyroid glands, leading to hypoparathyroidism (about 10% of cases). If the whole thyroid is removed (total thyroidectomy), then the patient will obviously become hypothyroid. Haematoma is a complication of any operation, but is more potentially dangerous in the neck as it can cause tracheal compression and laryngeal oedema, leading to significant stridor. If stridor is present, then the haematoma needs to be urgently evacuated.

OSCE answers

OSCE 1

a. Paget's disease of the nipple.

The typical features of Paget's disease are evident.

The nipple has been entirely covered by an eczematous rash which has spread onto the surrounding skin.

b. Triple assessment:
- clinical history and examination
- mammography
- cytology/pathology.

This is the key to assessment of all breast disease. In this case a biopsy of the nipple might also be necessary.

c. Carcinoma of the breast.

This tumour usually originates in the ducts beneath the nipple. In the early stages of the disease a lump may not be evident in the breast on examination.

d. Total mastectomy and axillary clearance.

This is the sole treatment option since it is necessary to remove the nipple and the underlying breast tissue en bloc in order to achieve tumour clearance.

OSCE 2

a. This is a mammogram.

b. The radiograph shows a stellate lesion which causes puckering and distortion of the surrounding breast

tissue. There are one or two areas of microcalcification.

c. Breast cancer.

An irregular radiodense breast mass with a spiculated border which contains areas of microcalcification is the hallmark of a breast cancer.

d. FNAC

OSCE 3

a. A steroid or moon face, excess facial hair.

b. Prolonged exogenous steroid administration or Cushing syndrome or Cushing's disease. All can produce the characteristic 'Cushingoid' face.

c. Hirsutism, abdominal striae, central abdominal obesity (a buffalo hump), menstrual irregularities and hypertension.

These features may be present in any combination.

d. The diagnosis is confirmed when excess or inappropriate steroid secretion is demonstrated by one or a combination of the following tests:
- loss of the normal diurnal plasma cortisol levels (morning peak, evening trough)
- elevated 24-h urinary cortisol levels dexamethasone suppression test.

OSCE 4

a. This radiograph shows areas of subperiosteal bone resorption in the phalanges.

b. Renal calculi, ectopic renal calcification.

c. Primary hypoparathyroidism is the most common cause.

d. The diagnosis would be confirmed by demonstrating elevated serum calcium levels in the presence of an elevated serum parathormone level.

Best of 5s answers

1. c. Total thyroidectomy with postoperative diagnostic radioiodine.

Papillary thyroid carcinoma is best treated by total thyroidectomy. Afterwards, a diagnostic radioactive iodine scan is used to assess whether there is any significant residual uptake within the thyroid bed or local lymph nodes. If there is, a therapeutic radioactive iodine dose is given to ablate the residual thyroid cancer cells.

2. c. Preparation with alpha blockade followed by adrenalectomy.

The hypertension and subsequent investigations all point to the diagnosis of a phaeochromocytoma. The hypertension should be well controlled with alpha blockers (*not* beta blockers), prior to removal by adrenalectomy.

Multiple choice answers

1. a. **False.** Axillary lymphadenopathy is uncommon. Its presence should raise the suspicion of malignancy.

b. **True.** The incidence of benign breast disease diminishes after the menopause.

c. **False.** Symptoms are often worse premenstrually, especially in patients with cyclical breast pain.

d. **True.** Gamma-linoleic acid (evening primrose oil) is useful; the mechanism is unknown.

e. **False.** The incidence of breast cancer is the same in patients with or without benign breast disease.

2. a. **True.** These patients may have an underlying cancer.

b. **False.** Often these patients are young with radiodense breasts. Mammography is best reserved for those patients over 35 years of age who have a localised area of nodularity or tenderness.

c. **True.** A stellate lesion on radiography may be an invasive carcinoma.

d. **True.** Any area of microcalcification needs to be biopsied to exclude a cancer.

e. **True.** Breast cancers may remain impalpable for up to 2 years. It is this group of tumours that are detected by mammographic screening programmes, enabling earlier treatment.

3. a. **False.** Gynaecomastia is usually a physiological change at puberty. Drug-induced gynaecomastia is the second most common cause.

b. **True.** Surgical treatment should be reserved for the few cases that do not resolve within 2 years.

c. **False.** The peak incidence is around puberty.

d. **True.**

e. **False.** Gynaecomastia is associated with hyperthyroidism.

4. a. **False.** The discharge associated with duct ectasia is yellow/green in colour.

b. **True.**

c. **False.** Fibroadenomas are not associated with nipple discharge.

d. **True.** An itching, excoriated bleeding nipple is the hallmark of Paget's disease.

e. **True.** A bloodstained nipple discharge is related to an underlying breast cancer until proven otherwise.

5. a. **True.** The risk is doubled in patients with a first-degree relative (mother, sister or daughter) who develops cancer before the age of 50 years.

b. **False.** Oophorectomy, particularly in young women (under 35 years of age), reduces the risk of breast cancer.

c. **True.** Endometrial and ovarian cancer appear to increase the risk of breast cancer.

d. **False.** There is no link between smoking and breast cancer.

e. **True.** A late first pregnancy, early menarche and late menopause are all associated with an increased risk.

6. a. **False.** There is usually an underlying intraduct breast carcinoma.

b. **True.** Itching and scaling of the nipple are usually the first signs of Paget's disease.

c. **False.** In the early stages of the disease, the underlying breast cancer is usually impalpable.

d. **False.** Nipple biopsy is the key diagnostic test. Microscopic examination will reveal large round Paget cells with clear cytoplasm and hyperchromatic nuclei.

e. **False.** The lesion should be treated as a breast cancer.

7. a. **False.** Radiotherapy is the treatment of choice for a painful bone metastasis.

b. **False.** Survival is less than 40% at 5 years for advanced breast cancer.

c. **True.** Mastectomy coupled with radiotherapy is probably the best way to deal with a locally extensive but resectable cancer that untreated may fungate or become attached to the chest wall.

d. **True.** Estrogen receptor positive patients are more likely to respond to hormonal manipulation.

e. **True.** Visceral metastases may be usefully palliated using chemotherapy.

8. a. **False.** Hoarseness suggests infiltration of the larynx or recurrent laryngeal nerves by thyroid malignancy.

b. **True.** Stridor or dysphagia is an indication for thyroidectomy.

c. **False.** A diffuse goitre is more likely to be physiological in origin during pregnancy or puberty. Iodine-deficient goitres are usually multinodular.

d. **True.** Hot nodules are caused by areas of thyroid overactivity. Malignancy is associated with cold nodules.

e. **True.** Hyperthyroidism uncommonly develops in a multinodular goitre.

9. a. **False.** Bone metastases arising from thyroid cancer are usually associated with follicular tumours.

b. **False.** Cancers infrequently develop in a multi-nodular goitre.

c. **True.** Cold areas on scanning are caused by either malignancy or simple cysts.

d. **True.** Follicular tumours avidly take up radio-iodine, which destroys the deposits.

e. **True.** Papillary cancers metastasise most often to the cervical lymph glands.

10. a. **False.** Radioiodine treatment is highly effective.

b. **False.** Agranulocytosis is a side effect of antithyroid drug treatment with agents such as carbimazole.

c. **False.** Many patients require thyroid hormone replacement after treatment. The incidence increases with time.

d. **True.** Surgery for recurrent thyrotoxicosis can be difficult and risks damage to the recurrent laryngeal nerves and parathyroid glands. Radioiodine or antithyroid drugs are the treatment of choice.

e. **True.** Although there is no increased risk of malignancy, almost all children treated with radioiodine will eventually become hypothyroid. For this reason, children should not have radioiodine treatment.

11. a. **True.** Of all cases of primary hyperparathyroidism, 90% are caused by a single adenoma.

b. **True.** Parathormone inhibits renal reabsorption of phosphate.

c. **False.** Subperiosteal bone resorption is a late sign in long-standing disease.

d. **True.** Chronic renal failure is more usually the cause of secondary hyperparathyroidism.

e. **False.** Most patients are diagnosed when asymptomatic, on routine biochemical screening.

12. a. **True.**

b. **False.** The biochemical diagnosis is made on an analysis of a 24-h urine collection for catecholamines.

c. **False.** A phaeochromocytoma is a tumour of the adrenal medulla.

d. **True.** A phaeochromocytoma can present dramatically as a hypertensive crisis that precipitates a stroke.

e. **True.** Although unilateral disease is more common.

13. a. **False.** Conn syndrome is characterised by hypokalaemia.

b. **True.** Hypertension and hypokalaemia are frequently the cause for the investigation of hyperaldosteronism.

c. **True.** Patients with a mild variant of the disease or those unfit or unsuitable for surgery can be maintained in the long term on an aldosterone antagonist such as spironolactone.

d. **False.** Patients with primary hyperaldosteronism have a low plasma renin. A high renin level is characteristic of secondary hyperaldosteronism caused by hepatic or renal disease.

e. **True.** 80% of patients with primary hyperaldosteronism have a solitary adrenal cortical adenoma. The remainder are associated with bilateral adrenal cortical hyperplasia.

14. a. **True.** Visual field defects are likely to develop as the pituitary adenoma enlarges and compresses the optic chiasm, classically causing a bitemporal hemianopia.

b. **False.** Cushing syndrome is 10 times more common in women than in men.

c. **False.** Serum cortisol levels are normally at their lowest in the evening. Loss of this circadian rhythm with a high evening cortisol (and ACTH) are in keeping with a diagnosis of Cushing syndrome.

d. **True.** Glucose intolerance and fasting hyperglycaemia are common in Cushing syndrome.

e. **False.** Adrenal medullary tumours (phaeochromocytoma) are linked with medullary thyroid cancers in patients with multiple endocrine adenomatosis in MEN type 2 syndrome.

Hernias

6

Chapter overview

Abdominal hernias are among the most common minor surgical ailments. The majority are inguinal and affect males. Numerous techniques of repair are described. Current refinements such as an open mesh repair or laparoscopic repair aim to reduce postoperative pain to a minimum, enabling most procedures to be undertaken as a day case. Few patients are unfit for surgery, and operation will avoid the development later of serious complications such as intestinal obstruction and strangulation.

6.1 Hernia formation

Learning objectives

You should:
- understand how a hernia develops and know the anatomical features that cause hernia complications.

Abdominal hernias can be classified as external or internal. External hernias are much more common. They consist of a protrusion, usually of normal intra-abdominal contents, through the investing fascial and muscle layers of the abdominal wall. Most present externally as a lump and can contain omentum, small bowel or large bowel. Internal hernias develop if any of the viscera protrude through a defect in the mesentery or diaphragm or beneath an adhesive band within the abdomen. They usually present with intestinal obstruction (see section 3.5)

The four commonest types of hernia are:

- inguinal or femoral (groin hernias)
- incisional hernia
- umbilical hernia/paraumbilical
- epigastric hernia.

Most hernias are reducible, i.e. the contents can be returned to the abdominal cavity and the hernial sac emptied by either posture or pressure.

Many hernias are painless and patients will present primarily because they have discovered a lump. Others will complain of a dragging pain associated with the hernia. Surgical repair is indicated in both groups to relieve symptoms and to prevent or treat the development of the following complications:

- irreducibility
- obstruction
- strangulation.

As the hernia develops, it takes with it a protrusion of peritoneum, which forms a sac that invests the hernia contents. The neck of the sac as it passes through the abdominal wall is a narrow point, which will constrict the hernia contents and cause complications. A hernia becomes irreducible when the contents swell secondary to the constriction at the neck of the sac or if they adhere to the sac itself. If the hernia contains a loop of bowel that is irreducible, obstruction can develop (Figure 56) and strangulation will supervene if the blood supply to the bowel becomes compromised.

6.2 Types of hernia

Learning objectives

You should:
- be able to diagnose a groin hernia confidently and differentiate between inguinal and femoral hernias
- understand the principles and options in surgical hernia repair.

Groin hernias

Inguinal and femoral hernias are considered together as both present as a lump in the groin. Inguinal hernias are 10 times more common than femoral hernias, and together account for 80% of all hernias.

A simplified view of the anatomy of the inguinal canal is shown in Figure 57.

Inguinal hernias

There are two types of inguinal hernia:

- indirect
- direct.

Indirect inguinal hernia These hernias are congenital and develop when the processus vaginalis (the peritoneal

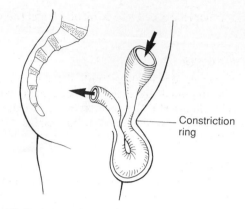

Figure 56 An obstructed inguinal hernia.

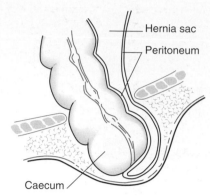

Figure 58 Sliding type inguinal hernia.

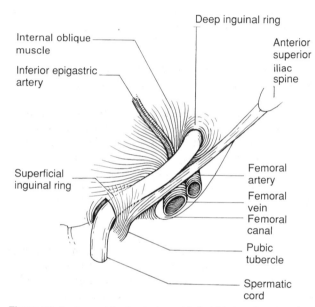

Figure 57 Anatomy of the inguinal canal (left side) deep to external oblique muscle.

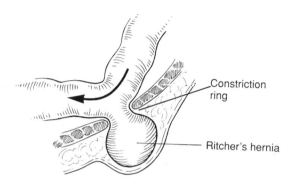

Figure 59 Richter's hernia.

Unusual types of groin hernia

Sliding inguinal hernia In this hernia, part of the wall of the hernial sac is formed by the caecum (right side), pelvic colon (left side) or bladder (both sides) which has slid down extraperitoneally into the inguinal canal (Figure 58). It is vitally important to recognise this variant at operation in order to prevent injury to the sliding component during ligation of the hernial sac.

Richter's hernia In this hernia, part of the intestinal wall has become incarcerated in the neck of the hernial sac and may strangulate. The bowel will not be obstructed and the diagnosis may be overlooked (Figure 59).

Clinical features

Both direct and indirect inguinal hernias present as a lump in the groin. The various physical signs used to differentiate these two hernias are frequently unreliable. The relationship of the hernia to the pubic tubercle is more important and is the key to differentiating an inguinal from a femoral hernia. An inguinal hernia always emerges above and medial to the tubercle whereas a femoral hernia lies below and lateral (Figure 60).

The differential diagnosis of a groin lump includes:

- direct or indirect inguinal hernia
- femoral hernia
- inguinal lymphadenopathy
- undescended testicle
- saphena varix (a dilatation of the long saphenous vein as it enters the femoral vein just below the inguinal ligament)
- femoral artery aneurysm (an expansile swelling).

sac through which the testicle descends into the scrotum) remains patent. Although they can occur at any age, they are the most frequent form of hernia found in children and young adults. The processus vaginalis develops into the hernial sac when an increase in intra-abdominal pressure and/or a weakening in the abdominal wall musculature allows abdominal contents through the deep inguinal ring into the inguinal canal and sometimes into the scrotum (inguoscrotal hernia).

Direct inguinal hernia These are usually smaller than indirect hernias and are less prone to complications. They are formed from a protrusion through the posterior wall of the inguinal canal medial to the inferior epigastric artery (Figure 57). Occasionally, a combination of both types of hernia can affect the same inguinal canal (pantaloon hernia). Direct inguinal hernias develop in an older age group; they rarely extend into the scrotum. They are associated with a weakness in the abdominal wall musculature and are frequently bilateral.

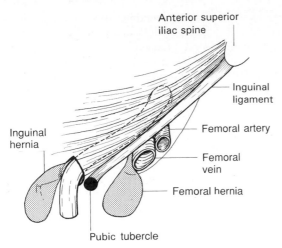

Figure 60 Femoral hernia – relationship to inguinal hernia.

six

Treatment

Age is no bar to hernia repair. Most symptomatic hernias can be repaired even in the elderly, using local or regional anaesthetic techniques. Repair should always be considered in order to prevent the risk of complications developing at a later date. Perhaps the only exception is a small obviously direct inguinal hernia, which can be left alone or managed with a truss.

Hernia repair can be undertaken using open or laparoscopic surgery. The key steps are:

1. reduction or ligation of the hernia sac
2. strengthening of the posterior inguinal wall with a non-absorbable mesh or sutures.

Earlier repair techniques involved a muscle repair either suturing the conjoint tendon/internal oblique muscle to the inguinal ligament behind the spermatic cord (a Bassini repair) or a suture repair of the transversalis fascia in addition to the muscle repair (the Shouldice repair). Both have been superseded by techniques which create a 'tension-free' repair implanting a non-absorbable mesh. The most commonly used open method (the Lichtenstein technique) sutures a flat piece of polypropylene mesh to the posterior inguinal wall behind the spermatic cord. Sometimes the technique is used in combination with a mesh 'plug' to bridge any major areas of weakness in the inguinal canal.

Laparoscopic hernia repair techniques use either the transperitoneal or the totally extraperitoneal approach to place a prolene mesh over the defects in the floor of the inguinal canal. The method is especially useful in patients with bilateral or recurrent inguinal hernias.

'Tension-free' open surgery and laparoscopic surgery cause less postoperative pain and enable an earlier return to full ambulation and work.

Prognosis

Up to 1 in 20 (5%) hernias will recur. Early recurrence within 2 years is usually a result of an inadequate primary operation. Late recurrence reflects a progression of the underlying neuromuscular weakness that caused the original hernia. Recurrent hernias can be difficult to repair and

laparoscopic surgery may be of particular benefit to these patients.

Femoral hernia

A femoral hernia descends through the femoral canal beneath the inguinal ligament to lie medial to the femoral vein (Figure 60). The neck of the sac is extremely tight and because of this femoral hernias are prone to complications.

Clinical features

Femoral hernias are more common in women than in men because of the width of the female pelvis. In contrast to inguinal hernias, the neck of the sac is below and lateral to the pubic tubercle in a position corresponding to the femoral canal. These hernias are often irreducible and frequently the primary presentation is with a complication such as obstruction or strangulation.

Treatment

The femoral canal can be approached from above or below the inguinal ligament or even through the posterior wall of the inguinal canal.

Reduction of the hernia, particularly if it is obstructed, is often difficult because of the tight neck. The surgical aim is to obliterate the femoral canal using either non-absorbable sutures or, preferably, a 'plug' of non-absorbable prolene mesh inserted into the femoral canal. A repair of the hernia will sometimes have to be combined with a resection of gangrenous small bowel or omentum.

Incisional hernia

Incisional (or ventral) hernias develop through a previous operation scar. They are more common in vertical incisions than in transverse incisions. In each case there is usually one or more of the following predisposing factors:

- poor surgical technique
- poor perioperative nutritional status
- postoperative wound infection or haematoma
- underlying disease
  - *intra-abdominal sepsis*
  - *malignancy*
- postoperative cough
- obesity.

Clinical features

Untreated, these hernias will gradually increase in size. The omentum and intestines are often adherent to the scar tissue associated with these hernias and episodes of obstruction are frequent if these hernias are neglected.

Treatment

Incisional hernias are best repaired with a non-absorbable mesh to bridge the defect which will provide a 'tension-free' closure of the abdominal wall. Small defects can be simply repaired with non-absorbable sutures.

Laparoscopic surgery can be used to place a mesh across the defect from inside the peritoneal cavity. This avoids a large open abdominal wound allowing a faster and less painful recovery.

Umbilical and paraumbilical hernia

Umbilical hernia True umbilical hernias, which develop through the centre of the umbilical cicatrix, are a disorder of childhood. Usually they disappear as the child grows and the rectii muscles develop.

Paraumbilical hernia In adulthood, a paraumbilical hernia develops through the interlacing fibres of the linea alba that have become weakened with age and obesity. This hernia is much more common in women than men and develops just above the umbilicus. As it enlarges the hernia incorporates the umbilicus in the hernial swelling. The hernial sac is often multiloculated with a tight neck and is prone to complications.

Clinical features

Patients present with a localised swelling through or around the umbilicus that is often irreducible.

Treatment

The defect can be repaired by overlapping and suturing together the rectus sheath that forms the border of the defect (Mayo's repair). Sometimes the umbilicus will need to be excised. For larger defects a mesh repair or laparoscopic techniques can be used.

Epigastric hernia

This hernia often occurs in well-built, muscular men. The protrusion develops through the interlacing fibres of the linea alba (in the midline) in the epigastrium.

Clinical features

These hernias are usually small but painful and are tender on examination. Although larger hernias may contain omentum and occasionally loops of intestine, most small hernias only contain extraperitoneal fat.

Treatment

These defects are usually small and wherever possible are repaired with non-absorbable sutures. Larger hernias will require a mesh repair.

Self-assessment: questions

Extended matching items questions (EMIs)

EMI 1

Theme: Groin hernia

A. Richter's hernia

B. direct inguinal hernia

C. pantaloon hernia

D. obturator hernia

E. sliding hernia

F. indirect inguinal hernia

G. Spigelian hernia

H. femoral hernia

Which of these types of hernia are best characterised by the following descriptions?

1. A single hernia sac which protrudes through the deep inguinal ring and the posterior wall of the inguinal canal.

2. A hernia where part of the wall of the hernia sac is formed by an adjacent viscera.

3. Any hernia which contains just part of the circumference of the intestine.

4. Any hernia where the neck of the sac lies below and lateral to the public tubercle.

EMI 2

Theme: A groin swelling

A. inguinal hernia

B. saphena varix

C. femoral hernia

D. femoral artery aneurysm

E. groin lymphadenopathy

F. undescended testis

G. hydrocoele

H. psoas abscess

Select from the above list the diagnosis that best matches the following clinical presentations.

1. A middle-aged woman with varicose veins in both legs and a painless groin swelling which reduces on lying down. There is a positive 'tap sign'.

2. An elderly lady with a small rounded swelling in the groin which is difficult to reduce and is below and lateral to the pubic tubercle.

3. A young man with a history of pain in the right groin on exertion; in addition he has noticed a swelling in the groin. On examination the right side of the scrotum is empty.

4. A young woman with a history of malaise, weight loss and night sweats has a non-tender, firm, irreducible swelling in the left groin.

5. An expansile irreducible swelling in the left groin of an elderly man.

6. A 40-year-old man with a swelling in the right groin which extends above and below the inguinal ligament. He complains of a 'throbbing' pain within it. His right hip is slightly flexed and any extension is extremely painful. His right loin is tender and he has a raised white cell count.

Objective structured clinical examination questions (OSCEs)

OSCE 1

A 54-year-old woman presents with a 2-day history of colicky abdominal pain and vomiting. She has a small painful lump in the left groin. Examine her plain abdominal radiograph (Figure 61) then answer the following questions.

a. What is the radiological diagnosis?

b. What is the most likely cause?

c. What is the correct treatment?

OSCE 2

A 50-year-old lady presents with a swelling in the central abdomen which has existed for many years. It has recently increased in size and has become irreducible. She has no other gastrointestinal symptoms and has not had any previous abdominal surgery. It is not tender and is dull to percussion. Bowel sounds are absent on auscultation of the swelling.

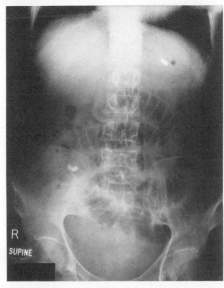

Figure 61 Plain abdominal radiograph.

a. What is the diagnosis?

b. What do you think it may contain and why?

c. What treatment options are there?

Multiple choice questions

1. The following points relate to hernias in general:
   a. all hernias that strangulate are obstructed
   b. most hernias are irreducible
   c. hernias are nearly always acquired; they are rarely congenital
   d. chronic constipation and prostatic outflow symptoms can aggravate a hernia
   e. every hernia is invested with a layer of parietal peritoneum

2. Direct inguinal hernias:
   a. are frequently bilateral
   b. are usually congenital
   c. generally occur in an older age group than indirect inguinal hernias
   d. often extend into the scrotum
   e. have a neck that lies medial to the inferior epigastric vessels

3. A femoral hernia:
   a. is more common in a woman than an inguinal hernia
   b. lies lateral to the femoral vein
   c. can be differentiated from an inguinal hernia by the position of its neck, which lies below and lateral to the pubic tubercle
   d. rarely strangulates
   e. rarely recurs

4. Incisional hernias are more common under the following circumstances:
   a. in thin patients
   b. in patients with underlying malignancy
   c. in vertical incisions
   d. after a major wound infection
   e. in severely septic patients

5. A sliding type inguinal hernia:
   a. can usually be diagnosed preoperatively
   b. will rarely recur
   c. may contain bladder
   d. if unrecognised can lead to bowel injury
   e. is usually associated with direct inguinal hernias

Self-assessment: answers

EMI answers

EMI 1

Theme: Groin hernia

1. C. Pantaloon hernia.

In this hernia the peritoneal sac protrudes on either side of the inferior epigastric vessels. By definition these patients have a combination of an indirect and a direct hernia. Often the indirect inguinal component is very wide necked and can be difficult to repair.

2. E. Sliding hernia.

These hernias have a higher recurrence rate than an uncomplicated inguinal hernia. Most often the sliding component contains caecum or bladder in a right-sided hernia and sigmoid colon or bladder in a left-sided hernia.

3. A. Richter's hernia.

This unusual type of hernia is more commonly associated with a femoral hernia, in which a segment of the circumference of the intestine can become trapped in the narrow neck which is characteristic of a femoral hernia.

4. H. Femoral hernia

The site of the neck, below and lateral to the pubic tubercle, is the distinguishing feature of a femoral hernia.

EMI 2

Theme: A groin swelling

1. B. Saphena varix.

A saphena varix can be differentiated from a hernia because it is a painless swelling which lies below the inguinal ligament and always disappears when the patient lies down. Also, most patients have obvious varicose veins. While the patient is lying down a venous 'thrill' can often be detected on palpation when the patient gives a cough. With the patient standing, a transmitted pulsation can be detected over the varix by tapping the long saphenous vein some distance from the groin while simultaneously palpating the varix (the tap sign).

2. C. Femoral hernia.

The neck of a femoral hernia lies below and lateral to the pubic tubercle. This is the key diagnostic feature. Additionally, this condition is most frequent in elderly women.

3. F. Undescended testis.

Always remember to examine the scrotum in any male patient who presents with a groin swelling. An undescended testicle may have been missed at examination early on in life and can present later with a swelling in the groin which may be painful. Without surgical correction these patients are at increased risk of developing cancer in the undescended testicle.

4. E. Groin lymphadenopathy.

This patient has systemic symptoms – malaise, weight loss and night sweats – which should make you think of an underlying disease such as lymphoma. These patients may present with peripheral lymphadenopathy. Check also other sites, e.g. axilllae and neck, and look for hepatosplenomegaly.

5. D. Femoral artery aneurysm.

An expansile swelling is the hallmark of an aneurysm in any vessel. A true femoral aneurysm develops with atherosclerotic degeneration of the vessel wall. A false aneurysm may be the sequel to deliberate puncture of the vessel wall during an arteriogram.

6. H. Psoas abscess.

A psoas abscess (an abscess which overlies the psoas muscle) may develop as the sequel to any retroperitoneal infection or even a neglected appendicitis or diverticulitis. The pus tracks along the psoas muscle (which passes behind and below the inguinal ligament) and may eventually present as a swelling in relation to the inguinal ligament.

OSCE answers

OSCE 1

a. Small bowel obstruction.

The ladder pattern of central distended loops of intestine with complete mucosal folds across the full width of the intestinal lumen is characteristic of small bowel obstruction. From the appearance of the radiograph, with multiple loops of distended small bowel, it is probably a distal obstruction.

b. Femoral or inguinal hernia.

From the history, examination and radiological findings, the small bowel obstruction is likely to be secondary to either a femoral or inguinal hernia.

c. The obstruction should be relieved by operative repair of the hernia and release of the trapped intestine. A laparotomy may be necessary to resect the segment of intestine involved if it has been strangulated.

OSCE 2

a. An umbilical hernia.

The position of the swelling and the long history are characteristic. As the patient has not had any previous abdominal surgery an incisional hernia can be ruled out.

b. Omentum.

Omentum and small intestine are the commonest contents of an umbilical hernia sac. Occasionally it contains the large intestine. This hernia is dull to percussion and bowel sounds were not heard on auscultation. These features plus the lack of any gastrointestinal disturbance (no colic or obstructive symptoms) suggest that the omentum is the major component in this hernia.

c. Mayo's or mesh repair.

This patient's hernia has increased in size and cannot be reduced – both are indications for surgical repair. The larger the hernia the more likely a mesh type repair will be required.

Multiple choice answers

1. a. **False.** Strangulation implies that the blood supply to a loop of bowel or omentum has been compromised. If the hernia contains omentum only or only a part of the circumference of the bowel (i.e. a Richter's type hernia) then strangulation will occur without obstruction.

   b. **False.** Most hernias are reducible. The onset of irreducibility indicates that the hernial contents are trapped by the neck of the sac and cannot return to the abdomen. This will predispose to obstruction and strangulation.

   c. **False.** Indirect hernias are almost always congenital and are caused by failure of the processus vaginalis to obliterate. Although some will present in the neonatal or childhood period, many do not develop until later in life.

   d. **True.** Any condition that intermittently or chronically raises the intra-abdominal pressure can predispose to hernia development.

   e. **True.** As the hernia contents leave the abdominal cavity and enter the fascial defect that constitutes the hernia, they take with them a sac that is formed from the parietal peritoneum.

2. a. **True.** Direct hernias are frequently associated with lax abdominal wall muscles. The weakness is usually symmetrical and results in bilateral muscular defects.

   b. **False.**

   c. **True.** The muscular defects associated with direct hernias are frequently an effect of ageing.

   d. **False.** Direct hernias are usually small and almost never extend into the scrotum. Inguoscrotal hernias usually have a massive sac and are indirect in origin.

   e. **True.** The inferior epigastric vessels are a vital anatomical landmark. By definition, hernias whose neck lies medial to them are direct and hernias where the neck lies lateral to the vessels are indirect in origin.

3. a. **False.** Although femoral hernias are more common in women than men, the overall incidence of inguinal hernias (in both sexes) is far greater. Hence a groin hernia in a woman is still more likely to be inguinal than femoral in origin.

   b. **False.** A femoral hernia passes beneath the inguinal ligament along the femoral canal, which lies medial to the femoral vein.

   c. **True.** The pubic tubercle is an important anatomical landmark. The neck of a femoral hernia lies below and lateral to it whereas the neck of an inguinal hernia lies above and medial to the pubic tubercle.

   d. **False.** The neck of a femoral hernia is small and tight. These hernias are particularly prone to strangulation.

   e. **True.** A recurrence is rare provided the defect is carefully closed.

4. a. **False.** Obesity predisposes to incisional hernia formation by straining the wound during the healing phase.

   b. **True.** Malignancy, particularly when the disease is found to be inoperable, impairs wound healing.

   c. **True.** Vertical incisions are more prone to incisional hernia development than transverse incisions.

   d. **True.** A major wound infection or a postoperative wound haematoma impairs the healing process and predisposes to incisional herniation.

   e. **True.** These patients are usually catabolic and wound healing is impaired.

5. a. **False.** The diagnosis is made at operation when the hernial sac is opened and is found to contain a portion of the viscus or the bladder forming part of the wall and neck of the hernial sac.

   b. **False.** This type of hernia can be technically quite difficult to repair and recurrence is more common compared with an uncomplicated inguinal hernia.

   c. **True.** The bladder, sigmoid colon, caecum and ovary are the most common contents of a sliding type inguinal hernia.

   d. **True.** If this hernia variant is not recognised at operation, the sliding component can be damaged during ligation of the neck of the hernial sac.

   e. **False.** Sliding hernias are a variant of an indirect inguinal hernia.

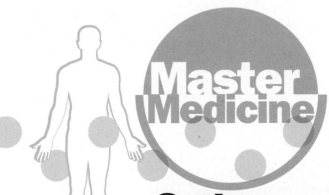

Orthopaedic surgery

Trauma

Musculoskeletal trauma in adults

Chapter part overview

This chapter outlines how to safely identify and manage diseases and injuries of bones, joints, muscles, tendons and ligaments. Rather than organising things by disease process or anatomical region, you are going to learn how these problems will present to your surgery, clinic or A&E department. The system of orthopaedic examination which is used to come to a diagnosis can be summarised as follows:

- listen (take a history)
- look
- feel
- move.

7.1 Clinical examination in major trauma

Learning objectives

You should:
- be familiar with the advanced trauma life support (ATLS) system's approach to the management of major trauma
- be able to describe a systematic approach to the management of open fractures
- recognise the clinical features which suggest that compartment syndrome may be developing.

To prevent the arrival of a patient with multiple injuries being accompanied by much ill-coordinated activity, a uniform approach such as that advocated by the ATLS system is recommended. This routine method of efficiently managing such patients facilitates the delivery of lifesaving measures and should become second nature to the medical and nursing staff who may be called upon to attend patients with musculoskeletal trauma.

After initial assessment of injuries and appropriate resuscitation, the importance of a 'second-look' examination should be emphasised because it is at this stage that additional incidental injuries will be discovered.

During every patient interaction, the clinical skills of 'listen', 'look', 'feel' and 'move' should be followed.

Emergency treatment

The first few hours after injury is the time in which life can be saved if emergency measures are effectively applied. This emergency treatment of the multiply injured patient is best achieved if the members of the resuscitation team follow the ATLS principles:

- airway and cervical spine control
- breathing
- circulation

followed by:

- dysfunction (neurological disorder)
- exposure/environmental control.

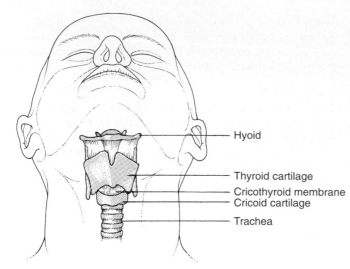

Hyoid

Thyroid cartilage
Cricothyroid membrane
Cricoid cartilage
Trachea

Figure 62 A cricothyroidotomy can be made through the cricothyroid membrane between the cricoid and thyroid cartilages.

Airway and cervical spine control

The airway should be cleared of any obstructions such as dentures or vomit and in the comatose patient the tongue should be prevented from blocking the pharynx by holding the jaw forwards. An oropharyngeal or nasopharyngeal tube is often necessary but endotracheal intubation, cricothyroidotomy (Figure 62) or a tracheostomy may be required if the upper airway is obstructed. The cervical spine must be manually steadied until it can be immobilised with a semirigid cervical collar, sandbags to either side of the head and stout pieces of sticky tape across the forehead and chin.

Breathing

Observe chest expansion, spontaneous ventilation and any abnormal movements of the chest wall, such as paradoxical movement, flail segment or a penetrating wound. Percuss and auscultate the chest to detect pneumothorax or haemothorax and to assess air entry. Palpate the trachea for deviation away from the affected side in tension pneumothorax.

Circulation

Bleeding should be controlled by pressure dressings and elevation. Improvised tourniquets are too dangerous. A fast flowing intravenous infusion should be instituted in a large peripheral vein; a cut-down on a peripheral vein may be required. A volume challenge with 2 l of an intravenous crystalloid is the initial treatment of hypotension. If the patient fails to respond, blood may also be required; but no amount of blood transfusion will save the patient unless the bleeding vessel is found and stopped. This means that the patient might have to go for a laparotomy before the initial assessment is complete. Later cross-matched blood may be required. Passing a urinary catheter allows accurate monitoring of fluid balance and relieves the agitation caused by bladder distension.

Disorder (neurological disorder)

A rapid but thorough examination for evidence of head injury is carried out. The Glasgow Coma Scale is commonly used. This records the patient's motor, verbal and eye opening responses to stimulation. Evidence of spinal cord or peripheral nerve injury can be sought at this stage.

Exposure/environmental control

The entire patient must be exposed for thorough examination to exclude the presence of any additional injuries. The extent and depth of burns can be charted at this stage. Do not forget to examine the perineum and the back. Once this is done, steps must be taken to keep the patient warm. Recording of vital signs should be commenced.

Radiographic examination

Radiographs of chest, pelvis and lateral cervical spine are always required. Radiographs of other regions can be delayed until resuscitation is completed.

Open fractures

Open fractures require urgent treatment if bacterial invasion of the wound is to be avoided. Open fractures are classified according to their degree of contamination and soft tissue damage.

Management

Management can be divided into several steps:

- initial management in A&E department
  - photograph, broad-spectrum intravenous antibiotics, iodine dressing
- wound excision
  - all devitalised tissue, especially muscle, is excised and dirt washed from the wound with copious saline
- reduction
  - the bony fragments are aligned into normal position
- stabilisation
  - this may be achieved with internal metalwork or an external fixator (Fig. 63)
- skin cover
  - the wound is initially left open with an iodine dressing. A second operation is performed 48 h later when any further devitalised tissue is removed. If the skin cannot be closed without tension, a skin graft or plastic surgical flap may be required. If a plastic surgeon is available on the day of injury, it is permissible to cover the wound primarily with a flap of muscle.

Complications

Complications of fractures are described later; those particularly associated with open fractures are:

- wound infection
- chronic osteitis
- non-union.

Compartment syndrome

Bleeding from a fracture and swelling of injured muscle may increase the pressure in the adjacent fascial compartments. In the leg, there are four compartments (Figure 64) and in the forearm two compartments.

Clinical features:

- **Listen** – pain more severe than would be expected from the injury alone.
- **Look** – tense swollen limb.
- **Feel** – altered sensation and diminished distal pulses will eventually be present but by then it will be too late.
- **Move** – pain on passive stretching of the muscle bellies in the involved compartment.

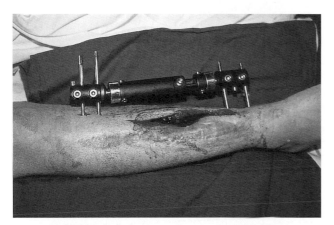

Figure 63 External fixator used to stabilise an open tibial fracture without hindering access to the wound.

Diagnosis

A pressure transducer can be introduced to monitor pressure within the compartment but clinical features remain the most important in making the diagnosis.

Management

The immediate removal of circumferential dressings and an urgent fasciotomy are required to relieve the raised compartment pressure. In the lower leg, the compartments are released as shown (Figure 64). The skin wounds are left open to be closed or covered with a split thickness skin graft a few days later when the swelling has subsided.

Complications:

- Volkmann's ischaemic contracture
- persisting nerve damage.

Second-look examination

After initial emergency assessment, it is important to carry out a second-look examination to identify any additional injuries.

7.2 Fractures

Learning objectives

You should:
- understand the importance of the history in determining the type and extent of the fracture and the soft tissue injury sustained and know how this may relate to the management and the outcome
- be able to describe a fracture in terms of its pattern and type of malalignment
- be aware of the potential complications of fractures and understand how early management can influence these.

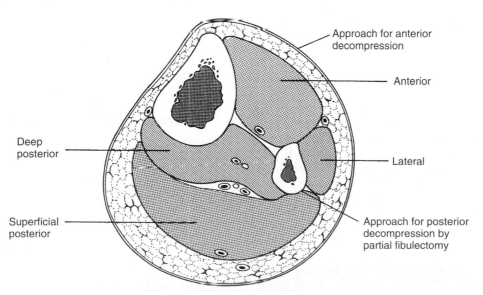

Figure 64 Fascial compartments in the leg.

Anterior

Lateral

Approach for anterior decompression

Approach for posterior decompression by partial fibulectomy

Deep posterior

Superficial posterior

Clinical features

The characteristic features of a fracture of any long bone are:

- **Listen**
  - a history of trauma
  - pain
- **Look**
  - bruising
  - deformity
  - swelling
- **Feel**
  - diminished pulses and altered sensation may be present
- **Move**
  - loss of function
  - crepitus.

In addition there may be local bruising, and examination of the periphery may show diminished pulses and areas of altered sensation.

The most important fact to establish is whether the fracture is open or closed. The presence of a skin wound that communicates with the fracture means that the fracture is open and the risk of infection is increased.

It is easy to think of the bone injury in isolation, especially when looking at a radiograph, but it must be remembered that the soft tissues will also have been damaged by the injuring force. An accurate history will tell something about the mechanism of the injury and about the amount of energy absorbed by the bone and soft tissues from the injuring force. The radiograph will show the pattern of the resulting fracture. Both the history and the radiograph will help in making a decision on the probable stability of the fracture and the extent of damage to be expected in the surrounding soft tissues.

Mechanism of injury

Direct violence

When direct violence is applied to a bone, the overlying skin and soft tissues are likely to be broken and damaged. A small force to a localised area, such as from a blow with a stick to the forearm, will bruise or break the overlying skin and cause a transverse fracture usually of the ulna (Figure 65).

A large force to a large area, such as from being hit by a car bumper, will produce a comminuted fracture with extensive soft tissue damage, crushing and devitalisation. A large force to a small area from a missile injury will produce severe damage to bone and soft tissues in a localised area.

Indirect violence

The injuring force is applied to the limb at a distance from where the fracture occurs. Examples are a twisting injury to the tibia (Figure 66), often caused when the foot is jammed (for instance in a football tackle) while the body twists and falls to the side. The fracture is less likely to be open than one caused by direct violence, but the soft tissue

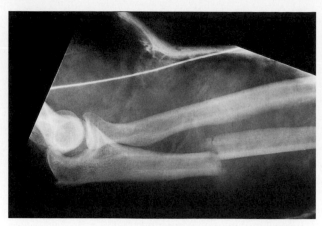

Figure 65 Transverse fracture of the middle third of the ulna following a direct blow on the forearm.

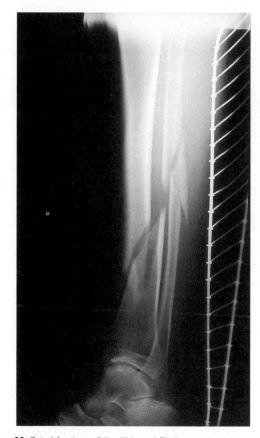

Figure 66 Spiral fracture of the tibia and fibula.

envelope is more likely to be extensively stripped from the bone.

When angulatory forces are directed to the limb, a transverse fracture results, which may have intact periosteum on the compression side but a tear in the periosteal sleeve on the distraction side.

Other mechanisms of injury include stress fractures from repetitive forces being applied to the bone, as seen in the 'march fracture' of the second metatarsal.

Fracture patterns

Transverse fractures These arise when angulatory forces are applied to the limb, for instance by levering it over a fulcrum (e.g. the leg caught between the rungs during a fall from a stepladder) or a fall on the outstretched hand. Direct blows to an isolated area of the bone can also cause a transverse fracture.

Spiral fractures Twisting forces create spiral fractures (e.g. the foot blocked in a football tackle while the player falls to the side).

Comminuted fractures These are high-energy fractures and are inherently unstable (e.g. the leg hit by a car bumper).

Crush fractures These occur as a result of longitudinal (axial) forces and are seen in areas of cancellous bone, such as the tibial condyles and vertebrae (e.g. a patient who falls from a height and lands on the feet may fracture the calcaneum and vertebrae) (Figure 67).

Oblique fractures These are caused by a combination of twisting, angulation and compression forces.

Malalignment

A fracture may be:

- displaced
- angulated
- shortened
- rotated.

Displacement In a displaced fracture, the distal fragment is displaced in a sagittal or coronal plane relative to the proximal fragment but without any angulation (Figure 68). The overall alignment of the limb is satisfactory. If the fracture is stable then healing will proceed without residual deformity as the fracture remodels.

Angulation The distal fragment may be angulated dorsal or volar, anterior or posterior, medial (varus) (Figure 69) or lateral (valgus). In children, remodelling may take place if the deformity is in the plane of movement of an adjacent joint. Varus/valgus deformities do not remodel except near the shoulder and hip.

Shortening In a completely displaced fracture, the bone fragments will override each other and the limb will shorten (Figure 70). Shortening also occurs in comminuted fractures where there is impaction of the articular surface into the metaphysis.

Rotation The distal fragment of a fracture may be rotated on the proximal fragment. A radiograph showing the full length of the injured limb will make it easier to recognise this deformity (Figure 71).

Complications

Complications can be considered under the following categories:

- early/late
- local/systemic
- bony/soft tissue.

Potential complications of fractures are:

- injury of adjacent nerves, vessels or viscera
- compartment syndrome
- infection
- heterotopic ossification (bone laid down in injured soft tissues)
- malunion (fracture heals in the wrong position)
- delayed union (fracture has failed to unite but still shows progress towards union)

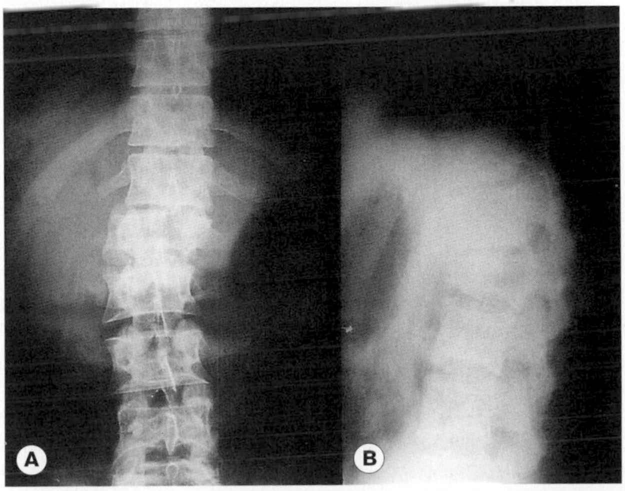

Figure 67 (A) Crush fracture of the body of the first lumbar vertebra. (B) View of the same injury showing the displacement associated with the crush fracture.

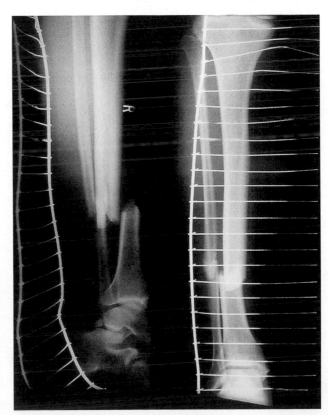

Figure 68 Transverse fractures of the distal tibia and fibula with 100% displacement but with no angulatory deformity.

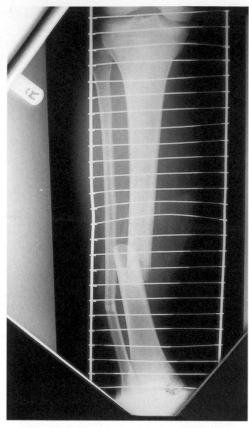

Figure 69 Transverse fracture of the distal tibia and fibula with marked varus angulation at the fracture site.

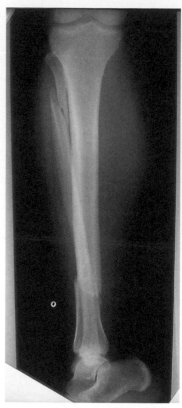

Figure 71 Rotary deformity of a fracture of the distal tibia and proximal fibula. The radiograph shows an antero-posterior view of the knee with a lateral view of the ankle.

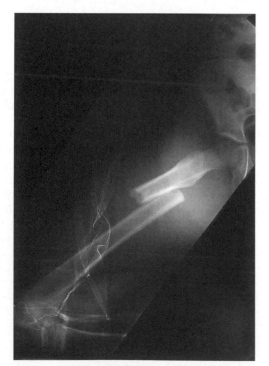

Figure 70 Transverse fracture of the upper third of the femur in a child with considerable shortening at the fracture site due to overriding of the bone ends.

- non-union (fracture fails to unite and shows no progress towards union)
- fat embolus (fat and coagulation products from the fracture site enter the circulation and cause an inflammatory reaction in the lung known as adult respiratory distress syndrome)
- deep vein thrombosis and pulmonary thromboembolism.

7.3 Methods of treatment

Learning objectives

You should:
- be able to describe methods of non-operative treatment of fractures and list their advantages and disadvantages
- be able to describe methods of internal fixation of fractures and list their advantages and disadvantages
- be able to describe the advantages and disadvantages of external fixation
- begin to be able to balance these approaches to the management of any particular fracture in a particular patient.

Fracture stabilisation may be achieved by external or internal techniques:

External:
- traction
- splint, e.g. plaster cast
- external fixator.

Internal:
- intermedullary rod
- plates
- screws
- wires.

Traction

Traction is used to overcome muscle spasm and so allow the bone fragments to realign in the soft tissue envelope. The use of a collar and cuff sling for fractures of the proximal humerus is a form of traction.

Skin traction to a maximum of 5 kg can be applied to the leg by fastening the weights to adhesive strapping around the limb. This is used only as a temporary measure in adults but is used for definitive treatment of femoral fractures in young children.

In skeletal traction, weights are applied to the limb via a pin passed through the tibial tuberosity for traction on the femur or through the os calcis for traction on the tibia. The limb can be nursed in a Thomas splint and the traction cords tied to its end. This is fixed traction. Alternatively, the patient can lie free in bed with the fracture supported in a cradle while traction applied distally is provided by weights which hang to the floor round a pulley at the foot of the bed. This is balanced traction (Figure 72).

Advantages:
- does not require a general anaesthetic
- safe to use.

Disadvantages:
- prolonged immobilisation with associated problems of pressure sores, osteoporosis, muscle wasting, joint stiffness, respiratory infection and thromboembolism
- distraction of the fracture
- pin track sepsis.

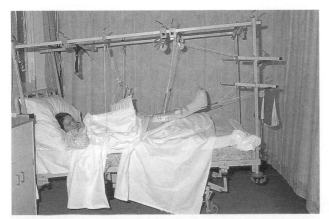

Figure 72 Balanced traction. The femoral fracture is nursed in the canvas cradle while traction is applied distally via the tibial tuberosity.

Plaster casts

Plaster of Paris immobilisation is the most common type of splintage to hold a fracture after it has been manipulated into a satisfactory position. Three-point fixation is required to prevent subsequent loss of the position achieved.

Advantages:
- cheap
- readily available
- usually does not require a general anaesthetic.

Disadvantages:
- rigid fixation is not possible so the bone fragments can slip
- pressure sores beneath the plaster
- stiff joints
- peripheral swelling.

External fixation

Threaded pins are drilled into the bone on either side of the fracture and fixed via universal joints to a rigid bar near the skin surface. In the Illizarov method, multiple 'spokes' transfix the proximal and distal fragments between circular or semicircular frames.

Advantages:
- quick and easy to apply
- allows access to wounds and observation of the skin surface
- allows subsequent manipulation and repositioning of the fragments.

Disadvantages:
- pin track infection and occasional osteitis
- requires general or regional anaesthesia
- patient acceptability.

Internal fixation

Internal fixation is used where an absolutely stable reduction in an exact position is required, such as in an intra-articular fracture. This level of stability can only be achieved by compressing the fragments together. Plates and screws (Figure 73) or loops of wire tend to be used under these circumstances and healing occurs by the slow process which is normally responsible for routine turnover of healthy bone. Internal fixation can also be used in extra-articular fractures where a relatively stable, as opposed to absolutely stable, construct is desirable. Here, the aim is to have a bit of movement at the fracture site; under these circumstances the body will rapidly convert the haematoma between the bone ends into an immature type of bone called callus. Intramedullary rods and wires are used to create this environment but this is also the type of healing which occurs with external fixation methods.

Advantages:
- anatomical reduction
- early mobilisation of joint, and patient
- allows access to wounds
- supports bone even if fracture fails to heal (e.g. pathological fractures).

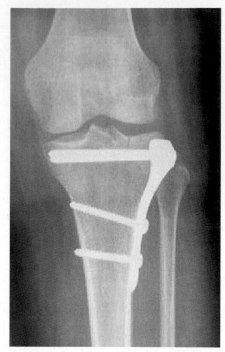

Figure 73 An intra-articluar fracture of the proximal tibia fixed with a plate and screws.

Disadvantages:

- requires general or regional anaesthesia
- infection
- non-union
- failure by cutting out or metal fatigue
- can be technically demanding.

Internal fixation gives the best chance of early rehabilitation and return to normal life and is especially useful for problem patients and problem fractures. Problem patients include those with:

- multiple injuries
- prolonged unconsciousness.

    Problem fractures include:

- intra-articular fractures
- unstable fractures
- pathological fractures.

7.4 Fractures and dislocations of the hip and pelvis

Hip injuries

> **Learning objectives**
>
> You should:
> - know that hip injuries in young people are different from those in the elderly population.
> - recognise the clinical appearance of a dislocated hip. Understand why this is a surgical emergency.
> - be able to identify a fractured pelvis radiologically.
> - differentiate stable from unstable pelvic fractures. Remember that the complications of hypovolaemic shock and urethral damage may be present.

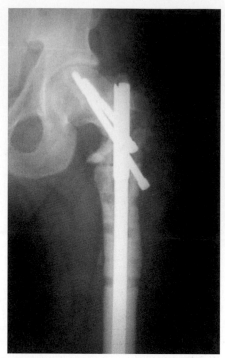

Figure 74 Reconstruction nail used in the treatment of a subtrochanteric fracture previously treated unsuccessfully with a sliding nail plate.

Hip injuries in young people

Whereas fractures of the femoral neck are commonplace low-energy injuries in elderly women, a similar fracture in a young adult is uncommon but, when present, indicates the involvement of a high-energy injuring force. Fractures are, therefore, commonly comminuted and may extend into the upper third of the femur (subtrochanteric fractures) or involve the femoral head.

Clinical features:
- pain
- excessive swelling of the hip and thigh
- leg externally rotated and shortened
- injuries to adjacent soft tissues
- injuries elsewhere.

Diagnosis
Plain radiographs will show the fracture fragments.

Management
High fractures of the femoral neck are stabilised by screw fixation, but subtrochanteric fractures can be more difficult. Operative stabilisation with an intramedullary device such as the 'reconstruction nail' is used and allows early active movement and weight-bearing (Figure 74).

Complications:
- of the injury
  - shock
  - damage to adjacent soft tissues
- of surgery
  - wound infection

– delayed union
– non-union.

Dislocation

A high-energy injury is required to dislocate the hip. Involvement in a road traffic accident is a common history. Dislocations can be classified as:

• posterior dislocation
• anterior dislocation.

Posterior dislocation

As the hip has dislocated posteriorly, there may be an associated fracture of the posterior wall of the acetabulum or of the head of the femur itself.

Clinical features:

• **Listen** – There is a history of a direct blow to the knee while seated, often from the car dashboard in a road traffic accident.
• **Look** – The leg lies in a characteristic position of adduction and internal rotation and appears short. There is often flexion of the hip and knee. There may be a telltale injury over the knee.
• **Feel** – Sciatic nerve compression from the displaced femoral head causes altered sensation in the leg.
• **Move** – Hip movements are resisted, and with sciatic nerve compression there may be weakness of ankle movement.

Diagnosis

Plain radiographs show the dislocation and any major fractures of the acetabular margin, but small fractures, especially displaced fragments of a femoral head fracture, will be best seen by CT scan (Figure 75).

Management

Urgent reduction of the dislocation under anaesthesia is required as avascular necrosis of the femoral head will occur if stretching of the capsular vessels to the femoral head is prolonged. Open reduction may be necessary if closed reduction is blocked by fracture fragments. Open reduction and internal fixation of associated fractures can be delayed a week or so to allow further imaging or recovery from other injuries.

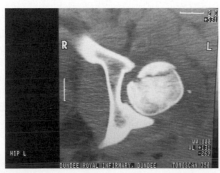

Figure 75 CT scan of a reduced dislocation of the hip showing an associated fracture of the femoral head.

Complications:

• sciatic nerve damage
• avascular necrosis
• secondary osteoarthritis.

Anterior dislocation

This injury is rare. The leg lies in external rotation, abduction and flexion. The dislocation can be reduced by manipulation under anaesthesia. Again, avascular necrosis is a complication.

Other acetabular fractures

Displaced fractures of the acetabulum require open reduction and internal fixation in order to try to reduce the chance of post-traumatic osteoarthritis. This treatment can be delayed a week or so and is usually carried out in specialist centres.

Fractured pelvis

Fractures of the pelvis can range from trivial to life threatening.

Fractured pubic rami

A minor fall in an elderly patient is often the cause of a fracture of one or two pubic rami.

Clinical features

After a minor fall, the patient complains of discomfort around the hip and groin. Clinical examination reveals no evidence of fracture of the femoral neck or greater trochanter (which are other likely sites of injury) but there is localised tenderness at the pubic rami and maybe bruising and swelling here later.

Diagnosis

Plain radiographs will confirm the diagnosis. Both pubic rami on the same side are usually injured.

Management

The patient rests until the discomfort has settled and then gradual mobilisation begins over the following few days.

Complications:

• none except those related to bed rest.

Fractures of the pelvic ring

Depending on the mechanism of injury, fractures may be classified as due to:

• AP compression – 'open book' and 'floating segment' fractures (Figure 76, Figure 77)
• lateral compression – a crush from the side involving the pubic rami and the sacroiliac region (Figure 78)
• vertical shear – vertical displacement in the region of the sacroiliac joints can be seen (Figure 79).

All types of pelvic ring fracture carry a risk of massive haemorrhage, disseminated intravascular coagulation (DIC) and urethral or bladder damage.

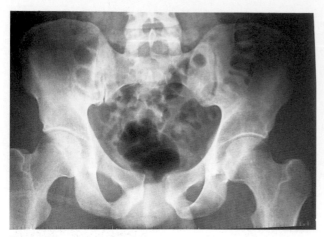

Figure 76

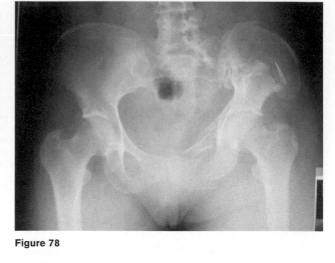

Figure 78

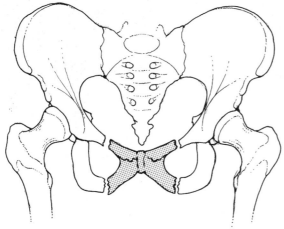

Figure 77 Fracture of all four pubic rami creating a floating segment.

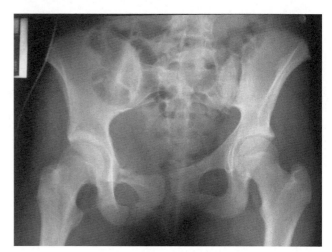

Figure 79

'Open book' fracture

The pelvic rim is disrupted both anteriorly and posteriorly and has 'hinged' open like a book. A binder or external fixator between the anterior iliac crests should be used in the emergency room to 'fold' the pelvis together and so control bleeding.

'Floating segment' fracture

Clinical features A direct blow from the front may fracture all four pubic rami, creating a floating segment incorporating the fragments attached to the pubic symphysis, the bladder and the urethra (Figure 77). There is a boggy swelling and bruising in the perineum. There may be extraperitoneal extravasation of urine, haematuria or blood at the urinary meatus.

Diagnosis Plain radiographs show the fracture but the presence of urinary tract rupture must be sought by retrograde urethrograms.

Management Initially, circulating volume must be restored as internal bleeding may be extensive. A single attempt is usually made to pass a urethral catheter but, if this fails, suprapubic drainage must be commenced, usually by a urologist. Bladder and urethral repair may be

required. Definitive open reduction and internal fixation can be attempted later.

Lateral compression fractures

There are often minimally displaced and can be treated non-operatively. Open reduction and internal fixation is required where displacement leads to rotatory management of the lower limb or can be used to allow earlier mobilisation.

Vertical shear fractures

Clinical features Disruption of the pelvic ring with anterior and posterior injuries creates an ipsilateral segment of one-half of the pelvis. There may be fractures of two ipsilateral pubic rami, together with a posterior fracture of the ilium or a separation of the sacroiliac joint. Stressing the pelvis produces pain. One-half of the pelvis is obviously higher than the other, creating a difference in leg length.

Diagnosis Radiographs show the extent of the disruption.

Management Early stabilisation with an external fixator and longitudinal traction on the limb restores haemodynamic stability but definitive internal fixation will be necessary later.

Complications:
- circulatory collapse
- sacral nerve root disruption
- leg length discrepancy.

7.5 Spinal cord injuries

Spinal cord injuries usually occur in road traffic collisions or in falls from a height but can occur in falls from standing height in the elderly or in sporting injuries. They must always be suspended in major trauma patients and in those who have evidence of injury above the clavicles.

Cervical spine

The bony injury to the cervical spine may be complicated by damage to the cervical cord.

Clinical features:
- **Listen** – there may be a history of a fall from a height or other type of deceleration injury
- **Look** – abdominal respiration without thoracic expansion
- **Feel** – numbness to touch sensation in dermatomes below the level of the injury
- **Move** – the patient is unable to move the arms or legs voluntarily.

Diagnosis
Radiograph of the cervical spine shows the level of the injury, which may be a subluxation, a dislocation or a fracture (Figure 80). The extent of the bony injury can be further defined by CT scan and the soft tissue injury by MRI.

Management
Emergency treatment involves stabilisation of the spine with a collar, sandbags and tape while other life-threatening injuries are identified and treated. A urethral catheter is passed and ventilatory support may be required as the remaining respiratory muscles tire. Definitive management of the fracture or dislocation may be operative with internal fixation or non-operative with traction or an external fixation device. After a period of time, the definitive level of neurological deficit becomes apparent. Expert nursing care and multidisciplinary rehabilitation are

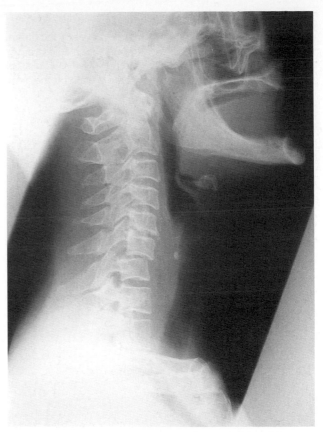

Figure 80 Lateral radiograph of the cervical spine showing all the cervical vertebrae. There is a subluxation of C6 on C7.

required to avoid complications. Reconstructive surgery can sometimes restore some function to the hand and elbow by tendon transfers from functioning muscles.

Complications:
- renal calculi
- urinary tract infection
- pressure sores
- impotence
- respiratory infection
- constipation
- depression.

Thoraco-lumbar spine

High-velocity injuries can cause fractures of the thoracic or lumbar spine without neurological damage, but in cases of fracture dislocation the spinal cord is often damaged, resulting in paraplegia.

Clinical features:
- **Listen** – history of a fall or road traffic accident
- **Look** – swelling and bruising over the spine at the site of the injury
- **Feel** – local tenderness
- **Move** – loss of voluntary movement below the spinal level of the injury.

Bladder function is impaired causing urinary retention.

Diagnosis

Radiological examination confirms the level of the spinal injury and shows the configuration of the fracture. As before, computed tomography (CT) and MRI will show the extent of cord and nerve root compression by the bony fragments.

Management

Particular care is required to prevent further damage to the cord and to avoid bed sores. Urethral catheterisation is required. The permanent level of the neurological deficit becomes apparent over a short period of time. Surgical stabilisation of the bony injury may be appropriate for local pain relief, but it does not reverse the neurological damage.

Patients will require a wheelchair for mobility, but with enthusiastic support a great deal of independence can be enjoyed.

Complications:

- renal calculi
- urinary tract infection
- pressure sores
- impotence
- constipation
- depression.

Fractures in children

Chapter part overview

How are children different?
- Bones are less brittle leading to different fracture patterns.
- Secondary ossification centres can cause problems with diagnosis.
- Children heal more quickly.
- Children's bones remodel.
- Physeal injuries.
- Non-accidental injury (child abuse).
- Primary bone tumours can be misinterpreted as injuries.

7.6 Clinical examination in children

Learning objectives

You should:
- know how to adapt your history taking and examination technique to the injured child
- be able to describe greenstick fractures and classify epiphyseal injuries
- be able to describe the management of these conditions.

A gentle and friendly approach is always required when examining children. Care must be taken not to cause any additional pain. It may be necessary to palpate in order to identify the likely fracture site prior to radiography but this should be done very gently. Early application of a plaster slab will relieve pain to allow testing of distal neurological function and circulation. Clinical comparison with the uninjured limb is valuable in identifying the injury but comparison radiography of the normal side should only be required in exceptional circumstances.

7.7 Fracture patterns

Because the growing bone has not yet fully ossified, skeletal injuries are different from those seen in adults. The bones are less brittle (more plastic) than those of adults. A moderate force will cause a child's bone to buckle on the compression side. With more force the distraction side of the bone will fracture causing the classic 'greenstick' fracture (Figure 81A). The growth plate of the bone (the physis) has not yet fused and can be seen between the epiphysis and the metaphysis (Figure 81B). Through this area particular injuries have been described.

Physeal injuries These injuries take place through the calcifying layer of chondrocytes in the growth plate or physis. Salter and Harris described various types of physeal injury (Figure 82). Types III, IV and V often cause partial or complete physical arrest.

Remodelling Children have the power to correct deformity as they grow. This is called remodelling. Remodelling is best when the patient is young, the fracture is near a physis and the deformity is in the plane of movement of an adjacent joint. Rotational deformity never remodels and varus/valgus deformity remodels poorly except near the shoulder and hip. Acceptable limits for various fractures are published.

7.8 Elbow fractures

Learning objectives

You should:
- be able to recognise a supracondylar fracture and institute emergency treatment
- know how to manage any early complications of this injury
- become familiar with the normal pattern of ossification at the elbow so that you can distinguish secondary centres of ossification from fractures.

Supracondylar fractures

This injury has the potential to be an orthopaedic emergency as it can cause compromise of the brachial artery leading to irreversible forearm ischaemia if treatment is delayed. The median nerve also may be compressed or injured.

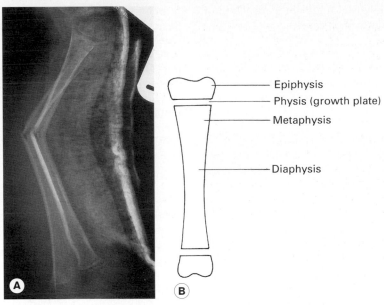

Figure 81 Greenstick fracture. (A) Fracture of both bones of the forearm. The compression side is still intact but the fracture is present through the cortex on the opposite side of the bone. (B) The immature skeleton grows longitudinally by the action of the growth plate situated between the epiphysis and the metaphysis.

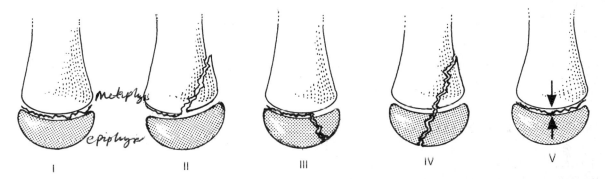

Figure 82 Salter and Harris classification of physeal injuries. I – The injury has separated the epiphysis from the metaphysis through the growth plate. II – The injury passes through a corner of the metaphysis. This is the most common injury. III – The injury passes through the epiphysis itself. IV – The fracture line crosses the physis from epiphysis to metaphysis. This type of injury can result in premature fusion of the epiphysis to the metaphysis. V – There has been a compression force on the physis. The radiograph appears normal.

Clinical features:

- **Listen** – a fall from a bicycle or a swing onto the outstretched hand in a young child is the usual presentation.
- **Look** – there is deformity and bruising at the elbow and a tense swelling develops quickly (Figure 83).
- **Feel** – the radial pulse must be palpated and if weak or absent the elbow should be gently extended to minimise any kinking of the brachial artery in the antecubital fossa. Symptoms and signs of median nerve compression may be apparent in the hand, and rarely the ulnar and radial nerves may be affected too.
- **Move** – all elbow movements are resisted.

Diagnosis

An antero-posterior radiograph shows varus or valgus angulation at the fracture site but a lateral view looks the most dramatic, especially in a completely displaced

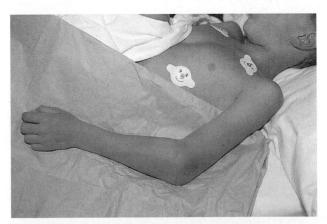

Figure 83 Supracondylar fracture of the elbow of an 8-year-old boy.

fracture (Figure 84A). The distal fragment is displaced or angulated posteriorly in nearly all cases.

Management

Undisplaced fractures can be treated in a cast. For displaced fractures, it is usually possible to correct the displacement by manipulation under anaesthesia but the

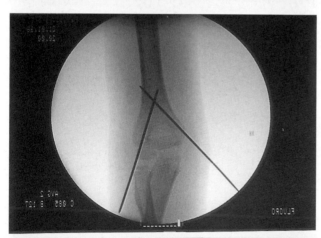

position will slip unless the elbow is held in extreme flexion. For this reason, the position is held with Kirschner wires (Figure 84B) allowing the elbow to be immobilised at 90°. Occasionally, it is necessary to open the fracture site to achieve the reduction. If the distal part of the limb is still ischaemic after fracture reduction then an arteriogram and/or exploration of the brachial artery will be required.

Complications:
- Early complications:
  - *acute occlusion of the brachial artery*
  - *median nerve damage*
  - *compartment syndrome.*
- Later complications:
  - *Volkmann's ischaemic contracture*
  - *myositis ossificans*
  - *malunion.*

Fractured lateral condylar mass

Avulsion fractures of the lateral aspect of the humerus may produce a displaced fragment that may be rotated and, therefore, will be impossible to correct by closed manipulation (Figure 85A).

Diagnosis

The radiograph may be difficult to interpret if there is no familiarity with the normal pattern of the centres of secondary ossification around the elbow. A comparison radiograph of the uninjured elbow is occasionally necessary.

Management

Accurate reduction by operative exposure and securing the fragment with a suture or Kirschner wire produces a secure anatomical position (Figure 85B).

Complications:
- non-union
- development of valgus deformity as a result of premature growth arrest
- tardy ulnar palsy (late ulnar nerve dysfunction secondary to the developing valgus deformity).

Medial epicondylar avulsion

A valgus injury to the elbow may avulse the medial epicondyle (Figure 85C). Sometimes it is only slightly displaced but on other occasions it is widely separated and becomes trapped in the joint space.

Diagnosis

Look carefully at the lateral view for any incongruity of the elbow joint indicating that a fragment is trapped between the surfaces. The fragment may be visible on either the AP or the lateral films. The medial epicondylar apophysis appears at between 5 and 8 years of age but does not fuse onto the rest of the bone until the mid-teens.

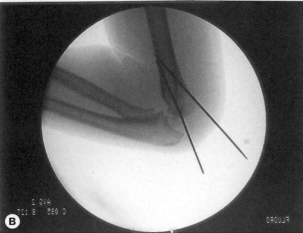

Figure 84 Supracondylar fracture. (A) Radiograph showing gross displacement at the fracture site. The associated kinking and compression of the brachial artery and median nerve can be imagined as they pass anterior to the bone fragments. (B) Kirschner wires used to secure a supracondylar fracture in the reduced position.

Management

Fractures with displacement of less than 5 mm are treated non-operatively. Those with incarceration of the fragment within the joint need an operation to remove the fragment

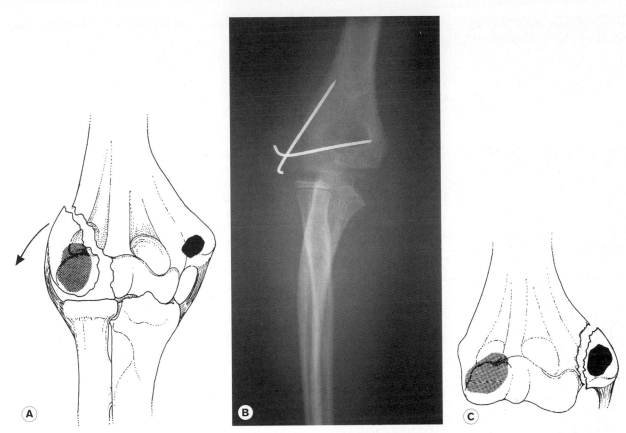

Figure 85 Fracture of the lateral condylar mass. (A) Diagram showing the mechanism of rotation and displacement caused by the fracture. (B) Kirschner wire fixation of the fracture seen in (A). (C) A fracture of the medial epicondyle may displace so that the fragment lies within the joint.

and fix it with Kirschner wires. There is disagreement about whether fractures between these extremes are treated operatively or non-operatively.

Complications:
- ulnar nerve dysfunction.

7.9 Femoral fractures

Clinical features

Significant trauma is required to break the femur. A fall down stairs or out of a tree is a typical history. On examination, the affected leg is shorter, swollen and externally rotated. There may be considerable blood loss into the tissues.

Diagnosis

Although the diagnosis is apparent clinically, a radiograph is necessary to assess the fracture pattern and the degree of displacement and angulation.

Management

Most femoral fractures in children are treated non-operatively in traction. Gallows traction (Figure 86) is used in children up to about 18 months old but after this age the height of the feet above the heart is too great and the toes become ischaemic. A Thomas splint is used in older children but pressure sores are a risk where the top of the splint rubs against the thigh. The number of weeks in traction is calculated as the child's age in years +1. You can see that traction treatment would be very prolonged for older children and may be unsuitable for other children such as those with attention deficit hyperactivity disorder. Adult nails are unsuitable because their insertion would destroy the physis, so plates, external fixators and flexible intramedullary nails are used instead.

Complications:
- shock
- malunion
- leg length discrepancy.

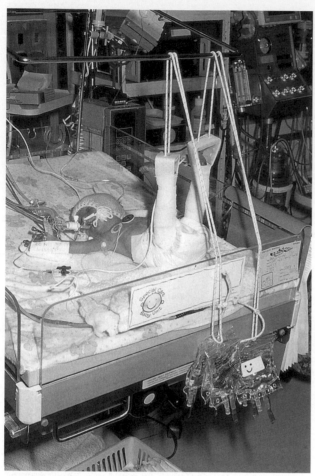

Figure 86 Gallows traction being used to manage a femoral fracture in a neonate.

7.10 Dysplasia, cysts and non-accidental injury

Learning objectives

You should:
- know when to suspect that a fracture may be caused by one of these
- know when to suspect non-accidental injury and what to do about it.

Fractures in the absence of a history of significant injury raise the possibility of these diagnoses.

Dysplasia

Fibrous dysplasia The bone is soft and weak with extensive areas of fibrous tissue. Fractures and deformity develop.

Osteogenesis imperfecta There is often a positive family history, but occasionally a case occurs as a result of a new mutation. A spectrum of severity can occur from multiple fractures causing deformity, stunted growth or death in infancy to mild cases with few fractures. Some

types are associated with blue sclerae or malformation of the teeth.

Management:
- simple immobilisation of fractures
- bisphosphonate treatment to reduce further fractures in osteogenesis imperfecta
- later surgery to correct deformity.

Bone cysts

A bone cyst is a fluid-filled cavity within a bone. It is seen on the radiograph as a lucent area within the bone that is ovoid or loculated with a clearly defined edge. If the edge is not clearly defined or the lucency looks ragged, suspect a malignant tumour instead. Benign and malignant cartilage tumours are distinguished by their speckled calcification.

Non-accidental injury

The group most at risk are pre-school children. Suspect non-accidental injury when the history does not fit the injury, e.g. femoral fracture attributed to a simple trip and fall. Be especially suspicious of fractures in children too young to walk. Other suspicious signs are

- fractures at various stages of healing
- history changes between witnesses or over time
- burns or bruises on other areas of the body
- abnormal affect of child or parent.

Management:
- Admit to hospital.
- Examine the whole child.
- Skeletal survey (a series of standard radiographs).
- Manage jointly with senior paediatrician.
- Inform child protection services.

Fractures in the elderly and other low-energy fractures

7.11 Clinical examination in the elderly

Learning objectives

You should:
- practice how best to communicate with an elderly patient who may be debilitated, deaf or suffering from dementia
- know how to look for medical comorbidities and malignancy
- demonstrate a holistic approach considering rehabilitation and prevention of other fractures.

When elderly people suffer a fracture, there is commonly both a medical cause for the fall and a reason why the bone is fragile enough to break. These must be actively investigated but history taking may be complicated by deafness, debility or dementia. Listen to relatives and talk to the patient's GP or nursing home staff. Remember that the medicines the patient brings in may not be the ones they are currently taking and that some patients are harmed by omission or incorrect prescription in hospital. The physical examination needs to be extensive enough to identify comorbidities such as atrial fibrillation or exacerbation of COPD causing hypoxia.

The physical examination of the injured part involves the usual 'look, feel and move', but in the presence of suspected malignancy do not forget the breasts, chest, abdomen, neck and rectum.

Remember that a multidisciplinary approach will be required to return the patient to their optimum function and that the team should include physiotherapist, occupational therapist, social worker, specialist nurses and geriatrician as well as the orthopaedic surgeon.

Osteoporosis

Osteoporosis presents in both men and women with advancing age but is much exacerbated in women by the drop in estrogen levels after the menopause. Immobility, smoking, alcoholism and dietary deficiency also contribute. It is caused at a tissue level by an excess of bone resorption over bone formation and, in contrast to osteomalacia, both mineral and non-mineral matrix are lost. Secondary prevention of osteoporosis (i.e. treatment which begins after a fracture has occurred) involves stopping smoking, reducing alcohol consumption, increasing weight-bearing exercise and the use of bisphosphonates. These drugs act to reduce resorption of bone by osteoclasts, allowing the osteoblasts to catch up.

7.12 Distal radius fractures

Learning objectives

You should:
- be able to recognise a Colles' fracture clinically
- remember the importance of a true lateral radiograph in assessing the direction and degree of angulation
- know that high-velocity fractures in younger people will be unlikely to behave as satisfactorily with plaster immobilisation alone as low-velocity fractures of the same area in older people.

The Colles' fracture is the classic injury seen in postmenopausal women usually in the seventh decade. The true Colles' fracture is extra-articular and there is dorsal displacement of the distal fragment.

Clinical features:

- **Listen** – there is usually a history of a fall on the outstretched hand.
- **Look** – the distal fragment of the radius and the attached carpal bones are usually displaced posteriorly to create the characteristic 'dinner fork' deformity of the wrist (Figure 87). There is often swelling and bruising. Radial deviation and supination of the distal fragment may also be present.

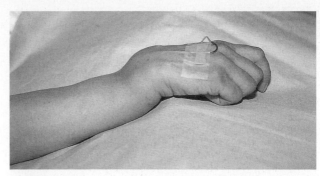

Figure 87 Classic dinner fork deformity of a Colles' fracture.

- **Feel**
  - tenderness
  - the median nerve may be compressed, producing altered sensation in the radial three and a half digits.
- **Move**
  - the patient is reluctant to move the wrist
  - crepitus may be apparent.

Diagnosis

An antero-posterior and a true lateral radiograph of the wrist are required to confirm the diagnosis (Figure 88A). There is often impaction at the fracture site as the distal fragment is displaced proximally. This produces shortening of the radius, and the ulna now appears relatively long.

Management

The casualty officer dealing with this injury needs to decide whether the fracture requires to be reduced. To do this the amount of displacement at the fracture site must be assessed to see if it is acceptable and can be simply splinted; otherwise an anatomical position should be sought by means of manipulation under anaesthesia.

If the fracture is not manipulated or 'reduced', the fracture will still unite but in an abnormal position. Moderate degrees of displacement may be acceptable, but more severe malunion will cause limitation of wrist function, especially flexion and supination. Figure 88B shows the method of measuring the degree of angulation present at the fracture site between the two fragments. The line AB has been drawn across the articular surface of the radius on the lateral radiograph. A perpendicular line to this transects the line drawn along the long axis of the proximal fragment of the radius; usually 15° of angulation is acceptable. Angulation greater than this is usually corrected by manipulation.

Manipulation of the fracture requires reversal of the direction of the deforming force that produced the original injury. After manipulating a fracture into an acceptable position, there are several ways available to hold it until the fracture has united.

Usually a Colles' fracture can be held in place with a plaster of Paris cast. This holds the wrist in the reduced position of flexion, ulnar deviation and pronation. This position is exactly the opposite from the displaced position of the Colles' fracture.

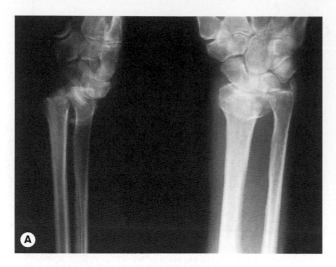

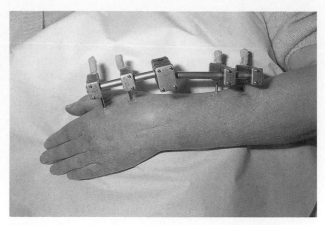

Figure 89 Comminuted fracture of the distal radius in a younger patient stabilised by an external fixator which holds the radius at its correct length and position.

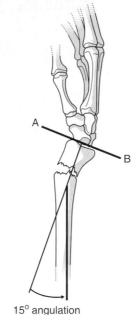

B 15° angulation

Figure 88 (A) Lateral and antero-posterior radiograph of a Colles' fracture, showing the posterior displacement of the distal radial fragment and shortening of the radius. (B) Method of measuring the degree of angulation present at the fracture site.

A minor degree of malunion is acceptable as the functional result may be unimpaired. In some cases, the fracture may be very unstable when manipulated and consequently difficult to hold in the correct position in relation to the ulna by plaster of Paris alone. In such cases percutaneous pins or an external fixator may be used to splint the fracture until union is achieved. The external fixator can be applied to the second metacarpal and the proximal radius (Figure 89).

Fractures with displaced intra-articular fragments or volar angulation and comminuted, high-energy injuries in high-demand patients are less likely to give satisfactory results with closed treatment. Here, open reduction and plate fixation or percutaneous reduction and pins along with an external fixator may be better.

After 4–6 weeks' immobilisation, the wrist will become stiff and a period of physiotherapy is often required to regain a full range of mobilisation. The patient is required to attempt active dorsiflexion, palmar flexion and supination/pronation exercises and also to exercise the elbow and shoulder.

Complications

Complications can be divided into those occurring early and late:

- early complications
  - *median nerve compression*
- late complications
  - *malunion*
  - *elbow and wrist stiffness*
  - *stiff shoulder*
  - *spontaneous rupture of extensor pollicis longus*
  - *reflex sympathetic dystrophy (Sudek's atrophy).*

7.13 Proximal humerus fractures

Learning objectives

You should:
- be able to distinguish extracapsular fractures of the surgical neck from intracapsular fractures involving the tuberosities and/or anatomical neck of the humerus
- be able to recognise the complications of axillary nerve or brachial artery damage
- be aware of the importance of early mobilisation in rehabilitating soft tissues and preventing shoulder stiffness.

A history of a fall on the outstretched hand in a woman in her seventies is a common presentation of a fracture of the upper humerus.

Classification:

- Intracapsular fractures occur at the anatomical neck with avulsion of one or both tuberosities.
- Extracapsular fractures occur at the surgical neck, the narrowest portion of the proximal humerus.

The blood supply to the humeral head may be disrupted in intracapsular fractures because of its separation from the greater and lesser tuberosities (and their soft tissue attachments) and because of the fracture in the shaft below it. The head is liable to undergo avascular necrosis in the same way as that seen in subcapital fractures of the head of the femur (see p. 170).

Clinical features

There is bruising and swelling over the shoulder with loss of abduction because of pain. Axillary nerve damage may be present and must be searched for by eliciting an area of decreased sensation in the 'badge patch' area at the point of the shoulder.

Diagnosis

An antero-posterior and lateral or axial radiograph of the shoulder are required. The bone fragments may be impacted into each other or widely displaced. The greater and lesser tuberosities may form separate fragments and the humeral head may appear to have 'capsized' in the joint (Figure 90A). Coexisting dislocation of the shoulder joint occurs rarely.

Management

Impacted fractures of the surgical neck of the humerus are usually rested for a few days in a collar and cuff sling and pendulum exercises begun early to avoid shoulder stiffness. Modern fixation methods allow fixation of displaced, extra-articular fractures if the patient's general health and local tissues are good enough.

Intracapsular fractures with marked displacement of the fragments may lead to avascular necrosis of the head. In these cases, a hemiarthroplasty is used (Figure 90B). Early mobilisation is essential with all treatment modalities.

Complications:
- early
  - *axillary nerve palsy*
- late
  - *stiff shoulder*
  - *malunion*
  - *impingement (see section 8.10, p. 192).*

7.14 Femoral neck fractures

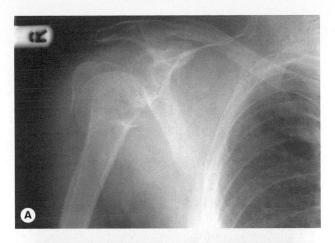

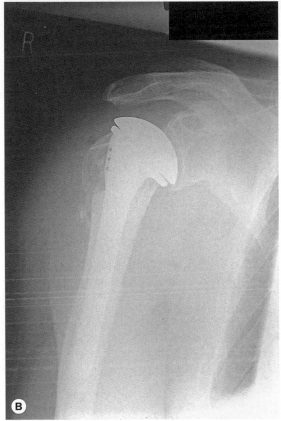

Figure 90 (A) Four-part fracture of the humerus in a 65-year-old man. The articular surface of the humerus is rotated away from the glenoid. (B) Fracture seen in Figure 90A treated by excision of the humeral head and insertion of a hemiarthroplasty.

Learning objectives

You should:
- be able to recognise the classic clinical appearances of external rotation and shortening
- be able to distinguish an extracapsular fracture from an intracapsular fracture on radiological examination
- anticipate when avasacular necrosis of the femoral head may be expected to occur
- appreciate the importance to the patient of early postoperative mobilisation and rehabilitation.

A fracture of the femoral neck is the most common fracture seen in elderly women and usually occurs in the eighth and ninth decade of life. The cause is usually a simple fall at home but it may be associated with another medical problem, such as a stroke, hypotensive crisis or poor vision. Whatever the cause, the result may be the ultimate loss of independence, especially for someone who was previously just managing to live alone safely.

Classification:

- Intracapsular fractures occur within the capsule and may be transcervical or subcapital.
- Extracapsular fractures occur outside the capsule and may be sited through the base of the femoral neck (basal) or through the trochanters (intertrochanteric).

Why is it so important to differentiate intracapsular fractures from extracapsular fractures? Figure 91 shows the blood supply to the femoral head, which comes through the diaphyseal vessels along the femoral neck, via the foveal artery to a small area of the articular surface and, most importantly, via the retinacular vessels, which are reflected from the capsule along the femoral neck to enter the head around its margin. If these vessels are damaged by a significantly displaced subcapital fracture then avascular necrosis of the femoral head will result.

Clinical features:

- **Listen** – a usual history of the event is that of a frail elderly woman who has fallen at home and been found by neighbours after she has been lying on the floor all night. Apart from pain at the hip, the patient is often confused and may be suffering from hypothermia.
- **Look** – the affected leg is shortened and externally rotated.
- **Feel** – tenderness over the greater trochanter.
- **Move** – pain on attempting movement of the hip.

A variety of medical problems are often present.

Intracapsular fractures

Diagnosis

An antero-posterior and lateral radiograph of the femoral neck are required (Figure 92). If the line of the cortex of the medial side of the femoral shaft is traced upwards towards the pelvis, it can be seen how this line continues along the inferior side of the neck of the femur until it comes to a sudden stop at the fracture site. The fracture in this case is intracapsular and in particular a subcapital fracture. If the fracture were not there, the line traced along the medial

side of the shaft of the femur and the inferior side of the femoral neck would continue in a smooth curve along the inferior side of the superior pubic ramus (Shenton's line). A break in continuity of this line helps to find a fracture in the femoral neck (Figure 93).

Management

Initial management includes rehydration, pain relief and treatment of underlying medical conditions.

An undisplaced intracapsular fracture is usually treated with internal fixation although avascular necrosis can still occur. Displaced intracapsular fractures have a significant rate of avascular necrosis and a hemiarthroplasty is used in the elderly and frail to reduce the requirement for a second operation. In younger patients, reduction and internal fixation can be attempted with the salvage option of total hip replacement if it fails.

Complications

Avascular necrosis of the femoral head is the main complication arising from an intracapsular fracture. Other complications may occur after hemiarthroplasty:

- dislocation
- erosion of acetabular floor
- need for revision surgery
- infection.

Extracapsular fractures

In Figure 94, you can see how the fracture line passes obliquely through the greater trochanter at the top left of the picture across towards the lesser trochanter. This is an extracapsular fracture. This fracture is distal to the capsule and is sited through the trochanters at the base of the femoral neck.

Management

General medical management is required initially as before.

Extracapsular fractures will unite without treatment, but malunion will be present unless external rotation and

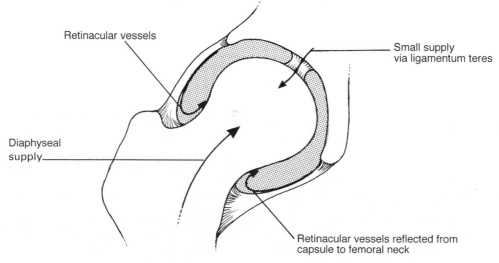

Retinacular vessels

Small supply via ligamentum teres

Diaphyseal supply

Retinacular vessels reflected from capsule to femoral neck

Figure 91 Blood supply to the femoral head.

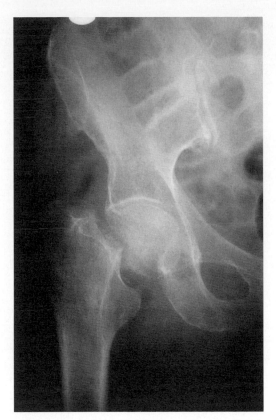

Figure 92 Intracapsular (subcapital) fracture of the femoral neck.

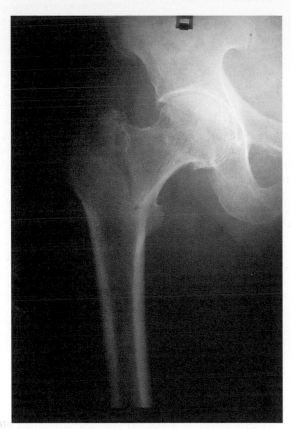

Figure 94 Extracapsular (intertrochanteric) fracture of the femoral neck.

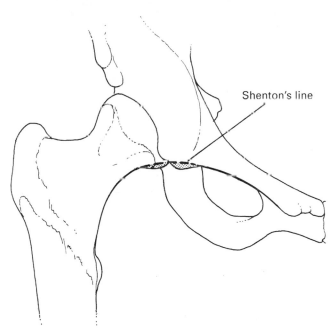

Shenton's line

Figure 93 Normal appearance of Shenton's line. Compare this with the radiograph of the fracture of the femoral neck in Figure 92.

shortening are corrected. Traction could be used to prevent this, but the prolonged period of bed rest involved would give rise to many other complications which together would probably be fatal. For this reason the fracture is usually treated by closed reduction and fixed with an internal fixation device such as the dynamic hip screw. The barrel and sliding screw portion are positioned in the neck and head of the femur with radiographic screening using an image-intensifier. The plate is then secured to the upper femoral shaft by screws.

The patient can begin weight-bearing within 2 or 3 days of surgery, allowing the screw to retract into the barrel as the fracture impacts. With this device, the patient has the best chance of regaining mobility and independence and of returning home.

Complications

Complications of internal fixation include:

- general complications of surgery
- infection
- implant failure
  - *cutting out*
  - *breaking*
- fracture through the porotic bone at the end of the plate.

7.15 Vertebral body fractures

Learning objectives

You should:

- be able to recognise these fractures on a lateral radiograph
- remember that, although osteoporosis is a common cause, secondary deposit in the vertebral bodies should be looked for.

Patients with osteoporosis may suffer spontaneous vertebral compression fractures of the vertical bodies. The thoracic vertebrae are most commonly affected but the lumbar vertebrae may also be involved.

Clinical features

An elderly woman gives a history of sudden onset of back pain after merely stooping or lifting a light object. Often there is a history of multiple similar events and, as a result, an increasing kyphosis becomes apparent in the thoraco-lumbar spine.

Characteristically, there are no neurological deficits in the limbs as there is no impingement of the spinal cord or nerve roots. The fractures are stable.

Diagnosis

Crush fractures of vertebrae characteristically form wedge shapes compressed anteriorly when seen on the lateral radiograph (Figure 95).

Management

Symptoms are relieved by a short period of bed rest. Mobilisation should be commenced as soon as possible. Implement a secondary prevention strategy.

Complications:

- increasing kyphosis
- pressure sores over the prominent spinous processes.

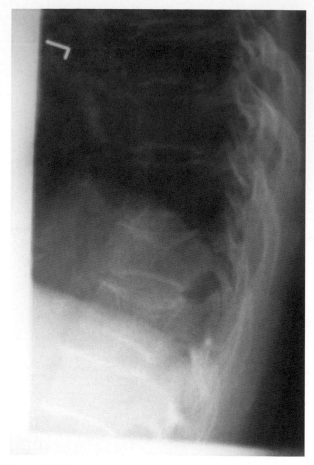

Figure 95 Both wedge-shaped and bi-concave compression fractures are seen in the lower thoracic vertebrae in this woman with osteoporosis.

7.16 Pathological fractures

Learning objectives

You should:
- be able to list the common primary tumours which metastasise to bone
- recognise features in the history which may suggest a pathological fracture
- remember that treatment may be required for hypercalcaemia, dehydration and the primary pathology as well as for the fracture.

Pathological fractures occur through areas of abnormally weak bone.

Classification

Bone may be weak because of:

- generalised disease
  - osteoporosis
  - osteomalacia and rickets
  - Paget's disease
  - osteogenesis imperfecta
- local disease
  - metastatic tumour
  - primary tumour (including multiple myeloma)
  - fibrous dysplasia
  - bone cysts
  - osteitis.

The most common tumour seen in the skeleton is a metastasis from a primary tumour elsewhere. Usual sites of the primary are:

- bronchus
- breast
- prostate
- thyroid
- kidney.

Clinical features

The key features of a pathological fracture are:

- pain at the site, which pre-dates the injury
- a fracture caused by minimal trauma.

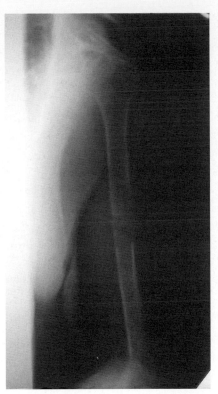

Figure 96 Pathological fracture in the humerus in a patient with a primary breast carcinoma.

Diagnosis

Pathological fractures are characteristically transverse and may be widely displaced (Figure 96).

Management

The local management of a fracture through a metastatic deposit in a long bone is with intramedullary nailing without reaming so as to reduce tumour embolisation. Adjuvant treatment with radiation or chemotherapy depends on the tissue type of the tumour. Primary tumours are often treated with wide excision and endoprosthetic reconstruction. They should be managed in specialist units.

Complications:

- hypercalcaemia
- dehydration
- occult primary
- second deposit elsewhere.

Seven

Self-assessment: questions

Musculoskeletal trauma in adults

Extended matching items questions (EMIs)

EMI 1

Theme: Treatment of fractures

A. functional bracing

B. balanced traction

C. intermedullary fixation

D. plate and screw fixation

E. tension band wire

F. fixed skin traction

G. plaster of Paris cast

H. external fixator

I. overhead traction

J. interfragmentary screws

From the list above identify the most suitable method for treating the fractures described below:

1. A fracture of both bones of the forearm in an adult.

2. A displaced fracture of the olecranon.

3. A femoral shaft fracture in a 3-year-old.

EMI 2

Theme: fracture management

A. traction

B. internal fixation

C. external fixator

D. manipulation and plaster cast

E. collar and cuff sling

F. prosthetic replacement

Match the following injuries with their usual treatment. Each option may be used once, more than once or not at all.

1. A displaced intracapsular fracture of the femoral neck in an 85-year-old.

2. A displaced fracture of the medial tibial plateau.

3. An undisplaced fracture of the proximal humerus.

4. A midshaft femoral fracture in a 4-year-old.

5. An angulated, extra-articular fracture of the distal radius.

6. A displaced fracture of the acetabulum.

EMI 3

Theme: Fractures of the femur

A. fractured shaft of femur

B. displaced intracapsular fractured neck of femur

C. intertrochanteric fracture

D. displaced intra-articular fracture of the distal femur

E. osteochondral fracture of the femoral head

Match the following statements with the most appropriate injury.

1. is usually treated with an intramedullary nail

2. is usually associated with an acetabular fracture

3. is usually treated with a sliding screw and plate

4. carries a risk of post-traumatic osteoarthritis of the knee

5. is usually treated with prosthetic replacement

EMI 4

Theme: Clinical presentation

A. external rotation and shortening of the leg

B. fixed flexion

C. adduction contracture

D. increase in true leg length

E. apparent lengthening

F. bruising down the iliotibial tract

G. bruising over the trochanteric bursa

H. perineal swelling and bruising with blood at the urinary meatus

I. abduction deformity

J. internal rotation and shortening of the leg

Identify the clinical presentation from the list above which is mostly commonly associated with the conditions described below:

1. A front seat car passenger involved in a head-on collision injures her knee on the dashboard. Her hip is painful.

2. Subtrochanteric fracture.

3. High-energy fracture of multiple public rami.

Constructed response questions (CRQs)

CRQ 1

A 20-year-old man has been thrown from his motorcycle in a collision with your car. He is lying on his back motionless at the roadside.

a. What is the first thing that you should do?

b. What is the next important thing to do for the victim?

c. The patient is conscious but has bleeding wounds over both thins; the legs below this level are obviously out of alignment. What should you assess next? *open/closed*

d. Subsequent examination in hospital reveals open, comminuted fractures of the upper third of both tibia and fibula. What would be a suitable method of managing these injuries for this patient?

CRQ 2

The ward nurse calls you to a patient complaining of pain beneath his plaster. He has had a closed fracture of the tibia manipulated and an above-knee cast applied earlier in the day. When you observe the patient, he has swollen, purplish toes and does not like to move them.

a. What do you think is the cause of the patient's symptoms?

b. What clinical manoeuvre could you carry out to reinforce this diagnosis?

c. What simple measure would you take next?

d. Despite this measure the patient's symptoms are unaltered. Describe the pathological process which is taking place.

e. If you do nothing now what will develop?

f. What should your next line of management be?

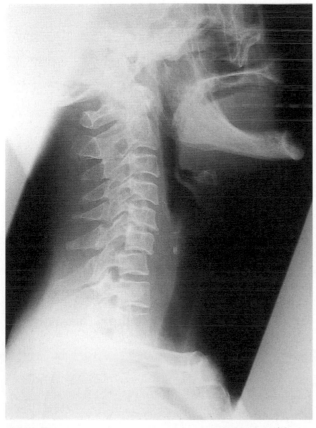

Figure 97

Objective structured clinical examination questions (OSCEs)

OSCE 1

Study the photograph of an radiograph of the cervical spine from a patient in a high velocity accident (Figure 97).

a. At which cervical vertebra level has there been an injury?

b. What symptoms would you expect the patient to be complaining of:
   i. in the neck?
   ii. in the arms?

c. You are uncertain whether the spinal column is stable. How could this be visualised more accurately?

d. What conservative management could be used?

   What other definitive treatment can you suggest?

OSCE 2

A young man has bilateral hip injuries from a motorbike accident. Study the photograph of a radiograph of the right hip (Figure 98A and B).

a. What injury is shown?

b. What further information would you require about this fracture?

c. On the left side he has had a posterior dislocation of the hip, which has been reduced urgently in the casualty department. CT scan of this site shows an abnormality. How has this occurred?

d. How should both these injuries be treated?

Best of 5s questions

1. A 24-year-old motorcyclist is brought into accident and emergency after a high-speed collision with a car. He has a grossly deformed, swollen thigh with an overlying wound. Your first priority is:
   a. give intravenous broad-spectrum antibiotics and put an antiseptic dressing on the thigh wound
   b. take a radiograph of the femur
   c. apply a Thomas splint
   d. assess the airway and protect the cervical spine
   e. give intravenous morphine

Fractures in children

Extended matching items questions (EMIs)

EMI 1

Theme: Complications

A. myositis ossificans

B. ischaemic contracture

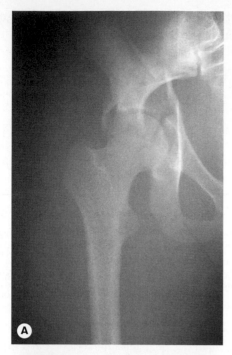

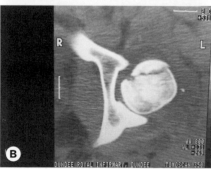

Figure 98

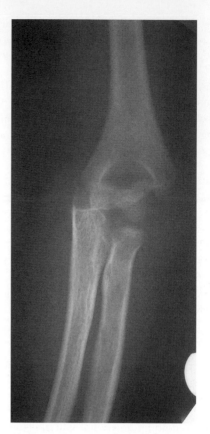

Figure 99

C. varus deformity developing with growth

D. loss of full flexion

E. valgus deformity developing with growth

F. initial bone length discrepancy

G. vascular injury

H. acute ulnar nerve dysfunction

I. risk of avascular necrosis

J. loss of full extension

Which of the complications listed above is most likely to be associated with the conditions below?

1. An overriding transverse femoral shaft fracture in a 4-year-old boy.

2. Fracture of the lateral condylar mass involving the growth plate.

3. Severe displacement or over-aggressive manipulation of a slipped femoral epiphysis.

Constructed response questions (CRQs)

CRQ 1

An 8-year-old boy presents to the accident and emergency department with a history of having fallen from a swing and hurt his elbow.

a. You are the casualty officer on duty. What would you expect to find on physical examination?

b. He is holding the elbow flexed in a sling. What additional damage may this be causing beyond the fracture site?

c. What would you do to remedy this situation?

d. You suspect a supracondylar fracture of the humerus. What radiographs would you request?

e. What is the name given to the condition caused by prolonged vascular occlusion with this injury?

Objective structured clinical examination questions (OSCEs)

OSCE 1

Study the photograph of the radiograph of an elbow of an 8-year-old (Figure 99).

a. What condition does this show?

b. What are the principles of treating this injury?

c. What is a long-term complication of this injury?

d. What is the effect of this on the ulnar nerve?

Multiple choice questions

1. When managing fractures in children:

    a. the presence of multiple fractures of different ages is suggestive of non-accidental injury (NAI)

    b. the presence of pain on passive extension of the toes after a closed tibial fracture is due to impingement of the muscle bellies at the fracture site

    c. failure to achieve a satisfactory reduction of a fracture at the elbow warrants open reduction and internal fixation

    d. conservative treatment is used less frequently than internal fixation for the stabilisation of femoral shaft fractures

    e. the initial treatment of impending compartment syndrome would be the release of all constricting plaster bandages

Fractures in the elderly and other low-energy fractures

Extended matching items questions (EMIs)

EMI 1

Theme: Fracture descriptions

A. a transverse fracture through a previously painful area

B. undisplaced Colles' fracture

C. multiple vertebral crush fractures

D. fracture of the surgical neck of humerus

E. subcapital femoral neck fracture

F. displaced Colles' fracture

G. fractured greater tuberosity

H. vertebral body fracture

I. lytic area in a vertebral body on radiograph

J. extracapsular femoral neck fracture

Which of the descriptions listed above most commonly matches the statements below:

1. This is a pathological fracture.

2. There is a substantial risk of avascular necrosis.

3. Further general investigations are needed.

Constructed response questions (CRQs)

CRQ 1

An 86-year-old woman is found lying on her kitchen floor. She is unable to bear weight on her right leg. She appears to have been lying overnight but has no other injuries.

a. What clinical features would confirm a diagnosis of a fractured femur?

b. What other general medical problems are likely to be present in this particular case?

c. Radiograph examination shows a fracture extending from the greater trochanter to the lesser trochanter. What type of fracture is this?

d. How is this injury usually managed?

e. List four postoperative complications associated with this line of management.

CRQ 2

An 84-year-old woman weighing 95 kg presents having fallen in her home. She is unable to bear weight on the right leg. There is little to see on physical examination but moving the hip is painful. You suspect a fracture of the femoral neck and arrange a radiograph. This is reported as negative.

a. What other fracture may she have sustained?

b. You decide to manage her conservatively with bed rest. What are the risks of bed rest for this patient?

c. After a week she is reluctant to recommence weight bearing but the nursing staff think she should be made ready for discharge. Who might help you with this patient at this stage?

CRQ 3

An emaciated 65-year-old woman, with a lifetime history of smoking and a recent non-productive cough, presents with a sudden exacerbation of back pain. She has had discomfort in the same area for some months, but while bending to pick something from the floor today experienced a sharp, severe and persisting pain in this region.

a. What do you expect to find on physical examination of her back?

b. Antero-posterior and lateral radiographs are taken. What would you particularly look for?

c. What is the site of the likely cause of these features?

d. Outline aspects of the management now required.

Objective structured clinical examination questions (OSCEs)

OSCE 1

Look at the photograph of the radiograph of the Colles' fracture (Figure 100).

a. What deformity does the distal fragment show?

b. Looking at the antero-posterior radiograph, what does this show has happened to the radius?

c. In this type of injury the patient may complain of pins and needles in the radial three digits. Why should this be?

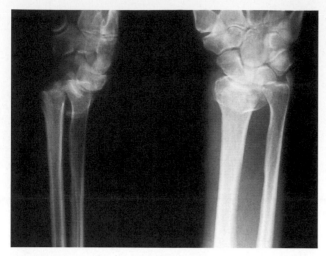

Figure 100

d. Manipulation and plaster of Paris immobilisation are the usual ways of treating this injury in an elderly patient. List four complications.

OSCE 2

Study the photograph of an radiograph of a fracture of the upper humerus in a 60-year-old woman (Figure 101).
  a. The fracture has divided the humerus into three large portions. What are they?
  b. Is this then an intracapsular fracture, an extracapsular fracture, or both?
  c. The rotator cuff muscles are attached to which of these portions?
  d. What is the risk to the humeral head in this fracture?
  e. If the axillary nerve has been damaged by the fracture, how could this be detected?

Multiple choice questions

1. Recognised complications of Colles' fracture include:
   a. median nerve compression
   b. loss of full supination
   c. loss of dorsiflexion

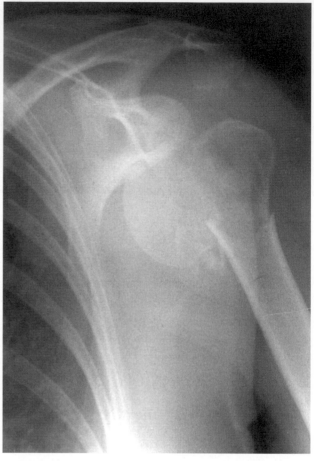

Figure 101

   d. reflex sympathetic dystrophy
   e. avascular necrosis of the lunate

2. The following complications are associated with a fracture of the surgical neck of the humerus:
   a. avascular necrosis of the humeral head
   b. non-union of the greater tuberosity
   c. axillary nerve damage
   d. loss of abduction
   e. non-union

Self-assessment: answers

Musculoskeletal trauma in adults

EMI answers

EMI 1

Theme: Treatment of fractures

1. D. Anatomical reduction with direct compression plate fixation or low contact direct compression plate is the treatment of choice for a fracture in an adult.

2. E. A displaced fracture of the olecranon requires to be held in place. Tension band wire is a recommended way of doing this.

3. F. Fixed traction using elastoplast attached to the skin provides satisfactory control of this fracture.

EMI .2

Theme: Fracture management

1. F
2. B
3. E
4. A
5. D
6. B

EMI 3

Theme: Fractures of the femur

1. A
2. E
3. C
4. D
5. B

EMI 4

Theme: Clinical presentation

1. J. This is a classic story of a posterior dislocation of the hip. The characteristic clinical presentation for this is internal rotation and shortening.

2. A. In a subtrochanteric fracture the leg will lie in external rotation with shortening.

3. H. In a high-energy injury with multiple fractures of the pubic rami, there will be a perineal swelling and bruising, with possible damage to the urethra presenting with blood at the urinary meatus.

CRQ answers

CRQ 1

a. Take measures to ensure the safety of yourself and the victim both from other vehicles and from petrol fire at the site of the accident.

b. Check airway and cervical spine control.

c. Peripheral pulses distal to the site of injury.

d. Wound excision and debridement. External fixation.

CRQ 2

a. Compartment syndrome.

b. Pain on passive dorsi-flexion of the toes.

c. Split the plaster down to the skin.

d. Swelling or bleeding within a fascial compartment causing flexor muscle compression and nerve ischaemia.

e. Continuing pain with progression to loss of peripheral sensation and circulation.

f. Surgical decompression of the fascial compartments in the leg.

OSCE answers

OSCE 1

a. Forward subluxation of C6 on C7.

b. The patient may complain of localised mechanical neck pain due to soft tissue and joint injury in this area. In the arms, the patient may have pain, tingling or numbness in the C7 dermatome on the ulnar side of the hand and forearm.

c. CT scan or MRI scan.

d. The patient's neck can be stabilised in a rigid cervical collar with metal supports between the occiput support and breast plate. Surgical treatment would be formal reduction of the dislocated vertebrae with posterior stabilisation using plates or wire loops.

OSCE 2

a. A comminuted fracture of the right acetabulum.

b. CT scan to determine the anatomy of the fragments.

c. This is a displaced fracture of the femoral head, which has been sheared off during the dislocation of the head by the posterior acetabular lip.

d. Open reduction and internal fixation is required on the right side. The femoral head fragment on the left side may require internal fixation if large.

Best of 5s answer

1. d.

Fractures in children

● ● ● ● ● ● ● ● ● ● ● ● ● ● ● ● ● ● ●

EMI 1

Theme: Complications

1. F. As the fracture heals with some overriding of the bone ends there will be *shortening* of leg length but this will correct as the limb grows. If the fracture were anatomically reduced there would be a risk of *increased* leg length in response to the hyperaemia of fracture healing.

2. E. Premature physeal growth arrest on the lateral side of the elbow allows the development of valgus angulation as the medial side grows.

3. I. The blood supply to the capital epiphysis may be disrupted causing chondromalacia and ultimately avascular necrosis of the femoral head.

CRQ 1

a. Bruising, swelling, deformity around the elbow.

b. Compromised blood supply to the forearm and hand. Absent radial pulse.

c. Straighten the arm and observe the return of the radial pulse.

d. Antero-posteral and true lateral (see Figure 84A).

e. Volkman's ischaemic contracture.

OSCE 1

a. Fracture of the lateral mass of the elbow.

b. Open reduction and internal fixation to secure anatomical position. K wires used to secure the fragment across the growth plate (see Figure 102).

c. Premature closure of the lateral condylar physis and development of cubitus valgus.

d. Tardy ulnar palsy.

Multiple choice answers

1. a. **False.** The child may have bone dysplasia such as osteogenesis imperfecta. Other features such as bruising are required to make the diagnosis of NAI.

b. **False.** The presence of pain on passive extension of the toes in this case is caused by ischaemia of the muscle bellies and not by impingement at the fracture site. The findings suggest compartment syndrome.

c. **True.** In general, operative techniques and anaesthetic procedures are now so safe and reliable that it is in the patient's best interests to change the fracture management to open reduction and internal fixation if a satisfactory position cannot readily be achieved or held by conservative measures.

d. **False.** Conservative treatment is the usual method of splinting femoral shaft fractures in children.

e. **True.** Compartment syndrome is suspected because of the presence of intractable pain in the limb exacerbated by passive extension of the digits. There may be associated paraesthesia or numbness in a peripheral nerve distribution. If symptoms are not relieved by releasing all constricting dressings, fasciotomy should be undertaken sooner rather than later.

Fractures in the elderly and other low-energy fractures

● ● ● ● ● ● ● ● ● ● ● ● ● ● ● ● ● ● ●

EMI 1

Theme: Fracture descriptions

1. A. The deposit in the bone has been a source of pain before the fracture occurs. Fractures are usually transverse with minimum trauma.

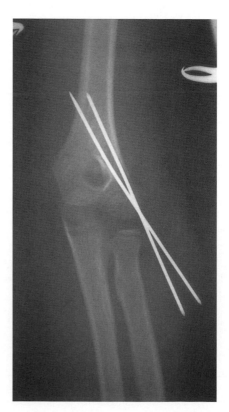

Figure 102

2. E. Loss of blood supply to the femoral head from a displaced subcapital fracture may lead to avascular necrosis.

3. I. Isolated lytic area in a vertebral body on a radiograph requires further investigation to determine its nature. It is probably best considered a secondary deposit until proved otherwise.

CRQ 1

a. local pain and deformity

shortened leg

external rotation

b. hypothermia and dehydration

c. extracapsular/intertrochanteric fracture

d. internal fixation under radiograph control using a dynamic hip screw or a nail and plate

e. chest infection

deep vein thrombosis

wound breakdown

loss of mobility

CRQ 2

a. Fracture of the greater trochanter or fracture of a pubic ramus.

b. pressure sores

DVT

urinary tract infection

chest infection

c. physiotherapist

walking aids

occupational therapist for home visit and assessment for any additional aids in the house

CRQ 3

a. Localised tenderness and swelling at the site of the pain with prominence of the spinus process suggest an underlying kyphosis.

b. Wedge fracture of a vertebrae at the site. Evidence of bone destruction nearby suggesting a metastatic tumour deposit.

c. bronchogenic carcinoma

d. bed rest until comfortable with analgesics and mobilisation

radiotherapy to the secondary deposits

investigation to find the site of the primary tumour and start appropriate therapy

investigations for hypercalcaemia and dehydration

OSCE 1

a. Dorsal angulation.

b. Impaction and shortening.

c. Median nerve compression from the deformity and associated swelling.

d. Loss of reduction.

Stiffness.

Swelling.

Reflex sympathetic dystrophy.

Loss of full range of movement.

OSCE 2

a. Humeral head, greater tuberosity, humeral shaft.

b. There are aspects of both an intracapsular and extracapsular fracture present in this injury.

c. Greater tuberosity.

d. Avascular necrosis.

e. Numbness in the 'badge-patch' area at the point of the shoulder.

Multiple choice answers

1. a. **True.** Median nerve compression is sometimes seen as a complication of a displaced Colles' fracture. Bony fragments or haematoma compress the median nerve in the carpal tunnel. It is not seen in the majority of cases in elderly patients. However, if compression is suspected, carpal tunnel decompression should be carried out early.

   b. **True.** Full supination may be lost as a result of malunion of a Colles' fracture. The distal fragment is displaced into pronation and unless corrected will not rotate normally into full supination as the distal radio-ulnar joint moves.

   c. **False.** The distal fragment in a Colles' fracture is displaced dorsally so loss of dorsiflexion is not seen in cases of malunion. However, palmar flexion may be lost as the normal arc of motion of the wrist joint is displaced dorsally. After reduction of a Colles' fracture, there may be residual stiffness of the wrist, causing some loss of dorsiflexion.

   d. **True.** Although some stiffness, pain and swelling may persist after treatment of a Colles' fracture, a full-blown reflex sympathetic dystrophy is rare. In these cases there is pain, swelling, stiffness in the hand and wrist, which is sweaty and cold.

   e. **False.** Avascular necrosis of the lunate (Keinbock's disease) is an uncommon condition affecting the lunate. It occurs spontaneously. The aetiology is unclear.

2. a. **False.** A fracture of the surgical neck of the humerus does not interrupt the blood supply to the humeral head. Avascular necrosis is not, therefore, seen.

b. **False.** A fracture of the surgical neck is below the tuberosities.

c. **True.** The axillary nerve winds round the neck of the humerus to supply the deltoid muscle and a small area of skin over its insertion onto the humerus.

d. **True.** Damage to the axillary nerve associated with the fracture results in paralysis of the deltoid and loss of abduction.

e. **False.** Fractures of the surgical neck of the humerus unite readily.

Upper limb

Hand injury and infection

Chapter part overview

Hand injuries and infections are common and present to both general practitioners and emergency departments. A suboptimal result can be devastating for the patient in terms of their ability to work or to do what they enjoy. Any delay in appropriate treatment can adversely affect the result.

8.1 Clinical examination – hand and wrist

Learning objectives

You should:
- know how to take an appropriate history from a patient with a hand injury
- ask for details of the patient's injury, occupation, hobbies and whether the patient is right- or left-handed
- be able to examine the injured hand and consider which underlying structures may have been damaged
- understand the importance of splintage and therapy for rehabilitation of the injured hand.

Because of their exposed position in the body and their busy prehensile activity, the hand and wrist are vulnerable to injury in a variety of ways:

- cuts and bites
- fractures/dislocations
- burns
- crushing
- infection
- high pressure injection.

Almost any combination of structures within the hand may be damaged in these ways so for any injured hand a checklist should be made of all the structures that could possibly be injured:

- skin
- tendons
- nerves
- vessels
- bone
- joints
- ligaments.

Much information can be gained from the careful examination of the hands not only for local pathology but also because the hands often manifest signs associated with remote or systemic diseases. Patients who have suffered a hand injury are very anxious and distressed about the effect this will have on normal hand function. Patients with infection in the hand will be in acute pain and resist the slightest attempts at examination. With so much information to be found from the hands, it is important to carefully follow the pattern of 'listen, look, feel, move'.

Listen Several important questions must be asked, concerning:

- details of the injury
  - *position the hand was in at the time*
  - *mechanism of injury*
  - *duration of contact of the hand with the injury force, e.g. crush from industrial rollers*
- right- or left-handed
- occupation
- hobbies
- other activities involving precision use of the hand.

Look Systematically look at each joint in the hand and wrist and remember to look at both palmar and dorsal surfaces. Do not forget to inspect the nails closely. In an exam, always describe what you are looking for and what you find to the examiner. Note any abnormal posture in the hand such as that associated with loss of function of a flexor or extensor tendon.

Feel Palpate the surface of any swelling and determine whether it is in the skin or beneath the skin. See if the lesion moves in relation to the flexor tendon. Try to locate areas of tenderness very precisely with single digit palpation. Areas of altered sensation should be assessed by light touch and especially the moving two-point discrimination test. Patients should be able to discriminate between the points of a pair of dividers or the ends of a paper clip two millimetres apart when they are being moved on the skin surface.

Move Observe the passive and active range of movement of the joint. Remember that at the wrist ulnar and radial deviation can be measured and compared with the opposite side. Examine the fingers for integrity of the flexor digitorum superficialis (FDS) and flexor digitorum profundus (FDP) tendons.

A careful history and examination should make it possible for you to predict exactly which structures have been injured.

Therapy

The worst complication of any injury to the hand is stiffness and contracture due to failure to prevent swelling or to encourage mobilisation. Sometimes, however, mobilisation is not possible and the hand must, therefore, be correctly splinted to avoid the development of joint contractures.

The correct position for splinting the hand is with the metacarpophalangeal joints in flexion and the proximal interphalangeal (PIP) joints in extension. In this position, the collateral ligaments of the joint are at their longest and, therefore, cannot contract. To aid this position, some dorsiflexion of the wrist is also used and can be maintained by a plaster back slab. A bulky dressing on the palm of the hand is made with layers of fluffed gauze. If only the wrist is to be immobilised, it is important that the dressing does not impede full flexion of the metacarpophalangeal joints.

8.2 Fractures and dislocations

• •

Learning objectives

You should:
- recognise what fracture patterns in the phalanges and metacarpals are likely to be unstable and require internal fixation or splintage rather than early mobilisation
- be able to recognise disruption of the ulnar collateral ligament of the thumb metacarpophalangeal (MCP) joint clinically and radiologically
- be able to recognise a scaphoid fracture or dislocation of the lunate but equally be aware that the absence of a bony injury does not exclude the absence of a ligamentous injury to the wrist, especially at the scapholunate junction.

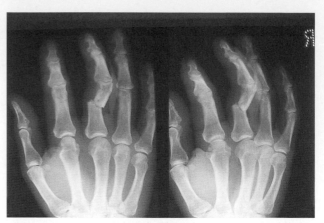

Figure 103 Unstable transverse fracture of the proximal phalanx of the middle finger with posterior angulation and displacement.

Phalanges

Clinical features

Fractures are caused by either twisting or angulating forces, may be stable or unstable and may be displaced or undisplaced (Figure 103). The pull of the interossei on the proximal fragment causes it to flex, resulting in dorsal angulation at the fracture site as the extensors pull on the middle phalanx.

Management

Stable, undisplaced fractures can be splinted by the adjacent finger or a short metal splint. Closed reduction and Kirschner wiring or open reduction and fixation with places and screws may be necessary for unstable fractures.

Dislocation of the interphalangeal joint

This common injury is usually easily reduced but is associated with either disruption of the collateral ligaments or volar plate. There may be an associated avulsion fracture from the base of the adjacent phalanx.

Management

Reduction and splinting to the adjacent finger are usually sufficient but a large intra-articular fragment will require accurate internal fixation.

Complications:
- stiffness caused by adhesion of extensor tendon at the fracture site
- malunion responsible for the rotated position of the finger, which becomes apparent with flexion
- flexion contracture due to scarring of the volar plate.

Metacarpals

Fifth metacarpal

The most commonly encountered fracture in the hand is a fracture of the neck of the fifth metacarpal (boxer's fracture). The metacarpal head is usually rotated and angled towards the palm.

Eight

Management

Unless this angulation is more than 40° from the long axis of the metacarpal shaft, it can be ignored so long as rotation is controlled by strapping the small and ring fingers together. Angulation of more than 45° often requires reduction and stabilisation of the fracture by percutaneous Kirschner wires.

Complications:

- extension lag
- stiff finger
- painful lump in the palm.

First metacarpal

Fractures of the first metacarpal may be:

- extra-articular: the fracture is usually transverse and above the level of the carpal joint
- intra-articular: the fracture is oblique, unstable, often displaced and involves part of the articular surface (Bennet's fracture; Figure 104).

Clinical features

There is usually a history of a staving or punching injury. The base of the first metacarpal is prominent.

Management

Undisplaced fractures can be held in a plaster cast that is well moulded to the base of the metacarpal and extended to the tip of the thumb. Displaced fractures require reduction and fixation either by an inter-fragmentary screw or by stabilising the position of the first metacarpal relative to the second by transverse Kirschner wires from one to the other.

Complications:

- malunion
- osteoarthritis.

Multiple metacarpal fractures

These fractures are usually unstable and if displaced will require internal fixation with minifragment plates or Kirschner wires.

Ulnar collateral ligament disruption at the MCP joint of the thumb

Acute abduction of the MCP joint of the thumb tears the ulnar collateral ligament and may avulse its origin on the base of the proximal phalanx. This injury commonly occurs in skiing or bike accidents. Chronic laxity, 'gamekeeper's thumb', is due to repeated ligamentous injury.

Management

A Bennet's-type plaster is appropriate for partial tears but open reduction and intraosseous fixation are required if the bony fragment is widely displaced or if the joint is very lax. In these cases the adductor aponeurosis will be interposed between the avulsed ligament and its insertion on the proximal phalanx.

Carpals

Scaphoid

Clinical features

Falls on the outstretched hand in young people, usually at sports, may result in a fracture to the scaphoid.

- **Listen** – today the injury is often associated with sports, although at one time it was due to the kickback from a motor-car starting handle.
- **Look** – swelling in the anatomical snuffbox.
- **Feel** – there is localised tenderness in the anatomical snuffbox.
- **Move** – pain is exacerbated by radial deviation of the wrist and on axial compression of the thumb.

Diagnosis

Radiographs of the wrist in ulnar deviation show the scaphoid best and the type of fracture (stable, oblique, displaced) can be observed. Occult fractures may be more apparent if re-radiographed a week later.

Management

Most scaphoid fractures can be treated conservatively in a plaster cast to immobilise the wrist while healing occurs. Unstable or displaced fractures are probably best treated by early open reduction and internal fixation with a screw or Kirschner wires.

   Non-union is a risk with these types and if present should be treated with bone graft either in isolation (Russe bone graft) or with an internal fixation device (Herbert screw).

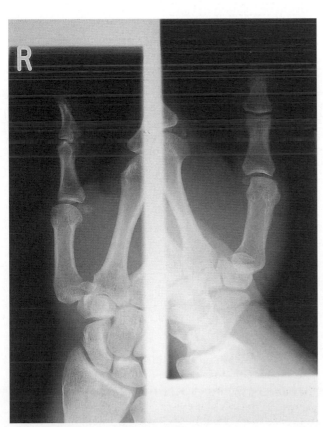

Figure 104 Bennet's fracture of the first metacarpal.

Complications:
- non-union
- avascular necrosis of the proximal fragment due to the retrograde blood supply to the scaphoid
- osteoarthritis and carpal collapse (SNAC wrist – scaphoid non-union advanced collapse)
- persisting pain
- weak grip.

Dislocation of the lunate

A hyperextension injury of the wrist may dislocate the lunate anteriorly (Figure 105) and produce acute symptoms of median nerve compression. Other more complex dislocations are associated with fractures of the scaphoid or capitate.

Management

Closed reduction may be possible followed by percutaneous wire stabilisation of the lunate, but often it is best to carry out an open reduction, repair the tear in the wrist capsule and decompress the carpal tunnel at the same time.

8.3 Soft tissue injuries

Sharp injuries

Cuts to the hand frequently occur from falls onto broken glass or from cuts on a knife or metal edge. The skin wound often looks trivial so the depth of the wound and hence the damage to the underlying structures are frequently missed when patients attend the casualty department.

Clinical features:

- **Listen** – an exact description of the mechanism of the injury should be elicited. The position of the hand at the time of the accident is important. For example, if the fingers were cut gripping the blade while trying to resist a knife attack then, when straightened, the position of the flexor tendon injury will be distal to the cut in the skin.
- **Look** – if a flexor or extensor tendon is divided, the affected finger will be out of cadence with the other fingers, which normally fall into a resting position of partial flexion that increases from the index to the small finger. The site of the skin wound should be noted. Injuries on the palmar aspect of the proximal phalanx may have divided both flexor tendons as they pass through the fibro-osseous tunnel in zone II (Figure 106).
- **Feel** – sensation on each side of the finger should be checked, although absence of touch sensation is not registered immediately by patients despite division of a digital nerve. Eventually the denervated side of the finger feels very dry because sudomotor innervation is lost.

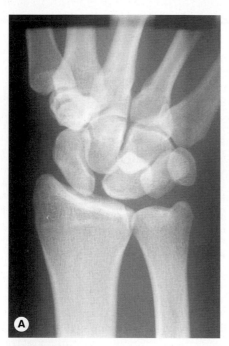

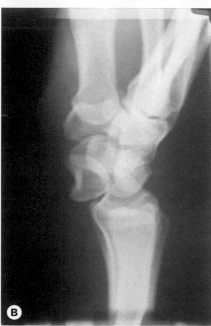

Figure 105 Antero-posterior (A) and lateral (B) radiographs of the wrist showing anterior dislocation of the lunate.

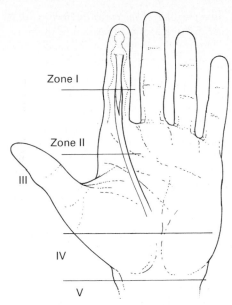

Zone I

Zone II

III

IV

V

Figure 106 Five zones of the hand showing the site of the fibro-osseous tunnel in zone II containing both flexor digitorum superficialis and flexor digitorum profundus in the fibrous flexor sheath.

- **Move** – complete division of FDS causes loss of proximal interphalangeal joint flexion. If the adjacent fingers are held straight, the injured finger is unable to flex at the proximal interphalangeal joint as this manoeuvre disables the mass action muscle, flexor digitorum profundus FDP, from flexing both joints of all fingers. FDS in contrast controls each finger independently. Complete division of FDP causes loss of distal interphalangeal joint flexion when the finger is held straight at the proximal interphalangeal joint. Partial division is associated with painful weakness of these movements. If an extensor tendon is divided, the finger hangs lower than its neighbours and cannot extend actively.

Diagnosis

The extent of injury to the underlying structures can be determined clinically in most cases. If the injury was caused by a radiopaque material, a radiograph is useful to exclude any particles remaining in the wound.

Management

Tendons, nerves and vessels can all be repaired. The principles of surgery on the hand include the use of a bloodless field (produced by a tourniquet on the limb), magnification and appropriately fine instruments and suture material. The patient's hand should be rested on a table that is wide enough to allow the surgeon to rest his elbows on it while operating. In this way hand tremor is reduced. If digital vessels and nerves are to be repaired, the operating microscope should be used, but operating loupes magnifying between two and three times are sufficient for most procedures. Postoperative splinting to protect the repair together with exercises supervised by a hand therapist are required if a good result is to be achieved after these injuries.

Complications:

- stiffness
- tendon adhesions
- cold intolerance
- numbness
- neuroma formation
- scar contracture.

Bites

Human or animal bites are usually seen at the knuckles or fingertips. The skin wound is ragged and the extensor tendon may be partially or completely divided. Occasionally the underlying joint capsule is open and in very severe injuries a digit may be partially or completely amputated.

Management

Infection is the main problem. Copious lavage, surgical debridement and best-guess antibiotics, usually co-Amoxiclav and metronidazole, are needed.

Wounds should be left open initially and reinspected at 24 h before being closed.

Crush injuries

With crush injuries, it is important to know the nature of the crushing object. Often the injury involves industrial machinery. The size, weight, temperature or velocity of the equipment responsible may be of relevance. The length of time the hand was crushed may also be relevant.

Clinical features

A hand crushed between blunt objects or rollers may be swollen and bruised without definite injury to any of the internal structures. However, the skin may have been sheared (degloving injury) from the underlying structures and become devascularised. Loss of capillary return helps to confirm this diagnosis. The defatted skin however, may be reapplied to the underlying raw tissue as a skin graft.

High-pressure injection injuries

Paint, lubricants or other solvents may be injected under pressure into the hand or digits.

Clinical features

The entry wound is small and the severity of the injury is easily underestimated initially. After a few hours, there is increasing pain and swelling. Hypodermic injection of irritant, fat-soluble chemicals such as fish vaccines can cause a similar clinical picture and need similar urgent treatment.

Management

Surgical opening of the area reveals the extent of spread of the injected substance. Mechanical lavage and surgical debridement are necessary. Closure should be delayed until swelling subsides.

Delay in surgical debridement leads to irreversible thrombosis of the digital vessels and loss of the finger.

8.4 Infection

Learning objectives

You should:
* be able to recognise infection in the hand and know how this should be managed as an emergency.

Clinical features

Staphylococcal infection in the hand presents as a web-space infection, paronychia (nail-fold infection) or a tendon-sheath infection. There is a collection of yellow pus, inability to move the affected finger and inflammation. Streptococcal infection is associated with a more insidious spreading infection, cellulitis, and ascending lymphangitis without the presence of pus at the original site.

Management

Pus under pressure must be released and the area washed out. Specimens are sent for bacteriological examination and intravenous antibiotics commenced. Flucloxacillin and Fucidin are the 'best guess' for staphylococcal infections, but penicillin must be used if streptococcal infection is suspected.

Complications:
* swelling
* contracture
* stiffness
* skin necrosis is seen in some cases of streptococcal infection
* a digit may be lost if its vessels become thrombosed following infection.

Non-traumatic hand pain and deformity

Chapter part overview

Patients present in the elective clinic because of pain, disability or a cosmetic deformity. Where a deformity is cosmetic, it is important to ensure that the patient's ideas of what can be achieved are realistic and that the danger of recurrence is satisfactorily explained.

8.5 Entrapment neuropathy

Learning objectives

You should:
* be able to describe the clinical features of carpal tunnel syndrome and differentiate these from ulnar nerve compression at the elbow.

Pressure on a peripheral nerve in its fibro-osseous tunnel causes pressure on a localised section of the nerve, which results in neuronal dysfunction causing characteristic features.

Carpal tunnel syndrome

Clinical features:
* **Listen** – the classic history is of pain at night in the radial three and a half digits (the distribution of the median nerve). There may be numbness, tingling, dysaesthesia and clumsiness.
* **Look** – there may be wasting of the muscles of the thenar eminence, especially abductor pollicis brevis, which is always innervated by the median nerve.
* **Feel** – there is altered or diminished sensation in the palmar aspect of the radial three and a half digits but not in the palm of the hand as the superficial branch of the median nerve supplying this area does not pass through the carpal tunnel.
* **Move** – there is weakness of abductor pollicis brevis. Tinel's sign, percussion over the median nerve at the carpal tunnel, exacerbates the symptoms, as does palmar flexion of the wrist (Phalen's sign).

Diagnosis

The diagnosis is usually made clinically but in equivocal cases nerve conduction studies are helpful, showing characteristic decreases in nerve conduction velocities at the wrist if the median nerve is significantly compressed.

Management

Conservative A dorsiflexion splint to wear at night prevents wrist flexion during sleep and relieves symptoms. Local infiltration of a steroid into the carpal tunnel may be effective.

Surgical Division of the flexor retinaculum achieves a dramatic improvement in symptoms. In cases of advanced thenar muscle wasting, an opponensplasty to restore thumb opposition to the other digits can be achieved using palmaris longus, if present, or flexor digitorum superficialis from the ring finger.

Cubital tunnel syndrome

Clinical features:
* **Listen** – pressure or traction on the ulnar nerve at the elbow causes pain and tingling in the distribution of the ulnar nerve.
* **Look** – there may be wasting of the hypothenar eminence and of the interossei. This is best seen in the first web space where the first dorsal interosseus is easy to see.
* **Feel** – there is altered sensation or numbness in both palmar and dorsal aspects of the ulnar one and a half digits.
* **Move** – there is weakness of abductor digiti minimi and of abduction and adduction of all the fingers. Adductor pollicis is also weak, resulting in a positive Froment's sign in which interphalangeal joint flexion of the thumb occurs to increase pinch grip.

Diagnosis

Nerve conduction studies will confirm the diagnosis and localise the constricting lesion – usually a fibrous band between the two heads of flexor carpi ulnaris at the elbow.

Management

The ulnar nerve can be decompressed in the cubital tunnel by dividing the fibrous band. Traction on the nerve can be relieved by an anterior transposition, which relocates the nerve on the anterior side of the medial epicondyle.

8.6 Ganglia

Learning objectives

You should:
- be able to describe the common sites of appearance of a ganglion and describe the usual clinical features.

The presence of a lump on the wrist or hand is a frequent presentation at the hand clinic. Ganglia are seen at the following sites:

- wrist: palm or dorsal aspects
- flexor tendon sheath
- distal interphalangeal joints.

The pathology causing a ganglion to develop is somewhat uncertain. Although ganglia communicate with a synovial-lined cavity, such as a joint or the flexor tendon sheath, the fluid they contain is more gelatinous than pure synovial fluid. Although a pedicle can often be found connecting them to a joint (at the wrist this is usually the scapholunate joint), abnormal areas of joint capsule are found near the base where mucoid degeneration is taking place. Intraosseous and intratendinous ganglia are occasionally found.

Clinical features

Patients complain of a lump on the dorsum of the wrist or on the line of the flexor tendon sheath or on the dorsum of the distal interphalangeal joints. The lumps characteristically come and go but when present can be quite large and painful. Grip strength is impaired and the wrist may ache after prolonged use. Flexor tendon sheath ganglia are small and hard. They remain static during finger movement and cause pain when gripping objects tightly. Ganglia at the distal interphalangeal (DIP) joints (usually referred to as mucous cysts) are unsightly. There is underlying osteoarthritis of the joint and the associated osteophytes are readily palpable.

Wrist ganglia are fixed to the underlying structures but not to the overlying skin. Their surface is smooth and they are often large and fluctuant but may be small and tense. On the palmar side, they are frequently in close conjunction to the radial artery.

Ganglia compressing the ulnar nerve as it passes through Guyon's canal, between the pisiform and the hook of the hamate may present with weakness of the muscles innervated by the ulnar nerve or altered sensation on the palmar aspect of the ulnar one and a half digits or with both motor and sensory abnormalities.

Diagnosis

Clinical examination is usually sufficient to make the diagnosis. A radiograph of the fingers will show the underlying changes of osteoarthritis associated with a mucous cyst.

Management

Wrist ganglia were classically treated by dispersion as they were ruptured by being hit with a heavy object. Recurrence, however, is frequent after this procedure. Small ganglia can be managed by aspiration and injection of hydrocortisone, and this method is sometimes effective in flexor tendon-sheath ganglia. The most reliable method is surgical excision but the recurrence rate is still 20%. At the wrist, ganglia must be carefully dissected from the radial artery and the stalk dissected back to the joint. Any abnormal areas of joint capsule must be removed at the same time. Flexor tendon-sheath ganglia must be removed with a similar surrounding area of abnormal flexor tendon sheath. Mucous cysts require to be carefully dissected from the overlying skin. Osteophytes can be trimmed and the skin repaired. Sometimes a small rotation flap is necessary to close the defect.

Complications:
- recurrence.

8.7 Dupuytren's contracture

Learning objectives

You should:
- be able to recognise the predisposing features associated with the development of Dupuytren's contracture
- know when a patient should be referred for surgery.

Dupuytren's disease is a progressive contracture of the palmar fascia of the hand or foot of uncertain aetiology but it is more commonly seen in people of north-west European ancestry than others. Factors associated with the development of Dupuytren's contracture are:

- positive family history
- alcohol abuse
- diabetes
- anticonvulsant medication.

Clinical features

The disease usually affects the hands symmetrically and the ring and small fingers are usually the most severely involved. The condition may begin as a pit or a nodule in the palm before spreading distally as a cord to the digit and proximally to the base of the palm. Contracture of the cord produces flexion of the MCP and proximal interphalangeal joints. The presence of knuckle pads, involvement of the plantar fascia and a positive family history are associated with a poor prognosis and an increased recurrence rate after surgery.

Management

Surgical excision of the contracted cord is indicated if the MCP joint is flexed more than 40° or if there is any flexion of the proximal interphalangeal joint. Great care must be taken to protect the neurovascular bundles during the excision of the Dupuytren's tissue, which often winds round the neurovascular bundle to produce a spiral cord. Postoperative extension exercise and splintage are required to keep the finger straight.

Patients with recurrence often require multiple operations. Full-thickness skin grafts are sometimes helpful to achieve healthy skin cover, but after several operations, amputation of the affected digit may be necessary.

Complications:

- recurrence in the same area after surgery
- extension to other parts of the hand
- maceration if left untreated
- cold intolerance ⎫ if the neurovascular bundles
- numbness ⎬ have been damaged.

8.8 Arthritis

> ### Learning objectives
>
> You should:
> - recognise the presenting features of arthritis in the hand
> - know when surgery should be recommended and what surgical options are available
> - recognise the classic sites of osteoarthritis in the hand and know the surgical procedures available.

Rheumatoid arthritis

The wrist and hand are common sites to be affected by rheumatoid arthritis.

Clinical features

Movements are restricted and painful.

- **Listen** – painful joints cause difficulty with tasks of everyday life.
- **Look** – swollen joints due to synovial hypertrophy and effusion are present. Muscle wasting may be seen in later stages. Characteristic deformities in the hand occur when the joints have become lax. They include radial deviation of the carpus and metacarpals, ulnar deviation of the phalanges, Z-shaped thumb, and Boutonnière and swan neck deformities of the fingers (Figure 107).
- **Feel** – synovial effusion and hypertrophy may be felt over the MCP joints.
- **Move** – joints may be immobile or very lax, allowing movement in any direction. If tendon ruptures have occurred then individual fingers will be floppy.

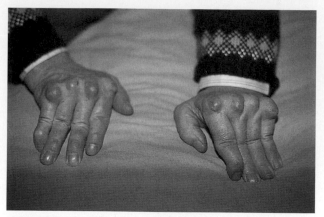

Figure 107 Rheumatoid hand showing dislocation of the MCP joints and swan neck deformity of the fingers.

Diagnosis

Radiological features of rheumatoid arthritis are:

- osteopenia
- joint space narrowing
- marginal erosions
- joint subluxation and dislocation

and in later stages

- confluent, spontaneous arthrodesis of the carpus.

Management

Conservative:
- splints
- analgesics, non-steroidal and disease-modifying agents
- intra-articular steroids.

Surgical:
- arthroplasty – replacement of the metacarpophalangeal joints and wrist
- arthrodesis – for any severely destroyed joints and for stabilisation of the interphalangeal joints
- excision arthroplasty – excision of the distal ulna allows pain-free supination and pronation, and prevents further extensor tendon ruptures
- tendon transfer – the distal ends of ruptured ulnar side extensor tendons can be 'piggy-backed' onto the adjacent intact tendons. Transfer of extensor indicis proprius is useful for rupture of extensor pollicis longus.

Indications for surgery:
- pain
- loss of function
- cosmetic deformity.

Complications:
- progressive deformity
- loss of function
- loss of independence.

Osteoarthritis

In the hand, primary osteoarthritis is often seen in women over the age of 60 years. The sites affected are:

- distal interphalangeal joints
- carpometacarpal joint of the thumb
- triscaphie joint (between the scaphoid, trapezium and trapezoid)
- the proximal interphalangeal joint is rarely affected.

Secondary osteoarthritis may develop because of:

- intra-articular fractures
- septic arthritis
- carpal collapse – seen following scaphoid non-union
- Keinbock's disease (avascular necrosis of the lunate)
- rheumatoid arthritis.

Clinical features:

- **Listen** – patients complain of pain, weak grip and loss of function.
- **Look** – the affected joints are swollen and stiff. There is deformity caused by osteophyte formation and eventually loss of function. At the distal interphalangeal joint, mucous cyst formation is seen as an eccentric dorsal swelling.
- **Feel** – tenderness and swelling.
- **Move** – movements are limited and painful. Crepitus may be present.

Diagnosis

Radiological examination shows features of osteoarthritis:

- joint space narrowing
- subchondral sclerosis
- cysts
- osteophyte formation.

Management
Conservative:

- analgesics, splints

Surgical The following surgical options should be considered:

- arthrodesis for the distal interphalangeal joint and triscaphie joint
- interposition arthroplasty for the carpometacarpal joint of the thumb
- excision arthroplasty for the carpometacarpal joint of the thumb
- joint replacement for the interphalangeal joint of the middle or ring finger.

Complications:
- adduction deformity of first metacarpal following subluxation of arthritic first carpometacarpal joint
- first web-space contracture
- weak pinch grip
- chronic pain.

Shoulder and elbow pain

Chapter part overview

Both the elbow and shoulder joint are relatively subcutaneous, so that during palpation it is possible to acquire quite a detailed picture of any pathology and relate it to a knowledge of the underlying anatomy. Shoulder pain is usually associated with loss of full range of movement but it is necessary to determine whether this is the result of inflammation, degeneration or tears in the rotator cuff or because of inflammation or degenerative changes in the joint. Rheumatoid arthritis (RA) is commonly seen in the upper limb and may eventually require surgery. A variety of operative procedures are available and the indications and limitations of each should be known.

Anterior dislocations of the shoulder are common presentations to the accident and emergency department but it is important not to miss the less common posterior dislocation. Patients who have had multiple dislocations are a special group and often need surgical management. Soft tissue problems around the elbow are a common presentation in general practice, where they can often be reliably diagnosed and treated.

8.9 Clinical examination

Learning objectives

You should:
- be able to relate your clinical examination to your knowledge of the underlying anatomy
- practice the 'listen, look, feel and move' approach to examination.

Examination of the shoulder and elbow provides plenty of opportunity to exercise the routine of 'listen, look, feel and move'.

Shoulder

Listen Is there a history of trauma or gradual onset of symptoms? Which movements aggravate the symptoms or are impossible? Can the patient reach to the back of the head and the buttock?

Look With the patient suitably undressed, the shoulders can be observed from all sides and compared. It is helpful to sit the patient down and observe the shoulders from above as well as from the front and sides. Loss of normal lateral contour is indicative of a dislocation of the shoulder or wasting of the deltoid. Scars, swelling and inflammation can also be looked for.

Feel Bony outlines of the pectoral girdle can be felt, beginning at the sternoclavicular joint, continuing along the clavicle to the acromioclavicular joint and tracing around the point of the acromion along the spine of the scapula. Finally the angle of the scapula can be palpated. The upper humerus and tuberosities may be felt in thin people. Tenderness over the joints can be noted.

Move The full extent of flexion and extension is observed. When assessing abduction, the angle of the scapula should be palpated to determine how much abduction is true glenohumeral movement and how much is scapulothoracic rotation. With the elbows tucked into the sides, external rotation and internal rotation can be noted. Because the abdomen gets in the way of internal rotation, this movement can be further assessed by observing how far the patient can reach up their back with each hand.

Elbow

Listen Did the onset follow a particular activity or injury? Are other joints similarly painful? Can the elbow stretch out and the hand be brought to the mouth?

Look An effusion in the elbow and swelling of the olecranon bursa are easily seen at the elbow. Rheumatoid nodules over the olecranon are a common finding.

Feel The bony prominences of the medial and lateral epicondyles and of the olecranon are readily palpable and form the points of an equilateral triangle. The radial head can be palpated; during pronation and supination of the forearm, crepitus may be felt here by the examining thumb.

Move Any loss of full extension of the elbow can be measured and the range of flexion noted. Supination and pronation must be examined with the elbows stabilised against the chest wall to eliminate any contributory movements from the shoulder. Varus or valgus laxity of the elbow should be sought.

8.10 Shoulder disorders

Learning objectives

You should:
- be able to recognise and treat acute symptoms of supraspinatus tendinitis
- be able to differentiate subacromial impingement from rotator cuff tear
- be able to recognise the features of shoulder instability
- know a procedure to reduce an anterior dislocation of the shoulder.

Shoulder pain

Pain in the shoulder is a common complaint. It may be referred pain from the cervical vertebrae, radicular pain from cervical nerve root entrapment or intrinsic pain caused by specific pathology in the shoulder joint itself.

Acute supraspinatus tendinitis

This condition is seen in early middle age and occurs commonly. Inflammation of the supraspinatus muscle in the rotator cuff produces a swollen area on the rotator cuff which becomes squashed beneath the acromion during abduction.

Clinical features:

- **Listen** – there is sometimes a history of unaccustomed heavy use of the shoulder prior to the onset of symptoms.
- **Look** – patients prefer to keep the shoulder still.
- **Feel** – there is tenderness over the anterior rotator cuff.
- **Move** – initially abduction is comfortable, but between 30° and 60° it becomes painful; beyond 60°, however, when the inflamed portion of the rotator cuff advances beyond the tight area beneath the acromion, pain is relieved.

Diagnosis

Radiological examination occasionally may show the presence of calcification in the supraspinatus tendon. The diagnosis is then 'acute calcific tendinitis', which is excruciatingly painful, unresponsive to analgesia, but relieved by 'needling' the deposit while injecting a steroid.

Management

Rest and non-steroidal analgesics are the first line of management. If symptoms are very severe or persistent, local infiltration of hydrocortisone and local anaesthetic into the subacromial bursa produces dramatic relief (Figure 108).

Complications:

- intratendonous injection with steroids may cause a tear in the rotator cuff.

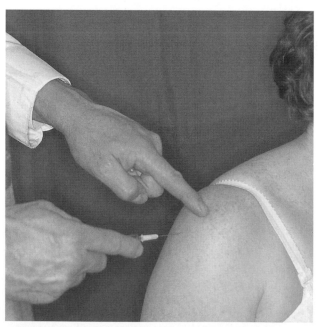

Figure 108 The subacromial bursa can be injected from the lateral side as shown or anteriorly. The needle is passed under the acromion into the bursa and not into the rotator cuff itself.

Subacromial impingement

In older patients (40–60 years) there is chronic thickening of the rotator cuff from repeated 'wear and tear'. Associated with this may be arthritic degeneration of the acromioclavicular joint with osteophytes causing further impingement on the rotator cuff.

Clinical features

Patients present with similar symptoms and signs to those with supraspinatus tendinitis, but:

- **Listen** – there is a long history of repeated episodes of shoulder pain. Reaching upwards with the arm exacerbates the pain.
- **Look** – patients tend to shrug the shoulder rather than abduct it.
- **Feel** – there is tenderness over the rotator cuff.
- **Move** – painful abduction can be demonstrated.

Management

The chronic impingement of a thickened rotator cuff in a narrowed subacromial space will not respond to anti-inflammatory agents and requires more space to be made by subacromial decompression of the rotator cuff. Arthroscopic acromioplasty or open procedure may be required including acromioclavicular joint excision.

Complications:

- rotator cuff tear.

Rotator cuff tear

Rotator cuff tears may be acute or degenerative, full thickness or partial thickness. Severe injuries to the shoulder in a young person produce an acute tear, but in an elderly person a trivial injury may be sufficient to produce an acute tear in a degenerative rotator cuff.

Clinical features

There is pain on attempting to move the shoulder. In full-thickness tears, active movement is impossible. Initiation of abduction, particularly, is absent, but further abduction is possible by the action of the deltoid. In partial thickness tears, movement is possible but there is pain and weakness.

Diagnosis

An arthrogram (Figure 109) or MRI scan will show the defect on the rotator cuff.

Management

In the young person, an acute rotator cuff tear can be treated by surgical repair. In the elderly, degenerative changes make repair unsuccessful, but a course of heat treatment until symptoms settle followed by strengthening exercises over a full range of movement will produce an acceptable result.

Complications:

- shoulder stiffness – disuse of the shoulder for whatever reason results in shrinking of the capsule and loss of movement in all directions.

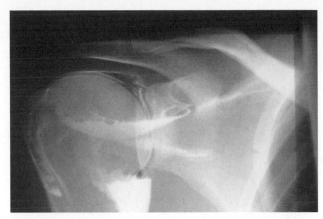

Figure 109 Arthrogram of the shoulder showing a partial thickness tear of the rotator cuff.

Frozen shoulder

An injury to the shoulder or elsewhere in the limb can result in shoulder stiffness but idiopathic adhesive capsulitis (true frozen shoulder) is a separate condition. Histological changes in the joint capsule are similar to those seen in the palmar fascia in Dupuytren's contracture.

Clinical features

The joint is initially very painful and movement becomes restricted in all directions, especially external rotation. This is followed by a period of continued stiffness without pain and eventually some movement returns. The whole process takes about 2.5 years.

Management

Analgesics, physiotherapy and manipulation under anaesthesia are each used in the various stages of this condition.

Sporting shoulder injuries

Dislocations and fractures of the shoulder can occur particularly in those involved in sports

Dislocations can be:

- anterior
- posterior
- inferior (luxatio erecta – very rare)
- associated with a fracture
- recurrent.

Anterior dislocation

This injury occurs with an abduction and extension force on the shoulder (Figure 110). It is associated with falls and with sports.

Clinical features:

- **Listen** – there is a history of a fall or a twisting injury of the shoulder.
- **Look** – the affected shoulder appears flatter than normal on the lateral aspect. The tip of the acromion is prominent and is in line with the lateral epicondyle of the elbow, giving a 'squared off' appearance to the shoulder on the affected side.

Eight

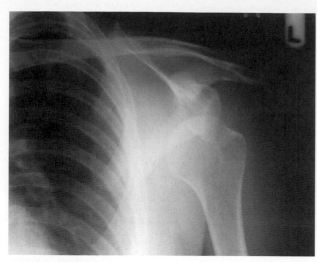

Figure 110 Anterior dislocation of the shoulder.

- **Feel** – the humeral head may be palpable anteriorly. Loss of sensation on the 'badge-patch' area must be sought because, if present, it denotes damage to the axillary nerve at the humeral neck.
- **Move** – normal shoulder movements are impossible.

Diagnosis

The diagnosis is usually obvious clinically but a radiograph should be taken to exclude an associated fracture. Radiographs can sometimes be difficult to interpret. Posterior dislocations are notorious for being overlooked as the humerus appears to be in joint. Close inspection, however, shows the characteristic 'lightbulb' shape of the humeral head as the tuberosities are not seen in their usual position.

Management

Occasionally, the shoulder may reduce spontaneously or by the 'hanging arm' technique, in which the patient lies prone allowing the affected arm to hang vertically over the side of the couch. More usually, however, reduction under anaesthesia is required. Kochner's manoeuvre is commonly used, in which the arm is externally rotated and abducted; the arm is then swung into internal rotation and adducted across the patient's chest to be nursed there in a broad arm sling for 3–4 weeks while the anterior capsule heals. Alternatively, traction on the arm against counter-traction from a colleague's hand in the axilla can be used.

Complications:

- Axillary nerve damage: this may occur during the injury or during the manipulation; the integrity of the nerve must always be checked prior to attempting reduction. Absence of sensation over the point of the acromion suggests the nerve is damaged and, if it is, there will be resulting paralysis in the deltoid.
- Associated humeral fracture.
- Arterial damage: the axillary artery may be damaged.
- Shoulder stiffness.

- Irreducible dislocation: this is present if the humeral head buttonholes through the rotator cuff. This happens only rarely but requires open reduction.
- Recurrent dislocation.
- Iatrogenic humeral fracture (especially a risk in osteoporotic patients).

Posterior dislocation

This condition is unusual but easily missed. Ligamentous laxity gives some patients the ability to voluntarily dislocate the shoulder posteriorly.

Diagnosis

The radiograph shows the characteristic 'lightbulb' shape of the humeral head.

Management

Manipulation under anaesthesia followed by 3 weeks' immobilisation and subsequent physiotherapy.

Recurrent dislocation

Recurrent anterior dislocation occurs with extension and external rotation movements, usually without any further trauma. Some patients report dislocating their shoulder while simply turning over in bed.

Diagnosis

Radiological examination shows flattening of part of the humeral head; the Hill–Sachs lesion. Elevation of the anterior glenoid rim and subscapularis muscle (the Bankart lesion) may be demonstrated by arthrography or MRI.

Management

Recurrent dislocation requires stabilisation of the shoulder by securing the soft tissues back to their anatomical positions. Reefing the subscapular tendon or providing a dynamic anterior support by the transfer of the conjoint tendon through the subscapularis are more extensive procedures with their own complications.

Fractured clavicle

This common injury is often associated with sports but can occur with any fall on the outstretched hand.

Clinical features

Pain and tenderness. The patient characteristically supports the weight of the arm with the opposite hand.

Diagnosis

The majority of injuries are in the middle third and occasionally there is overriding of the bone ends.

Management

The arm should be rested in a broad arm sling until pain subsiders. A figure-of-eight brace is commonly used in some countries.

Complications:

- malunion
- damage to the subclavicular vessels

- non-union: this may be asymptomatic but, occasionally, requires open reduction, internal fixation and bone grafting
- deformity
- brachial plexus damage.

Acromioclavicular joint disruption

A fall on the point of the shoulder, classically during a rugby game, produces this injury (Figure 111).

Clinical features

The injury may be a sprain, a subluxation or a dislocation. The clavicle springs upward at the acromioclavicular joint, producing a characteristic step on the shoulder.

Diagnosis

Radiographs comparing both shoulders while the patient carries weights in the hands are used to confirm a diagnosis and to differentiate between subluxations and dislocations.

Management

Conservative treatment is often all that is required, but occasionally fixation of the clavicle to the coracoid (Weaver–Dunn procedure) is carried out for those patients who require their shoulder for heavy work.

Complications:

- pain
- weakness.

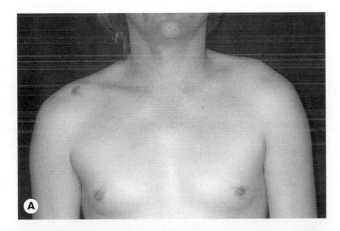
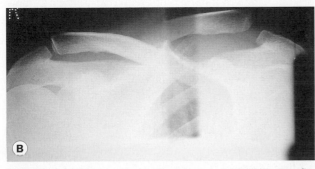

Figure 111 (A) 30-year-old man with acromioclavicular dislocation of his left shoulder. (B) Radiograph appearance of both acromioclavicular joints.

8.11 Rheumatoid arthritis

Learning objectives

You should:
- be able to list the radiological features of rheumatoid arthritis
- be able to describe the different contributions of medical (non-operative) management
- be able to describe various operative procedures which may be used and list the possible complications associated with each.

Rheumatoid arthritis (RA) is an inflammatory systemic disease of unknown aetiology, characterised by relapses and remissions, which may affect many joints simultaneously. An autoimmune inflammatory reaction in the synovium produces synovial hypertrophy and effusion. Eventually there is destruction of the articular cartilage, ligamentous laxity and erosion of the subchondral bone. These combine to result in mechanical derangement of the joint leading to subluxation and eventually permanent dislocation and deformity. The care of the rheumatoid patient progresses from medical treatment, often supervised by a rheumatologist, to combined care with an orthopaedic surgeon once surgical intervention is required.

Shoulder

Clinical features:

- **Listen** – morning stiffness is characteristic.
  The shoulder is painful and limits function. It is difficult to comb the hair and reach to the perineum comfortably. Patients complain that they are unable to lie on the affected side.
- **Look** – muscle wasting around the shoulder girdle.
- **Feel** – joint swelling is not easy to detect. There may be tenderness at the acromioclavicular joint.
- **Move** – movements of the joint are painful and restricted, especially abduction and external rotation.

Diagnosis

Features of systemic disease may be present, such as a raised ESR (erythrocyte sedimentation rate) and CRP. A positive RA latex may also be apparent, but in approximately 30% of patients this test is negative. Classically, radiographs of the wrists are used to look for early signs of rheumatoid arthritis. Radiological examination of the affected joint shows:

- joint space narrowing
- marginal erosions
- osteopenia
- irregular joint surface
- eventually features of secondary osteoarthritis develop (Figure 111).

Management

Medical management includes:

- drugs: simple analgesics and NSAIDs are commenced along with disease-modifying drugs such as

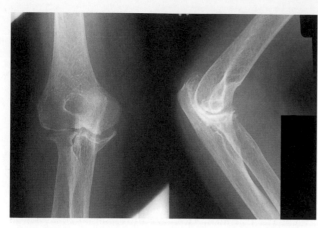

Figure 112 Common radiological features of rheumatoid arthritis include joint space narrowing, marginal erosions, irregular joint surface and osteopenia.

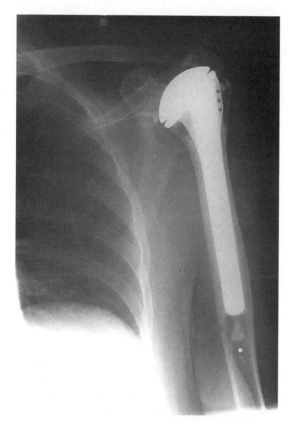

Figure 113 Hemiarthroplasty of the shoulder for rheumatoid arthritis.

sulphasalazine, methotrexate, penicillamine and gold; intra-articular injection of steroid and systemic steroids are used for acute exacerbations
* physiotherapy: preserves useful joint movement
* appliances to aid in the activities of daily living.

Surgical management includes:

* arthroscopic synovectomy
* hemiarthroplasty of the humeral head is usually sufficient (Figure 113)

* total shoulder replacement is required if the glenoid is severely eroded.

Complications
Complications of the disease:

* joint destruction
* dislocation
* rotator cuff degeneration.

Complications of prosthetic replacement:

* infection
* loosening.

Elbow

Clinical features

Patients with rheumatoid arthritis involving the elbow may have involvement of the humero-ulnar, humero-radial or proximal radio-ulnar joint or a combination of any of them. In addition, there may be disease at the distal radio-ulnar joint.

* **Listen** – patients complain of pain and loss of function in the elbow. There may be difficulty with eating and washing, and patients may complain of neck pain secondary to stretching forwards in an attempt to bring the mouth to the hand.
* **Look** – swollen joint from synovial effusion; deformity of the bony contours due to subluxation.
* **Feel** – crepitus and swelling.
* **Move** – when the humero-ulnar joint is involved, the patient loses full flexion and extension and is unable to get the hand to the face. If the humero-radial or distal radio-ulnar joints are involved, there is loss of supination and pronation.

Diagnosis
Radiological examination shows features of RA (see Figure 112), but in addition excess bone resorption may be seen, which allows the olecranon to migrate proximally between the supracondylar ridges of the distal humerus.

Management
Conservative treatment includes drug therapy as for the shoulder and splinting. Surgical management includes synovectomy, usually combined with radial head excision in cases of humero-radial joint involvement. Destruction of the humero-ulnar joint requires a total elbow replacement.

Complications
Complications of the disease include:

* progressive loss of function
* instability
* weakness.

Complications of surgery include:

* infection
* dislocation
* ulnar neuritis
* loosening of the prosthesis.

8.12 Elbow disorders

Elbow injuries associated with sport

Enthesopathy is the name given to discomfort at the site of origin of a muscle. It is caused by a tear in the muscle origin near the bone following repetitive activities involving lifting or stretching.

Tennis elbow/golfer's elbow

Clinical features

In tennis elbow there is pain over the lateral epicondyle of the elbow, which limits normal use. Local tenderness is found at the common extensor origin and symptoms can be exacerbated by stressing these muscles by forced palmar flexion of the wrist.

In golfer's elbow similar symptoms and signs are found on the medial side of the elbow at the common flexor origin. In this case, forced dorsiflexion of the wrist or resisted palmar flexion is painful.

Diagnosis

Radiological examination is unremarkable.

Management

Resting the elbow and avoiding particular activities may be all that is required. An above-elbow splint can be used to enforce this. Infiltration of the common extensor or flexor origin with local anaesthetic and steroid may produce some relief and can be repeated up to three times. Occasionally, surgical release is indicated, but the results are unpredictable.

Complications

Complications can arise from steroid injection:

- subcutaneous fat necrosis
- loss of skin pigmentation
- persisting symptoms.

Osteoarthritis

Arthritis in the elbow may be the result of heavy manual work or sports such as cricket.

Clinical features

There is pain, crepitus and loss of the full range of motion in the elbow.

Diagnosis

Radiological examination shows the features of osteoarthritis: joint space narrowing, osteophytes and subchondral sclerosis.

Management

Symptoms may be relieved by changing occupation and avoiding the use of the arm for strenuous activities. Occasionally, surgical debridement of osteophytes and release of joint capsule contractures can improve the range of movement but the results are often not maintained. In severe cases, total elbow replacement may be carried out, but the arm cannot be used for heavy activities after this procedure.

Complications:
- continuing pain
- loss of full range of movement.

Bursitis

Olecranon bursitis

This is either inflammatory or infective. Inflammatory bursitis is associated with rheumatoid arthritis, gout, other crystal arthropathies or direct trauma to the olecranon. Classically, this was described as resulting from pressure or friction on the olecranon, hence the original name of 'student's elbow'. Infective bursitis is usually due to staphylococcal infection.

Clinical features

There is a large fluctuant swelling at the olecranon associated with pain and redness. In infective bursitis, there is oedema, tenderness and spreading inflammation.

Diagnosis

Aspiration will help to identify the infecting organism and also to relieve the acute symptoms of inflammatory bursitis.

Management

A course of non-steroidal anti-inflammatory analgesics is sufficient for mild inflammatory disease. An appropriate antibiotic is necessary in addition for infected cases. Surgical excision of the bursa prevents recurrence.

Complications of surgery:
- poor wound healing
- sinus formation.

Self-assessment: questions

Hand problems

Extended matching items questions (EMIs)

EMI 1

Theme: Upper limb injury

A. radial nerve

B. flexor digitorum profundus

C. flexor digitorum superficialis

D. median nerve

E. ulnar nerve

F. brachial artery

Which of the above structures is most likely to be injured in the following situations? Each option may be used once, more than once or not at all.

1. A patient who has loss of sensation of the little finger and a positive Froment's sign.

2. A patient who has a cut on the volar aspect of the middle finger and is unable to flex the DIP joint.

3. A child with a supracondylar fracture and a white, pulseless hand.

4. An adult who sustained a shaft of humerus fracture in a traffic collision.

5. A patient who has wasting of the thenar eminence 6 months after a stab wound to the upper arm.

6. A patient who is unable to extend the wrist.

EMI 2

Theme: Diagnoses

A. carpal tunnel syndrome

B. rheumatoid arthritis

C. tendon-sheath infection

D. rheumatoid nodule

E. Dupuytren's contracture

F. cubital tunnel syndrome

G. osteoarthritis

H. ganglion

I. phalangeal fracture

J. trigger finger

Which of the diagnoses listed above is the most likely cause of the symptoms described below?

1. Pea-sized firm spherical mass in the line of the flexor tendon at the proximal interphalangeal joint.

2. Painless inability to fully extend the proximal interphalangeal joint of the index finger.

3. Paraesthesia on both dorsal and palmar surfaces of the ring and small fingers.

4. Pain and dorsal angulation in relation to the proximal phalanx.

5. Fixed flexion of the proximal interphalangeal joint and hyperextension of the distal interphalangeal joint in the ring finger.

6. Painful inability to flex or extend a red, swollen index finger.

Constructed response questions (CRQs)

CRQ 1

A 30-year-old female keyboard operator complains of pain in her right hand and fingers by the end of the week. Symptoms are becoming worse and the discomfort and altered sensation becoming permanent. Further questioning reveals that it is the radial three digits which are involved.

a. What other questions might you ask about her symptoms?

b. Physical examination reveals wasting of abductor pollicis brevis in the thenar eminence. Why should this be present?

c. What special clinical tests can be carried out?

d. These tests are all positive. What is your diagnosis?

e. Is it possible that her symptoms could be related to her occupation?

CRQ 2

A 60-year-old woman complains of pain in the radial side of her wrist and base of her thumb when knitting. On examination the first metacarpal is adducted and there is prominence at the carpometacarpal joint suggesting subluxation. Her thumb is developing a Z-shaped deformity, her other hand is satisfactory.

a. What diagnosis does this suggest?

b. On manipulating the joint and attempting to reduce the subluxation of the carpometacarpal joint, what symptoms would you expect to produce?

c. What conservative management could be tried initially?

d. Her symptoms fail to settle over the following few months, and you arrange a radiograph. What do you expect this to show?

e. Is a repeat of the management you suggested in 'c' likely to help at this stage?

f. What would be your next line of management?

Objective structured clinical examination questions (OSCEs)

OSCE 1

Study the clinical photograph below (Figure 114).

a. What action is this patient unable to do with his finger?

b. What structure do you think has been damaged?

c. The cut in the patient's hand is on the palmar aspect of the middle phalanx. Why is he still able to flex the proximal interphalangeal joint?

d. What other structures may be damaged?

OSCE 2

Look at the clinical photograph below (Figure 115).

a. What condition of the hand does it show?

b. List three predisposing factors for this condition.

c. What are the indications for recommending surgery?

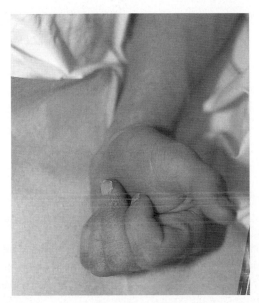

Figure 114

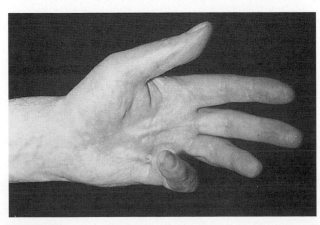

Figure 115

d. What structures are in jeopardy during the operation and what postoperative complications should the patient be aware of?

Multiple choice questions

1. The radial nerve supplies:
   a. the extensors of the wrist
   b. the radial flexors of the wrist
   c. abductor pollicis brevis
   d. extensor pollicis longus
   e. sensation to the tip of the thumb

2. In the hand:
   a. Boutonnière deformity results from rupture of the flexor digitorum tendon
   b. 'trigger finger' may be caused by tightness of the flexor tendon sheath
   c. 'mallet finger' is a flexion deformity of the proximal interphalangeal joint associated with trauma
   d. a functioning first dorsal interosseous muscle indicates intact motor function of the ulnar nerve
   e. stenosing tenosynovitis (de Quervain's) affects the extensor pollicis longus tendon

Best of 5s questions

1. A 39-year-old lady presents with a painful, swollen wrist which is stiff in the morning. Which one of the following findings makes rheumatoid arthritis unlikely?
   a. crystals seen on polarised light microscopy and a high serum urate
   b. negative rheumatoid factor (RA latex)
   c. reduced joint space on plain films
   d. subarticular cysts
   e. periarticular erosions

Shoulder and elbow pain

EMIs

EMI 1

Theme: Diagnoses

A. medial epicondylitis
B. osteoarthritis
C. rotator cuff tear
D. subacromial impingement
E. acute supraspinatus tendinitis
F. bursitis
G. rheumatoid arthritis
H. posterior dislocation of the shoulder

I. recurrent shoulder dislocation

J. fractured clavicle

Match the most appropriate diagnosis from the list above to each of the clinical histories below:

1. Pain in the mid-range of shoulder abduction.
2. Elevation of the anterior glenoid labrum and subscapularis seen on arthrogram or MRI scan.
3. Inability to initiate shoulder abduction.

EMI 2

Theme: The shoulder

A. frozen shoulder

B. supraspinatus tendonitis

C. anterior dislocation

D. rheumatoid arthritis

E. minimally displaced fracture of the humeral neck

Match the following statements with the pathologies above.

1. may be treated with hemiarthroplasty
2. runs a course of about 2.5 years
3. requires surgical intervention if recurrent
4. can be treated in a collar and cuff sling
5. produces a painful arc of movement in mid-abduction

Constructed response questions (CRQs)

CRQ 1

> A 70-year-old woman trips and falls onto her right shoulder. She complains of pain and inability to move the joint. She has localised tenderness around the humeral head. There is some swelling and bruising and localised tenderness around the greater tuberosity.

a. What might you expect to see on a plain antero-posterior radiograph?

b. The radiograph is reported as normal. What is a possible diagnosis now?

c. How could you visualise this lesion?

d. In a younger person how might this be treated?

e. Why might this treatment not be suitable in an older person and what would you suggest instead?

CRQ 2

> A 50-year-old accountant complains of pain in his dominant right shoulder after a weekend spent painting his house. Physical examination reveals well-localised acute tenderness, just lateral and superior to the coracoid process.

a. What diagnosis does this suggest?

b. What initial treatment would you suggest?

c. He attends two weeks later feeling no better. What would you expect to find on physical examination?

d. How would you treat him now?

e. Your treatment is satisfactory on this occasion. The patient presents some years later following several further episodes but now with a longer history of continued pain exacerbated by abduction. What would you expect to find on examination?

f. Your previous treatment does not help on this occasion. Radiography of the shoulder shows no evidence of arthritis. How would you manage this patient now?

OSCEs

OSCE 1

Study the photograph of a radiograph of the elbow (Figure 116).

a. Label the features marked A and B. What important structure passes near the eroded area of bone marked C?

b. What is abnormal about the radial head?

c. Looking at the elbow as a whole, what do you think is the likely diagnosis?

d. What are the classical features of this condition?

e. If you were to recommend a total elbow replacement for this patient, list two advantages and two complications to warn the patient about.

OSCE 2

Study the photograph of a radiograph of the left shoulder of a man who has suffered an injury in a fall at football (Figure 117).

a. What sensory examination should you carry out on a patient with this condition?

b. Describe the procedure used in the management of this condition.

c. What two contrasting complications are associated with this injury?

Best of 5s questions

1. Acute calcific tendonitis of the shoulder:

   a. can be effectively relieved by needling the lesion

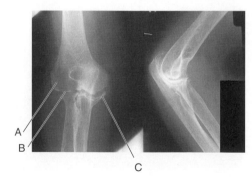

Figure 116

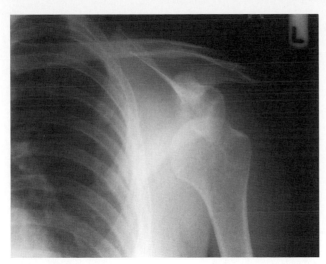

Figure 117

b. is not very painful
c. is associated with dramatic loss of passive external rotation
d. runs a course of about 2.5 years
e. usually needs arthroscopic surgery

Multiple choice questions

1. In the 'painful arc syndrome':
   a. calcification in the region of the supraspinatus tendon may be seen on plain radiographs
   b. the cause is a tear of the supraspinatus tendon
   c. typically there is severe pain on initiating abduction
   d. tenderness is generalised
   e. if untreated, shoulder stiffness often results

2. In rheumatoid arthritis:
   a. radiographic features of osteoarthritis may be superimposed on those of rheumatoid arthritis
   b. crepitus and pain may be produced by palpating the radial head while pronating/supinating the forearm
   c. joint laxity allows a full range of shoulder movement to be retained in most patients
   d. ulnar nerve dysfunction is rarely seen
   e. synovectomy and radial head excision may relieve symptoms in the early stages of disease

Self-assessment: answers

Hand problems

EMI answers

EMI 1

Theme: Upper limb injury

1. E
2. B
3. F
4. A
5. D
6. A

EMI 2

Theme: Diagnoses

1. H. This is a classic description of a tendon-sheath ganglion. The lesion is fixed to the tendon sheath and does not move with the tendon as the finger flexes and extends. They are always painful when squashed. Patients complain of discomfort when gripping objects.

2. E. Flexion and contraction of the proximal interphalangeal joint caused by Dupuytren's contracture causes a painless block to full extension.

3. F. Paraesthesia and numbness localised to the ulnar one and a half digits is the classic distribution of altered sensation seen in compression of the ulnar nerve at the cubital tunnel. Compression occurring more distally (i.e. in Guyon's canal) would not cause numbness on the dorsal surface of the fingers as the dorsal cutaneous branch leaves the main nerve more proximally.

4. I. A transverse fracture of the proximal phalanx is dorsally angulated by the pull of the extensor tendon on the middle phalanx and flexion of the proximal fragment by the interosseii. A fracture is painful.

5. B. The deformity described is a Boutonnière deformity characteristic of rheumatoid arthritis.

6. C. The finger is red and swollen and movements are painful and resisted. This is characteristic of a tendon-sheath infection; prompt decompression is required.

CRQ answers

CRQ 1

a. Does the patient wake up at night with an exacerbation of altered sensation, pins and needles or tingling with numbness in these digits? Is she aware of clumsiness or inability to distinguish articles by touch?

b. The recurrent motor branch of the median nerve comes off the main nerve distal to the carpal ligament so compression of the nerve causes muscle atrophy.

c. Phalen's test

   Tinel's test.

d. Carpal tunnel syndrome.

e. Possibly.

CRQ 2

a. Osteoarthritis of the carpometacarpal joint.

b. Pain and crepitus.

c. Splintage.

   Intra-articular steroid injection.

   Non-steroidal anti-inflammatory analgesics.

d. Joint space narrowing at the joint between the first metacarpal and the trapezium.

   There may be osteophytes and sclerosis.

   The joints between the trapezium, the scaphoid and the trapezoid may also be affected (pan-trapezoidal arthritis).

e. No.

f. Trapezectomy or prosthetic replacement of the trapezium.

OSCE answers

OSCE 1

a. Flexion at the distal interphalangeal joint of the left middle finger.

b. Flexor digitorum profundus to the middle finger.

c. Flexor digitorum superficialis has not been damaged at this level.

d. The digital nerve and vessel to the finger.

OSCE 2

a. Dupuytren's contracture.

b. Family history.

   Alcohol abuse.

   Diabetes or antiepileptic medication.

c. Metacarpophalangeal joint contracture more than 40°.

   Any proximal interphalangeal joint contracture.

d. Neurovascular bundles may wind around Dupuytren's cords and are at risk of injury during surgery.

Numbness and cold intolerance may be problems if they are damaged.

Recurrence and inability to regain full extension despite the surgery.

Multiple choice answers

1. a. **True.**
   b. **False.** Flexor carpi radialis is supplied by the median nerve.
   c. **False.** Abductor pollicis brevis is supplied by the median nerve.
   d. **True.**
   e. **False.** Sensation at the tip of the thumb is supplied by the median nerve.

2. a. **False.** The Boutonnière deformity is caused by rupture of the central slip of the extensor tendon over the proximal interphalangeal joint.
   b. **True.** Constriction at the mouth of the flexor tendon sheath at the level of the first annular pulley produces local swelling of the tendon, which prohibits its gliding into the mouth of the tendon sheath, producing a snapping movement called triggering.
   c. **False.** 'Mallet finger' is used to describe the inability to extend the distal interphalangeal joint following traumatic rupture of the extensor tendon or avulsion of a bony fragment from the base of the terminal phalanx.
   d. **True.** The first dorsal interosseous muscle is supplied by the ulnar nerve and its muscle belly can be readily seen in the first web space.
   e. **False.** De Quervain's tenosynovitis refers to symptoms related to the first dorsal compartment containing the tendons of abductor pollicis longus and extensor pollicis brevis.

Best of 5s answer

1. a.

Shoulder and elbow pain

EMI answers

EMI 1

Theme: Diagnoses

1. E. Pain in the mid-range of shoulder abduction is the classical painful arc of discomfort associated with acute supraspinatus tendinitits.

2. I. Elevation of the anterior glenoid labrum with a potential space extending beneath subscapularis is a classic finding on an arthrogram or MRI scan and is associated with a history of recurrent dislocation of the shoulder.

3. C. A significant tear in the rotator cuff will make it impossible to initiate abduction as this action is carried out by supraspinatus.

EMI 2

Theme: The shoulder

1. D.
2. A.
3. C.
4. E.
5. B.

CRQ answers

CRQ 1

a. Fractured tuberosity or complex intra-articular fracture.
b. Rotator cuff tear.
c. MRI scan, arthrogram or ultrasound scan.
d. Operatively by formal rotator cuff repair.
e. Surgical treatment is often not possible in an older person because the tear may be large and the rotator cuff muscles friable. This makes it impossible to reoppose the edges of the tear and suture them together. Instead conservative management is usually carried out with physiotherapy and ultrasound.

CRQ 2

a. Acute supraspinatus tendonitis.
b. Rest.
   Anti-inflammatory analgesics.
   Ultrasound treatment from the physiotherapist.
c. Painful arc of abduction.
d. If he is not getting any relief, it may be appropriate to consider long-acting steroid and local anaesthetic injection into the subacromial bursa.
e. Painful abduction in an older patient suggests a diagnosis of subacromial impingement as the rotator cuff is swollen and frayed beneath the arch of the acromion.
f. Subacromial impingement is best managed by an acromioplasty or acromioclavicular joint excision if associated with arthritis of this joint.

OSCE answers

OSCE 1

a. A – Lateral epicondyle.
   B – Radial head.
   C – Ulnar nerve.
b. It is flattened and eroded.
c. Rheumatoid arthritis.
d. Joint space narrowing.
   Irregular joints surface.

Margin erosions.

Osteopenia.

e. **Advantages:**

- pain-free joint
- increased functional use
- possible increased range of movement.

Complications:

- persistent ulnar neuritis
- infection, dislocation or loosening of the prosthesis.

OSCE 2

a. Examination for numbness over the 'badge-patch' area checking for damage to the axillary nerve.

b. General anaesthesia or muscular relaxation is required. Kocher's manoeuvre involves external rotation and abduction of the shoulder followed by adduction while internally rotating. Counter-traction with the help of a colleague's hand in the axilla may be required.

c. Shoulder stiffness.

Recurrent dislocation.

Best of 5s answer

1. a.

Multiple choice answers

1. a. **True.** 'Painful arc syndrome' is caused by inflammation in the supraspinatus area of the rotator cuff, and calcification may

occasionally be seen here on radiological examination.

b. **False.** A tear of the supraspinatus part of the rotator cuff causes loss of ability to initiate abduction; although there may be pain in the shoulder, the painful arc is not present.

c. **False.** The severe pain of painful arc syndrome is during the range from 30° to 60° as the inflamed, swollen area of the rotator cuff passes beneath the acromion. There is no pain during the initiation of abduction.

d. **False.** There is acute localised tenderness over the rotator cuff.

e. **True.** If the patient is inhibited in the use of the shoulder because of pain then the capsule contracts and a stiff shoulder results.

2. a. **True.** Once the joint is destroyed by rheumatoid arthritis, secondary osteoarthritis may develop.

b. **True.** Crepitus from motion between the two joint surfaces and pain on movement are readily found at the radial head during supination and pronation.

c. **False.** Usually the destruction of the joint and the long period of immobility resulting from the pain have resulted in a loss of full shoulder joint movement.

d. **False.** Ulnar neuritis is often associated with rheumatoid disease involving the elbow or wrist.

e. **True.** Excision arthroplasty of the radial head and synovectomy reduce the disease process and painful movement of the elbow. Dramatic relief can be achieved.

Lower limb

Hip pain in adults

Chapter part overview

Many clinical signs can be elicited by careful examination of a patient with either osteoarthritis or rheumatoid arthritis of the hip, but it is a detailed history of the extent and degree of their pain and the limitation of ability that will help you decide whether or not surgery is indicated.

9.1 Clinical examination – lower limb

Learning objectives

You should:
- in addition to listen, look, feel and move, remember to observe the patient lying, standing and walking, which may reflect an underlying disorder
- observe the patient standing to look for short leg length or a positive Trendelenberg sign
- observe the patient lying to measure true and apparent leg lengths.

In addition to the usual 'listen, look, feel, move', examination of the hip includes observation of the patient walking, standing and lying.

Walking Observe for short leg gait, antalgic gait or Trendelenburg gait.

Standing Observe the pelvic tilt while standing on each leg in turn. A positive Trendelenburg sign is present when the patient's pelvis dips to the opposite side while weight bearing on the affected leg (Figure 118). It indicates an inability to abduct the hip.

Lying With the patient lying supine, movements of the hip joint can be measured. These include flexion and extension, abduction and adduction, and internal and external rotation. Care must be taken to ensure that the pelvis does not move during these manoeuvres, and this can best be achieved by stabilising the pelvis with one hand while manipulating the leg with the other. Thomas's test, which unmasks a fixed flexion deformity of the hip, should be performed by flexing the unaffected hip up to the chest wall and observing whether the leg on the affected side rises off the couch during this manoeuvre. The test should be carried out with the examiner's hand under the lumbar spine to check that the secondary lumbar lordosis has been abolished by this manoeuvre. Finally, true and apparent leg lengths should be measured. True leg length is measured with the hips in the identical degree of adduction, measuring from the anterior superior iliac spine to the medial malleolus. Apparent leg length is measured with the legs parallel to each other measuring from the umbilicus to the medial malleolus.

9.2 Osteoarthritis

Learning objectives

You should:
- be able to carry out Thomas's test for fixed flexion deformity
- recognise the radiological features of osteoarthritis in the hip
- know the rare occasions when osteotomy, arthrodesis or excision arthroplasty of the hip may be indicated
- outline the technique for total hip replacement
- be able to list the general complications, the specific early complications and the specific late complications of this operation.

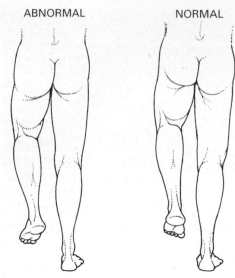

Figure 118 Normal test standing on the *unaffected* left hip. Positive Trendelenburg test when standing on the *affected* right hip.

Osteoarthritis of the hip is a common condition, affecting patients usually in their sixties and seventies. Primary osteoarthritis occurs idiopathically but is sometimes associated with a positive family history.

Secondary osteoarthritis can develop following previous insults to the joint from:

- trauma
- infection
- avascular necrosis
- Perthes' disease
- slipped upper femoral epiphysis
- acetabular dysplasia.

The sequence of pathological changes in the articular cartilage begins with fibrillation and cleft formation of the articular surface secondary to breaks in the normal arcades of collagen fibres. Clefts develop in the articular cartilage and the intracellular enzymes released cause synovial irritation. The resulting inflammation leads to contracture of the capsule. Eventually, articular cartilage is destroyed and subchondral bone becomes exposed. Cysts may develop in the subchondral bone and contribute to the femoral head collapse.

Clinical features

The main clinical features are:

- pain
- stiffness
- loss of function.

Listen The severity of pain should be graded to assess the severity of the condition. A useful scale is one ranging from pain that is present with vigorous activity, through pain that is present with weight bearing, to pain that is present at rest and, ultimately, pain that prevents sleep. Pain is often referred to the groin and thigh and sometimes the misleading symptom of isolated pain at the knee is the presenting feature of hip disease. Does the patient need regular analgesics and use a walking stick?

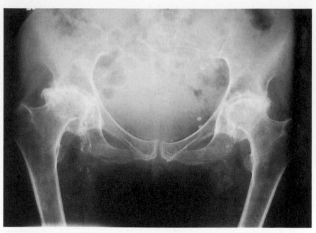

Figure 119 Bilateral osteoarthritis of the hips with loss of the joint space, subchondral sclerosis, osteophytes and subchondral cysts. Very extensive femoral head collapse.

Look Examination of the patient walking may show an antalgic gait, a Trendelenburg gait or a short-leg gait (see Figure 119).

Feel Because the hip joint is deeply situated, little can be felt by palpation, but tenderness may be elicited in the groin or by percussion over the greater trochanter.

Move There is limited range of movement and in particular there are flexion and adduction contractures with loss of internal rotation. Flexion contractures can be unmasked by Thomas's test, which corrects the secondary hyperlordosis of the lumbar spine.

Diagnosis

Radiological examination shows joint space narrowing, subchondral sclerosis, osteophyte formation and subchondral cysts (Figure 119).

Management

General Some simple advice may be helpful. The patient may be able to live within the limits of their discomfort without further treatment. Weight reduction may help. The use of a walking stick in the opposite hand decreases the load crossing the painful hip. If there is leg length inequality, a shoe raise is used to correct the gait and so relieve secondary back pain. Physiotherapy has a role in keeping other joints mobile.

Medical management Analgesics and non-steroidal anti-inflammatory drugs are useful, although there is a risk of gastrointestinal haemorrhage with these.

Surgical management The mainstay of surgical management has become a total joint replacement, but this is not always the most appropriate option. Other procedures to be considered include:

- osteotomy
- arthrodesis
- excision arthroplasty.

Osteotomy

Cutting the femur in the area of the trochanters and displacing the fragments can be used to rotate the head and realign the joint (Figure 120). This has the effect of altering

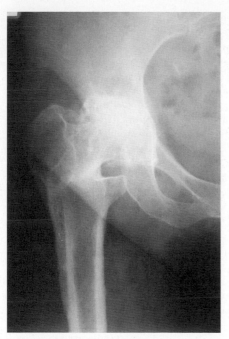

Figure 120 Osteoarthritis of the hip, which has previously been treated by an intertrochanteric displacement osteotomy.

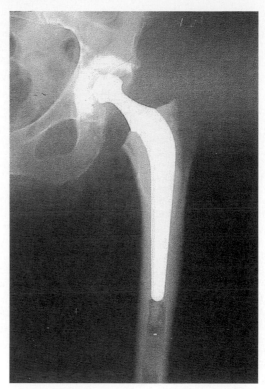

Figure 121 Arthritis of the hip treated by a Charnley total hip replacement.

the weight-bearing surface, reducing the load across the hip joint and achieving vascular decompression of the bone. Symptoms may be relieved and joint function improved. Osteotomy is appropriate for a young patient with only an isolated point of arthritis in the joint.

Arthrodesis

Fusion of the hip joint with a bone graft achieves pain relief but at the expense of loss of movement. The knee, back and contralateral hip must have free painless movement to compensate for the arthrodesed joint. This debilitating operation may be considered in severe arthritis in a young patient.

Excision arthroplasty

If the affected joint is excised, the 'gap' fills with fibrous tissue. The leg is several centimetres shorter after this procedure but painless movement is possible. This is usually reserved as a revision operation following removal of an infected joint replacement.

Total joint replacement

A total joint replacement involves replacement of both the acetabular and femoral parts of the joint. An acetabular cup made of high-density polyethylene and a metal femoral component are used (Figure 121). These are cemented into the bone with acrylic cement. Prophylactic antibiotics and precautions against deep venous thrombosis and pulmonary embolism are usually required. Reliably good results can be achieved but there is a long-term risk of recurrence of hip pain if the implant becomes loose or infected. Revision surgery is then required.

Complications of surgery:
- infection
- dislocation
- venous thromboembolism, myocardial infection, stroke and gastrointentestinal (GI) haemorrhage together contribute to a 0.5% risk of death
- eventual failure and need for revision.

9.3 Avascular necrosis

> **Learning objectives**
>
> You should:
> - list the predisposing causes of avascular necrosis of the hip.

Avascular necrosis of the femoral head may be idiopathic but is also associated with alcohol abuse and deep sea diving. Sometimes it is secondary to infection or to intracapsular fractures or dislocations of the hip. The avascular bone dies, collapses and appears sclerotic on radiograph.

Clinical features

The hip joint is stiff and painful and the patient walks with a limp.

Diagnosis

Plain radiographs will eventually show collapse and sclerosis of the avascular femoral head with osteoporosis of the surrounding bone but MRI will show the changes much earlier.

Management

Treatment of the early painful phase of avascular necrosis is difficult. Osteotomy and core excision of the femoral neck and head have been used in an attempt to stimulate revascularisation. An operation to insert a vascularised iliac crest bone graft has also been used in an attempt to bring a new external blood supply to the femoral head. Once osteoarthritic changes have developed total joint replacement is necessary.

Complications:

• secondary osteoarthritis.

Knee pain

Chapter part overview

The knee lends itself to physical examination as many of its anatomical landmarks are palpable and pathological features may readily be detected on physical examination. The presentation of a painful swollen knee is common in both elective orthopaedic practice, where it may be associated with rheumatoid or osteoarthritis, and trauma surgery, where haemathrosis is commonly seen in sports players and signifies some internal derangement in the joint.

Arthroscopic surgery has revolutionised the approach to knee surgery for many patients and the applications of this treatment should be understood. Both rheumatoid and osteoarthritis remain common and total knee replacement has become the treatment of choice for advanced disease. The indications for surgery and postoperative management should be clearly understood. Intra-articular fractures, especially of the tibal plateau, remain a technical challenge for orthopaedic surgeons. Loose bodies and infection in the knee are less common but, as with many other knee problems, much can be gained by careful attention to history and physical examination.

9.4 Clinical examination – knee

Learning objectives

You should:
• be able to examine the knee and relate your findings to the underlying anatomy
• know how to detect an effusion of the knee joint
• know how to carry out tests for ligamentous laxity.

The knee joint is very superficial, so much of its structure can be observed and palpated. Examination can be very precise, and if done carefully will help extensively in making a diagnosis. Being asked to examine the knee is a common question in undergraduate clinical examinations as patients with specific clinical findings are readily available. It is very important, therefore, to be proficient at the examination technique involved. This, as always, includes 'listen, look, feel and move'. Do not forget to observe the patient walking and standing as well as lying down.

• **Listen** – Key features in the history include:
 – mechanism of injury
 – pain
 – instability
 – swelling or locking.
• **Look:**
 – quadriceps muscle wasting
 – varus/valgus alignment
 – effusion in the suprapatellar pouch
 – scars from previous injury or surgery
 – do not forget to look behind the knee for a popliteal cyst.
• **Feel** – with the knee extended, feel for retropatellar tenderness or a small effusion. With the knee flexed to 90°, the medial and lateral joint lines are easily palpated. The origins and insertions of the medial and lateral collateral ligaments may be tender if they have been stretched or torn.
• **Move** – carry out the anterior drawer sign to check for anterior cruciate laxity. Observe for the presence of a posterior sag suggestive of posterior cruciate ligament rupture. Apply varus and valgus stresses to the partially flexed knee to check the integrity of the medial and lateral collateral ligaments. Observe the knee for evidence of locking (a block to full extension) and demonstrate that full flexion is possible.

9.5 The 'sportsman's knee'

Learning objectives

You should:
• be able to recognise a history suggestive of a meniscal lesion
• be able to differentiate the clinical findings of a torn miniscus from a collateral ligament injury
• know the emergency management of a haemarthrosis.

Knee injuries are often caused by sporting activities.

Meniscus

Meniscal tears are the most common injury to the knee. They are caused by twisting injuries while weight bearing on the affected leg. Those associated with sports are usually vertically orientated (Figure 122) and may form part of a triad of injuries which includes damage to the medial collateral and anterior cruciate ligaments. In an older patient the meniscus becomes degenerate and minor twisting forces may be enough to cause meniscal tears, which are usually orientated horizontally.

Clinical features

The key features of meniscal damage are:

• pain
• instability
• swelling
• locking.

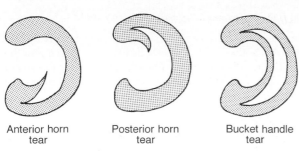

Figure 122 Three types of vertical tears seen in the meniscus.

Anterior horn tear   Posterior horn tear   Bucket handle tear

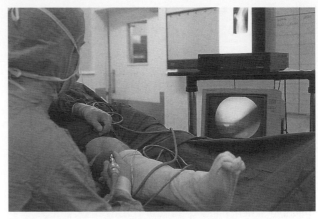

Figure 123 Arthroscopic examination of the knee.

Listen Patients complain of pain in the knee and instability, especially on stairs. There is often a history of an injury while playing sports.

Look A swelling may be seen in the parapatellar recesses or, if large, in the suprapatellar pouch. The effusion must be very large before the patella rises away from the femoral condyles and a patellar tap can be elicited by balloting it back down. A swelling occurring within hours of an injury is usually due to bleeding and is a haemarthrosis. A swelling which occurs slowly is usually due to synovial fluid from the inflamed or irritated synovial lining.

Feel There is well-localised jointline tenderness usually on the medial side.

Move A block to full extension is called 'locking' and is due to trapping of an intra-articular structure, usually the displaced meniscus, within the joint. Twisting and compression manoeuvres may reproduce the pain and 'lock' or 'unlock' the joint (McMurray's test).

Diagnosis

MRI scan will show a torn meniscus but careful clinical examination will make the diagnosis in the majority of cases. Examination under anaesthesia followed by arthroscopy will make it possible to proceed to a therapeutic procedure on the same occasion. Other knee conditions with some of the same clinical features can also be seen arthroscopically. These include loose bodies, discoid meniscus and cystic meniscus.

Management

A large haemarthrosis should be drained to relieve pain although this carries a small risk of introducing infection. Only the peripheral portion of the meniscus is well enough vascularised to allow healing, so repair of the meniscus is only occasionally possible. In most cases, the torn portion is removed to allow free joint movement. Both these procedures are done arthroscopically (Figure 123).

Complications

The articular surface of the knee may be damaged by repeated trauma from long-standing fragments of displaced meniscus.

Anterior cruciate ligament

The anterior cruciate ligament (ACL) arises at the anterior tibial spine and passes backwards across the knee joint to be inserted on the medial side of the lateral femoral

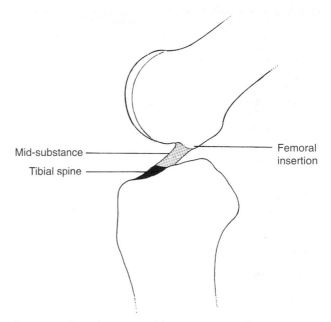

Mid-substance
Tibial spine
Femoral insertion

Figure 124 Sites of disruption of the anterior cruciate ligament.

condyle. It prevents the tibia sliding off the front of the femur.

Clinical features

A tear of the ACL is a common sporting injury (Figure 124). Rupture of the ACL accounts for 75% of haemarthrosis associated with sports.

Listen There is a history of a twisting injury, a direct blow behind the upper tibia or a hyperflexion injury. The patient often describes a snapping sound and sensation from the knee.

Look/Feel A haemarthrosis develops quickly.

Move In the presence of a large haemarthrosis, detailed examination will be difficult. Drainage of the haemarthrosis may enable a positive anterior drawer sign to be elicited but hamstring spasm may still lead to a false negative. The Lachman test involves the examiner grasping the femur and tibia in opposite hands and attempting to slide the tibia forwards on the femur with the knee at 20° to 30° flexion. This test is more at right angles to the hamstring

Nine

209

pull and can therefore be more useful. The diagnosis is often much easier a few weeks later.

Diagnosis

A lateral radiograph may show an avulsion of the anterior tibial spine but usually the tear is in the mid-substance of the ligament and requires MRI to visualise it.

Management

Initial treatment involves aspiration of the knee and early physiotherapy to regain stability by hamstring function. As a rough guide, one-third of patients become asymptomatic with this regime. Another third remain symptomatic but adjust their lifestyle to having a knee which is unstable when making sudden changes of direction at speed. Sports that involve cutting and turning movements, such as squash, are not possible but other types of physical exercise can comfortably be carried out.

The final third require a reconstruction to regain a knee which is more stable for sporting activities. The usual method is with a composite bone – patellar tendon – bone transfer or a hamstring autograft. In the rare cases of an avulsion of the anterior tibial spine, open reduction and internal fixation can be carried out.

Complications:

- osteoarthritis
- meniscal tear.

Reconstruction within a year of injury reduces the incidence of meniscal tear but it is controversial whether it reduces the incidence of osteoarthritis in the long term.

Posterior cruciate ligament

The posterior cruciate ligament (PCL) arises on the posterior aspect of the tibia and passes anteriorly to be inserted on the lateral side of the medial femoral condyle. This ligament holds the tibia forward under the femur and prevents it dropping backwards. Injuries to the PCL are less frequently seen than ACL injuries.

Clinical features

There is a history of hyperextension or forced posterior displacement of the tibia on the femur. There is a haemarthrosis and an obvious posterior sag to the knee.

Diagnosis

MRI confirms the diagnosis.

Management

Conservative management involves aspiration of the joint and physiotherapy to the quadriceps muscles to stabilise the knee.

Surgical management will involve open reduction and internal fixation of any avulsed bony fragment from the PCL insertion. Mid-substance PCL tears require autograft reconstruction.

Complications:

- chronic instability.

Medial collateral ligament

Damage to the medial collateral ligament is usually associated with both a medial meniscus tear and damage to the anterior cruciate ligament. Injuries are usually the result of twisting forces on the knee. Isolated, pure valgus injury is unusual.

Clinical features

Clinical presentation will include:

- bruising
- swelling
- tenderness
- laxity.

Tears may be in the mid-substance of the ligament or at its origin or insertion on the femur or tibia.

Diagnosis

Radiological examination may show an avulsed bony fragment at either end of the ligament. Stress radiographs may be helpful.

Management

Conservative Splinting in an orthosis protects the collateral ligament but allows flexion and extension.

Surgical Reconstruction of an associated anterior cruciate ligament rupture may help to regain stability if a complex derangement of the knee is present.

Complications:

- Pellegrini–Stieda syndrome (calcification and discomfort in the medial collateral ligament)
- chronic ligamentous laxity.

Lateral collateral ligament

Isolated injuries can be treated non-operatively in a hinged brace but repair or reconstruction is required when the injury is part of a complex knee injury or dislocation.

Management

A functional brace protects the ligament while allowing flexion and extension.

Complications:

- chronic ligamentous laxity.

Knee dislocation

This can only occur if multiple ligaments are disrupted. Injury to the popliteal artery is common and emergency reduction of the knee is required followed by emergency arteriography. Repair of a damaged artery is an emergency and operative reconstruction of the damaged ligaments will be required.

Complications:

- popliteal artery injury
- tibial or common peroneal nerve injury
- chronic instability or stiffness.

9.6 Osteoarthritis

You should:

- know the typical features of osteoarthritis and rheumatoid arthritis of the knee
- list the radiographic features of osteoarthritis and rheumatoid arthritis
- know the principles of management for both these conditions and their indications.

Rheumatoid arthritis and osteoarthritis are both frequently seen in the knee.

Osteoarthritis

Primary osteoarthritis may develop in the knee spontaneously and is sometimes associated with a positive family history.

Secondary osteoarthritis may follow trauma, infection or intra-articular derangement of the knee, such as a ligamentous disruption or meniscectomy.

The medial side of the joint is more frequently involved than the lateral side.

Clinical features

Listen There is knee pain ranging in severity from being associated only with walking, especially on stairs, to being present at rest.

Look Classically, there is varus alignment of the joint with synovial thickening and effusion. In late cases there is a flexion contracture.

Feel There is a swelling in the suprapatellar pouch due to effusion. Marginal osteophytes can be felt at the tibial plateau.

Move There may be loss of full extension due to flexion contracture. Any varus deformity will usually not be correctible. Moving the knee produces crepitus.

Diagnosis

Radiographs show:

- joint space narrowing
- sclerosis
- subchondral cysts
- osteophytes
- varus alignment.

Management

Conservative management:

- physiotherapy
- NSAIDs
- walking stick
- weight reduction
- limitation of activities.

Operative management

Upper tibial osteotomy A laterally based wedge of bone at the upper tibia is removed (Figure 125). This realigns the tibia on the femur and redistributes load

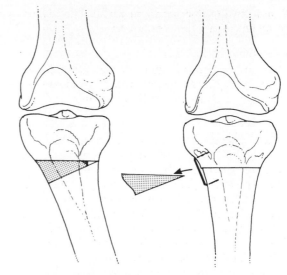

Figure 125 Procedure of a tibial osteotomy.

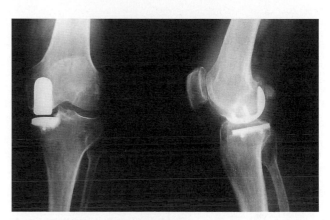

Figure 126 Unicompartment arthroplasty.

across the joint, diverting high pressures from the damaged medial compartment to the undamaged lateral compartment. The osteotomy is secured with a staple. This operation is suitable for early disease in young patients.

Unicompartmental joint replacement This replaces both the femoral and tibial sides of one-half of the joint, usually the medial compartment (Figure 126). Disease needs to be confined to the one compartment and the ACL must be intact.

Total knee replacement A semi-constrained surface replacement by a metal convex femoral component and a metal-backed high-density polyethylene concave tibial component is used. The prosthesis can be cemented or uncemented to the bone. The stability of the joint depends on correct tensioning of the medial and lateral collateral ligaments and on the contour of the high-density polyethylene tibial component (Figure 127A and B).

Arthrodesis Surgical fusion of the joint may be appropriate for a young patient with arthritis but may also be used to salvage a knee after infection.

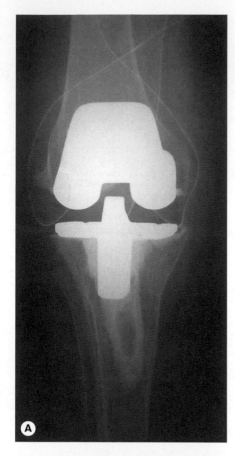

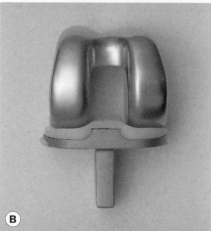

Figure 127 (A) Total knee prosthesis in flexion. (B) Total knee prosthesis cemented in place with the knee extended.

Complications of total knee replacement:
- infection
- venous thromboembolism, myocardial infection, stroke and GI haemorrhage contribute to a 0.5% risk of death
- eventual loosening and need for revision.

Rheumatoid arthritis (also see other sections on rheumatoid arthritis)

Rheumatoid arthritis begins as inflammation of the synovium as part of an autoimmune response. The inflam-mation ultimately spreads to the articular cartilage and destroys it. The presence of persisting synovial effusions stretches and damages the ligaments and capsule of the joint. The joint surface becomes destroyed and the joint itself lax. This results in subluxation, deformity and painful movement.

Clinical features
- **Listen** – the joint is unstable; during exacerbation of the disease it becomes warmer and more painful.
- **Look**
  – *swelling*
  – *valgus alignment.*
- **Feel** – a joint effusion may be apparent.
- **Move** – laxity of the lateral collateral ligament.

Diagnosis
Radiographic features of rheumatoid arthritis include:

- joint space narrowing
- irregular joint surface
- marginal erosions
- valgus alignment.

Management
Medical management includes the use of both analgesics and disease-modifying drugs. Synovectomy may prevent the progression of the disease. This can be done by injection of intra-articular radioactive yttrium or as an arthroscopic or open procedure.

Operative management All rheumatoid patients listed for surgery must have radiographs taken of the cervical spine in flexion and extension. This assesses the extent of subluxation of the odontoid process as there is a risk of cord compression with cervical spine manipulation during anaesthesia.

Arthroscopic synovectomy or total joint replacement may be indicated.

Complications:
- as listed for knee surgery in osteoarthritis but in rheumatoid arthritis the bone is softer and the skin thinner and more easily damaged
- systemic manifestations: ligamentous laxity of the cervical spine may cause spinal cord compression by the odontoid process during intubation.

Gout and pseudogout

These conditions are due to deposition of crystals within the joint; urate in the case of gout and pyrophosphate in pseudogout. The first presentation can be difficult to dif-ferentiate from septic arthritis. Gout can be precipitated by certain drugs such as thiazide diuretics.

Clinical features
- **Listen** – there will be a history of an acutely painful, swollen knee and the patient may describe previous similar episodes.
- **Look** – swelling and possibly redness.
- **Feel** – a large, hot effusion.
- **Move** – painful restriction of joint movement.

Diagnosis

ESR and C-reactive protein (CRP) will be raised but the serum urate may be normal, even in acute gout. Radiographs show calcification in the menisci in pseudogout. Microscopy of fluid aspirated from the knee under polarised light will reveal the crystals.

Management

The acute episode is managed with non-steroidal antiinflammatories. In gout, frequency of further episodes can be reduced by the uricosuric drug allopurinol but this should not be started until symptoms settle. Drugs that precipitate gout should be withdrawn if possible.

9.7 Infection

Learning objectives

You should:
- know how to identify infection in the knee by physical examination
- know the emergency management of an infected knee.

Knee infection may occur as a result of surgery and tuberculous arthritis is still occasionally seen.

Clinical features

Clinical features include:

- pain
- swelling
- heat
- tenderness
- resistance to active or passive movement.

Diagnosis

There is a raised temperature, white cell count and CRP. Radiographs are normal in the early stages. Immediate Gram stain of the aspirate can be falsely negative but the organisms can eventually be cultured and identified.

Management

Children with less than a 24-h history and patients who are not fit for anaesthesia can be treated with aspiration and antibiotics. Best-guess antibiotics are started as soon as an aspirate has been taken for bacteriology. All other patients should be taken urgently to theatre. In early cases an arthroscopic debridement is possible, but in later cases the tissues are too stuck and an open operation is required. Arthrodesis may be necessary as a late procedure to salvage a painful, arthritic knee or the knee may spontaneously ankylose.

Complications:
- destruction of articular cartilage leading to a painful, stiff knee
- bony or fibrous ankylosis.

9.8 Intra-articular fractures

Learning objectives

You should:
- be able to recognise different types of tibial plateau fracture from the radiological appearance
- know which of these require further imaging for assessment and which will require elevation of the tibial plateau and bone grafting.

Osteochondral fractures

In young adults, shearing forces or direct trauma will produce an osteochondral fracture that may separate entirely from its bed. Such a fragment may grow in the joint as it receives nutrition from the synovial fluid.

Management

A small fragment should be removed arthroscopically, but a large fresh fragment should be reattached.

Tibial plateau fractures

Valgus forces directed to the knee will tear the medial collateral ligament and damage the lateral tibial plateau.

Clinical features:
- **Listen**
  - *history of an angulatory or twisting force to the knee*
  - *pain on either side of the joint*
- **Look**
  - *medial bruising*
  - *swelling*
  - *haemarthrosis may be present*
- **Move**
  - *valgus laxity on stressing the joint.*

Diagnosis

Radiological examination may show:

- vertical split
- depression fracture (die punch)
- comminution of the whole lateral tibial plateau
- combination of split and depression fractures.

The different types of tibial plateau fracture are shown in Figure 128.

Management

Cleavage fractures require screw fixation to restore the stability of the articular surface.

Depression fractures require elevation of the defect with a bone graft. A portion of the lateral meniscus may be found driven into the crater by the injury.

More complex fractures require elevation of the plateau and stabilisation by a buttress plate on the tibia. Bone graft is always necessary. Postoperatively, the knee is nursed in a functional brace, which allows the joint to mobilise, but weight bearing has to be avoided for 6 to 8 weeks.

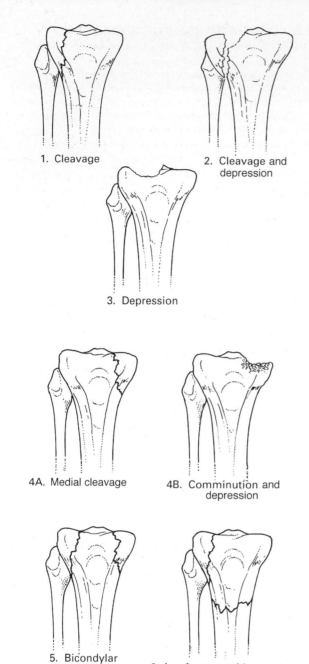

1. Cleavage

2. Cleavage and depression

3. Depression

4A. Medial cleavage

4B. Comminution and depression

5. Bicondylar

6. Any fracture with discontinuity between diaphysis and metaphysis

Figure 128 Classification of types of tibial plateau fracture.

Complications:

- osteoarthritis requiring later total conversion to a total knee replacement
- valgus laxity
- stiff joint.

Condylar fractures of the femur

Axial angulatory forces directed across the knee may fracture the distal femur.

Clinical features

Clinical features include:

- haemarthrosis
- joint laxity.

Diagnosis

Radiological examination shows a split fracture of a single condyle or a Y-shaped fracture of both condyles. There may be a comminuted fracture involving both condyles.

Management

The haemarthrosis is aspirated. Plaster immobilisation may be sufficient for an undisplaced unicondylar split fracture, but accurate anatomical reduction with screw fixation to prevent subsequent displacement is preferable for more complex fractures. Postoperatively, the knee is mobilised in a functional brace.

Complications:

- valgus/varus angulation
- osteoarthritis.

9.9 Extensor mechanism injury

Learning objectives

You should:
- know how to diagnose an extensor mechanism injury
- know the principles of management.

Resisted extension of the knee may disrupt the extensor mechanism anywhere from the tibial tuberosity to the quadriceps. Direct trauma to the patella can cause a stellate (star-shaped) fracture and a blow to the side of the patella or a genetic predisposition can cause a dislocation. Disruption of the extensor mechanism results in inability to maintain extension of the knee against gravity and there may be a palpable gap.

Avulsion of the tibial tuberosity

This rare injury is treated with open reduction and internal fixation.

Ruptured patellar tendon

Radiographs show proximal migration of the patella. Open repair is required and this is supported with a loop of wire between the patella and tibial tuberosity.

Transverse fractures of the patella

Undisplaced fractures can be treated by splinting the leg straight in a cylinder cast until union is achieved. Most fractures require open reduction and internal fixation to achieve a congruent joint surface and restore extensor function.

Stellate fractures of the patella

These can often be treated in a cylinder cast but sometimes require fixation.

Rupture of quadriceps tendon

These usually occur in the elderly with minimal trauma and the diagnosis is frequently missed. There will be a palpable gap but the radiographs may not show any obvious signs. Open repair followed by a period of protection in a cast or splint is required.

Dislocations of the patella

These injuries are common in teenagers and young adults. The dislocation occurs to the lateral side; if the patella is still dislocated at the time of presentation, the diagnosis will be obvious. Urgent relocation under analgesia or sedation will relieve the acute pain. Frequently, the dislocation will reduce spontaneously and there will be a swollen knee with tenderness medial to the patella where the retinaculum has been torn. Some patients have a deficient lateral femoral condyle or very valgus knees and can dislocate with minimal force.

Radiographs should be inspected to detect any associated osteochondral fracture. The first episode should be treated with immobilisation in a cylinder cast to allow the retinaculum to heal, followed by physiotherapy to strengthen the medial quadriceps. If the dislocation recurs, the retinaculum is already deficient and immediate physiotherapy is more appropriate. Consideration can be given to operative realignment of the extensor mechanism for recurrent dislocation.

Complications of extensor mechanism injuries

Complications include:

- weak quadriceps and loss of straight leg raising
- a painful ossicle in the patellar tendon may follow tibial tuberosity avulsion.

Foot and ankle pain

Chapter part overview

Developmental degenerative and inflammatory conditions are often seen in the feet, presenting as bunions, hallux valgus, hallux rigidus, gout or rheumatoid arthritis. In addition, the feet are involved in the serious changes of progressive peripheral vascular disease. Fractures of the foot and ankle are commonly seen in the accident and emergency department, where it is important to be able to differentiate between those that will require further investigation and operative treatment and those that can be managed conservatively.

9.10 Clinical examination – foot and ankle

Learning objectives

You should:
- remember to examine the patient's shoes and watch them walking
- observe the patient barefoot from behind both fully weight-bearing and standing on tiptoe
- examine the various joints individually: ankle, subtalar, midtarsal, metatarsophalangeal and interphalangeal.

Examination of the foot and ankle must include an examination of the patient walking and standing. It is important to remember to examine the patient's shoes for signs of wear on the sole and of damage to the uppers.

The patient's feet are observed while walking. With the patient standing with the feet together, the posture of the foot is examined. Looking from behind, the alignment of the calcaneum can be seen and any degree of calcaneovalgus noted. The posture of the longitudinal arches can be observed. If apparently absent, the arch will often reconstitute when the patient stands on tiptoe. With the patient seated and the foot cradled on the examiner's knee, the peripheral pulses, capillary circulation and peripheral sensation can be examined. Movements of the foot and ankle should be examined in turn. Movement occurs in the following joints:

- ankle
- subtalar
- midtarsal
- metatarsophalangeal
- interphalangeal.

At the ankle joint, only flexion and extension is possible. Subtalar movement is assessed by cupping the heel in the palm of the hand and inverting and everting the foot.

With the calcaneum immobilised on the talus, inversion and eversion at the midtarsal joint can be elicited. Flexion and extension are possible at the metatarsophalangeal and interphalangeal joints.

9.11 Foot disorders

Learning objectives

You should:
- be able to examine the foot for hallux valgus deformity and differentiate this from hallux rigidus
- differentiate the pathology and management of the common form of hallux valgus in a middle-aged woman from that seen in an adolescent girl
- recognise the deformity of claw toes in the rheumatoid foot and know the different ways of managing this condition
- be able to recognise critical limb ischaemia in the lower limb.

Bunions and hallux valgus

This is the most commonly occurring deformity in the foot, but it is not always symptomatic. Two distinct groups of patients usually present.

The adolescent girl There is a strong family history of hallux valgus. The underlying abnormality is varus deformity of the first metatarsal.

The middle-aged woman There is forefoot splaying because of ligamentous laxity. Constricting footwear may provide an additional deforming force. There may be degenerative changes in the first metatarsophalangeal joint and abnormalities of the adjacent toes. Hallux valgus is often seen in association with rheumatoid arthritis in this age group.

Clinical features:

- **Listen** – patients complain of rubbing or pressure over the first metatarsophalangeal joint and that their shoes feel tight.
- **Look** – there is a prominent exostosis at the first metatarsal head covered with a protective bursa. This may become inflamed or even infected. The big toe is displaced laterally and pronated, and crowds the second toe so that one may override the other. There may be callosities to see.
- **Feel** – if inflamed the bunion may be painful to touch.
- **Move** – once established the valgus deformity cannot be corrected.

Diagnosis

Weight-bearing radiographs will show the extent of the deformity, the degree of subluxation of the joint and any secondary arthritic degeneration (Figure 129).

Management

Initially all patients should consider accepting the deformity and adapting their footwear to accommodate it. If this is not acceptable to the patient, surgery can be discussed.

Adolescents Management is usually with surgery. An osteotomy of the first metatarsal, which realigns the first ray and narrows the forefoot (Figure 130), will correct the valgus deformity of the big toe but it may recur if the foot is still squashed into pointed shoes.

Adults

Orthoses Comfortable, wide shoes that accommodate the splayed forefoot are the easiest solution. The shoe uppers should be soft over the bunion and have moulded insoles to support the metatarsal heads.

Surgery:
- First metatarsal osteotomy as described above is suitable where there is no secondary degeneration.
- Realignment of the hallux can be achieved in patients with mild disease by a capsulorrhaphy of the first metatarsophalangeal joint and release of the adductor hallucis; an excision of the exostosis at the first metatarsal head can be included.
- Arthrodesis of the first metatarsophalangeal joint is indicated in more severe disease with secondary arthritis.
- Excision arthroplasty is suitable for older people who are less active; the base of the proximal phalanx and the exostosis are removed (Keller's operation; Figure 131); the alignment is corrected but the big toe is now floppy and fails to provide a strong 'push-off' when walking.

Complications:

- local pressure effects
- bursitis.

Complications of surgery:

- infection
- poor wound healing

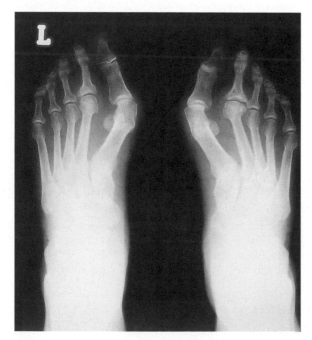

Figure 129 Radiograph of the feet showing bilateral hallux valgus deformity. On the right there has been a previous excision of the exostosis but the underlying metatarsus primus varus remains.

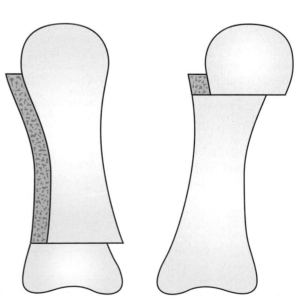

Figure 130 Two types of osteotomy of the first metatarsal which will correct the underlying varus deformity and allow the big toe to become straighter.

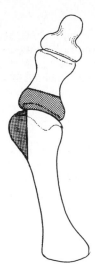

Figure 131 Keller's arthroplasty of the first metatarsophalangeal joint.

- hallux varus or hallux erectus deformity from overcorrection
- recurrence
- altered sensation.

Hallux rigidus

Some forgotten minor trauma may be the precipitating cause of this condition, which affects men more than women. There is osteoarthritis of the first metatarsophalangeal joint, which causes pain and stiffness of the big toe (hallux rigidus). The changes are isolated and not part of widespread osteoarthritis.

Clinical features:
- **Listen**
  - pain on walking, especially up hills
  - patients notice reduced stride length
  - women complain of pain when wearing high-heeled shoes
- **Look**
  - dorsal osteophyte
- **Feel**
  - local tenderness
- **Move**
  - first metatarsophalangeal joint is stiff
  - dorsiflexion is painful, resisted and limited.

Diagnosis
The familiar radiological features of osteoarthritis are present: sclerosis, joint space narrowing, osteophyte formation (Figure 132).

Management
Conservative A carbon fibre insole or rigid sole with a rocker bottom allows the patient to roll over the metatarsophalangeal joint. Low heels are comfortable.

Operative In early cases, the dorsal osteophyte causes most of the symptoms and its excision (cheilectomy) can relieve symptoms while preserving joint motion. Where disease affects the whole joint, arthrodesis is the gold standard for pain relief but can be unpopular with women

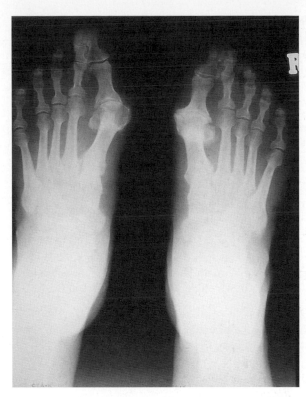

Figure 132 Hallux valgus on the left foot and hallux rigidus on the right with radiological features of joint space narrowing, sclerosis and osteophyte formation.

because it restricts the patient to one heel height. Joint replacement has its enthusiasts but the early failure of several devices makes this a controversial option.

Complications of surgery:
- infection
- failure of cheilectomy to relieve symptoms
- non-union of arthrodesis
- restricted choice of footwear with arthrodesis
- early failure of joint replacement.

Fasciitis

Fasciitis is pain at the origin of the plantar fascia where it arises from the calcaneum.

Clinical features
The main clinical features are pain on walking and localised tenderness at the calcaneum.

Diagnosis
Radiological examination sometimes shows a spur on the calcaneum.

Management
Management includes:

- heel pad
- steroid injection
- AFO (ankle–foot orthosis) to wear at night
- Achilles tendon stretching.

Rheumatoid feet

The foot, like the hand and wrist, is often involved in rheumatoid arthritis. Ligamentous laxity following synovitis allows dorsal dislocation of the proximal phalanges on the metatarsal heads. This causes the weight-bearing pad of thick plantar skin to be drawn distally; weight bearing, therefore, takes place through the unprotected metatarsal heads, which cause pain in the sole of the foot (Figure 133).

Clinical features:

- **Listen** – patients classically complain that they are 'walking on pebbles'.
- **Look** – there are pressure signs over the dorsum of the proximal interphalangeal joints of the toes. The metatarsal heads can be seen prominently in the sole.
- **Feel** – the metatarsal heads can be easily felt.
- **Move** – eventually the toes cannot be corrected to their normal straight alignment.

Diagnosis

Radiological examination shows the extent of joint subluxation and of bone destruction (Figure 134).

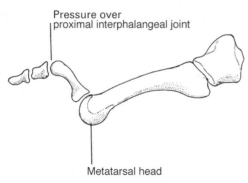

Pressure over proximal interphalangeal joint

Metatarsal head

Figure 133 Mechanism of metatarsophalangeal joint displacement in rheumatoid arthritis.

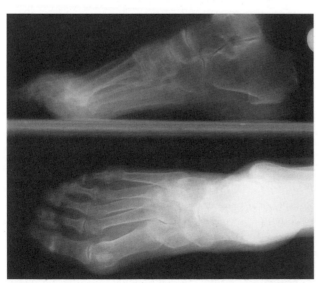

Figure 134 This true lateral view of the foot shows the extent of the dislocation of the metatarsophalangeal joint. The metatarsal heads are touching the ground but the toes are displaced upwards and do not contribute to weight bearing.

Management

Conservative Wide, deep shoes with soft uppers and moulded insoles accommodate the foot comfortably.

Operative In more severely affected patients, a forefoot arthroplasty is required. The metatarsal heads are excised, the toes realigned and the weight-bearing pad of skin, which has been drawn distally, is replaced under the metatarsal heads by excising a proximal ellipse of normal skin.

Complications

Persisting painful pressure areas in the sole are usually the result of failure to remove sufficient length from the distal metatarsals. Wound healing is occasionally prolonged.

Peripheral vascular disease

Usually the cause of peripheral vascular disease (PVD) is proximal large-vessel atheroma, but sometimes distal small-vessel disease due to diabetes is the cause. In these patients the condition is often complicated by persisting infection and ulceration, although either type of PVD may give rise to peripheral gangrene.

Clinical features:

- **Listen** – in large-vessel disease, the patient complains of intermittent claudication and eventually of severe constant ischaemic pain in the limb. The patient is usually a smoker.
- **Look** – there are peripheral trophic changes, including thinning of the skin and loss of skin hair. The skin is pale and ulceration and incipient or frank gangrene may be apparent (Figure 135).
- **Feel** – the leg feels cold below the knee and peripheral pulses are absent

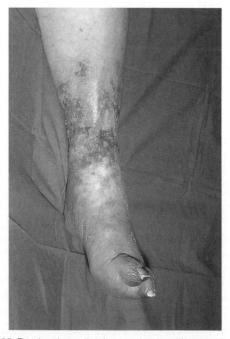

Figure 135 Peripheral vascular disease showing rubor, trophic changes and incipient gangrene in the toes and forefoot.

• **Move** – elevation of the limb produces further pallor but dependency causes rubor due to reactive hyperaemia (Buerger's test).

In diabetes, the proximal findings are not seen but peripheral infection, ulceration and dry or wet gangrene of individual toes may be present.

Diagnosis

The diagnosis can be confirmed and the level of vascular obstruction demonstrated by doppler ultrasound and arteriography.

Management

Prevention Patients who smoke must stop to have any chance of halting progression. The control of diabetes mellitus and care of the feet to avoid infection are important in diabetics.

Surgery Patients with proximal atheroma are investigated by arteriogram of the affected limb, and the circulation to the foot may be improved initially by a sympathectomy or in later cases by an appropriate bypass graft.

Toes affected by dry gangrene can be allowed to demarcate and separate. In the presence of intractable pain and progressive wet gangrene, an amputation is required. Diabetic patients are well served by a below-knee amputation, which usually heals more reliably than a midtarsal amputation, especially in the presence of coexisting large-vessel disease. The majority of patients with large-vessel disease can be treated by a below-knee rather than an above-knee amputation (Figure 136). Well-supervised prosthetic fitting and physiotherapy are required postoperatively.

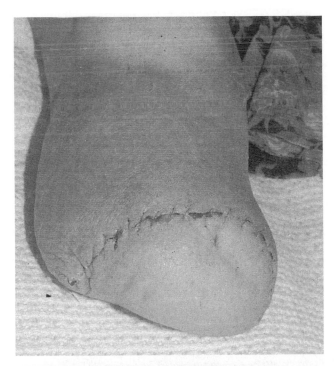

Figure 136 A right below-knee amputation with a long, posterior myocutaneous flap to provide good wound healing and weight distribution.

Complications:
• advancing gangrene
• death.

Complications following surgery:
• stump breakdown occurs if the limb has been amputated too distally
• phantom limb pain (a feeling that the amputated limb is still there and is still painful).

9.12 Fractures

Ankle fractures

Injuries to the ankle are frequently seen. They are usually caused by twisting forces or angulating forces. Falls from a height often cause more severe injuries involving the distal tibial plafond, the calcaneum and, more proximally, the vertebral column or base of skull. At the ankle, a combination of ligamentous and bony injury is seen.

The ligaments involved are:
On the lateral side:

• inferior tibiofibular ligament
• anterior and posterior talofibular ligaments
• calcaneofibular ligament.

On the medial side:

• deltoid ligament.

The bony margins involved are:

• medial malleolus
• lateral malleolus
• posterior surface of the tibia.

The forces that give rise to the injury can be grouped as:

• pronation and external rotation
• pronation and abduction
• supination and external rotation
• supination and adduction.

Clinical features

There is pain and swelling over one or both sides of the ankle with bruising and sometimes fracture blisters. If there is associated dislocation of the joint, there will be gross deformity, stretching of the overlying skin and loss of normal peripheral circulation and sensation. In this circumstance an attempt at reducing the dislocation should be made immediately without waiting for radiograph confirmation.

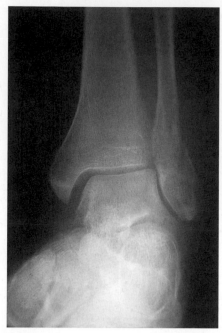

Figure 137 Fracture of the lateral malleolus of the ankle of a young man with lateral displacement of the talus.

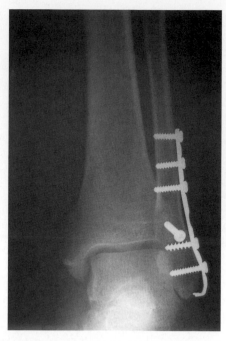

Figure 138 The fracture has been treated with a neutralisation plate on the fibula, which restores it to normal alignment and length and reduces the displacement of the talus.

Diagnosis

A lateral and an antero-posterior radiograph centred on the ankle mortice are required to assess the injury and to demonstrate any lateral displacement of the talus (Figure 137).

Management

Conservative Dislocation should be reduced urgently to reduce pain, relieve pressure on the peripheral vessels and nerves and prevent ischaemia of the overlying skin. Manipulation under anaesthesia in such a way as to reverse the direction of the injuring forces will correct a displaced fracture. An above-knee plaster or patella-bearing cast is required for those injuries where rotatory control is necessary; in other patients, a well-moulded below-knee plaster is sufficient. After initial swelling has settled, partial weight bearing can be allowed. Radiological follow-up is necessary to ensure that the fracture does not redisplace while in plaster. Immobilisation is required until the fracture heals, usually between 6 and 8 weeks.

Operative Open reduction and internal fixation is indicated for unstable fractures. This is best done before swelling develops and must not be done through very swollen tissues because of the risk of wound dehiscence. This technique restores the anatomical position of the articular surfaces and, by providing rigid fixation, allows early active mobilisation.

Lag screws are inserted across the fractures and the fibula is further kept out to length and stabilised by a neutralisation plate (Figure 138). Tension band wiring may be used in porotic bone in preference to screws to avoid cutting out.

Complications of conservative treatment:

- malunion
- talar shift leading to
- secondary osteoarthritis.

Complications of operative treatment:

- infection
- wound dehiscence
- non-union.

Foot fractures

Talus

Forced dorsiflexion injuries to the foot can result in a fracture of the talus through either the body or the neck of the bone. Osteochondral fractures can also occur, which may eventually become loose bodies in the joint.

Clinical features

Clinical presentation is with pain, swelling and bruising. If a portion of the fractured talus is displaced, it may cause pressure effects on the overlying skin.

Diagnosis

Radiological examination shows the site of the fracture but CT will give more detail.

Management

Displaced fractures require open reduction and internal fixation if avascular necrosis of the proximal fragment is to be avoided. Even with adequate treatment, there is still a substantial risk of this happening.

Complications:

- avascular necrosis of the body of the talus due to its retrograde blood supply being cut off by the fracture
- osteoarthritis of the subtalar, talonavicular or ankle joints

- formation of loose bodies from osteochondral fractures.

Calcaneum

A fall from a height is the usual cause of this injury and if present features in other sites must be sought, especially in the vertebrae, pelvis and base of the skull.

Clinical features

These include:

- pain
- deep bruising
- inability to bear weight
- fracture blisters
- swelling.

The heel may appear wider and shorter than the opposite one.

Diagnosis

Lateral and axial radiographs (Figure 139) are required. Fractures are usually described as:

- extra-articular
- intra-articular.

A CT scan will show the fracture pattern more precisely. 'Beak' fractures at the insertion of the Achilles tendon and fractures of the sustentaculum tali are usually then seen to be part of a more extensive intra-articular fracture.

Management

Elevation and exercise of the ankle and subtalar joints is appropriate management for many of these fractures. In some cases, open reduction and internal fixation with a bone graft is possible, but adequate fixation is technically difficult

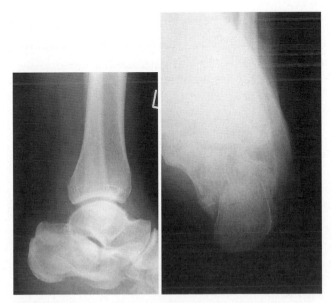

Figure 139 Fracture of the calcaneum.

and wound breakdown is common. After either procedure weight bearing is prohibited for at least 8 weeks.

Complications:

- persisting pain
- subtalar arthritis, requiring subsequent fusion of the subtalar joint.

9.13 Achilles tendon rupture

Learning objectives

You should:
- be able to examine the calf and Achilles tendon and recognise the features of an Achilles tendon injury.

Rupture of the Achilles tendon usually occurs in patients in middle age during the course of some strenuous activity such as running or playing squash.

Clinical features:

- **Listen** – a sudden movement of the ankle is followed by acute severe pain. Patients frequently think they have been hit in the back of the calf.
- **Look** – the gap in the tendon may be visible beneath the skin before swelling develops.
- **Feel** – palpation reveals a gap in the tendon at the ankle.
- **Move** – there may be loss of normal plantar flexion when the calf is squeezed (Symons' test).

Diagnosis

The clinical features are usually convincing, but sometimes tenderness is located in the mid-calf, in which case a partial rupture of the medial head of the gastrocnemius or a rupture of the plantaris tendon is a possible diagnosis. Clinical findings must be differentiated from those of deep venous thrombosis.

Management

Conservative There are many different regimes but all involve an initial cast with the ankle in full equinus followed by progressively more plantegrade casts and finally a heel raise in the patient's shoe.

Operative Direct repair of the tendon is performed surgically but the repair still needs to be protected with a cast or orthosis initially. Operative repair is indicated in those wanting to return to high level sport, where presentation is delayed or where re-rupture occurs after non-operative management.

Complications:

- re-rupture
- poor spring during toe-off
- poor wound healing and scar sensitivity after operative repair.

Self-assessment: questions

Hip pain in adults

Constructed response questions (CRQs)

CRQ 1

A 40-year-old labourer presents with a 12-month history of increasing pain in his right hip. He is having annoying side effects from the analgesics he has been using. He has read about the benefits of total hip replacement and wishes to have surgery.

a. How would you define how severe his pain is?

b. You begin your examination with him standing up. He has a positive Trendelenberg test. Why should this be?

c. On examining him on the couch he has a fixed flexion deformity of the affected hip. What test would you do now?

d. You place his legs parallel to each other and measure from the midline to the medial malleolus on each side. You record a discrepancy of 4 cm in this measurement. What is the name of this type of shortening and why should it occur?

e. What other treatment option may be appropriate? Why may a total hip replacement be unsatisfactory for him?

Best of 5s questions

1. A 43-year-old alcoholic man presents with severe hip pain and his plain radiographs are normal. Your reaction is:

   a. oh dear, I don't know what's going on
   b. thank goodness, his radiographs are normal and I can discharge him
   c. good, we have caught him in time to do something
   d. I'll send off some blood tests
   e. I can't help him. I'll send him to the pain clinic

Multiple choice questions

1. Which of the following radiographic features are commonly seen in osteoarthritis?

   a. subchondral cysts
   b. marginal erosions at the joint
   c. osteophytes
   d. Looser's zones
   e. heterotopic calcification

Knee pain

Extended matching items questions

EMI 1

Theme: Clinical presentation

A. chondromalacia
B. degenerative meniscus
C. osteochondritis dissecans
D. chronic osteitis
E. osteoarthritis
F. separation of articular cartilage
G. fibrous ankylosis
H. synovial chondromatosis
I. septic arthritis
J. rheumatoid arthritis

Which of the diagnoses listed above most closely fits the clinical presentations described below?

1. An 8-year-old boy complaining of intermittent pain and swelling has occasional inability to fully extend the knee to different extents on different occasions.

2. A 70-year-old patient with various other joint problems has symmetrical genu valgus and knee pain with a moderate effusion.

3. A 65-year-old man with a year-long history of knee pain has well-localised medial joint line tenderness, a small effusion and loss of full range of movement. His knee radiograph shows no abnormalities.

EMI 2

Theme: The sportsman's knee

A. anterior cruciate ligament tear
B. posterior cruciate ligament tear
C. meniscal tear
D. lateral collateral ligament tear
E. medial collateral ligament tear

Match each feature below with the most appropriate injury.

1. hyperextension injury
2. positive Lachman test
3. medial pain on valgus stress
4. medial joint line tenderness
5. laxity on varus stress

EMI 3

Theme: Arthritis

A. rheumatoid arthritis
B. osteoarthritis

C. gout

D. ankylosing spondylitis

E. septic arthritis

Match the presentations below with the most likely diagnosis.

1. Osteophytes and subchondral cysts on the radiograph.

2. Back pain and raised ESR in a young man.

3. Valgus deformity of the knee.

4. Crystals on polarised light microscopy.

5. Fever and raised CRP with abnormal Gram stain of joint fluid.

Constructed response questions

CRQ 1

A 55-year-old man attends your surgery with a year-long history of increasing pain on the medial side of his knee at the site of previous surgery. There is diffuse tenderness around the joint, a small swelling, loss of full range of movement and some crepitus in the joint. He reminds you that he is a farmer and wishes to continue working.

a. What is the likely diagnosis at this stage?

b. How would you visualise this?

c. Your investigation shows abnormalities limited to the medial compartment. Is there a connection between this and his previous surgery?

d. You discuss treatment options with him. What medical (non-operative) things may be helpful?

e. He returns 6 months later. His symptoms have not been improved. The pathology remains limited to the medial compartment. What surgical procedure is considered in this situation?

Objective structured clinical examination questions

OSCE 1

Study the photograph of a radiograph of a patient's knees (Figure 140).

a. What abnormalities can be seen here?

b. What is the diagnosis?

c. The patient is otherwise well but you have to obtain her consent for surgery. What complications should she be made aware of?

Best of 5s questions

1. A 74-year-old man presents with osteoarthritis of the knee. Which of the following is most important in determining whether he should be offered joint replacement surgery?

   a. range of movement in the joint

   b. social support at home

   c. previous surgery for bowel malignancy

   d. severe varus deformity

   e. pain which wakes him at night

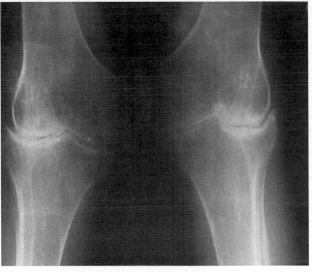

Figure 140

Multiple choice questions

1. In acute septic arthritis:

   a. *Staphylococcus aureus* is the usual infecting organism

   b. movement of the infected joint is restricted by adhesions

   c. antibiotics are withheld until the appropriate sensitivities are confirmed

   d. treatment includes joint irrigation

   e. small joints are more commonly affected than large joints

Foot and ankle pain

Extended matching items questions

EMI 1

Theme: Clinical presentation

A. Achilles tendon rupture

B. metatarsalgia

C. phantom pain

D. dry gangrene

E. fractured lateral malleolus

F. peripheral vascular disease

G. fractured medial malleolus

H. metatarsophalangeal joint subluxation from rheumatoid arthritis

I. calcaneal fracture

J. hallux rigidus

Which of the diagnoses listed above most closely fits the clinical presentations described below:

1. A 49-year-old man playing squash suddenly experiences sharp ankle pain. He can bear weight but can only walk with difficulty.

2. A 50-year-old woman with generalised joint pain has pressure effects from her shoes over the dorsum of all her toes. She says that her feet feel as though they are walking on pebbles.

3. A 45-year-old woman complains of pain in the first metatarsophalangeal joint. This is worst when walking uphill or wearing high heels.

Constructed response questions (CRQs)

CRQ 1

A 20-year-old youth is admitted in police custody to the accident and emergency department with a history of having jumped from a first-floor window. He is complaining of *bilateral* foot and ankle pain and swelling and cannot bear weight.

a. What would you expect to find on physical examination?

b. How would you investigate the patient at this stage?

c. On the left side the fibula is fractured at the ankle joint. What other deformity should be looked for on the antero-posterior radiograph?

d. A radiograph of the opposite foot shows an intra-articular fracture of the calcaneum with many fragments. What further information is needed?

e. What ways of treating this are possible?

Objective structured clinical examination questions

OSCE 1

Study the picture of a radiograph of a young man's ankle fracture (Figure 141).

a. How would you describe the fractures?

b. In what direction has the injury force been applied?

c. The fracture is unstable and lateral migration of the talus can be seen. How should this fracture be treated?

d. Postoperative management is essential to avoid prolonged stiffness. What would you ask the patient to do?

OSCE 2

Study the clinical photograph of an ankle and foot of a 70-year-old man with a long history of smoking and cardiovascular disease (Figure 142).

a. What features of peripheral vascular ischaemia should be looked for?

b. What other body systems may be affected in a patient with peripheral vascular disease?

c. What other systemic disease would you want to know about?

d. How would you investigate the patient further?

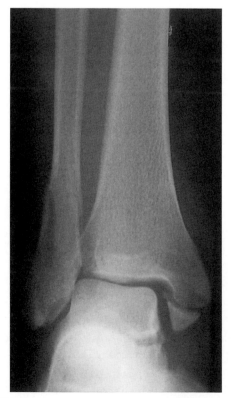

Figure 141

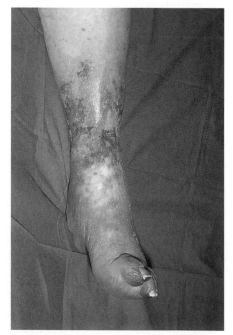

Figure 142

Best of 5s questions

1. A 45-year-old lady presents with a severely symptomatic hallux valgus deformity with a bunion but no degenerative disease of the joint. Which of the following is appropriate advice?

   a. Keller's excision arthroplasty of the proximal phalanx is an excellent procedure which will allow her to return to sport

   b. all bunion procedures have complications

   c. arthrodesis of the metatarsophalangeal joint is the most suitable operation

   d. joint replacement of the first metatarsophalangeal joint is a tried and trusted procedure

   e. there is no suitable surgical procedure and she will have to have special shoes

Self-assessment: answers

Hip pain in adults

CRQ answers

CRQ 1

a. Severity of pain can be graded according to how much it interferes with activities and rest. How much is his ability to work and his walking distance limited?

b. He has limited or absent ability to abduct the right hip.

c. Thomas's test.

d. Apparent shortening because of an adduction contracture of the affected hip.

e. Hip arthrodesis only if his other hip and spine are satisfactory. Total hip replacement in a young working man has an increased chance of loosening, thus requiring revision at an early date.

Best of 5s answer

1. c. Diagnosis is likely to be avascular necrosis. Outcome after core decompression is best when changes are only on MRI.

Multiple choice answers

1. a. **True.**
   b. **False.** These are associated with rheumatoid arthritis.
   c. **True.**
   d. **False.** These are associated with osteomalacia.
   e. **False.** This can be the sequela of an intramuscular haematoma.

Knee pain

EMI answers

EMI 1

Theme: Clinical presentation

1. C. A loose body in the joint produced by osteochondritis dissecans causes intermittent locking in different degrees of flexion and extension.

2. J. Genu valgus is characteristically seen in rheumatoid arthritis together with a knee effusion. Other joint problems are often seen symmetrically in the body.

3. B. A degenerative meniscus causes joint effusion and pain and may limit knee movement.

EMI 2

Theme: The sportsman's knee

1. B.
2. A.
3. E.
4. C.
5. D.

EMI 3

Theme: Arthritis

1. B.
2. D.
3. A.
4. C.
5. E.

CRQ answers

CRQ 1

a. Osteoarthritis.

b. plain radiograph
   weight-bearing antero-posterior views

c. Increased point loading due to absence of the medial meniscus particularly if he had a total meniscectomy.

d. NSAIDs
   walking stick
   weight reduction
   intra-articular steroid injection

e. High tibial (valgus) osteotomy – the result may be unpredictable so a total knee replacement may be considered if he will reduce his activity appropriately.

OSCE answers

OSCE 1

a. bilateral genu valgus
   marginal erosions
   joint space narrowing
   generalised osteopaenia
   irregular joint surfaces

b. Rheumatoid arthritis with secondary osteoarthritic changes.

c. Wound infection and breakdown; loosening of components and instability.

Best of 5s answer

1. e.

Multiple choice answers

1. a. **True.**
   b. **False.** Movement is restricted by acute pain.
   c. **False.** 'Best-guess' antibiotics should be prescribed as soon as specimens have been taken for bacteriological examination.
   d. **True.** Thorough irrigation of the joint, often using the arthroscope, will reduce the infection.
   e. **False.** The knee and hip are the most common sites of acute septic arthritis.

Foot and ankle pain

EMI answers

EMI 1

Theme: Clinical presentation

1. A. A rupture of the Achilles tendon classically presents in this fashion in this age group.

2. H. Subluxation of the metatarsophalangeal joints produces clawing of the toes, which rub on the shoes. The prominent metatarsal heads are painful to walk on.

3. J. In hallux rigidus, dorsiflexion of the metatarsophalangeal joint is painful.

CRQ answers

CRQ 1

a. bruising

   swelling

   deformity

   fracture blisters

   The heel may be appear wider than normal when viewed from behind.

b. Antero-posterior and lateral radiographs of the foot and ankle with axial view of the heel if clinically suspect.

c. Talar shift.

d. CT scan.

e. Internal fixation with bone graft may be required to restore normal anatomy of the subtalar joint.

OSCE answers

OSCE 1

a. Bimalleolar fracture.

b. Supination, external rotation injury.

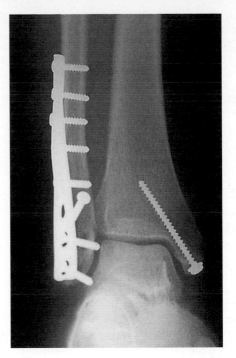

Figure 143

c. Open reduction and internal fixation using a lag screw or fully threaded cancellous screw in the medial malleolus and a third tubular neutralisation plate to control the length and position of the lateral malleolus (see Figure 143).

d. elevate the limb

   early active mobilisation

   no weight-bearing until the fracture is healed

OSCE 2

a. peripheral trophic changes

   changes in the skin

   loss of skin hair

   pale, thin, ulcerated skin

   frank gangrene

b. coronary artery occlusion

   vertebrobasilar insufficiency

   renal failure

c. The presence of diabetes mellitus.

d. thermography

   pressure studies

   skin pO_2 measurements

Best of 5s answer

1. b.

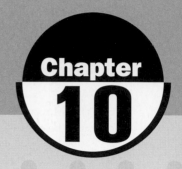

Back and neck pain

Chapter 10

Chapter overview

This chapter describes both cervical spine and lumbar spine problems and shows how the methods of differentiating mechanical pain from radicular pain due to nerve root compression are similar for both locations. The important diagnoses of cervical spinal cord compression and cauda equina compression are described. There is a brief description of spondylolisthesis, ankylosing spondylitis and spinal column problems caused by tumour or infection.

10.1 Clinical examination

Learning objectives

You should:
- be able to carry out a local examination of the cervical and lumbar spine looking for abnormalities and limited range of movement
- be able to carry out a neurological examination of the arms and legs to determine symptoms caused by dysfunction of any particular nerve root
- know the pattern of dermatome distribution in the limbs and which myotomes are associated with different movements.

Examination includes both a local examination of the axial skeleton and a neurological examination of the limbs.

Local examination

Cervical spine Observe any abnormal posture of the neck and the presence of muscle spasm. Localised tenderness can be elicited with one-finger palpation of the verte-bral spines. The full range of flexion, extension, lateral flexion and rotation should be attempted.

Lumbar spine The patient should be examined standing. The lumbar spine is observed from behind and from the sides for loss of the normal lumbar lordosis and the presence of paravertebral muscle spasm. The full range of spinal extension, flexion and lateral flexion and rotation should be elicited. Pain associated with spinal extension classically suggests facet joint or posterior column pathology, while pain associated with forward flexion suggests intervertebral disc or anterior column pathology. A patient with sciatica often shows a scoliosis to one side in an attempt to relieve traction on the compressed nerve root.

Neurological examination

Where there is compression of a nerve root in the neck (cervical radiculopathy) you may find muscle wasting, abnormal sensation in a dermatomal pattern, loss of reflexes or muscle weakness.

Similar findings may be present with nerve compression in the lumbar spine (sciatica) but, in addition, you should look for nerve root tension signs. To test the nerve roots of the sciatic nerve, the patient is placed supine and you lift the leg up with the knee straight until the patient complains of leg pain (not back pain). Flexion of the knee from this position relieves the pain and dorsiflexion of the ankle exacerbates it. A similar test for the roots of the femoral nerve is done by hip extension with the patient prone and the knee flexed. Some patients, sometimes those with abnormal pain behaviour, will resist the sciatic stretch test or make it difficult to interpret. It can be useful to lean the patient forward while their legs are straight in front or extend the knee when you test the reflexes with the patient seated. These both achieve stretch on the sciatic nerve roots. A rectal examination is mandatory when the history suggests central disc prolapse (10.3) to detect loss of voluntary anal contraction ('squeeze my finger') or loss of perianal sensation.

10.2 Mechanical back pain

Learning objectives

You should:
- know which features of the history and clinical examination indicate that symptoms are mechanical (arising in joints, muscles and ligaments) rather than neurogenic (due to nerve root involvement).

Backache is the cause of many lost hours from work and many visits to orthopaedic clinics. The vast majority will be due to mechanical backache and only a small minority will result from prolapse of an intervertebral disc or other specific abnormality.

Clinical features

Patients complain of acute or chronic back pain, which is exacerbated or relieved by certain movements or rest. It may radiate to the buttock or knee but not beyond. There may be an episode of lifting which the patient blames for their symptoms. There are no neurological deficits in the legs.

Diagnosis

Radiographs are not required unless you suspect a tumour or osteoporotic collapse. If done, they may show disc space narrowing or osteophytes but these features are also present in patients without back pain.

Management

Management of mechanical back pain involves:

* analgesics
* early return to normal activities and avoidance of bed rest
* reassurance that the pain is not a sign of spinal damage
* learning correct posture and lifting techniques.
* exercises – there is controversy about which ones work.

Surgery for back pain is usually inappropriate.

Complications

Patients' interpretation of their symptoms may be complicated by:

* functional overlay
* an outstanding claim for compensation.

10.3 Nerve root entrapment

Learning objectives

You should:
* be able to obtain an accurate history of nerve root compression and be able to deduce from this and subsequent examination which nerve root is affected
* describe the investigations used to detect a prolapsed intervertebral disc
* know how to differentiate this from bony nerve root entrapment and spondylolisthesis.

Prolapsed intervertebral disc

The lumbar disc is composed of the annulus fibrosus, which surrounds the nucleus pulposus. As the disc loses its water content as part of the degenerating process, the annulus fibrosus softens, allowing the nucleus pulposus to bulge posteriorly towards the spinal canal. Compression of a nerve root may result. Extruded fragments of degenerate disc may become lodged in a nerve root canal (Figure 144).

Clinical features

Patients complain of the local effects of pain in the back and of lower motor neuron symptoms in the legs.

* **Listen** – pain is more severe in the leg than the back and radiates to below the knee. In classical sciatica, pain is felt on the dorsum of the foot in the dermatome distribution of L5 or S1.
* **Look** – examination of the spine shows spasm in the paravertebral muscles, loss of lumbar lordosis and possibly scoliosis at the involved level.
* **Feel** – sensation may be diminished in the dermatomes supplied by the involved spinal nerves (Figure 145).

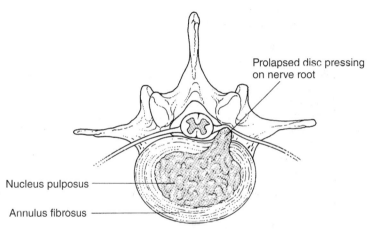

Figure 144 Pressure on a lumbar nerve root due to herniation of the nucleus pulposus through the annulus fibrosus of the intervertebral disc.

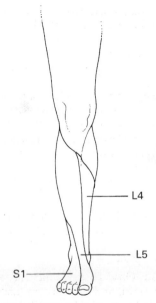

Figure 145 Dermatome distribution in the leg.

- **Move** – straight leg raising is diminished, tendon reflexes may be absent or depressed and power is weakened in the appropriate myotomes.

Patients with a central disc prolapse may develop urinary retention and a neurogenic bladder from compression of the sacral nerve roots of the cauda equina. Physical examination shows loss of anal tone and perianal anaesthesia.

Diagnosis

An MRI scan will show the nerve roots and the site of compression. L4/5 and L5/S1 are the most frequently affected levels for disc prolapse (Figure 146).

Management

Cauda equina lesions need emergency decompression if permanent bowel and bladder dysfunction are to be avoided.

In 80% of patients with sciatica, the pain will start to ease within 6 weeks. A caudal epidural injection of steroid and local anaesthetic may be used for temporary relief. Disc excision can be offered to those in whom conservative treatment fails.

Complications:

- persisting back pain
- interfacet joint degeneration
- arachnoiditis
- missed diagnosis of spinal tumour.

Other causes of nerve root entrapment

Two conditions must be considered:

- bony nerve root entrapment
- spinal stenosis.

Bony nerve root entrapment

In bony nerve root entrapment there is impingement of osteophytes on a spinal nerve root in the root canal (Figure 147).

Clinical features

Usually the patient is older than those with prolapsed intervertebral disc. There is pain in a dermatome distribution but, in addition, there is an ill-defined pain from osteoarthritic degeneration of the facet joints. Pain is usually less severe than with prolapsed intervertebral discs.

Diagnosis

An MRI is the most useful investigation for identifying the site of nerve root compression.

Management

Simple methods of local pain relief are used initially. In selected patients decompression of the nerve root canal may help.

Spinal stenosis

Even a mild degree of osteophytosis will cause impingement in the spinal canal if this is already narrow. In such patients, a minor degree of congestion in the spinal canal produces symptoms.

Clinical features

Exercise-induced pain in the buttocks and legs, especially when walking, gives rise to the description of symptoms as 'spinal claudication'. Symptoms are exacerbated by standing and extending the spine and relieved by sitting and flexing.

Diagnosis

A narrow spinal canal can be diagnosed from the MRI scan.

Management

Weight reduction and limitation of activities that involve extension of the spine may help. A multilevel decompression is required in some patients to decompress the spinal cord.

Complications:

- arachnoiditis
- missed diagnosis of spinal tumour
- spinal instability after laminectomy.

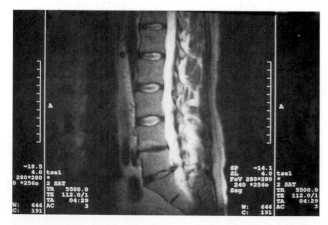

Figure 146 MRI scan showing posterior prolapse of the disc at L5/S1.

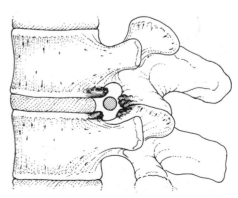

Figure 147 In bony nerve root entrapment the spinal nerve is compressed by osteophytosis from the adjacent joints.

10.4 Spondylolisthesis

This is a forward slip of one vertebra on the one below. It is most common at L4/5 and L5/S1. Minor degrees of spondylolysthesis are commonly seen as a result of degeneration of the facet joints but the more significant form is a result of a defect (spondylolysis) in the pars interarticularis in younger patients. This is the part of the vertebra between superior and inferior articular facets.

Clinical features

The patient is classically a young active person who complains of low back pain radiating to the buttocks. On examination, a step may be felt in the tender area at the base of the lumbar spine.

Diagnosis

Oblique radiographs are required and show either a lucent area in the pars interarticularis or a slip of one vertebrae on the other at this point (Figure 148).

Management

Rest during acute episodes, a spinal support and extension exercises may all help. A lumbo-sacral fusion is indicated for progressive slips.

Complications:
- persisting back pain
- nerve root impingement.

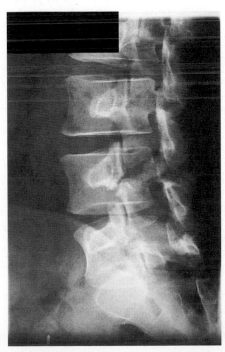

Figure 148 Oblique radiograph of a 20-year-old showing a spondylolysis at L4 but without any forward slip of the vertebrae.

10.5 Ankylosing spondylitis

This inflammatory disease is more common in men and tends to present in young adults.

Clinical features

There is stiffness in the lumbar spine and low back pain. There is often a positive family history. In severe cases, gross flexion and fusion of the entire spinal column is seen and chest wall expansion becomes limited. Other joints may also be involved.

Diagnosis

The ESR will be raised. Radiographs in patients presenting early may show loss of definition of the sacroiliac joints. Eventually the characteristic 'bamboo spine' develops (Figure 149).

Management

Non-steroidal anti-inflammatory agents can give symptomatic relief. Multidisciplinary management is best coordinated by a rheumatologist who may choose to use sulphasalazine or other disease-modifying drugs. The thoracic and cervical spine tend to fuse in flexion so the patient can only see the floor. Sometimes an extension osteotomy of the cervical spine is done to allow the patient to look forwards.

Complications:
- quadriplegia either from falling onto the face fracturing the rigid cervical spine or from surgery
- colitis
- uveitis.

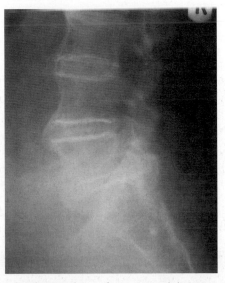

Figure 149 Calcification of the soft tissues in ankylosing spondylosis producing the characteristic 'bamboo spine'.

Ten

10.6 Tumour and infection

Tumours

The spine is a common site of bony metastasis. The most common tumours to metastasise to bone are:

- breast
- bronchus
- prostate
- bowel
- kidney.

Multiple myeloma and lymphoma are the most common primary tumours but primary tumours of bone or neuro-developmental tissue may occur. Occasionally, primary spinal canal tumours such as neurofibroma and meningioma are encountered.

Clinical features ('Red Flag Signs')

Patients typically present with back pain which gets progressively worse over time and has no exacerbating or relieving factors (non-mechanical pain). Progressively deteriorating neurological function is very suggestive when present but not necessary for the diagnosis. Tumour should be positively excluded in patients presenting with back pain for the first time over the age of 55 and also in children. Tumour should be considered when patients present with thoracic back pain.

Diagnosis

Plain radiographs may show lytic or sclerotic lesions, typically starting in the pedicle but are not sensitive enough to pick up all tumours. An MRI scan is necessary to definitively exclude tumour in the bone or spinal canal. An isotope bone scan will be positive for most tumours but not for myeloma. A monoclonal band on serum electrophoresis and Bence Jones proteins in the urine are diagnostic for multiple myeloma.

Management

This depends on tumour type. Some are amenable to chemotherapy, hormone manipulation or radiotherapy. Surgery to decompress the spinal cord and stabilise the spine is sometimes of benefit. Benign intraspinal tumours can be excised.

Complications:

- vertebral collapse
- nerve root invasion
- spinal cord compression resulting in paraplegia.

Infection

Patients with acute infective discitis are usually children or are immunosuppressed. Blood-borne infection may involve the disc and an adjacent vertebra. Tuberculous discitis presents more insidiously.

Clinical features

Back pain is typically severe and unrelenting but pyrexia may be absent. ESR and CRP are elevated, but leucocytosis may be absent.

Diagnosis

MRI scan will reveal the diagnosis and show whether an abscess is present. An isotope bone scan will show a 'hot spot' in the affected bone or in the bone adjacent to the infected disc. CT-guided aspiration is not normally done for uncomplicated discitis but can be useful when there is an abscess or when the patient fails to respond to empirical treatment.

Management

High doses of 'best-guess' antibiotics agreed with the local microbiologist. Clindamycin is often used.

Complications:

- kyphosis
- spinal cord compression.

10.7 Cervical spondylosis

Cervical spondylosis is the name given to chronic degeneration of the cervical spine involving the intervertebral discs and the ligamentous and osseous structures associated with them. It can be responsible for a spectrum of problems ranging from mechanical neck pain to cervical cord compression.

Figure 150 shows the normal anatomical relationship between the intervertebral foramen and the two adjacent vertebral bodies. The intervertebral disc lies anteriorly and the facet joint posteriorly. The emerging nerve root is shown end-on.

Figure 151 shows how degeneration of the cervical disc and the associated osteophyte formation around the vertebral end-plates can press on the nerve roots and on the spinal cord itself. With increasing age, the intervertebral disc loses its water content and shrinks. In doing so, its height decreases and movement at the interfacet joints is altered. Osteoarthritic degeneration of these joints can then occur (Figure 152).

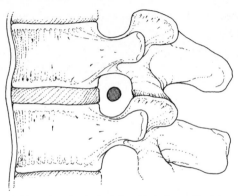

Figure 150 Normal anatomical relationship between the intervertebral foramen and the two adjacent vertebral bodies. The nerve root exits through the intervertebral foramen.

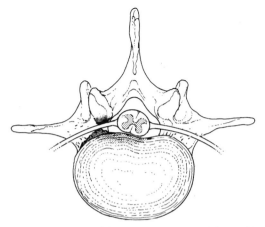

Figure 151 Compression of the spinal nerve root and the cord itself following cervical disc degeneration and associated osteophytosis of the adjacent joints.

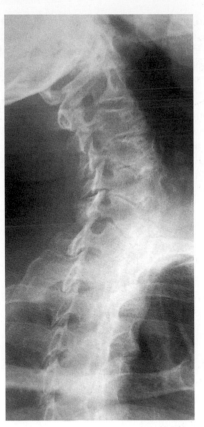

Figure 152 Oblique view of the cervical spine showing osteophytes narrowing the intervertebral foramen at C5/6 especially.

Radiological evidence of degeneration of the cervical discs is seen in 50% of the population over the age of 50 and 75% of the population over the age of 65. However, this may be an incidental finding and the patient may have no symptoms. However, if the spinal canal measures less than 13 mm on CT scan, its contents are more at risk from compression and symptoms will ensue.

Acute cervical disc prolapse is uncommon (unlike lumbar disc prolapse). Severe trauma to the cervical spine is necessary to produce this injury. When it occurs, it is usually in young patients. More commonly, cervical disc herniation is an acute-on-chronic phenomenon seen in older patients.

The following syndromes are associated with cervical spondylosis:

- mechanical neck pain
- radiculopathy
- myelopathy.

Mechanical neck pain

This is the most common presentation of cervical spondylosis.

Clinical features:
- **Listen** – neck pain and associated muscle spasm originating from facet joint degeneration radiate to the occiput and shoulders but there is no pain radiating down the arms. Symptoms are worse with activity and in the morning.
- **Look** – the neck may be held to one side.
- **Feel** – localised tenderness in the paravertebral muscles.
- **Move** – there is only slightly decreased range of movement in the cervical spine because 50% of rotation takes place at the atlanto-axial joint, which is not usually affected.

Management
The majority of patients respond to simple treatment.

A cervical collar may give temporary symptomatic relief but should be avoided as dependence on the collar rapidly develops. Symptomatic treatment with analgesics followed by exercise are used and the symptoms will settle in the majority of patients.

Radiculopathy
Clinical features
Radiculopathy is the name given to the symptoms produced when a nerve root is compressed by or stretched around an osteophyte or prolapsed intervertebral disc.

233

The settling down of one facet joint on another following shrinking of the intervertebral disc causes narrowing of the intervertebral foramen, which also contributes to compression on the nerve root. Patients complain of lower motor neuron symptoms in the arms.

- **Listen** – patients complain of pain in a dermatome distribution in the arm (brachalgia) (Figure 153).
- **Look** – wasting of the muscles in the myotome involved.
- **Feel** – there may also be decreased sensation in the appropriate dermatome.

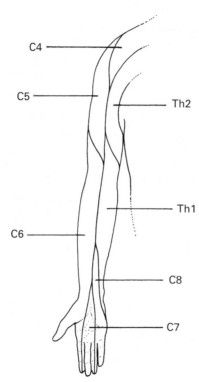

Figure 153 Pattern of dermatomes in the upper limb.

- **Move** – muscle weakness and depressed tendon reflexes.

Diagnosis
MRI scan will confirm the diagnosis but is usually only done to confirm the level of the affected nerve root when surgery is contemplated.

Management
Conservative:
- analgesics
- tricyclic antidepressants such as amitryptiline can be useful for any nerve mediated pain.

Surgical When conservative measures fail, decompression of the compressed nerve root by excising the adjacent osteophytes (see below) can be carried out electively.

Myelopathy

Clinical features
Pressure from a protruding cervical disc or the associated osteophytes may cause pressure on the spinal cord itself. This is present when patients exhibit upper motor neuron signs in the legs and lower motor neuron signs in the arms. Patients complain of the insidious onset of weakness, clumsiness and dysaesthesia in the hand; they may develop difficulty in walking because of spasticity and weakness of the lower limbs, and retention of urine due to a neurogenic bladder.

Diagnosis
MRI.

Management
Surgical decompression is urgently required for patients who develop symptoms of cervical cord compression. In the classic operation of anterior cervical decompression, a core of vertebral body and intervertebral disc is drilled out and prolapsed material removed. Osteophytes can be trimmed through the same approach to decompress the spinal cord and the nerve root canal.

Self-assessment: questions

Extended matching items questions (EMIs)

EMI 1

Theme: Pathology

A. S1 nerve root entrapment

B. spondylolisthesis

C. central cord compression

D. T1 root entrapment

E. C 5/6 root entrapment

F. L3 root compression on the left

G. infection in the L4/5 disc

H. spinal tumour

I. cauda equina lesion

J. L3 root compression on the right side

Match the clinical presentations below to the most appropriate pathology listed above:

1. Neck pain and wasting of the interossei muscles in the hand.

2. Depressed right knee-jerk reflex and weakness of knee extension.

3. Pain shooting from the back down the side of the leg to the lateral side of the foot.

4. Back pain in a 60-year-old without radiation associated with pyrexia, high white cell count and 'hot spot' on bone scan.

5. Bilateral leg pain with back pain and urinary retention.

6. Loss of ankle jerk on examination.

EMI 2

Theme: Back pain

A. metastatic tumour

B. mechanical back pain

C. prolapsed intervertebral disc

D. spinal stenosis

E. spondylolysthesis

F. scoliosis

G. osteoporosis

Match the following patients with the most likely diagnosis. Each option may be used once, more than once or not at all.

1. A 14-year-old girl with intermittent back pain which is worse on spinal extension and exacerbated by sports.

2. A 45-year-old man with a few weeks of intermittent back pain.

3. An 80-year-old woman with constant, thoracic back pain and 2 stones' weight loss in the last 6 months.

4. A 60-year-old lady with sudden onset back pain after falling onto her bottom and a past history of fractures to distal radius and proximal humerus.

5. A 30-year-old man with lancinating pain down the left leg to below the knee after a day digging the garden.

Constructed response questions (CRQs)

CRQ 1

A 58-year-old man consults you complaining of a 4-week history of pain in the back of his neck experienced down the outside of the same arm into the hand, thumb and index fingers.

a. What dermatome distribution is being described?

b. What physical finding would you expect to find on examining this area?

c. You continue your examination of myotomes. Which movement would you expect to be weak?

d. You proceed to examination of the reflexes. Which reflex would you expect to be diminished?

e. You decide to radiograph the patient's neck. What views would you ask for and why?

CRQ 2

A 40-year-old offshore worker injures his back while lifting heavy weights. He is seen by the medic on the oil rig and a diagnosis of mechanical back pain is made. There are no neurological symptoms.

a. What would be the appropriate management at this stage?

b. He subsequently arrives home and attends your surgery. What would you expect to find when you examine his back?

c. In addition he tells you that there is now pain radiating down the legs to the heel and lateral sides of both feet. Which dermatome is he describing?

d. What is the significance of this bilateral symptom?

e. What else must you examine or ask at this stage?

f. What is the emergency management of this?

Objective structured clinical examination questions (OSCEs)

OSCE 1

Study the diagram of a prolapsed lumbar invertebral disc (Figure 154).

a. Name the portions indicated by the lines.

b. What investigation could be used to show the lesion like this?

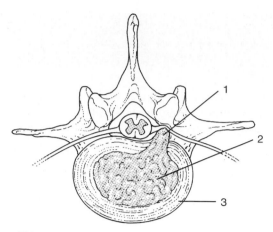

Figure 154

c. What is the route of approach for decompression and excision of the prolapsed disc?

OSCE 2

A 70-year-old patient complains of low back pain which has been going on for some time but has been more intense for the last 2 weeks. Plain radiographs show minor degenerative changes only (Figure 155).

a. What is the main finding on the bone scan?

b. What three possible conditions could cause this finding?

c. The patient also complains of urinary outflow obstruction. Blood tests reveal an elevated prostatic specific antigen. What is the most likely diagnosis now?

d. How would you confirm this?

Best of 5s questions

1. A 57-year-old lady presents with 2 weeks of lacerating pain down the right arm and an absent triceps jerk. She has a long history of neck pain and stiffness. The most likely diagnosis is:
   a. spinal malignanacy
   b. C5 radiculopathy
   c. brachial plexus lesion
   d. myelopathy
   e. encroachment on the C7 exit foramen

2. A 56-year-old lady on long-term prednisolone for severe asthma presents with acute low back pain. Which of the following is never appropriate?
   a. plain radiograph of the lumbar spine
   b. DXA scan
   c. serum protein electrophoresis
   d. referral to physiotherapy without investigation
   e. isotope bone scan

Multiple choice questions

1. In a 40-year-old patient with a prolapsed intervertebral disc affecting S1 root, the

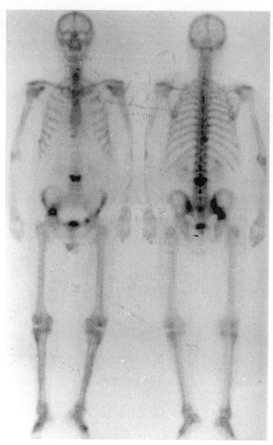

Figure 155 Bone scan of a 70-year-old man with lower back pain. (Courtesy of Dr N. Kennedy, Nuclear Medicine Unit, Ninewells Hospital and Medical School, Dundee.)

following signs and symptoms are classically found:
   a. limited straight leg raising in the affected leg
   b. absent knee jerk
   c. absent ankle jerk
   d. weakness of extensor hallucis longus
   e. weakness of plantar flexion of the ankle

2. In cervical spondylosis:
   a. the majority of patients respond to conservative treatment
   b. pressure on a cervical nerve root causes upper motor neuron signs to be present in the arms
   c. assessment of the lower motor neuron deficits helps to identify the level of the cervical lesion
   d. wasting of the interossei muscles in the hand suggests a C5/6 disc prolapse
   e. unlike a prolapsed lumbar intervertebral disc, a prolapsed cervical disc does not merit surgical intervention

Self-assessment: answers

EMI answers

EMI 1

Theme: Pathology

1. D. The first thoracic nerve root controls the interossei. Wasting of these muscles is eventually seen in T1 root entrapment.

2. J. The knee jerk reflex and knee extension are both usually innervated by the third lumbar spinal nerve root.

3. A. The first sacral nerve root dermatome extends in this distribution.

4. G. A septic discitis will produce reactive hyperaemia in the adjacent vertebral body, which will show as an area of increased isotope uptake on the bone scan.

5. I. A central disc prolapse at the L5/S1 level may cause cauda equina compression and a neurogenic bladder. Bilateral S1 dermatome signs are a warning feature.

6. A. The ankle jerk reflex is controlled by the first sacral nerve root.

EMI 2

Theme: Back pain

1. E.
2. B.
3. A.
4. G.
5. C.

CRQ answers

CRQ 1

a. C6.

b. Diminished touch sensation.

c. Wrist dorsi flexion and elbow flexion.

d. Supinator reflex.

e. An oblique view of the cervical spine gives the clearest view of the intervertebral (neural) foramena. Osteophyte formation here will show as a 'figure-of-eight' deformity indicating that there is nerve root compression.

CRQ 2

a. Early return to normal activities. Rest from heavy work, and analgesia until symptoms subside.

b. muscle spasm

   scoliosis

   paravertebral tenderness

   restriction of lumbar spine movement

c. S1.

d. It suggests central disc prolapse causing cauda equina compression.

e. The patient may have altered perineal sensation and urinary retention.

f. urinary catheterisation

   emergency MRI scan

   neurosurgery to decompress the nerve roots and cauda equina

OSCE answers

OSCE 1

a. 1. Prolapsing disc.
   2. Nucleus pulposus.
   3. Annulus fibrosus.

b. MRI scan.

c. Fenestration of the lamina to again access for excision of the prolapsed disc.

OSCE 2

a. Increased uptake of radioactive technitium in the third lumbar vertebra.

b. vertebral body crush fracture

   vertebral body or disc infection

   secondary deposit in a vertebral body

c. Secondary deposit from prostatic carcinoma.

d. Core biopsy from the lesion under radiograph control to get a histological diagnosis.

Best of 5s answers

1. e.
2. d.

Multiple choice answers

1. a. **True.** Symptoms from S1 nerve root compression are exacerbated by traction on the nerve to which this root contributes. Stretching the sciatic nerve by flexing the hip with the knee fully extended, therefore, exacerbates the symptoms.

   b. **False.** The knee jerk is supplied by nerve roots L3 and 4. The ankle jerk is supplied by S1.

   c. **True.** The ankle jerk is absent as it is supplied by S1.

   d. **False.** Extensor hallucis longus is supplied by L5 and is, therefore, functioning.

e. **True.** Plantar flexion of the ankle is controlled by S1 and is, therefore, weak.

2. a. **True.** In most patients, simple analgesics, heat, rest and sometimes longitudinal traction will relieve symptoms of cervical spondylosis.

b. **False.** Pressure on a nerve root produces lower motor neuron signs, but if the cervical cord is compressed in the spondylitic process then upper motor neuron signs may be present in the lower limbs.

c. **True.** The pain and paraesthesia in a particular dermatome will help to elicit the level of the cervical nerve root compression. The neurological level can be confirmed by looking for weakness or loss of tendon reflexes in the appropriate myotome.

d. **False.** The interossei muscles are supplied by the T1 root and are, therefore, weak or wasted when the compression is at this level.

e. **False.** Surgical decompression at the appropriate level is required in the presence of unremitting pain, progressive motor weakness or evidence of cord compression.

Children's complaints

The limping child

Chapter part overview

A limping child is a common presentation both in general practice and in the emergency room. The source of the limp will often be the hip but not always. Remember to consider unwitnessed trauma and non-accidental injury.

11.1 Clinical examination

Learning objectives

You should:
- know which conditions to suspect in different age groups
- know how to differentiate transient synovitis from septic arthritis
- know when to suspect a child might have a bone or soft tissue tumour

Clinical examination in children aims to get the same information as in adults but rushing in to touch a painful area or move a painful limb will result in an uncooperative child and no information. Find out as much as you can by watching the child in the play area and commence the examination on a parent's knee rather than the examination couch. Observe the child standing, lying and walking. Assess leg lengths and examine each joint in turn. Examination of the hips while prone is the easiest way to detect rotational joint restriction at the hip and will also show if a torsional deformity is above or below the knee.

11.2 Developmental dysplasia of the hip

Developmental dysplasia of the hip (DDH) covers a spectrum of disease from a shallow acetabulum with a located hip through to a complete dislocation. Clinically significant DDH affects between 1 and 2 per 1000 babies. Risk factors are:

- positive family history in a parent or sibling
- breech presentation
- foot deformity
- white or native American race
- female gender.

Clinical features:
- **Listen** – for risk factors. An older child will present with a limp ever since they started walking. Walking age is not delayed.
- **Look** – limp with externally rotated, short leg. Bilateral cases will present with a waddling gait There may be asymmetrical joint creases.
- **Feel and move** – there is restricted abduction when the hips are in 90° of flexion. The hip may be felt to 'clunk' back into joint as the hips are further abducted while the index finger exerts forward pressure over the greater trochanter (positive Ortolani test). Backwards pressure with the hips adducted and flexed reveals loss of resistance on the affected side and dislocates a reduced but dislocatable hip (Barlow manoeuvre). The Ortolani test can then be done as before. Figure 156 demonstrates the Barlow manoeuvre followed by a positive Ortolani test. The 'clunk' of the Ortolani test is quite different from the high-pitched soft tissue clicks which are common in neonates.

Diagnosis
The Ortolani and Barlow tests will only be positive in the neonate. The diagnosis can be confirmed on ultrasound and many centres use this as a screening test. Over the age

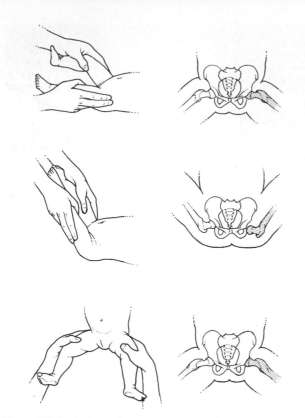

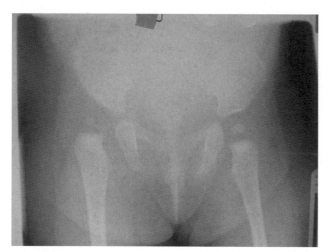

Figure 156 Ortolani's test (see text for description).

Figure 157 Late presenting developmental dysplasia of the right hip in a 6-month-old girl.

of 6 months, radiographs can be used as the capital femoral epiphysis will have appeared (Figure 157).

Management
Treatment is easier the earlier the condition is diagnosed. Up to 6 months of age, splintage in abduction and flexion with the hip reduced can result in satisfactory remodelling of the acetabulum (Figure 158). Above this age a formal closed or open reduction under anaesthesia followed by several months in cast are required. If these measures fail, or in children presenting even older, osteotomies of the

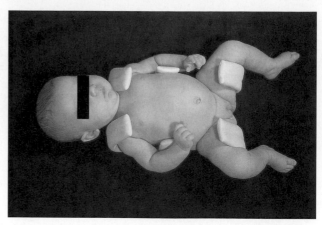

Figure 158 A von Rosen splint used to keep the dislocated hip in the reduced position.

femur and/or acetabulum may be required and the chance of a satisfactory result is reduced.

Complications:
- osteoarthritis in early adulthood
- avascular necrosis as a result of splintage or surgery.

11.3 Infection

Learning objectives

You should:
- be able to recognise the clinical features of infection in a bone or joint
- know how to begin appropriate urgent treatment.

Acute osteitis and septic arthritis are not as common as they once were but can still cause devastating complications. *Staphylococcus aureus* is the most common infecting organism but others, including salmonella, can cause the disease. *Haemophilus influenzae* used to be a common cause but is much rarer since a vaccine was developed.

Clinical features:
- **Listen** – pain or a limp lasting hours or days. The child will be off his or her food and will have lost interest in play.
- **Look** – the child will be listless and reluctant to move, and with septic arthritis will be unable to bear weight.
- **Feel** – a hot, swollen, tender joint or bone.
- **Move** – in septic arthritis, the child will not allow joint movement and will scream in pain. In osteitis, the signs may be less marked.

Diagnosis
The four cardinal signs of septic arthritis are

- inability to bear weight
- fever >38°C
- ESR >40 mm/h
- white cell count (WCC) >12 × 10^9/l

ESR, CRP and WCC will also be raised in osteitis. Radiographs are normal in both initially but will eventually show joint destruction in septic arthritis and periosteal elevation with islands of dead, infected bone (sequestrum) in osteitis. Blood cultures may be positive.

Management

Septic arthritis is treated with aspiration of the joint, usually under anaesthetic, followed by large doses of 'best-guess' antibiotics, modified once culture results are available. If the history is greater than 24 h or is uncertain, as is often the case in babies under 1 year, open washout of the joint is indicated. Osteitis is treated with large doses of best-guess antibiotics, modified if the results of blood culture indicate. If a sequestrum or an abscess develops, or if the child is getting worse despite antibiotics, then surgical debridement is indicated.

Complications:
- joint destruction
- chronic osteitis
- growth arrest.

11.4 Transient synovitis

This is a form of self-limiting reactive arthritis of the hip. It is sometimes associated with an upper respiratory infection. It can be differentiated from septic arthritis as the child is not unwell and, although they may limp, they can usually bear weight. Some cases are equivocal and require a period of observation and measurement of the CRP, ESR and WCC to distinguish them from early septic arthritis. The condition eases within a few days although the limp may persist for a few weeks. Non-steroidal anti-inflammatories may help but no specific treatment is required. If symptoms persist, Perthes' disease should be suspected.

Management

After a short period of bed rest, the child's symptoms usually settle. There are no long-term complications but the child may have another episode in the future.

11.5 Osteochondritis

Osteochondritis is caused by interruption of the blood supply to an area of bone. It has many eponymous names depending on the anatomical site.

Perthes' disease

This usually presents with weeks to months of limping in a child between the ages of 3 and 12. It is an osteochondritis of the capital femoral epiphysis. The prognosis worsens with age of onset and it takes many months to years before the femoral head regains its blood supply and heals.

Diagnosis

Hip movement will be restricted, particularly in internal rotation and abduction. Radiographs can be normal initially but after a few months will show sclerosis and collapse of the capital femoral epiphysis (Figure 159).

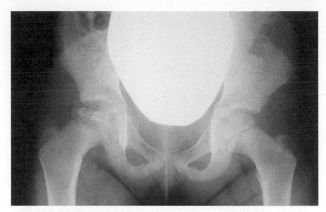

Figure 159 Perthes' disease of the right hip compared with the opposite normal side. The capital epiphysis is flattened, sclerotic and fragmented.

Management

Milder cases in younger children can be managed non-operatively. It is traditional to limit activities but it is doubtful how much this is possible in young children. Older children at risk of serious femoral head deformation are treated by containing the affected part of the head within the acetabulum. This can be achieved with abduction plasters but it is more common to perform a femoral or acetabular osteotomy.

Other sites of osteochondritis

Osteochondritis dissecans In the knee the lateral side of the medial femoral condyle is the usual site for an area of avascularity to develop. An island of bone demarcates and eventually may separate and become a loose body in the joint causing intermittent locking and pain.

Traction apopyhysitis Osgood–Schlatter's disease is a common example of a traction apophysitis. Idiopathic aseptic necrosis of the tibial tuberosity causes knee pain in adolescence, which is usually exacerbated by vigorous activity. The tibial tuberosity is elevated and tender. Radiographs show elevation, sclerosis and fragmentation of the tuberosity and, in older patients, a fragment of bone is sometimes seen in the patellar tendon. Management consists of avoiding sports when symptoms are severe. Sometimes a splint or plaster cylinder is used to enforce this (Figure 160).

Kienbock's disease This condition presents in young adults with pain and stiffness of the wrist caused by avascular fragmentation and collapse of the lunate. Radiographs show increased density.

11.6 Slipped upper femoral epiphysis

This is another diagnosis not to miss as the treatment of early small slips gives a much better result than that in large ones. The condition is a pathological fracture through the capital femoral physis. The typical patient is an overweight adolescent but the condition can present in children as young as 8, especially if they have Down syndrome or an endocrine disorder. Presentation may be acute, after an injury, or chronic and insidious. There are stable forms

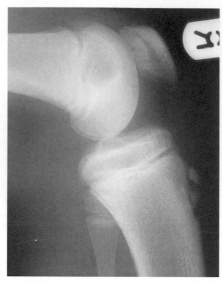

Figure 160 Osgood–Schlatter's disease. The tibial tuberosity is elevated, sclerotic and fragmented.

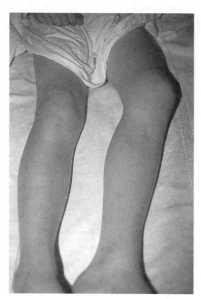

Figure 161 This 15-year-old presented with sudden pain in the left hip after a sporting event; the leg is externally rotated and shortened.

in which the child can walk and unstable ones in which they cannot.

Clinical features:
- **Listen** – pain is often referred to the knee.
- **Look** – the leg is externally rotated and appears short (Figure 161).
- **Feel** – local tenderness.
- **Move** – pain on attempted hip rotation.

Diagnosis
The diagnosis may not be obvious on antero-posterior radiographs; a frog lateral (antero-posterior of the pelvis with both hips in external rotation) is required (Figure 162).

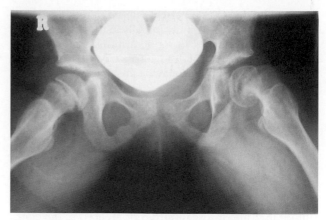

Figure 162 The radiograph of the pelvis shows that the capital epiphysis has slipped off the femoral neck on the left side. On the right side there is a suggestion of an early slip.

Management
Manipulation of the slipped epiphysis runs the risk of causing avascular necrosis of the head. Pinning of the capital epiphysis in the slipped position is, therefore, favoured. In cases of severe slip, an intertrochanteric oste-otomy can be performed later to correct the varus of the femoral neck. Some surgeons advocate prophylactic pinning of the opposite side as sequential slips are common.

Complications:
- avascular necrosis
- chondrolysis
- contralateral slip
- late osteoarthritis.

11.7 Tumour

Primary bone tumours are not confined to childhood but are commonest in the second and third decades of life. They may be benign or malignant. Clinical presentation is with a mass which is often painful in malignant tumours. Malignant tumours can clinically look like infection and a radiograph is wise if an infection in a limb is not reacting to antibiotics as expected. Benign cysts and cartilage tumours can present with pathological fracture.

Childhood deformity

Chapter part overview

The appearance of a child's body or the way they walk is a common cause of parental concern but many of the apparent abnormalities are either developmental phases or variants of normal. Splints and insoles were often inappropriately used in the past for these conditions, which does not help in con-vincing parents that their child is normal. Others conditions, such as club foot and scoliosis of the spine, may need orthotic or surgical treatment.

11.8 Normal variants

Eleven

Learning objectives

You should:
* know the spectrum of normal appearance in children at different ages.

In-toeing Parents complain that a toddler's feet point inwards and that they are always falling. Examination shows that it is the femur which is internally rotated and the child may be found to have lax ligaments. It is the lax ligaments which cause the child to fall as they send less proprioceptive information to the brain. This improves in later childhood. The in-toeing may also improve towards the age of 12 but is no handicap if it does not.

Knock-knee Normal physiological development of the lower limbs shows a progression from genu varus in the first 2 years of life through normal alignment at the age of 3 to genu valgus with a characteristic gap between the malleoli at the age of 4 (Figure 163).

Flat feet A combination of lax ligaments and a podgy foot leads to the apparent loss of the medial arch on standing. As long as the arch reappears on tiptoe or on dorsiflexing the first metatarsophalangeal joint, there is no need to worry. Occasionally, the foot is painful and an insole can help. An older child may present with a flat foot that does not correct in tiptoeing. These children may have a tarsal coalition, an abnormal connection between the calcaneum and the talus or navicular, which can be treated surgically.

11.9 Talipes equinovarus

Learning objectives

You should:
* be able to distinguish positional talipes equinovarus (TEV) from fixed TEV
* know what to tell the parents about the eventual outcome.

Clinical features

True (fixed) talipes equinovarus (TEV) is a condition which is present at birth and results in a foot which is pointed down (equinus) and then folded in medially on itself (varus and adductus) (Figure 164). At least some of the affected children have an underlying abnormality of the peripheral nerves but the exact cause remains uncertain. A similar appearance can be caused by compression of the foot in the later stages of pregnancy. This is called positional talipes equinovarus. The two are distinguished by the fact that the positional deformity can easily be manually corrected whereas the fixed deformity cannot. A similar positional deformity results in the foot being held dorsiflexed and everted (talipes calcaneovalgus).

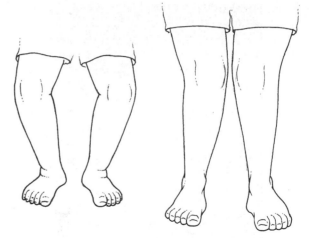

Figure 163 During the first years of life, a child's knees change from a genu varus position through normal alignment to a genu valgus position by the age of 4 years.

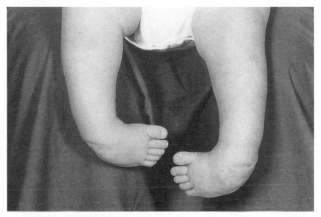

Figure 164 Bilateral talipes equinovarus.

Diagnosis

Radiographs are not useful as most of the calcaneum and talus are cartilaginous at birth. Clinical examination should be thorough enough to exclude spina bifida, congenital absence of the sacrum and arthrogryposis (a congenital condition with contractures in many joints), all of which can cause foot deformities similar to TEV.

Management

Initial management consists of using plaster casts to progressively correct the deformity over a couple of months. Sometimes, it is necessary to cut the Achilles tendon under local anaesthetic but at this age it reconstitutes well. Once the correct position is achieved, it is held at night in a splint until the child is about 4 years old. In some babies, this treatment cannot correct the deformity; in others, it recurs, and a second round of casts is unsuccessful. These babies need a surgical procedure to correct the deformity. Parents should be warned at the beginning that the calf on the affected side will always be thinner and the foot shorter by up to a couple of shoe sizes. Children with corrected club foot can walk and run with their peers but will not be of a competitive standard in sport.

Complications:
- recurrence
- short foot
- thin calf
- stiffness (usually only after surgery)
- overcorrection after surgery.

11.10 Scoliosis

Learning objectives

You should:
- be able to describe the different types of scoliosis.
- know the principles of radiological monitoring of a spinal curve.

Scoliosis is a twisting deformity of the spine in three dimensions, although it is simpler to visualise as a C- or S-shaped curve on an antero-posterior radiograph. There are idiopathic forms which are due to differential growth on opposite sides of the spine, neuromuscular ones secondary to weakness of the supporting muscles and rare congenital ones due to an absent or extra half-vertebra.

Clinical features
The cosmetic deformity is usually noticed by a parent or gym teacher. There may be back pain but this does not correlate well with the degree of deformity. The commonest idiopathic form occurs in teenagers but younger children tend to run into more severe problems because of the large amount of growth which is left and the capacity for damage to the immature lungs.

Diagnosis
Radiology confirms the diagnosis by showing the presence of rotated vertebrae. The degree of curve is classically measured as the angle between the end plates of the normal vertebrae above and below the abnormal section (Cobb angle) (Figure 165).

Management
The common adolescent idiopathic form is usually just observed or treated with an orthosis, depending upon its severity. If the deformity is progressing rapidly or reaches a Cobb angle of 40°, then surgery is considered to fuse

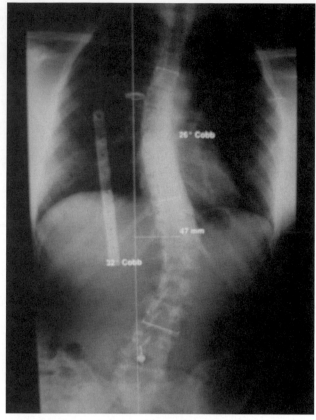

Figure 165 Adolescent idiopathic thoracic scoliosis with major thoracolumbar curve (apex L1, Cobb angle 32°) and minor thoracic curve (apex T8, Cobb angle 26°).

sections of the spine and support them with metal rods. Neuromuscular scoliosis inevitably progresses and surgery needs to be performed before respiratory function is compromised.

Complications:
- curve progression
- respiratory compromise in infants or neuromuscular patients.

Complications of surgery:
- death
- paraplegia
- incomplete correction
- implant failure.

Self-assessment: questions

Extended matching items questions (EMIs)

EMI 1

Theme: Diagnosis

A. Osgood–Schlatter's disease

B. osteochondritis dissecans

C. developmental dysplasia of the hip

D. transient synovitis

E. Perthes' disease

F. bow legs

G. flat feet

H. knock-knee (genu valgum)

I. in-toeing

J. infective arthritis

Which diagnosis from the list above is most likely to be indicated by the clinical findings below?

1. Intermalleoli distance of 20 cm in a 4-year-old.

2. Upper respiratory infection followed by pain and resistance to internal rotation of the hip.

3. Pain around the knee in an adolescent made worse by football.

4. Intermittent pain and locking of the joint during normal knee movement in an adolescent.

5. Asymmetrical buttock creases and a block to full hip abduction in a 6-month-old baby.

EMI 2

Theme: The limping child

A. malignant primary bone tumour

B. Perthes' disease

C. septic arthritis

D. developmental dysplasia of the hip

E. Osgood–Schlatter's disease

F. slipped upper femoral epiphysis

Match the following presentations with the most likely diagnosis. Each option may be used once, more than once or not at all.

1. An overweight 13-year-old boy with a limp for 3 weeks.

2. A 14-year-old boy with a warm, hard mass just above the knee.

3. A 2-year-old girl who has been limping since she started walking.

4. A 6-year-old boy with a limp for 2 months.

5. A newborn child whose mum had to wear a harness when she was born.

6. A 3-year-old girl with a swollen knee who has a fever and can't walk.

Constructed response questions (CRQs)

CRQ 1

A teenage sportsman complains of pain in his left knee which has been getting worse since training. He had a similar episode last year but this has been getting worse now for 3 weeks and is causing limping. He has localised tenderness at the tibial tuberosity but no swelling or hotness.

a. What is the most likely diagnosis?

b. Of what group of conditions is this an example?

c. What radiological findings are associated with this condition?

d. What is the initial treatment?

e. How can this be enforced?

CRQ 2

An athletic 12-year-old boy presents after school sports with an injury to his hip following a high jump. You suspect a slipped upper femoral epiphysis.

a. What would you expect to find on physical examination of the hip?

b. What radiograph view would you request?

c. You decide to suggest surgery. What two methods of treatment are appropriate depending on the degree of severity?

d. What are the complications of aggressive manipulation?

e. Why might a radiograph of the pelvis showing both hips be relevant in this case?

Objective structured clinical examination questions (OSCEs)

OSCE 1

Study the clinical photograph of a 2-year-old child (see Figure 166).

a. What abnormality of posture can you see?

b. What manoeuvre would you ask the child to carry out while you observe the feet and what would you expect to find in the majority of cases?

c. What is contributing to the appearance of the foot?

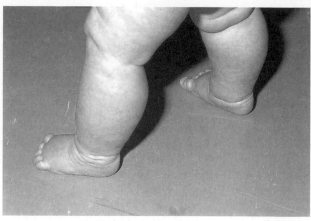

Figure 166 Feet of a 2-year-old child.

d. The parents are concerned that the child's shoes are wearing down quickly on the medial side. What could you suggest to help?

Best of 5s questions

1. Which of the following statements about bone and joint infection is true?
   a. tuberculous osteitis is not seen in Caucasians resident in the UK
   b. septic arthritis in children can be treated with joint aspiration and antibiotics
   c. septic arthritis in adults is best treated with antibiotics alone

d. a normal plain radiograph excludes the diagnosis of acute osteitis
   e. a WCC of $11.0 \times 10^9/l$ is one of the cardinal signs of septic arthritis

2. A 10-year-old child presents with a long-standing flat foot deformity which persists on tiptoeing. The most appropriate next step is:
   a. reassurance that all is well
   b. admission for emergency joint washout
   c. DXA scan
   d. plain radiographs of the foot
   e. steroid injection

Multiple choice questions

1. The following are possible sequelae of acute osteitis:
   a. Looser's zones found on radiograph
   b. sequestrum formation
   c. septic arthritis
   d. fracture of the affected bone
   e. myositis ossificans

2. A boy aged 12 presents with pain and a limp in the right leg of 2 months' duration. Likely diagnosis includes:
   a. late presentation of congenital dislocated hip
   b. transient synovitis of the hip
   c. Perthes' disease
   d. acute septic arthritis
   e. slipped femoral epiphysis

Self-assessment: answers

The limping child

EMI answers

EMI 1

Theme: Diagnoses

1. H. Knock-knee (genu valgum) is common in children around the age of 4 years until it gradually corrects with growth.

2. D. Transient synovitis (irritable hip) may occur following an intercurrent infection. It causes a reactive joint effusion in the hip. The capacity of the hip joint is greatest in external rotation. Internal rotation tightens the joint capsule, compresses the joint fluid and increases pain.

3. A. Osgood–Schlatter's disease is a traction apophysitis of the tibial tuberosity. The bone in this growing area is partially avulsed by the patellar tendon so is more painful during resisted knee extension movements.

4. B. Osteochondritis dissecans is characterised by separation of a portion of the intra-articular surface of the knee. The loose body formed causes mechanical locking of the knee by intermittently jamming between the joint surfaces during movement.

5. C. A dislocated hip in a baby causes a block to full abduction in flexion. It may subsequently reduce with a 'clunk' and then permit full abduction (positive Ortolani test).

EMI 2

Theme: The limping child

1. F.
2. A.
3. D.
4. B.
5. D.
6. C.

CRQ answers

CRQ 1

a. Osgood–Schlatter's disease.

b. Osteochondritis.

c. Lateral radiograph will sometimes show elevation of a small portion of the tongue of the tibial apophysis or occasionally a separate ossicle.

d. Rest and lighter sports.

e. By a splint to maintain the leg in extension and prevent flexion.

CRQ 2

a. The leg is held in external rotation, partial flexion and appears shorter. It is painful.

b. Frog-leg lateral shows the degree of displacement of the capital epiphysis most accurately.

c. Pinning the displaced femoral head in situ. If severely displaced an osteotomy of the femoral neck can be planned later.

d. Chondrolysis and avascular necrosis of femoral epiphysis.

e. There may be an early slip in the opposite, unaffected hip.

OSCE answer

OSCE 1

a. Flat feet.

b. Ask the child to stand on tiptoes. The medial plantar arch should reform and the calcaneo-valgus deformity correct so that the heel lines up with the Achilles tendon.

c. A large medial fat pad in the plantar arch ligamentous laxity around the ankle.

d. wedged insoles

   shoes with firm uppers

   a heel seat insert

Best of 5s answers

1. b.
2. d.

Multiple choice answers

1. a. **False.** Looser's zones are associated with osteomalacia.

   b. **True.** A portion of cortex may lose its blood supply as a result of the surrounding infection and become sequestrated as an island of dead bone.

   c. **True.** Osteitis in the metaphysis may spread to involve the adjacent joint, if the area of infection is within the joint capsule.

   d. **True.** The architecture of the infected bone is less strong than normal bone.

   e. **False.** Myositis ossificans is associated with calcification of an intramuscular haematoma and is, therefore, associated with fractures particularly around the elbow.

2. a. **False.** A case of congenital dislocation of the hip (CDH) missed on routine screening in infancy would have presented early in childhood when

the patient began walking. It is unlikely that the first presentation of CDH would be as late as the age of 12.

b. **False.** Transient synovitis of the hip has a short duration and usually resolves within 3 to 4 days.

c. **True.** Perthes' disease develops spontaneously, causing pain and limp that may persist for episodes of several weeks. Symptoms are relieved by rest but recurrent relapses are characteristic until the area of avascular necrosis heals.

d. **False.** Acute septic arthritis is characterised by acute severe pain in the hip and loss of movement.

e. **True.** Λ gradual slip of the upper femoral epiphysis presents with a prolonged history of pain and loss of movement. The condition is associated with hormonal imbalance in the adolescent. Acute slips have a shorter history and may be associated with direct trauma.

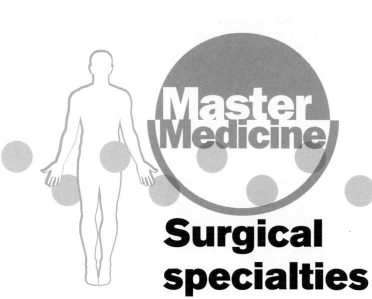

Master Medicine

Surgical
specialties

Cardiothoracic surgery

Chapter overview

Cardiothoracic surgery is concerned with the surgical management of intrathoracic diseases and chest trauma and is conventionally split into adult cardiac, paediatric cardiac, thoracic and transplant sub-specialities. In general terms, adult cardiac surgery is concerned with the treatment of acquired heart and great vessel disease whereas paediatric cardiac surgery almost exclusively involves the treatment of congenital cardiac and vascular malformations. Some children with congenital cardiovascular disease may require revisional surgery in later life whereas others may evade diagnosis and present for initial corrective surgery as adults.

Thoracic surgery deals with all other intrathoracic pathology. At present, the surgical management of oesophageal diseases is shared between thoracic and upper gastrointestinal surgeons with work patterns tending to reflect historical referral pathways and the interests of the surgical groups concerned.

Oesophageal diseases are discussed in Chapter 3 and cardiothoracic transplantation in Chapter 16.

12.1 Cardiac surgery

Learning objectives

You should:
- understand the indications and techniques for coronary artery revascularisation
- be aware of the possible complications of ischaemic heart disease that might benefit from surgical intervention
- appreciate the differences between biological and mechanical heart valves
- understand the different pathological states caused by native cardiac valve disorders
- understand the pathophysiology of cardiac tamponade.

Assessment of operative risk in cardiac surgery

Estimation of procedural mortality and morbidity (predominantly stroke) and communication of these risks to the patient have become essential elements in the preoperative discussion between the surgeon and the patient.

Mortality

This is estimated by using a scoring system in which a variable number of points is given for specified findings and the sum of these is used, either directly or via a correction graph, to indicate the operative risk as a percentage mortality rate. Predicted mortality rates range from 2% for routine and relatively straightforward procedures to over 50% for emergency and complex procedures.

Morbidity

The risk of stroke varies from 1% to over 10% depending on the procedure used. This is a catastrophic complication that occurs more frequently in patients with intracardiac thrombus, severe carotid disease or atheromatous disease of the proximal aorta. Other complications include:

- low cardiac output
- dysrhythmias
- fluid accumulation
- short-term memory impairment
- wound infection
- pulmonary infection.

Ischaemic heart disease

Medical treatment for coronary attacks (aspirin, beta blockers, ACE inhibitors and angioplasty) has reduced the immediate coronary death rate. Consequently, there is an increasing requirement for coronary revascularisation.

The main factors contributing to atheromatous disease are:

- smoking
- hypertension
- diabetes
- hyperlipidaemia
- family history of ischaemic heart disease.

Pathology

Atheromatous plaques narrow the coronary artery lumen. A 40% reduction in cross-sectional diameter has a significant effect on blood flow. Localised, proximal coronary atheroma is amenable to bypass surgery whereas disease that is diffusely spread along the coronary artery is not. Sometimes the intima and inner media of an artery obstructed by diffuse atheroma may be removed (coronary endarterectomy).

Classification of coronary artery disease

There are three coronary vessel systems, each based on one of the major coronary arteries:

- the right coronary artery
- the left anterior descending coronary artery
- the circumflex coronary artery (Figure 167).

Patients are put into categories according to the number of diseased vessel systems. Patients with disease in the initial segment of the left coronary artery (Figure 167) are referred to as having left main stem disease. These categories have prognostic implications for survival without surgery (Table 17).

Coronary revascularisation

Coronary revascularisation is the combined term for procedures used to improve myocardial blood flow (and relieve angina) in patients with atherosclerotic coronary heart disease. There are two main categories:

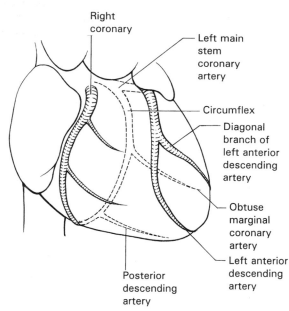

Figure 167 Coronary vessel systems.

Table 17 Coronary artery disease survival rates without coronary artery surgery

Diseased vessels	Annual mortality rate (%)
One vessel	2
Two vessels	4–6
Three vessels	8–11
Left main stem	9–11

- coronary artery bypass grafts (CABG)
- percutaneous transluminal coronary angioplasty (PTCA).

Major advances in angioplasty have led to a shift from simple balloon angioplasty to the routine use of coronary artery stents. This has dramatically reduced the complication and restenosis rates. Further refinements have included coating stents with a drug-containing polymer (drug-eluting stents), which reduces recurrent narrowing (restenosis) after angioplasty.

Angioplasty and surgery should now be considered equivalent methods of coronary revascularisation. The choice of technique should be based on patient preference and medical and other cardiac comorbidities. Often, the benefits of the less-invasive percutaneous procedure have to be balanced against the reduced likelihood of requiring further revascularisation procedures after CABG.

Assessment

Preoperative evaluation is based on the anatomical extent of coronary disease demonstrated by angiography (Figure 168) and the assessment of left ventricular function by echocardiography and/or left ventricular angiography combined with intracardiac pressure measurement.

Selection for revascularisation

Elective surgery is advised for patients who are not adequately controlled by medical therapy and for those with main stem or three-vessel disease. Urgent intervention is indicated in patients with crescendo (preinfarctional) angina and when a major vessel is in jeopardy after failed angioplasty.

Surgery

Coronary artery bypass grafts are frequently constructed using reversed segments of long or short saphenous vein, which are anastomosed proximally to the ascending aorta

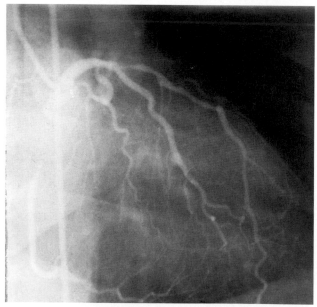

Figure 168 Coronary angiogram: left coronary injection showing multiple stenoses.

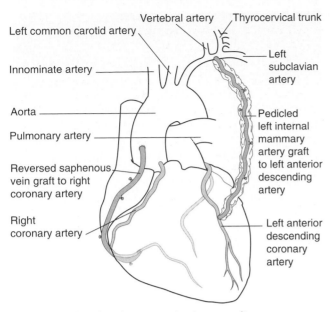

Figure 169 Examples of coronary artery bypass grafts.

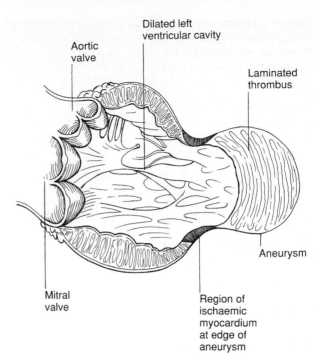

Figure 170 Ventricular aneurysm.

and distally to the diseased coronary artery beyond the stenosis. The long-term survival of vein grafts is limited to about 70% at 5 years and 50% at 10 years. This finding has led to the use of arterial conduits on the basis that these might have better long-term survival. The commonest arterial graft is the left internal mammary artery. This is normally used as a pedicled graft, which is left attached proximally to the left subclavian artery and sutured distally to the left anterior descending coronary artery. The long-term patency rate of over 70% at 10 years has led to this being the graft of choice for the left anterior descending artery. The right internal mammary artery can also be used as either a free or pedicled graft and there is now an increasing trend to use radial artery free grafts (Figure 169).

Although most coronary surgery is performed on an arrested heart with the patient on cardiopulmonary bypass, there is increasing interest in operating on the beating heart without bypass, which may reduce the risk of complications related to cardiopulmonary bypass such as stroke. Over the past 10 years the use of angioplasty has increased fourfold. The current ratio of PTCA/CABG in the UK is greater than 3:1.

Results

Operative mortality after elective revascularisation is less than 2%. Emergency revascularisation following recent myocardial infarction or failed angioplasty has a higher mortality rate (6%). Up to 3% of patients will have a perioperative cerebrovascular accident. In total, 80% of patients are symptom free at 1 year; the rest are significantly improved. Some degree of angina recurs in 5% of patients per year.

Surgery for the complications of ischaemic heart disease

Left ventricular aneurysm

Healing of a myocardial infarction may be accompanied by stretching of the scar, which assumes a sack-like shape

(Figure 170) termed a 'ventricular aneurysm'. The aneurysm usually contains a laminated thrombus, which may cause systemic embolisation. Left ventricular function is impaired and long-term survival is poor, with 80% of patients dying within 5 years.

Clinical features

Patients present with impaired exercise tolerance, left ventricular failure and dysrhythmias.

Diagnosis

Investigations involve:

- electrocardiogram (ECG): persistent ST-segment elevation
- chest radiograph: enlarged cardiac silhouette
- echocardiography: confirms aneurysm, thrombus
- cardiac catheterisation: demonstrates concurrent coronary artery disease, the aneurysm and raised left ventricular end-diastolic pressure.

Management

Management can be by:

- medical therapy: ACE inhibitors, diuretics
- surgery: excision of aneurysm, CABG.

Mitral valve incompetence

Rupture of a papillary muscle can be an acute complication of myocardial infarction. Acute pulmonary oedema develops and urgent valve replacement is required. Mitral reflux may also result from chronic papillary muscle ischaemia.

Myocardial failure

Severe myocardial ischaemia can result in myocardial fibrosis and progressive cardiac failure. Cardiac transplan-

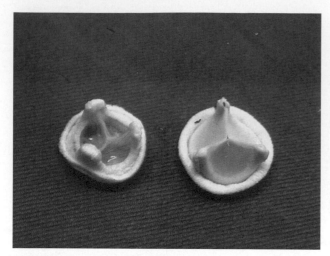

Figure 171 Biological valve prosthesis.

tation is an option in patients who would not benefit from revascularisation.

Valvular heart disease

Heart valve implants

There are two types of heart valve substitutes:

- prosthetic devices
- homografts.

Prosthetic devices

Prosthetic valves have inherent limitations:

- risk of endocarditic infection
- relative obstruction to blood flow (compared with human valves)
- haemolysis (caused by turbulence).

There are two main types:

Biological prosthesis This is constructed from porcine aortic valves or from bovine pericardium. The tissue is preserved in glutaraldehyde and mounted on a frame with a dacron sewing ring (Figure 171). The main advantages of a biological prosthesis are:

- anticoagulation is not required
- the valve is silent.

The main disadvantages are:

- valve failure 6–14 years after implantation
- the potential need to replace the valve.

A bioprosthesis is the implant of choice in women who intend to have a family, as the teratogenic risks of warfarin and the need for heparinisation during pregnancy are avoided. They are also useful in the elderly or in others in whom anticoagulation is contraindicated.

Mechanical prosthesis This is constructed from synthetic materials. The first design, a ball-in-cage valve, is still in use. Single or double leaflet flap valves are alternative designs (Figure 172). The main advantages of a mechanical prosthesis are:

- the valve is unlikely to need replacing
- it is less obstructive to blood flow.

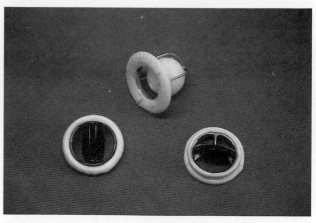

Figure 172 Mechanical valve prosthesis.

The main disadvantages are:

- the valve is audible
- it requires lifelong anticoagulation
- the possibility of haemolysis.

Mechanical valves are now the device of choice for most patients.

Homografts

Cadaveric human aortic valve tissue preserved in antibiotic solution can be used for aortic valve replacement. The main advantages are:

- excellent haemodynamics
- no anticoagulation required.

The main disadvantages are:

- it still wears out (over a longer period)
- theoretical risk of virus contamination
- harvesting difficulties and short storage time.

Homografts are not commonly used because of significant problems with harvesting and storage.

Acquired disease

Valvular heart disease is decreasing in the UK because of the virtual abolition of rheumatic heart disease. The few rheumatic cases that remain are seen in late middle-aged or elderly patients. In developing countries where rheumatic valvular disease predominates, all ages are afflicted.

Diseased cardiac valves restrict blood flow (stenosis) or fail to seal correctly (incompetence, regurgitation or reflux). Some valves exhibit stenosis and reflux ('mixed' valve disease). Abnormal heart valves are susceptible to subacute bacterial endocarditis (SBE) and patients require prophylactic antibiotic cover at the time of any surgical or dental intervention. Acute valve replacement surgery may be needed if valve destruction from SBE causes sudden cardiac decompensation.

Aortic stenosis

This may be congenital or acquired (rheumatic valve disease). The most common cause in the adult is calcification of a bicuspid aortic valve. It is characterised by fatigue, syncope, an ejection systolic murmur radiating to the neck and a slow rising pulse.

Diagnosis

Investigation involves:

- ECG: sinus rhythm (occasionally atrial fibrillation), left ventricular hypertrophy, ST depression in V leads
- chest radiograph: large left ventricle, dilated ascending aorta
- echocardiography: hypertrophic stiff left ventricle, restricted valve opening
- cardiac catheterisation: gradient of oxygen saturation across the aortic valve.

Management

Valve replacement is required for all significant stenoses. Valvotomy (division of the fused valve commissures) or resection of an obstructing membrane is appropriate in some children.

Aortic regurgitation

Abnormal valve leaflets and a dilated aortic valve ring are the chief causes of aortic regurgitation. The condition is often asymptomatic. Clinical features are a collapsing pulse, cardiac apex deviation to the left and a diastolic murmur at the left sternal edge.

Diagnosis

Investigation involves:

- ECG: sinus rhythm, eventual left ventricular hypertrophy
- chest radiograph: normal or dilated left ventricle
- echocardiography: dilated left ventricle, regurgitant aortic blood flow
- cardiac catheterisation: free aortic reflux, left ventricular dilatation.

Management

Aortic valve replacement is indicated when there is evidence of cardiac decompensation. Patients with dilatation of the ascending aorta may require replacement of the ascending aorta and aortic valve with a combined prosthesis into which the coronary arteries are reimplanted.

Mitral stenosis

This is usually caused by rheumatic heart disease. Patients have a history of rheumatic fever and embolism, exertional dyspnoea, orthopnoea, episodes of acute pulmonary oedema and right heart failure. Most patients have atrial fibrillation and a mid-diastolic murmur. There is a risk of embolisation of a left atrial clot.

Diagnosis

Investigation involves:

- ECG: atrial fibrillation, right ventricular hypertrophy
- chest radiograph: upper lobe blood diversion, small left ventricle, large pulmonary artery and left atrial appendage
- echocardiography: restricted valve opening
- cardiac catheterisation: elevated pulmonary artery and capillary wedge pressure.

Management

Medical therapy Drugs used are digoxin, diuretics and warfarin (to reduce the risk of embolisation).

Surgery This is indicated when pulmonary hypertension becomes marked. Balloon valvuloplasty or open mitral valve commissurotomy are options in occasional patients with mobile non-calcified valves. Mitral valve replacement is necessary for mixed valve disease and/or valvular calcification.

Mitral regurgitation

Mitral regurgitation is caused by:

- rheumatic fever
- annular dilatation from cardiomyopathy
- chordal rupture, papillary muscle dysfunction
- infective endocarditis.

Patients are dyspnoeic, orthopnoeic and fatigue easily. The cardiac apex is deviated laterally with a pansystolic murmur radiating to the apex.

Diagnosis

Investigation involves:

- ECG: atrial fibrillation, right ventricular hypertrophy
- chest radiograph: enlarged heart
- echocardiography: dilated, hyperactive left ventricle
- cardiac catheterisation: high left atrial pressure with regurgitation of contrast medium.

Management

Surgery is indicated in patients with progressive left ventricular dilatation. Results are better with earlier intervention. Mitral valve replacement is usual but valve repair and reconstruction is sometimes possible.

Tricuspid regurgitation

Tricuspid regurgitation is caused by:

- right ventricular dilatation secondary to pulmonary hypertension or myocardial infarction
- bacterial endocarditis
- rheumatic heart disease.

Patients have an elevated venous pressure with hepatomegaly, which is sometimes pulsatile. There is a pansystolic murmur at the right sternal edge.

Diagnosis

A chest radiograph will show an enlarged right atrium.

Management

Diuretic therapy is helpful. Surgical correction is only appropriate for cases that are secondary to mitral valve disease. Tricuspid regurgitation is dealt with by reconstructing the dilated valve annulus (ring). Valve replacement is rare.

Pericardial disease

Tamponade occurs when there is sufficient intrapericardial fluid to decrease cardiac output. The pericardial fluid prevents the heart from filling in diastole by compressing the cardiac chambers and by occluding the venous return.

The main causes are:

- blood: knife wounds, cardiac surgery, aortic dissection
- fluid: uraemia, malignancy, connective tissue disease.

Clinical features

Acute tamponade This is characterised by a reduced cardiac output, decreased blood pressure, narrow pulse pressure, elevated venous pressure and muffled heart sounds.

Chronic tamponade This is similar but shows less marked changes: refractory 'right heart failure'.

Diagnosis

Investigation involves:

- chest radiograph: no specific features in acute cases, smoothly enlarged pericardial contours in chronic cases
- echocardiography: small compressed active heart with surrounding fluid.

Treatment

Acute tamponade Temporary relief may be obtained by pericardial aspiration, but definitive open surgical drainage is mandatory.

Chronic tamponade Some respond to aspiration but surgery is required if fluid reaccumulates. Continuing pericardial drainage is provided by creating a pericardial 'window' into the pleural cavity or through the diaphragm into the peritoneum.

12.2 Aortic disease

> ### Learning objectives
>
> You should:
> - understand the difference between aortic aneurysm and dissection
> - be aware of the treatment options for these conditions
> - be aware of the specific risk of paraplegia associated with surgery to the descending aorta.

Aortic aneurysm

An aortic aneurysm is a localised dilatation of the aorta that is either tubular (fusiform) or saccular (Figure 173). The main causes are:

- hypertension
- atheroma
- syphilis
- cystic medial necrosis (Marfan syndrome).

The aneurysm is often an asymptomatic finding on a chest radiograph. It may cause chronic back pain or present acutely after a leak that causes collapse or a haemothorax.

Diagnosis

Investigation includes:

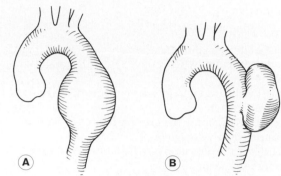

Figure 173 Thoracic aortic aneurysm. (A) Tubular. (B) Saccular.

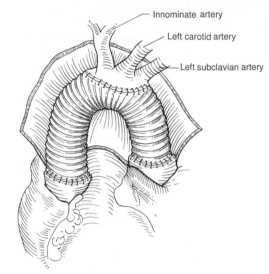

Innominate artery
Left carotid artery
Left subclavian artery

Figure 174 Dacron tube graft replacement of ascending aortic arch and proximal descending aorta for thoracic aortic aneurysm.

- chest radiograph: the aneurysm is usually visible; there may be a haemothorax
- computed tomography (CT) scan with i.v. contrast enhancement: confirms extent
- aortogram: defines arterial anatomy and relationships.

Management

In view of the risk of rupture and death, surgery is advised in all patients unless advanced age or coexisting medical conditions make survival unlikely. Aneurysms are treated by local resection and reconstruction with a dacron tube graft (Figure 174).

Aneurysms of the ascending aorta are repaired with the aid of cardiopulmonary bypass to sustain body perfusion. Aneurysms of the aortic arch require interruption of the cerebral circulation; cardiopulmonary bypass is used to achieve total body cooling, which allows hypothermic circulatory arrest during the operation. Aneurysms of the descending aorta are repaired using left heart bypass or a local diversionary shunt. Operations on the descending aorta are associated with a risk of paraplegia (2–5%) resulting from inadequate perfusion of the spinal cord.

Aortic dissection

A tear in the aortic intima usually located just above the aortic valve or adjacent to the left subclavian artery allows

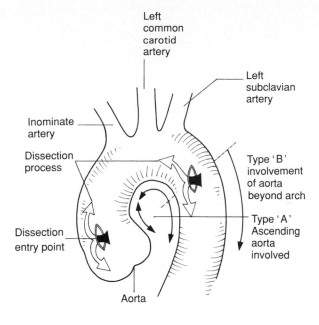

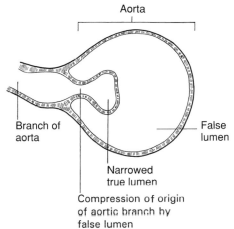

Figure 175 Aortic dissection.

blood to enter the media and create a false passage along the media layer. The false lumen spirals around the aorta (Figure 175) and can occlude branches of the aorta, including the carotid and coronary arteries, causing a stroke or a myocardial infarction. The false lumen may burst into the pericardial cavity causing tamponade or into the left pleural cavity resulting in exsanguination.

The main causes are:

- hypertension
- atheroma
- cystic medial necrosis.

Clinical features

Classically, patients will complain of a severe 'tearing' acute chest pain that may radiate to the back. They may be hypotensive with variably absent pulses.

Diagnosis

Investigation includes:

- ECG: to exclude a myocardial infarction, which can accompany dissection

- chest radiograph: widened mediastinum and/or left pleural effusion
- CT scan with i.v. contrast: confirms double aortic lumen
- aortogram: demonstrates luminal connections.

Management

Immediate surgery and graft replacement are required to control a dissection involving the ascending aorta and/or aortic arch. Surgery is performed using cardiopulmonary bypass. It may be necessary to replace the aortic valve and reimplant the coronary arteries and/or replace the aortic arch. If the dissection only involves the descending aorta, surgical and conservative management (controlling hypertension) are equally effective. Conservative treatment is favoured unless there is bleeding into the left chest or the vascular branches to the abdominal organs have been compromised. The surgical technique is similar to that used for a descending aortic aneurysm (see p. 100).

In some cases with a leaking descending aortic dissection it may be feasible to place an endovascular stent, which can reoppose the intimal layers and occlude the intimal tear thereby sealing the dissection origin.

Traumatic aortic rupture

This occurs at the junction of the descending aorta and the aortic arch. It is a deceleration injury that accompanies a major accident, e.g. a road traffic accident or a major fall. The disruption is caused by a transverse shearing force created at the junction of the relatively mobile aortic arch and the fixed descending thoracic aorta. The intimal and medial layers rupture and aortic integrity depends upon the adventitia. There are usually associated multiple injuries. If the diagnosis is missed, patients die from massive haemorrhage or they develop a false aneurysm.

Clinical features

There is a history of severe major injury. General examination is dominated by other concurrent injuries. It is *essential* to have a high index of suspicion.

Diagnosis

Investigations of use are:

- chest radiograph: wide mediastinum
- aortogram: shows intimal separation.

Treatment

Operation is undertaken through a left thoracotomy using a local shunt or left heart bypass to allow resection of the damaged area and tube graft repair. There is a risk of paraplegia.

12.3 Congenital heart disease

Learning objectives

You should:

- understand the difference between cyanotic and acyanotic congenital heart disease
- be able to describe the structural and pathophysiological abnormalities present in atrial and ventricular septal defect, tetralogy of Fallot, aortic coarctation and patent ductus arteriosus.

Twelve

Although congenital heart disease is customarily regarded as referring to diseases presenting in early life, a variety of defects may not require attention until later life.

Classification

Congenital heart defects are divided into two groups: those with and those without central cyanosis. Some conditions start acyanotic and later become cyanotic. This occurs with conditions causing large shunts of blood from the left to the right side of the heart. The massive increase in pulmonary blood flow eventually causes pulmonary hypertension. As the pulmonary artery pressure exceeds the systemic pressure, the shunt of blood reverses and produces cyanosis (Eisenmenger syndrome).

Atrial septal defect

Left to right shunting of blood occurs at the atrial level, increasing the right ventricular work and causing right ventricular hypertrophy and pulmonary congestion. Emboli ejected from the right ventricle may lodge in the systemic circulation because of paradoxical embolisation across the defect.

Clinical features

Atrial septal defect is often asymptomatic. Exertional dyspnoea and progressive pulmonary hypertension develop in adulthood. Examination reveals a right ventricular heave, widely fixed split second heart sound and a pulmonary ejection flow murmur.

Treatment

The defect is repaired with a patch of pericardium or dacron.

Ventricular septal defect

Ventricular septal defects (VSDs) mostly occur in the membranous septum (Figure 176). Small defects close spontaneously. Significant left to right shunting occurs across larger defects with consequent pulmonary congestion.

Clinical features

Infants with large defects may present with frequent chest infections. Others are often asymptomatic. A pansystolic murmur is audible, maximal at the left sternal edge. The second heart sound may be loud.

Diagnosis

Investigation involves:

- ECG: biventricular enlargement
- chest radiograph: pulmonary plethora
- echocardiography: demonstrates the defect.

Treatment

Asymptomatic defects are kept under observation. Early operation is preferred for large defects to prevent irreversible pulmonary hypertension. Isolated VSDs are closed with a dacron patch.

Patent ductus arteriosus

This defect results from a failure of the ductus arteriosus to close after birth. It can cause pulmonary blood flow and

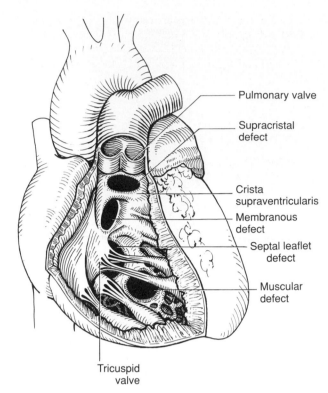

Pulmonary valve

Supracristal defect

Crista supraventricularis

Membranous defect

Septal leaflet defect

Muscular defect

Tricuspid valve

Figure 176 Ventricular septal defect.

pressure to significantly increase, leading to pulmonary congestion and hypertension. Growth is often retarded and there is a continuous 'machinery' type murmur.

Diagnosis

Investigation includes:

- chest radiograph: pulmonary congestion
- echocardiography: excludes concurrent intracardiac defect.

Treatment

In premature children, the duct may close with indomethacin infusion, but clipping or division through a left thoracotomy is often needed. Endovascular passage of an occluding umbrella is an option in older children.

Aortic coarctation

Coarctation is a narrowing of the thoracic aorta usually at the level of the ligamentum arteriosum. It causes upper body hypertension and may lead to heart failure in infancy, although children and young adults can be asymptomatic. Extensive chest wall collaterals develop as a means of delivering blood around the obstruction into the distal aorta.

Clinical features

The femoral pulses are absent or weak and delayed. Upper limb hypertension is present. A systolic murmur may be audible over the back.

Diagnosis

Investigation includes:

- ECG: left ventricular hypertrophy
- chest radiograph: enlarged left ventricle, reduced aortic knuckle, rib 'notching' resulting from the enlarged and tortuous intercostal arteries eroding the ribs.

Treatment

Open surgical correction is required. In infants, an onlay patch graft is created from the left subclavian artery. A dacron bypass graft is used in older children and adults. The proximal hypertension does not resolve in adult cases.

Tetralogy of Fallot

This complex defect (Figure 177) is the most common cause of cyanotic congenital heart disease. It is characterised by:

- a high VSD
- an aorta that overlies the septum
- right ventricular outflow obstruction
- right ventricular hypertrophy.

The obstruction to right ventricular outflow causes right to left shunting across the ventricular septal defect and, consequently, cyanosis.

Clinical features

The clinical features depend upon the severity of the right ventricular outflow obstruction. This may not be significant when the child is at rest but may be precipitated by adrenergic events. Consequently, the child may become blue and faint during feeding or crying.

Diagnosis

Investigation involves:

- ECG: right ventricular hypertrophy
- chest radiograph: small pulmonary artery
- echocardiography: demonstrates anatomy

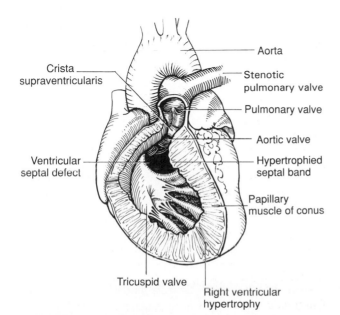

Figure 177 Tetralogy of Fallot.

- cardiac catheterisation: demonstrates pulmonary artery size.

Treatment

Correction is achieved by closing the VSD with a patch, resecting the right ventricular muscle bands, which contribute to the outflow obstruction, and enlarging the right ventricular outflow tract, usually with a patch graft. In children unfit for this procedure, a shunt from the subclavian artery to the pulmonary artery will increase pulmonary blood flow and buy 'time', allowing the child to grow with a view to definitive correction at a later date.

12.4 Thoracic surgery

> **Learning objectives**
>
> You should:
> - acquire a thorough overview of the frequency, clinical features and surgical management of bronchogenic carcinoma
> - understand the pathophysiology of the various types of pneumothorax and their appropriate management
> - be conversant with the difference between pulmonary abscess and empyema
> - recognise the common potential sequelae of thoracic trauma.

Bronchogenic carcinoma

Bronchogenic carcinoma is the most common cause of cancer death in men and women in the UK. It usually presents after the fifth decade. Cigarette smoking is the dominant risk factor. Exposure to asbestos, radioactive dust, bichromates or nickel ore is also important.

Tumours may be central (at the hilum) or peripheral (coin lesions; Figure 178). Cavitation is not uncommon and invasion of adjacent structures (chest wall, pericardium, trachea, phrenic nerve and superior vena cava) can occur (Figure 179).

The main tumour cell types are:

- squamous: 45%
- small cell: 25%
- adenocarcinoma: 15%
- large cell: 15%.

Approximately 70% of tumours are inoperable at presentation. Lymphatic spread is via intrapulmonary nodes to the hilar nodes and finally to the mediastinal nodes. Eventually, the scalene nodes may be involved. Distant haematogenous spread is to the brain, adrenals, liver and bones.

Clinical features

Cough, haemoptysis and pneumonia are typical, with occasional chest pain. Often, the tumour is an asymptomatic finding on a chest radiograph. Weight loss and tiredness are common.

Examination may be normal or reveal finger clubbing, signs of consolidation or collapse (Figure 180) or a pleural effusion.

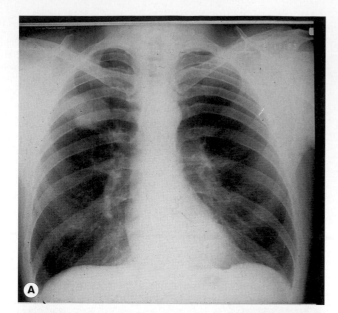

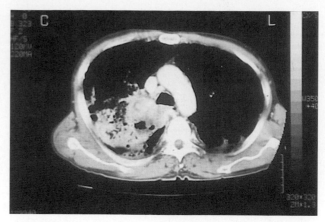

Figure 179 CT scan of the thorax showing an advanced bronchogenic carcinoma. Note the right hilar mass invading the mediastinum. There is collapse and cavitation of the lung parenchyma distal to the tumour.

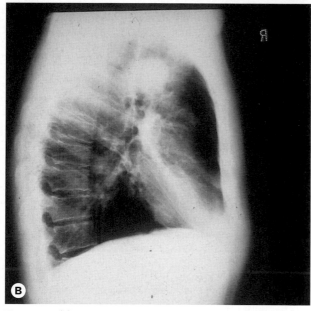

Figure 178 (A) Pulmonary coin lesion: 4-cm mass in right upper zone. (B) The same lesion seen on lateral view, which shows the lesion to be in the apical segment of the upper lobe.

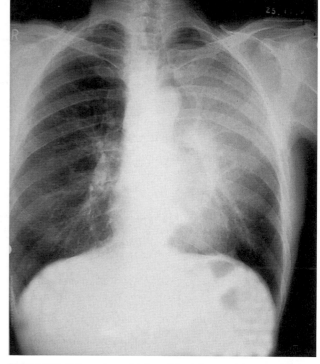

Figure 180 Collapse/consolidation of the left upper lobe associated with a bronchial neoplasm.

The following features indicate inoperability:

- scalene lymphadenopathy
- hepatomegaly
- superior vena caval obstruction
- Horner's syndrome (sympathetic chain involvement).

Diagnosis

Investigation involves:

- chest radiograph: peripheral opacity/cavity or hilar mass, consolidation or collapse
- CT/MR scan: identifies mass plus any mediastinal lymphadenopathy, images any liver metastases
- sputum cytology: may reveal carcinoma cells

- fine needle aspiration: may confirm tissue diagnosis
- bronchoscopy: used to assess operability, may provide tissue diagnosis
- mediastinoscopy: used to exclude/confirm involvement of mediastinal nodes.

Treatment

Resection is indicated in all fit patients with localised non-small cell cancer. Detailed assessment of cardiac and respiratory function is essential. CO_2 retention is an absolute contraindication to surgery because of the risk of postoperative respiratory failure. Overall, approximately 15–20% of patients presenting with a bronchogenic carcinoma are suitable for surgery. Resection (lobectomy or pneumonectomy) is performed through a posterolateral thoracotomy. Small peripheral cancers may be resected by excision of a wedge or segment of a lobe in patients with poor respiratory function. Radiotherapy is reserved for inoperable or unfit patients.

The treatment of small cell cancer is controversial. Surgery is probably best for early tumours but is less likely to benefit advanced lesions. These tumours often respond well initially to chemotherapy.

Postoperative radiotherapy does not enhance survival but reduces local recurrence. Postoperative chemotherapy improves survival in patients with very advanced local disease.

Prognosis

The overall operative mortality rate is 5%. Survival varies according to cell type (squamous > adenocarcinoma > large cell > undifferentiated > small cell), blood vessel invasion and disease stage (based on a TNM system) (see p. 123). One-third of resected patients will be alive 5 years postoperatively.

Pulmonary infection

Bronchiectasis

This condition is characterised by dilatations of the bronchial tree containing infected pools of secretion. Bronchiectasis usually results from childhood pneumonia or chronic bronchial obstruction, e.g. after foreign body inhalation.

Clinical features There is a history of a chronic productive cough with frequent exacerbations. Intermittent haemoptysis can be severe. One-third of patients have finger clubbing.

Diagnosis Investigation involves:

- bronchoscopy: excludes chronic obstruction
- bronchography: outlines bronchiectatic areas with a contrast medium
- CT/MR scan of thorax: most common method of delineating disease.

Treatment Conservative treatment with postural drainage and antibiotics for acute episodes or to control infection in winter is the rule. Surgery is indicated if disease is localised to one lobe or to control massive haemorrhage.

Lung abscess

This condition usually complicates pneumonia but may follow infection of a pulmonary cyst or bulla or central necrosis in a bronchogenic cancer or pulmonary infarct. In cases with a pneumonic origin, the initial cause is often aspiration in patients who are unable to protect their airways. It is a feature of debilitated or unconscious patients and after inhalation of gastric contents during anaesthesia.

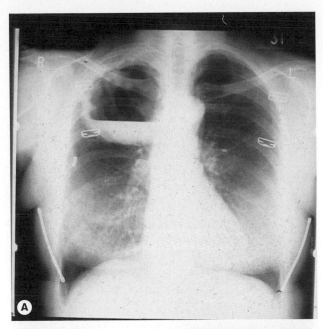

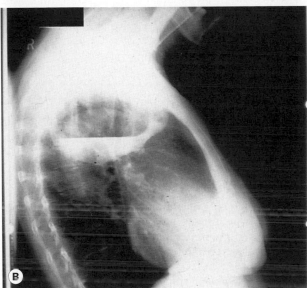

Figure 181 Lung abscess. (A) Posteroanterior view of lung abscess in the right upper zone. (B) Lateral view shows abscess is in the upper lobe.

Clinical features Symptoms include cough, fever and haemoptysis.

Diagnosis Investigation involves:

- chest radiograph: cavity with an air–fluid level (Figure 181)
- bronchoscopy: excludes an underlying carcinoma.

Treatment Broad-spectrum antibiotic therapy is the cornerstone of treatment. Resection is indicated if there is an associated carcinoma or severe haemorrhage.

Pneumothorax

Air in the pleural space is termed a pneumothorax. A pneumothorax is spontaneous if it is caused by an air leak with no external cause, iatrogenic if it occurs after

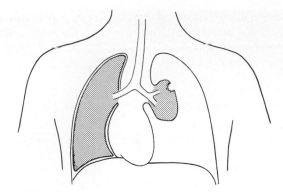

Figure 182 Left tension pneumothorax.

instrumentation of the chest and traumatic if it occurs following chest trauma. Air may arise from an internal air leak from some part of the respiratory system (closed pneumothorax) or from the oesophagus. A pneumothorax may also result from communication between the pleural cavity and the outside atmosphere through a defect in the chest wall (open pneumothorax). The intrapleural pressure remains constant and a mediastinal shift does not occur. A tension pneumothorax develops when the pleural air in a closed pneumothorax is under sufficient pressure to deviate the mediastinum to the opposite side and compress the ipsilateral lung (Figure 182). This results from a valve-like effect at the leakage site, where each successive breath increases the intrapleural pressure.

Spontaneous pneumothorax

Spontaneous pneumothorax occurs in two quite different groups of patients:

Primary pneumothorax This typically affects young, tall, asthenic individuals, and occurs more often in men than women. The lung looks normal and has small apical air blisters. The prognosis is excellent.

Secondary pneumothorax This usually develops in elderly patients with a background of bronchitis and emphysema. The air leak stems from a large air sac or bulla in the lung. Mortality is high because of poor lung function, slow healing and the risk of pneumonia.

Clinical features

Sudden onset of dyspnoea with hyper-resonance and reduced breath sounds are the hallmarks of a pneumothorax. In a tension pneumothorax, dyspnoea is severe; patients may be cyanosed with tracheal deviation and reduced blood pressure and pulse volume.

Diagnosis

Investigation by chest radiograph will show a pneumothorax and any bullous lung disease and emphysema in the other lung.

Treatment

Unless the pneumothorax occupies less than one-third of the periphery of the lung on a chest radiograph or is loculated, an intercostal drain, which is connected to an underwater seal drain, should be inserted. This should be sited at the lateral border of the pectoralis major. This location

is safer as it avoids the risk of damage to the internal mammary artery and is cosmetically more acceptable in a young woman.

A patient with a tension pneumothorax may not be able to wait for a confirmatory radiograph and should have a wide-bore needle placed into the pleural cavity as a first aid measure to relieve the intrapleural pressure. Patients with minute pneumothoraces can be treated conservatively.

In most cases, lung re-expansion occurs within 24–48 h and, provided that there is no ongoing leak, the drain can be removed. Surgery is indicated for:

* recurrent unilateral pneumothorax
* bilateral pneumothorax
* continued air leak
* any occupation where pneumothorax would be a hazard.

Operative management is based on securing any air blisters or bullae and achieving pleural fusion (pleurodesis) using chemicals or abrasion techniques or by stripping the parietal pleura (pleurectomy).

Pleural effusion

A pleural effusion may be a transudate (protein content <3 g/dl) or an exudate (protein content >3 g/dl). Transudates are usually bilateral and relate to underlying cardiac, renal or hepatic disease. Exudates are associated with malignancy, pneumonia, connective tissue disease, tuberculosis, pancreatitis and ovarian tumours.

Clinical features

Features suggesting any of these underlying causes should be sought from the history and examination. The classic features of a pleural effusion are dullness to percussion with reduced or absent breath sounds.

Diagnosis

Investigation includes:

* fluid biochemistry: the amylase content is diagnostic in a pancreatitis-related effusion
* culture and microscopy: identifies infection and sometimes malignant cells
* chest radiograph: a post-drainage film may reveal an underlying tumour
* sputum cytology
* bronchoscopy ⎫
* pleural biopsy ⎬ may provide a tissue diagnosis.

Treatment

The effusion should be drained for diagnostic and therapeutic reasons. If the preceding investigations are negative, thoracoscopy is indicated and any pleural or pulmonary abnormalities are biopsied. If the biopsies confirm a malignancy, a sclerosing agent can be inserted via a chest drain to prevent reaccumulation of the effusion.

Pleural empyema

An empyema is an intrapleural collection of pus, usually as a consequence of pneumonia. Other causes are a lung abscess, a complication of thoracic surgery or the sequel to chest drainage.

Clinical features

A swinging fever and weight loss with a preceding history of pneumonia characterise empyema. A large empyema may be associated with breathlessness.

Diagnosis

Investigations involve:

- chest radiograph: a basal effusion may be present
- aspiration: diagnostic; pus should be cultured.

Treatment

A recent empyema with thin pus (usually postpneumonic) may be drained fully using an intercostal tube and under-water seal drain. More often, the diagnosis is delayed and follows several courses of antibiotic therapy, resulting in a densely fibrous capsule around the empyema with little prospect of the underlying lung re-expanding. In a young fit patient, the empyema cavity is excised and the fibrous tissue removed from the underlying lung (decortication) through a thoracotomy. This allows the lung to re-expand. Tube drainage may be all that is possible in the elderly unfit patient.

Thoracic trauma

Rib fractures

A moderate impact injury will cause a simple fracture of one or several ribs. Double fractures of ribs create a free-floating or flail segment that moves paradoxically with respiration (Figure 183). This effect can tip elderly patients into respiratory failure. Fractures of the ninth to the eleventh ribs are often associated with splenic or renal injury. Fractures of the first rib denote a high energy injury and may be associated with a neurovascular injury. Bilateral rib fractures imply a major transmediastinal force, which can be associated with injuries to the heart, great vessels and trachea.

Pulmonary injury

Pulmonary contusion is associated with all rib injuries. If contusion is extensive, the lung becomes consolidated causing impaired blood and gas exchange. A penetrating pulmonary injury (even by fractured rib ends) may produce a haemopneumothorax. Massive rates of air loss suggest a bronchial injury.

Treatment

Treatment depends on the severity of the injury:

- uncomplicated rib fractures
  - oral analgesia with or without intercostal nerve block
  - physiotherapy
  - monitor arterial saturation, blood gases
- flail segment, major chest injury
  - as for uncomplicated injury
  - may need positive pressure ventilation
- penetrating injury (e.g. stab wound)
  - intercostal drainage and observation
  - thoracotomy if bleeding is >150 ml/h or >1 l initially (bleeding is usually from chest wall vessels)
- major airway injury
  - immediate thoracotomy and repair.

Cardiovascular injury

Great vessel injury This is usually associated with a transmediastinal or a deceleration injury. The aorta and subclavian vessels are most often affected. Injury to the subclavian vessels and brachial plexus can follow fractures to the first rib. Decreased pulse pressure and perfusion are evident in the affected limb with a soft tissue swelling in the supraclavicular area. There may be sensorimotor abnormalities.

Cardiac injury This should be considered in blunt sternal fractures or penetrating anterior chest wounds. Sternal fractures are often the sequel to a seat belt injury. Myocardial contusion may be present. Clinical features are similar to right ventricular infarction, with reduced cardiac output and elevated venous pressure. All patients with a fractured sternum should be admitted for observation. The management of any underlying myocardial contusion is supportive, as with myocardial infarction. Penetrating wounds cause cardiac tamponade (see p. 256).

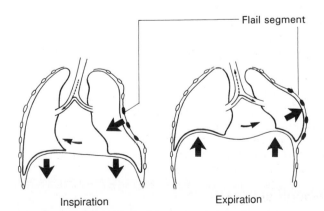

Figure 183 Flail segment. Movement of the mediastinum and paradoxical motion of the flail segment in a patient with flail chest injury.

Inspiration   Expiration

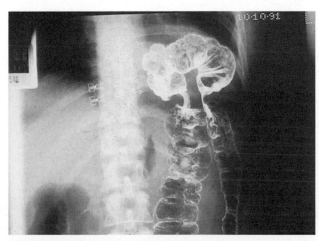

Figure 184 Traumatic diaphragmatic hernia.

Diaphragmatic rupture

Abdominal squash injuries lead to a sudden bursting pressure that may cause diaphragmatic rupture. The patient complains of dyspnoea, air entry is decreased and bowel sounds may be audible in the chest.

Diagnosis

Investigation involves:

- chest radiograph: may show bowel loops in chest
- ultrasound: may confirm diagnosis.

Treatment

Repair is undertaken via a thoracotomy; associated injuries to the viscera should be sought. Sometimes the diagnosis is missed and patients present years later with symptoms referable to bowel herniation into the chest (Figure 184).

Self-assessment: questions

Multiple choice questions

1. Factors contributing to the development of coronary artery disease include:
   a. hypertension
   b. family history of ischaemic heart disease
   c. diabetes mellitus
   d. hyperlipidaemia
   e. smoking

2. Coronary artery bypass surgery improves survival in:
   a. severely symptomatic patients
   b. patients with three-vessel coronary artery disease
   c. patients with a strong family history of coronary artery disease
   d. patients with impaired ventricular function
   e. patients with left main stem disease

3. Coronary artery bypass may be performed using:
   a. the internal mammary artery
   b. a synthetic small calibre graft
   c. the long saphenous vein
   d. the short saphenous vein
   e. the right gastroepiploic artery

4. Mechanical heart valves:
   a. require anticoagulation
   b. are liable to infection
   c. last for about 6–14 years
   d. are most commonly implanted in the UK for rheumatic heart valve disease
   e. are relatively obstructive to blood flow

5. Causes of thoracic aortic aneurysm include:
   a. hypertension
   b. atheroma
   c. syphilis
   d. age
   e. Marfan's syndrome

6. Atrial septal defect:
   a. causes increased pulmonary blood flow
   b. characteristically causes cyanosis
   c. is associated with a pulmonary ejection flow murmur and a fixed split second heart sound
   d. is a complication of myocardial infarction
   e. can be associated with mitral regurgitation

7. Bronchial carcinoma:
   a. is most commonly a small cell carcinoma histologically
   b. spreads via the bloodstream to the brain, adrenals and bone
   c. is often an asymptomatic finding on a chest radiograph
   d. is always associated with clubbing
   e. may result in a normal chest radiograph

8. In the management of bronchial carcinoma:
   a. surgery is only suitable for patients with malignant disease confined to the ipsilateral lung
   b. lung resection is only feasible if FEV_1 (forced expiratory volume in 1 s) is >1 l
   c. radiotherapy produces the best results
   d. survival after surgical resection depends on tumour size and node status
   e. a small cell carcinoma is always best managed by chemotherapy

9. Spontaneous pneumothorax:
   a. occurs in two different patient age groups
   b. can cause mediastinal deviation and compression of the contralateral lung
   c. if suspected, should always be confirmed by chest radiography prior to treatment
   d. is best managed by immediate pleurectomy
   e. is usually associated with structural abnormalities of the lung

10. In patients with pleural effusion:
    a. surgically relevant cases are usually unilateral
    b. a sample of pleural fluid should be sent for culture and microscopy
    c. an intercostal drain should be inserted
    d. sclerosants are useful in malignant cases
    e. surgical exploration and biopsy may be necessary

11. An empyema:
    a. is an intrapleural collection of pus
    b. tends to occur at the apex of the chest
    c. commonly follows an episode of pneumonia
    d. is always pulmonary in origin
    e. is best managed by decortication in all cases

12. In patients with multiple rib fractures:
    a. an associated pneumothorax should be excluded
    b. pulmonary contusion always occurs
    c. splenic and renal injuries may be present
    d. artificial ventilation may be required
    e. surgical repair of ribs is helpful

Extended matching items questions (EMIs)

EMI 1
Theme: Cardiothoracic emergencies

A. primary pneumothorax
B. secondary pneumothorax

C. empyema

D. right flail chest

E. aortic dissection

F. left diaphragmatic rupture

G. right pleural effusion

I. right tension pneumothorax

J. haemothorax

K. left tension pneumothorax

For each of the following patients select the most likely diagnosis from above:

1. A 26-year-old marathon runner collapses during a training session. He is rushed to the nearest A&E department. On arrival he is cyanosed and hypotensive. His trachea is deviated to the right and he has diminished breath sounds in his left hemithorax.

2. A 56-year-old woman with a long history of hypertension is admitted with severe chest pain and collapse. She has a normal ECG. A chest radiograph shows a widened mediastinum with a small left pleural effusion.

3. A 70-year-old man with long-standing chronic obstructive airway disease and emphysema self-presents in his local casualty department with a sudden increase in breathlessness. He is afebrile and the casualty officer notes a hyper-resonant left hemithorax with reduced breath sounds. There is no tracheal deviation.

4. A 66-year-old woman is admitted after being treated at home for pneumonia. Her GP has given her a 1-week course of antibiotics. Her condition has not improved and she complains of increasing breathlessness. On examination she has diminished air entry in the right lung base and over a period of 24 h observation her temperature has fluctuated widely. Her chest radiograph shows an opaque right lung base with obliteration of the costophrenic angle.

EMI 2

Theme: Heart valve implants

A. high risk of endocarditic infection

B. silent

C. require lifelong anticoagulation

D. will wear out

E. excellent haemodynamics

F. audible

G. do not require anticoagulation

H. can cause haemolysis

I. will usually last a lifetime

From the above list pick out the features that are characteristic of the following heart valves (one or more of the features may be correct for each type of valve):

1. Cadaveric human valve tissue

2. Mechanical heart valves

3. Porcine valve tissue.

Constructed response questions (CRQs)

CRQ 1

A 57-year-old male patient with a 3-year history of chronic stable angina presents with worsening symptoms despite maximal medical therapy. An exercise ECG demonstrates widespread ischaemic changes at a low exercise level. Cardiac catheterisation reveals significant stenoses in the right coronary artery, the left anterior descending coronary artery and the circumflex coronary artery, with good distal vessels and good left ventricular function. Surgery is discussed with the patient.

a. What probability of relief of symptoms could he be offered?

b. Would he derive any survival benefit from surgery?

c. What risks would he face with surgery?

d. What likely combination of conduits would be used to construct his coronary artery grafts?

CRQ 2

A 73-year-old previously fit male patient is admitted to hospital through the casualty department having sustained a syncopal episode. He has a past history of a 'murmur' noted at medical examination many years ago. On examination, he has recovered completely but a slow rising pulse and an apex beat that is deviated to the left are discovered. A loud ejection systolic murmur is audible, best heard in the second right interspace and radiating to the neck.

a. What is the probable diagnosis?

b. What would be the likely results of a chest radiograph and ECG?

c. What other investigations would be relevant?

d. What treatment would you recommend?

e. What risks would you quote to the patient regarding treatment?

CRQ 3

A 64-year-old woman is brought to the casualty department having collapsed with severe chest pain radiating through to her back. There is a past history of hypertension. She complains of weakness in the left limbs and a cold right arm. On examination she is sweaty, distressed and has a tachycardia of 115 beats/min. Her right radial pulse is very weak and the right arm blood pressure is 80/60 mmHg compared with the left arm pressure of 160/60 mmHg. An early diastolic murmur is audible.

a. What is the most likely diagnosis?

b. Why does she have reduced pulse pressure in the right arm and left-sided neurological symptoms?

c. What investigations would you order?

d. Why might she have an aortic diastolic murmur?

e. What are the treatment options for this condition and which would apply in this case?

CRQ 4

An 18-year-old motorcyclist is admitted to the casualty department following a road traffic accident in which he was thrown from his bike. On examination he is semiconscious but moving all limbs and has shallow respiration. His pulse is 100 beats/min of moderate volume and his blood pressure is 95/60 mmHg. He is tender over the left chest and pelvis. There is an obvious compound fracture of the left lower leg. Chest radiography shows multiple rib fractures, a widened mediastinum, left pleural fluid and a right pneumothorax; skull radiography shows no fractures; and pelvic radiography shows a left fractured pubic ramus. His leg radiograph confirms a fractured left tibia and fibula.

a. What intrathoracic injury would you suspect?

b. How would you investigate this?

c. Would you wish to perform any procedure prior to further investigation?

d. What therapy would be appropriate if the investigation is positive?

e. What warning should be given to the patient's family?

CRQ 5

An 18-year-old man is admitted collapsed to the casualty department having been stabbed in the anterior left fifth interspace adjacent to the left sternal edge. On examination he smells strongly of alcohol and is drowsy, irritable and uncooperative. He has shallow respiration at a rate of 20 beats/min. He has a tachycardia of 130 beats/min with a very low pulse volume and a blood pressure of 70/60 mmHg. His venous pressure is elevated to his ear lobes.

a. What is the likely diagnosis?

b. What form of treatment is required?

CRQ 6

A 64-year-old male patient complains of cough, haemoptysis and weight loss. He has noticed some aching joints over the preceding weeks. He has a 40-year history of smoking 25 cigarettes per day and has mild stable angina for which he has occasional nitrate therapy. He admits to long-standing mild shortness of breath on exertion. On examination he is clubbed and has slightly swollen fingers, but there are no other findings. A postero-anterior chest radiograph shows a 6-cm mass in the right upper zone, which is confirmed on a lateral radiograph to lie in the upper lobe.

a. What is the presumptive diagnosis?

b. What is the likely cause of his joint symptoms?

c. What further radiological investigation would you order and why?

d. What diagnostic procedures could you try?

e. If surgery is to be considered, what further assessment procedures would be necessary?

CRQ 7

A 69-year-old woman is admitted to the medical unit with pneumonia. She has been a lifelong smoker and has mild bronchitis but is otherwise independent and fit. Her chest radiograph shows shrinkage and consolidation of the entire left lung. Her systemic symptoms improve with antibiotic therapy and she is mobile but not breathless when up and about in the hospital. Her chest radiograph remains unchanged and her respiratory function tests show an FEV_1 of 1 l compared with a predicted value of 1.6 l for her size and age. Her gas transfer tests are approximately 66% of the predicted values.

a. What is bronchoscopy likely to show?

b. What possible choice of therapy is available?

c. Would her respiratory function tests influence your decision?

d. What would you advise her regarding further tests prior to therapy?

e. What would you say to her regarding her survival prospects?

CRQ 8

A 19-year-old male student is admitted to the casualty department as an emergency. He is acutely short of breath and has difficulty speaking. He experienced a sudden onset of right chest pain whilst bending over to pick up a book and rapidly developed severe difficulty with breathing and felt faint. A friend called an ambulance. There is a past history of a small left spontaneous pneumothorax, which was treated by observation alone 2 years ago. On examination he is tachypnoeic, centrally cyanosed and in distress. His pulse is 120 beats/min and his blood pressure 85/60 mmHg. His trachea and apex beat are displaced to the left and his right chest is hyper-resonant with absent breath sounds.

a. What condition would you diagnose?

b. What immediate action should you take?

c. What subsequent actions should you take?

d. What long-term treatment should be considered and what would you advise as the optimum treatment?

e. How would you explain this emergency?

267

CRQ 9

A 66-year-old woman was initially admitted to a medical unit some 3 weeks previously with a right lower lobe pneumonia. This was treated with intravenous antibiotics and her symptoms resolved over several days, but a right basal effusion was noted to evolve. This appeared to be reducing and aspiration 3 days after her admission revealed only straw-coloured fluid. She was discharged to convalescence but readmitted 3 days ago with a spiking fever and general malaise. She has been off her food for a week and her condition is generally deteriorating. She has a neutrophil leucocytosis. Her chest radiograph shows a large postero-basal collection in the right pleural cavity. Repeat aspiration reveals frank pus.

a. What is the diagnosis?

b. What are the possible causes and how might you separate them?

c. What initial treatment is necessary?

d. What long-term management would be appropriate in her case?

Objective structured clinical examination questions (OSCEs)

OSCE 1

a. What does this radiograph (Figure 185) show?

b. What possible complication could result?

c. What investigations would be relevant?

d. What treatment is appropriate?

OSCE 2 (see Figure 186)

a. What is this device?

b. What general principles apply to the use of this device?

c. How do you connect it once it has been utilised?

OSCE 3

A 44-year-old man presents to his GP with headaches and is found to have severe hypertension (blood pressure 180/120 mmHg) and reduced and delayed femoral pulses.

a. What abnormality is seen on the chest radiograph (Figure 187)?

b. What is the diagnosis?

c. What form of treatment is required?

d. Will this cure his hypertension?

OSCE 4

A 58-year-old man is involved in a road traffic accident and sustains blunt trauma to his upper abdomen. He complains of shortness of breath.

a. What abnormality is evident on the chest radiograph (Figure 188)?

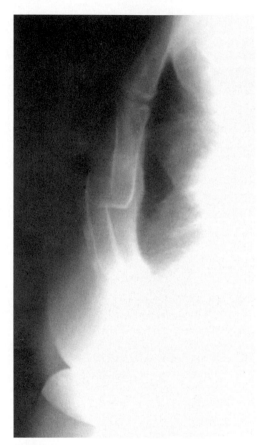

Figure 185

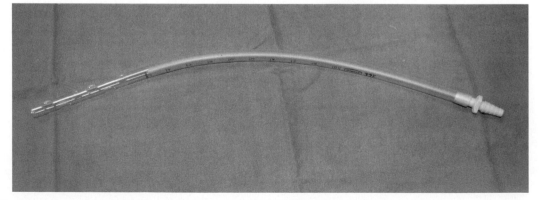

Figure 186

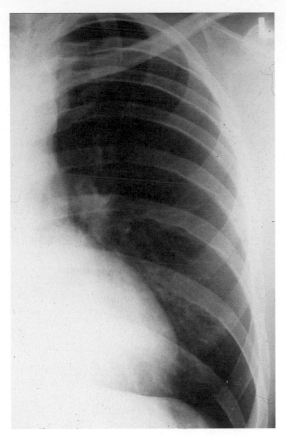

Figure 187

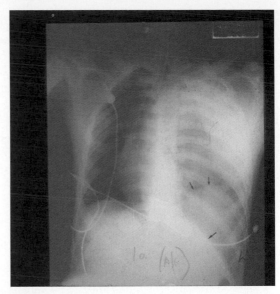

Figure 188

b. What is the diagnosis?

c. What other organ injury may exist?

d. What treatment is required?

OSCE 5

A 24-year old man is admitted to the casualty department with acute left chest pain and severe shortness of breath.

a. What abnormality is seen on the chest radiograph (Figure 189)?

b. What immediate treatment is necessary?

c. What long-term treatment is required?

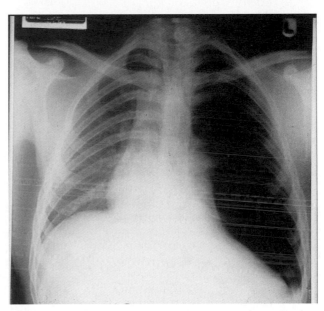

Figure 189

Self-assessment: answers

Multiple choice answers

1. a–e. **True.** These are the most important risk factors for coronary artery disease.

2. a. **False.** Although patients with severe symptoms require urgent bypass surgery, the effect of surgery on survival is determined by the pattern of disease that is present.
   b. **True.** Three-vessel disease is an index of extensive disease.
   c. **False.** The effect on survival is determined by the pattern of disease that is present.
   d. **True.** Survival is improved, particularly if left ventricular function is impaired before surgery.
   e. **True.** Left main stem disease is an index of extensive disease.

3. a, c–e. **True.** These are the most frequently used coronary artery grafts.
   b. **False.** Artificial grafts do not remain patent.

4. a. **True.** Because they are made from synthetic materials.
   b. **True.** Endocarditic infection is always a potential risk. Antibiotic prophylaxis is essential in patients undergoing invasive surgical or dental procedures.
   c. **False.** Mechanical heart valves should last indefinitely; bioprosthetic valves have a lifespan of 6–14 years.
   d. **False.** Because of the fall in incidence of rheumatic fever, surgery for rheumatic valve disease is no longer the most common reason for valve replacement. Its place has been taken by bicuspid calcific aortic stenosis.
   e. **True.** Compared with a human valve, all prosthetic valves restrict blood flow.

5. a–c, e. **True.** These are the main causes of a thoracic aortic aneurysm.
   d. **False.** Age is not causative, although advancing age is often associated with aneurysm development.

6. a. **True.** The left to right shunt increases pulmonary blood flow.
   b. **False.** Atrial septal defects only rarely cause cyanosis. This usually occurs late in adult life when long-standing pulmonary hypertension may cause shunt reversal as the pulmonary artery pressure begins to exceed the systemic pressure (Eisenmenger syndrome).
   c. **True.** These are classic features of an atrial septal defect.

d. **False.** A ventricular septal defect is a complication of myocardial infarction.
   e. **True.**

7. a. **False.** The most common type is a squamous cell carcinoma.
   b. **True.** Together with the liver, these are the most common sites of haematogenous spread.
   c. **True.** A routine chest radiograph may reveal the disease unexpectedly.
   d. **False.** Clubbing is not always present and may result from other causes.
   e. **True.** Occasionally the chest radiograph may be clear, with the diagnosis being made on bronchoscopy or sputum cytology.

8. a. **True.** Contralateral malignant disease represents metastatic disease and, therefore, surgery is contraindicated.
   b. **False.** The minimum acceptable FEV_1 varies according to the patient's predicted value, pulmonary gas transfer and the extent of functioning lung to be removed.
   c. **False.** The results of radiotherapy are not as good as those of surgery.
   d. **True.** Along with histological type, these are the key factors that predict outcome.
   e. **False.** Most cases of small cell carcinoma present at an advanced stage and are managed by chemotherapy. The few cases that are caught at an early stage are better resected.

9. a. **True.** Primary pneumothorax affects young patients with grossly normal lungs apart from apical air blisters. Secondary pneumothorax occurs in an elderly age group with underlying lung disease and usually large bullae.
   b. **True.** This is the hallmark of a tension pneumothorax.
   c. **False.** In patients with a tension pneumothorax, any delay (as in waiting for a radiograph) may cause death from cardiorespiratory embarrassment. Urgent chest drainage may be needed. The decision to perform radiography or not depends on the clinical assessment of severity.
   d. **False.** Surgery is reserved for young patients with a recurrent or bilateral tension pneumothorax or for those whose occupation makes a pneumothorax especially dangerous.
   e. **True.** Usually apical air blebs or bullae.

10. a. **True.** Bilateral effusions are usually medical in origin, e.g. cardiac failure, uraemia.
    b. **True.** This is a key analytical step.
    c. **True.** Intercostal drainage provides symptomatic relief and a large volume of fluid for analysis. A

post-drainage chest radiograph may reveal previously hidden underlying pathology.

d. **True.** They may prevent reaccumulation of a malignant effusion.

e. **True.** Surgical exploration is normally achieved by 'thoracoscopy'. Occasionally, a minithoracotomy is needed to obtain a pleural biopsy.

11. a. **True.** The pus collects within the pleural space.

b. **False.** An empyema develops as a basal or posteromedial collection under the influence of gravity.

c. **True.** Pneumonia or a lung abscess are the most common underlying causes of empyema.

d. **False.** Although most are pulmonary in origin, other important causes include oesophageal leak, subphrenic and liver abscesses, surgery and repeated pleural aspiration.

e. **False.** This is the procedure of choice in a young fit patient. In others, tube drainage may be adequate.

12. a. **True.** The fractured rib ends may puncture the lung parenchyma and cause an air leak.

b. **True.** Contusion is inevitable if the injury force is sufficient to cause multiple rib fractures.

c. **True.** The spleen is an anterior relation of the left rib cage. Injuries of sufficient force to cause multiple rib fractures may also be sufficient to produce major visceral injury.

d. **True.** Patients with a large flail segment or deteriorating gas exchange may require positive pressure ventilation.

e. **False.** Surgical repair of rib fractures has been abandoned in favour of ventilation.

EMI answers

EMI 1

Theme: Cardiothoracic emergencies

1. K. A tension pneumothorax is a dire emergency and causes the deaths of many young people each year. In addition to respiratory difficulty, the mediastinal shift may cause significant embarrassment of venous return and hence cardiac output. In this case, the patient has a left tension pneumothorax that pushes the mediastinum and trachea over to the right. The diminished gas exchange and reduced venous return cause cyanosis. Initial treatment is to insert a large-bore (14-guage) needle into the left chest. This will return the pneumothorax to a non-tension state, improve the patient's condition and allow elective insertion of a chest drain in a stabilised patient.

2. E. This history includes some of the key features of an aortic dissection. The patient is hypertensive – one of the three risk factors for aortic dissection – and has the classic history of severe chest pain and collapse coupled with a normal

ECG. The chest radiograph displays the typical features of dissection (a widened mediastinum and left pleural effusion) and the diagnosis would be confirmed either by an i.v. contrast CT scan or aortography.

3. B. A secondary pneumothorax usually develops in an older patient with underlying lung disease. These patients are more likely to have an air leak that does not respond to simple drainage and have a raised mortality because of pneumonia and cardiovascular problems.

4. C. An empyema is an intrapleural collection of pus that is usually a consequence of pneumonia, as in this case. This patient has several additional features that are typical of empyema – a swinging fever and an effusion on her chest radiograph. The diagnosis would be clinched by a needle aspiration in her right base.

EMI 2

Theme: Heart valve implants

1. B, D, E, G. These valves are silent, will wear out, have excellent haemodynamics and do not require anticoagulation.

2. A, C, F, H, I. These valves have a high risk of endocarditic infection, require lifelong anticoagulation, are audible, can cause haemolysis and will usually last a lifetime.

3. A, B, D, G, H. These valves have a high risk of endocarditic infection, are silent, will wear out, do not require anticoagulation and can cause haemolysis.

There are advantages and disadvantages of each type of implant. The choice will be dictated by issues such as the need to avoid warfarin therapy – for example in a young woman who requires surgery but who may wish to become pregnant later and avoid the teratogenic affects of warfarin – or the wish to avoid surgery in later life. In the latter case, patients may prefer to opt for a mechanical prosthesis.

CRQ answers

CRQ 1

a. He would have an 80% chance of being symptom free at 1 year and a 15–20% chance of having residual but improved symptoms. He should be told that symptoms recur at a rate of about 5% per year.

b. This patient has three-vessel disease and would be likely to gain a survival advantage with surgery.

c. He should be told that there is an operative mortality rate of 2% and a risk of cerebrovascular accident of up to 3%. As with all surgical patients, the possibility of wound infection and postoperative pulmonary infection exists. Deep venous thrombosis is remarkably infrequent after coronary artery surgery and is an insignificant risk. Many patients experience considerable discomfort from the leg vein donor site, sometimes added to by injury to the saphenous nerve, which causes numbness on the medial aspect of the lower leg and front of the foot.

d. Unless there were contraindications, it would be customary for him to have an internal mammary graft to the left anterior descending coronary artery and saphenous vein grafts to the right and circumflex coronary arteries.

CRQ 2

a. He is likely to have had a syncopal episode associated with severe aortic stenosis, resulting from a dysrhythmic episode. A cerebrovascular accident can be ruled out by the fact that he has no lasting disability. It is possible that he had a transient ischaemic episode; however, this is unlikely because some residual cerebral disturbance usually persists for a few hours after the event.

b. The chest radiograph would show an enlarged ventricular outline and might show valvular calcification. The ECG would probably be in sinus rhythm with evidence of left ventricular hypertrophy and strain.

c. Echocardiography and cardiac catheterisation should be performed. Echocardiography using Doppler can provide an estimate of the aortic valve gradient. Cardiac catheterisation would quantify the gradient and demonstrate the presence of any concurrent coronary artery disease.

d. Aortic valve replacement should be undertaken urgently in any patient with significant aortic stenosis and syncope.

e. Operative mortality would be about 4% and the risk of a cerebrovascular accident should be discussed.

CRQ 3

a. Aortic dissection should be considered in any patient with a history of collapse and acute chest pain radiating to the back. The principle differential diagnosis is myocardial infarction. Other possibilities include a leaking aortic aneurysm, oesophageal rupture and thoracic vertebral collapse.

b. In this patient, the false lumen of the dissection process has closed down the brachiocephalic artery, the first of the three aortic arch vessels, and has, therefore, interrupted flow into the right subclavian artery and right common carotid artery. This manifests as decreased arm perfusion and contralateral weakness resulting from decreased cerebral perfusion.

c. She should have an urgent contrast-enhanced CT scan to confirm the diagnosis. This investigation may also allow the radiologist to comment on the dissection entry site. Aortography will usually demonstrate this and also which femoral artery is connected to the true aortic lumen. This is important information as the patient will have to be perfused

retrogradely via a femoral artery during surgical repair.

d. This patient probably has damage extending into the aortic root. Separation of the aortic wall layers often occurs at this level.

e. Treatment is principally determined by which section of the aorta is involved. In this case, surgery is required to replace the entry point and the damaged proximal aorta. It is likely that this patient would need replacement of the ascending aorta and aortic arch and possibly also the aortic valve.

CRQ 4

a. With the nature of the accident and the combination of thoracic rib-cage injury, widened mediastinum and left pleural effusion, a ruptured thoracic aorta must be suspected.

b. Aortography is the investigation of choice.

c. The pneumothorax is an immediately life-threatening condition and an intercostal drain should be inserted before embarking on further investigation.

d. Urgent left thoracotomy and synthetic graft replacement of the ruptured portion of the aorta would be appropriate therapy.

e. They should be aware that (apart from the risk of death if the aorta ruptures completely before completion of surgery) there is a 5% risk of paraplegia associated with this procedure.

CRQ 5

a. The likely diagnosis is cardiac tamponade.

b. Emergency surgery is required to drain the pericardial collection and to allow the cardiac injury to be repaired. If surgical facilities or expertise are not immediately available, the tamponade may be transiently improved by aspirating the pericardium (pericardiocentesis). This is not always a good option because the heart may be further damaged by the manoeuvre. Also, it does not remove pericardial clots and fresh bleeding will continue to occur.

CRQ 6

a. The presumptive diagnosis is bronchogenic carcinoma.

b. The likely cause of the joint symptoms is hypertrophic pulmonary osteoarthropathy.

c. A contrast-enhanced CT scan should be performed. This would establish whether there were any lesions in the other lung and would screen the liver and adrenal glands for metastatic disease. Any enlarged mediastinal glands would also be detected.

d. Sputum cytology, bronchoscopy and fine needle aspiration.

e. If there are any abnormalities in plasma calcium, phosphate or alkaline phosphatase levels, a bone scan should be arranged. A liver ultrasound scan would be a useful complement to the initial CT. Mediastinoscopy would be needed to confirm that the mediastinal glands are free of disease. Preoperative respiratory function tests, arterial blood gas estimation and cardiac assessment by ECG and echocardiography would be helpful in determining the patient's ability to tolerate surgery.

CRQ 7

a. Bronchoscopy is likely to show a lesion obstructing the left main bronchus, as neither lobe is aerated. This could result from inspissated secretions or even a foreign body but is most likely caused by a tumour.

b. Secretions or a foreign body would need to be removed. A tumour would have to be further staged with consideration given to either radiotherapy or surgery.

c. No, the left lung is totally non-functional at present and so her respiratory function tests are largely irrelevant. She will still have a small residual right to left shunt through the left lung and pneumonectomy would, therefore, actually improve her respiratory status.

d. She will need a mediastinoscopy, screening for metastatic disease and assessment of her cardiac status to enable a decision to be made.

e. Radiotherapy would be palliative and probably increase survival by 8–12 months at best. If the lesion is removable surgically, survival would depend upon tumour stage and final cell type (cell type in the tumour mass does not always correlate with that reported in a biopsy).

CRQ 8

a. The diagnosis would be a tension right pneumothorax.

b. One or two large-calibre intravenous cannulae (14-gauge or below) should be inserted into the right chest to depressurise the tension element of the pneumothorax.

c. He requires an intercostal drain and a chest radiograph to verify re-expansion of the right lung.

d. He should have a procedure to achieve pleurodesis of the right lung. There are two reasons for this: first, this was a tension pneumothorax, which is life-threatening; and, second, he has had a contralateral pneumothorax, which would make pleurodesis desirable in any event. A right pleurectomy would be the procedure with the highest long-term success rate and this would allow the lung to be inspected for blebs or bullae that could be ligated at the same time.

c. The right lung has leaked air through a flap valve mechanism, probably in an apical bleb. This process allows air to be pumped into the right pleural cavity causing the lung to be totally flattened and the mediastinum to be displaced to the left. The left lung becomes compressed and cardiac output is reduced as the great vessels become distorted.

CRQ 9

a. The diagnosis is empyema.

b. This is most likely to be postpneumonic but it could result from contamination of her right basal effusion at the time of the initial aspiration. Some clue would be obtained from the organism grown from the empyema; for example, staphylococci are a frequent contaminant (unless the original pneumonia was staphylococcal in origin). Sometimes, a mixed culture of organisms will be obtained.

c. She should have a chest drain inserted into the collection to provide drainage and relieve her toxic symptoms.

d. Rib resection and open tube drainage would be the likely long-term management in someone of her age.

OSCE answers

OSCE 1

a. A fractured sternum

b. Cardiac contusion

c. The consequences of cardiac contusion are similar to those of myocardial infarction. It would be appropriate to obtain a 12-lead ECG to look for ST-segment elevation. Serial creatinine kinase enzyme assays should also be obtained as an indicator of myocardial damage. In some instances when there are features of cardiac embarrassment, a transthoracic echo may identify an akinetic area of myocardium, a pericardial effusion or, rarely, a localised ventricular rupture.

d. Treatment is supportive. Pain relief and physiotherapy are the most common requirements. If myocardial damage has occurred, it may be helpful to provide supportive therapy including inotropic agents; if a large pericardial effusion develops, aspiration may be required. Myocardial rupture is an exceptionally rare complication that would require emergency (and probably unsuccessful) surgery.

OSCE 2

a. This is an intercostal drain catheter, i.e. a 'chest drain'.

b. The general principles are as follows. The drain is inserted into the upper chest to drain air and into the lower chest to drain fluid. In either case, the insertion technique involves aseptic technique and the infiltration of local anaesthetic (e.g. 15 ml of lignocaine 1%) into the skin, subcutaneous tissue, muscle and pleura overlying the intended insertion site. The drain is most conveniently placed in the anterior axillary line so that the pectoral muscle is avoided. The two most important principles are:

(i) to make sure that air and/or fluid is beneath the intended entry site as anticipated by preliminary needle aspiration and (ii) to ensure that the drain will enter the pleural cavity by first inserting a finger tip to ensure that the lung is not adherent and that the pleural cavity has, in fact, been entered.

c. The drain should be connected to an underwater seal drain. In its simplest form this involves connecting the drain tube to a tube that lies in water about 5 cm below the surface. This system uses hydraulic principles to provide a one-way valve system that offers little resistance to the expulsion of air or fluid from the chest but prevents reflux of atmospheric air up the tube back into the chest. Alternatively, a 'flutter' valve may be used. This is useful in out-of-hospital situations and basically comprises a one-way valve system that is created using a thin rubber tube with a slit end. The slit end is kept flat by atmospheric air pressure but will allow drainage of chest fluid or air expelled under pressure, e.g. by a tension pneumothorax.

OSCE 3

a. The chest radiograph shows rib notching.

b. Coarctation of the aorta.

c. Left thoracotomy and construction of a bypass graft to take blood around the coarctation.

d. No. The bypass graft will result in a lower blood pressure but the patient will remain hypertensive. The response to drug therapy is much better after bypass of the coarctation.

OSCE 4

a. Opacification of the left chest with air fluid levels suggestive of bowel loops.

b. Ruptured diaphragm.

c. Spleen (which was also ruptured in this case).

d. Thoracotomy, splenectomy, if necessary, and repair of the diaphragm.

OSCE 5

a. Tension left pneumothorax.

b. Insertion of a chest drain; a large-calibre i.v. cannula may be required to relieve the tension while this is being prepared.

c. Left pleurodesis, probably by pleurectomy with ligation of any pulmonary blebs.

Urology

Chapter overview

Disease of the urinary tract accounts for a substantial proportion of primary care consultations and emergency and elective surgical admissions. The central role of the urinary system is the maintenance of fluid and electrolyte balance by the kidneys. The ureters, bladder and urethra together are responsible for continent storage and disposal of urine. Knowledge of the structure and function of the urinary system, the congenital anomalies of structure that may exist and the symptoms with which urinary disorders present is essential to understanding urinary tract disease. The most important disorders of the urinary system are infection, urinary stones, urinary tract obstruction, disorders of urine storage and malignant tumours.

13.1 Structure and function of the urinary tract

Learning objectives

You should:
- have a clear understanding of the anatomy of the urinary tract
- be able to relate this to function and dysfunction
- be aware of important congenital structural anomalies and their effects on function.

Kidneys

The two kidneys lie against the posterior abdominal wall musculature in a retroperitoneal position, flanking the abdominal aorta and vena cava. Important anatomical relations include the adrenals, the duodenum, the retroperitoneal colon, the spleen and the liver. The kidneys receive a very substantial blood supply – about 20% of the cardiac output. The functional renal unit is the *nephron*, each consisting of glomerular vessels and Bowman's capsule, the vasa recta and the renal tubule. There are about one million nephrons per kidney. Filtration of blood at the glomerulus followed by selective reabsorption and secretion of certain electrolytes and solutes by the renal tubule results in the production of urine.

The *renal parenchyma* is in two parts: the *cortex* consists of the glomeruli, the convoluted parts of the tubules and the short tubular loops (of Henle); the *medulla* consists of the long loops of Henle and the collecting tubules, which are grouped together to form the renal pyramids (Figure 190). The collecting system of the kidneys is formed by the calyces (each calyx cupping one or more renal papillae) and the renal pelvis.

Important congenital anomalies:

- renal agenesis or hypoplasia
- simple or crossed ectopia
- infantile polycystic disease
- adult polycystic disease
- horseshoe kidney.

Ureters

The ureters are completely retroperitoneal in their course. Important bony landmarks of the normal course of the ureters are the tips of the transverse processes of the lumbar vertebrae, the sacroiliac joints and the ischial spines. The ureters transport urine to the bladder by peristalsis, and reflux of urine from the bladder is normally prevented by a valvular mechanism at the vesicoureteric junction.

Important congenital abnormalities:

- pelviureteric junction obstruction
- complete or incomplete ureteric duplication
- vesicoureteric reflux
- megaureter.

Bladder

The empty bladder lies within the true pelvis but rises into the abdomen with filling. The bladder provides a highly compliant reservoir for urine, with the internal pressure rising only very slightly during normal filling and not normally exceeding urethral pressure except during voluntary voiding. Like the ureter and the pelvicalyceal system of the kidney, the bladder is lined with a transitional cell epithelium.

An *important congenital abnormality* of the bladder is extrophy, in which the anterior abdominal wall, anterior bony pelvis and bladder fail to close properly.

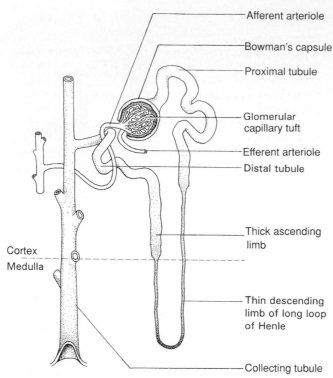

Afferent arteriole

Bowman's capsule

Proximal tubule

Glomerular capillary tuft

Efferent arteriole

Distal tubule

Cortex
Medulla

Thick ascending limb

Thin descending limb of long loop of Henle

Collecting tubule

Figure 190 A nephron.

Prostate

The prostate is a male organ that has no normal female counterpart. It is a pale firm structure, part muscular and part glandular, lying posterior to the lower part of the symphysis pubis at the neck of the bladder where it surrounds the proximal part of the urethra (the prostatic urethra). The fibromuscular part of the gland is complex and is concerned with seminal emission, ejaculation and urinary continence. The prostate also has an exocrine secretory function, which is incompletely understood.

Urethra

The proximal urethra and bladder neck form part of the continence mechanism.
Congenital anomalies (of the male urethra):

- posterior urethral valve, which causes bladder outflow obstruction in men
- hypospadius, where the ventral part of the anterior urethra fails to close properly.

Testis

Although strictly not part of the urinary tract, disorders of the male gonad and its associated structures, the epididymis and vas deferens, are considered part of urology.

The most *important congenital disorders* are those of infant hydrocele and maldescent. Two main types of maldescent are recognised:

- incomplete descent: the testis is arrested at some point in the normal path of descent
- ectopic testis: the testis has left the normal path of descent.

13.2 Urinary symptoms

Voiding symptoms

Patients may admit to having difficulties passing urine:

- poor flow: stream is prolonged and weak
- hesitancy: there is a delay before stream begins
- feeling of incomplete bladder emptying.

Storage symptoms

Patients may complain of:

- urgency: the urgent need to pass urine
- frequency: increased frequency of passing urine during the day
- nocturia: the need to get up to pass urine at night.

Pain

Dysuria Lower urinary tract pain during or just after voiding, which suggests inflammation in the bladder or urethra.

Loin pain Renal or ureteric pain may radiate to the scrotum, whereas testicular pain may radiate to the loin.

Ureteric colic The pain is very severe and the patient cannot remain still.

Incontinence of urine

Involuntary loss of urine:

- may be due to bladder outlet and pelvic floor weakness, provoked by factors that abruptly increase abdominal pressure – ask about coughing, sneezing, running, etc; this is suggestive of *stress incontinence*
- may be due to bladder over-activity (*urge incontinence*) – ask about frequency and urgency of micturition and leakage associated with a desperate urge to pass urine, which may be provoked by standing up, the sound of or contact with water or putting the key in the front door
- may be continuous, dribbling, insensible (no urge to void) – suggestive of fistula, or *overflow incontinence*, especially if wet at night.

Haematuria: blood in the urine

Haematuria may be:

- *painless* or accompanied by abdominal or flank pain or pain while voiding
- *microscopic* (undetectable to the naked eye)

- *frank*: blood can be seen with the naked eye and clots may also be seen (bladder pathology is more likely to be found).

If haematuria is frank, it may be *initial* (blood is seen only in the first part of the stream), *terminal* (blood is seen in the last part of the stream) or *total* (blood is seen throughout the stream). Initial and terminal haematuria suggest that the bleeding has occurred distal to the kidneys, possibly from the urethra or bladder neck. *Urethral* bleeding, where blood passes from the urethral meatus when urine has not been voided, can usually be distinguished from true haematuria.

13.3 Urinary tract infection

Learning objectives

You should:
- appreciate how the site and extent of urine infection influences symptoms and severity
- understand how to treat the acute episode
- be able to appropriately investigate the cause and advise on preventative measures.

Urinary infection

Bacterial infection in the urinary tract is common. It may be localised (cystitis, epididymitis) or may pass along the urinary tract as a diffuse urinary infection. The effects depend on the extent and site of infection and range from asymptomatic to life-threatening.

Acute bacterial cystitis

Occasional infection of the bladder urine occurs in otherwise healthy women but, in men and children, some other urinary abnormality is likely.

Symptoms

Symptoms are those of vesical inflammation: dysuria and frequency, sometimes with fever or haematuria. The urine may be cloudy or have a strong odour.

Treatment

Treatment should be started only after obtaining a midstream urine specimen for culture. Fluids are encouraged and a 'best guess' antibiotic prescribed (guided by knowledge of the common organism sensitivities) pending culture results. Bowel flora (e.g. *Escherichia coli*, the most common, *Streptococcus faecalis*, *Klebsiella* or *Proteus*) are usually involved.

Recurrent urinary infection

Recurrent urinary infection requires investigation to look for a causative urinary abnormality although, in women, a structural abnormality is not often found. Important aetiological factors include those that induce local stasis of urine:

- incomplete bladder emptying caused by obstruction
- urinary calculus
- urothelial tumour.

Pyelonephritis

Acute pyelonephritis

Acute renal infection may result from the ascent of a lower urinary tract infection or, less frequently, from haematogenous spread from elsewhere in the body. Destruction of renal tissue occurs and is especially severe if there is renal obstruction.

Symptoms Symptoms include loin pain and tenderness, high fever and tachycardia, which may obscure the symptoms of the associated bacterial cystitis. There may be a sympathetic pulmonary effusion or abdominal guarding.

Differential diagnosis Several differential diagnoses should be considered:

- pulmonary infection
- acute cholecystitis
- appendicitis
- diverticulitis.

Treatment Aggressive treatment is required (to prevent or treat septicaemia and to minimise renal damage), including intravenous fluids and parenteral antibiotics once blood and urine have been obtained for culture. An intravenous urogram (IVU) or renal ultrasound with a plain abdominal radiograph to include the kidneys, ureters and bladder (KUB) is required to exclude obstruction or calculus. An obstructed infected kidney should be drained promptly, usually percutaneously.

Outcome of an acute infection Commonly:

- resolution – no damage
- scarring – especially when there was an obstruction. Less often:
- suppuration – abscess or pyelonephrosis
- granuloma formation.

Chronic pyelonephritis

Chronic pyelonephritis is the cyclic sequence of post-infective scarring in the renal parenchyma and recurrent infection leading to further scarring. Accumulating damage leads to a serious loss of renal function and accounts for one-fifth of all cases of end-stage renal failure. Predisposing causes should be treated and infection eradicated with appropriate antibiotics, including long-term low-dose antibiotics. In children, *vesicoureteric reflux* is a treatable cause, which should be excluded by performing a micturating cystourethrogram and treated by surgical means to re-establish the ureterovesical valve mechanism.

Epididymitis

Epididymitis is the commonest cause of the 'acute scrotum' and presents as a painful hot scrotal swelling, often associated with systemic symptoms of infection and dysuria. It is an important cause of infertility.

Causes:

- in older men, often secondary to urinary tract infection
- in younger men, a sexually transmissible agent should be excluded, especially *Chlamydia*.

Thirteen

Management:
- sexual contact history, contact tracing if appropriate
- urine microbiology, including *Chlamydia*
- antibiotics and rest.

13.4 Urolithiasis

Learning objectives

You should:
- understand the factors that increase the risk of stone formation
- appreciate the stages involved in the management of stones
- be able to use investigations in logical sequence when a patient presents with loin pain.

Incidence:
- increasing
- more common in men
- more common with refined diet.

Pathogenesis

Urinary calculi form by the crystallisation of urinary solutes. Certain systemic conditions and local anatomical changes in the urinary tract predispose to stone formation. The main factors are increased concentration of solute, local urine stasis and an abnormal surface to form a nucleus on which crystallisation can begin.

Idiopathic For many calcium oxalate and calcium phosphate stones, no cause can be found. Alternatively, hypercalciuria may be found with no identifiable cause of the hypercalciuria.

Infective *Proteus mirabilis* converts the urea in urine to ammonia; this increases urinary pH and favours the crystallisation of magnesium ammonium phosphate ('triple phosphate stone'). Such stones can enlarge massively to fill the pelvis and calyces ('staghorn' calculus) and may be bilateral. Other infections encourage stone formation by providing infective debris as a nucleus for crystallisation.

Metabolic Certain conditions result in urinary solutes exceeding saturation. Though none are common and some are rare, they are important because treatment reduces recurrence.

Uncommon conditions:
- hypercalcaemia caused by hyperparathyroidism
- hyperuricosuria – uric acid stone (may be radiolucent).

Rare conditions:
- hyperoxaluria
- xanthinuria
- cystinuria.

Management of the acute episode

The pain of ureteric colic can be very severe and should be treated promptly. The size and position of the stone are then determined, the obstruction treated and removal of the stone planned if spontaneous passage is unlikely.

Analgesia Prostaglandin synthetase inhibitors such as diclofenac or indomethacin are more effective than opiates but both may be required, sometimes with an antiemetic.

Imaging:
- plain KUB film shows most (90%) calculi
- ultrasound may show renal tract dilatation
- non-contrast computed tomography (CT) or IVU give the most information in the acute phase. CT is more sensitive at detecting ureteric stones and may also demonstrate stones that are radiolucent on plain imaging (such as urate stones). CT is usually much quicker than IVU but gives approximately twice the radiation dose. Both tests are equally good at detecting ureteric dilatation.

If imaging shows no obstruction or obstruction with a small stone (less than 5 mm), conservative management is reasonable initially, because most small stones will pass spontaneously. Indications for intervention are:

- fever (suggesting infection and obstruction)
- persisting pain
- persisting obstruction without progress of stone.

Decompression of the obstruction Decompression relieves symptoms and minimises further renal damage. It is achieved by:

- direct percutaneous drainage of the obstructed system
- bypassing the obstruction with a ureteric stent, or
- displacement or removal of the obstructing stone.

Stenting Plastic self-retaining tubes (stents) can be passed endoscopically into the ureter to prevent reobstruction with a pelvic stone or to encourage passage of a ureteric stone. These can be left in place for several weeks while treatment of the stone is planned but will themselves eventually become encrusted with stone.

Removing stones

Small stones may pass spontaneously but larger stones often require intervention.

Open surgery Classic open surgery for renal and ureteric stones is still occasionally required but has become infrequent with the development of less invasive methods.

Percutaneous nephrolithotomy (PCNL) Direct puncture of the renal collecting system and dilatation of the puncture tract allows endoscopic disintegration and removal of renal stones.

Extra-corporeal shock-wave lithotripsy (ESWL) ESWL uses focused shock waves to disintegrate renal stones without requiring anaesthesia; the fragmented stone is left to be passed. Treatment of large stones requires combined techniques with PCNL and stenting.

Ureteric calculi A calculus that is stuck in the ureter can be snared and removed under direct vision with a ureteroscope or fragmented using an ultrasound probe or a pulsed-dye laser via a fibre passed along the ureteroscope. Alternatively, an upper ureteric stone can be 'pushed back' into the kidney for ESWL.

Bladder calculi Although renal stones may pass into and remain in the bladder, enlarging there to cause bladder symptoms, some stones arise in the bladder and are often multiple. There is usually bladder outflow obstruction and stasis, perhaps complicated by diverticula or even squamous cell carcinoma arising in the chronically irritated urothelium. The stone can be crushed and removed through the urethra but the associated pathology must also be treated.

Investigation after the acute episode

Once a renal stone has been dealt with, investigation is directed at identifying treatable causes of recurrence. Investigation includes:

- measurement of serum calcium, urate and phosphate levels
- measurement of urea and creatinine levels
- urine microscopy, culture and pH
- 24-h urine collection for calcium and phosphate measurements
- stone analysis.

The most important abnormality to exclude is hypercalcaemia. In most patients, however, no metabolic abnormality is found. All patients should be advised to maintain a high fluid intake to dilute urine.

13.5 Obstruction and incontinence

Learning objectives

You should:
- recall urinary tract structure and function in understanding the effects of obstruction at different levels in the urinary tract
- understand how the rate of onset of obstruction influences symptoms and outcomes
- understand the different mechanisms that cause incontinence and how these influence symptoms and treatment.

Upper urinary tract obstruction

Upper urinary tract obstruction occurring at points between the renal medulla and the bladder lumen is usually unilateral, except with extrinsic causes. The renal pelvis and ureter above the level of the obstruction become distended (hydronephrosis and hydroureter). Acute obstruction usually causes loin pain but chronic obstruction can be 'silent'. If obstruction is bilateral or in a solitary kidney, it may present with signs of renal failure.

Causes

The causes of obstruction can be classified as follows:

Intraluminal causes:

- calculus: by far the most common
- clot
- renal papillary necrosis.

Intramural causes:

- urothelial tumour of the ureter or bladder
- congenital pelviureteric junction obstruction
- ureteric stricture
- ureterocele.

Extrinsic causes:

- lymphadenopathy, most commonly caused by metastatic disease
- ureteric injury, most often iatrogenic
- direct invasion from carcinoma of the cervix, uterus, prostate or bladder
- retroperitoneal fibrosis, which may be malignant, inflammatory or idiopathic
- pregnancy.

Treatment

Treatment depends on the cause but the dilated collecting system proximal to the obstruction can be drained with a percutaneous cannula (nephrostomy), under ultrasound or radiographic control, to provide temporary relief of the obstruction. This protects renal function while the level and cause of the obstruction is determined and definitive treatment planned. It also permits antegrade urography, which may be very useful in diagnosis. If the cause is known to be untreatable pelvic malignancy, the decision to relieve obstruction needs to be taken with care, to avoid compromising best palliation.

Lower urinary tract obstruction

Obstruction occurring distal to the bladder (infravesical obstruction) causes voiding difficulty initially. Such bladder outflow obstruction is very common and of great importance in urology.

Causes

Acquired causes in the adult may be structural or functional:

Structural:

- urethral stricture
- benign prostatic hyperplasia
- carcinoma of the prostate
- other pelvic tumour
- bladder neck hypertrophy.

Functional:

- bladder neck and sphincter dysynergia.

Clinical features and treatment

The clinical features of bladder outflow obstruction will be discussed below in the section on benign prostatic hyperplasia (the most common cause in men). Treatment of this and the other causes are discussed in the relevant sections.

Urinary incontinence

Urinary incontinence is very common. Involuntary loss of urine per urethra occurs when the pressure in the bladder exceeds urethral resistance. This occurs during normal voiding but should not occur at other times in healthy individuals. Incontinent loss of urine can also occur if iatrogenic or childbirth injury to the bladder results in a urogenital fistula.

Thirteen

Stress incontinence

Stress incontinence is the result of a deficiency in the mechanisms that maintain urethral resistance. The incontinence is abrupt and typically occurs after a cough or sneeze.

Causes

The main cause is pelvic floor weakness secondary to childbirth. This is exacerbated by:

- obesity
- smoking and chronic cough
- detrusor overactivity (mixed incontinence).

Management

Management is first conservative:

- pelvic floor physiotherapy
- weight reduction.

  Then surgical:

- colposuspension is most effective
- placement of a tension-free vaginal tape (TVT) is a less invasive procedure but it is a newer treatment and its efficacy in the long term remains unproven.

Urge incontinence

Inappropriate contraction of the detrusor causes an urgent need to void, which results in incontinence if the urethral resistance is also insufficient. Incontinence is preceded by an urgent sensation of imminent wetting.

Causes:
- most often idiopathic
- neurological abnormality
- temporary – bladder irritation due to infection or stone.

Management:
- treat identifiable cause
- anticholinergic drugs
- bladder retraining
- surgical treatments:
  - cystoplasty: the augmentation of the bladder with a segment of bowel (usually ileum), which increases bladder volume and reduces the overactivity of the detrusor
  - botulinum toxin injections to the detrusor: a promising new treatment for detrusor overactivity.

Overflow incontinence

Slow-onset bladder outflow obstruction or neurological disorder cause chronic urinary retention. Eventually the resting bladder pressure exceeds the outflow resistance. This results in:

- continuous dribbling incontinence, which is worse at night
- a risk of upper tract damage (high pressure chronic retention – see later).

Management
Urgent:

- relieve obstruction (catheterise).

  Less urgent:

- treat obstructive cause
- rehabilitate bladder by intermittent self-catheterisation if possible.

Investigation of incontinence

All patients with urinary incontinence should be investigated using questionnaires and frequency volume charts to objectively identify their voiding patterns. In patients in whom surgical intervention is considered, urodynamics or cystometry (the measurement of bladder pressures during bladder filling and voiding) can accurately diagnose the type of incontinence present.

13.6 Benign disorders

> **Learning objectives**
>
> You should:
> - appreciate the importance of benign prostatic hyperplasia and urethral stricture as treatable causes of urinary tract obstruction
> - be aware that insidious onset can result in irreversible upper tract changes
> - know how to differentiate between benign scrotal swellings and testicular neoplasm
> - know how to manage the 'acute scrotum'.

Prostate: benign hyperplasia

Benign prostatic hyperplasia (BPH) is detectable in nearly all men over the age of 40 years and, in later years, some degree of bladder outflow obstruction will often develop as a result. Currently, only one in 10 men require surgical treatment but, with the advent of potentially effective drug therapies, both symptomatic presentation and treatment rates are rising.

Clinical features

Benign prostatic hyperplasia is the most common cause of bladder outflow obstruction in men. The clinical presentation of bladder outflow obstruction is very variable.

Early symptoms These are frequency, nocturia, hesitancy and poor stream, or symptoms of secondary urinary infection. Such symptoms may be tolerated for many years and patients may not complain at all until retention of urine occurs.

Retention of urine This may be acute retention, with an apparently sudden and distressing inability to pass urine. The bladder is tender and tensely distended, and the patient is well aware of a desperate urge to pass urine. Alternatively, the bladder may undergo gradual progressive dilatation and this results in painless chronic retention and eventually overflow incontinence. The stretched and weakened detrusor gives way in places to form diverticula, which come to contain stagnant infected urine and sometimes urinary stones. This insidious presentation is more serious because bladder function may not recover completely. If the chronic retention is low pressure, renal function is not affected.

High pressure chronic retention More importantly, though, untreated obstruction can lead to high pressure within the upper tracts, bilateral upper tract obstruction with hydronephrosis and consequent renal impairment (obstructive uropathy). Patients may then present for the first time with signs of established chronic renal failure with polyuria, anorexia, vomiting, hypertension and impaired consciousness.

Investigation

This depends on the stage at which the patient presents. Patients presenting with *early outflow symptoms* require careful assessment to exclude other causes of similar symptoms (described below), especially bladder cancer and prostate cancer:

- urinalysis and digital rectal examination are essential
- uroflowmetry gives an objective measure of poor flow
- ultrasound can sensitively measure incomplete bladder emptying
- a plain film is useful to exclude stones.

If there is incomplete bladder emptying, serum creatinine should be measured and an upper tract ultrasound examination performed because conservative management may be contraindicated.

Treatment

Patients presenting with *acute retention* require relief with urethral (or percutaneous suprapubic) catheterisation. Most will subsequently require surgical treatment but, if there is no preceding history of outflow symptoms, a trial removal of the catheter may be followed by a return to voiding, allowing elective assessment of the bladder outflow.

Medical treatment Alpha-adrenergic blockers inhibit contraction of the prostate capsule and bladder neck, which can improve mild symptoms. They can also be prescribed to men who have presented with acute retention of urine and increase the chances of a successful trial removal of the catheter. 5α-Reductase inhibitors cause gradual shrinkage of the prostate and reduce the progression of men with larger prostates to retention of urine or prostatic surgery. It may take 4–6 months before symptomatic improvement is seen. There is a move towards combination treatment with both agents.

Surgery Transurethral prostatic resection (TURP) is the gold standard treatment but is used increasingly following a trial of medical therapy.

Early complications of TURP include:

- haemorrhage
- septicaemia
- 'TUR syndrome' (when irrigant fluid enters circulation).

Late complications include:

- secondary haemorrhage
- retrograde ejaculation
- urethral stricture
- incontinence.

Retropubic (open) prostatectomy is reserved for very large glands. Bladder neck incision is used for bladder neck hypertrophy.

Alternative 'minimally invasive' treatments:

- transurethral laser coagulation/resection
- transurethral microwave thermotherapy (TUMT)
- prostatic stents.

Urethral stricture

Causes

Stricture results from contraction and fibrosis occurring during healing of a urethral injury or after an episode of inflammation.

Traumatic causes are:

- major pelvic fracture: urethral rupture
- perineal trauma: a 'fall astride'
- iatrogenic: instrumentation or catheterisation.

Infective and inflammatory causes are:

- gonococcal urethritis (now less common than in the past)
- non-specific urethritis.

Diagnosis

Urethral stricture should be suspected in a young man with poor urine flow. The urine flow rate has a characteristic 'plateau' appearance. The diagnosis is confirmed by urethroscopy and further assessed by contrast urethrography.

Complications of urethral stricture Complications are generally those of long-term bladder outflow obstruction:

- common
  - urine infection
  - epididymitis
- rare
  - squamous cell carcinoma.

Treatment

Urethral dilatation has been in use for centuries but provides temporary relief only and has to be repeated at intervals. Endoscopic incision (optical urethrotomy) may be curative but often has to be supplemented by intermittent self-dilatation by the patient. Formal urethroplasty (open urethral repair) is required for long, recurrent or dense strictures and can be curative for some short (<1 cm) strictures.

Benign scrotal disorders

Testicular torsion

The testis can occasionally twist on its vascular pedicle and become ischaemic. Torsion should be considered in any acute tender scrotal swelling, especially before puberty, and early exploration is needed to save the testis. Both testes should be sutured to prevent further episodes.

Differential diagnosis:
- acute epididymitis
- torsion of testicular appendage.

Hydrocele

Accumulation of fluid in the tunica vaginalis may be idiopathic but may also be secondary to inflammation or tumour.

Diagnosis

The fluid is limited to the scrotum, is fluctuant and can be transilluminated. Ultrasound can be useful to ensure that the underlying testis is normal.

Treatment

Treatment of secondary hydrocele is that of the underlying cause. For the idiopathic hydrocele, simple aspiration may be used but there is a risk of bleeding and infection and the fluid tends to reaccumulate. Surgical excision or eversion and plication of the hydrocele sac offers the best chance of a lasting cure.

Epididymal cyst

These are often small and symptomless and found on self-examination. Small cysts may cause discomfort and can occasionally enlarge sufficiently to warrant treatment.

Diagnosis

The cyst is felt separate from the testis and can usually be transilluminated.

Treatment

Surgical excision can compromise fertility by interfering with epididymal sperm transport and so should be avoided in young men unless significantly symptomatic.

13.7 Neoplasms

> ### Learning objectives
>
> You should:
> - recall how investigation of haematuria is directed primarily to the exclusion of renal and urothelial neoplasms
> - be able to apply the TNM staging system
> - be aware of other staging systems
> - appreciate how treatment is determined by tumour factors (stage and grade) and by patient factors (age, co-pathology)
> - be aware how much prognosis varies with the type and extent of tumour.

Renal – nephroblastoma

Wilms' tumour (nephroblastoma) accounts for 10% of child malignancies. The prognosis is now much improved as a result of multicentre cooperation.

Clinical features

Patients may present with signs and symptoms of the primary tumour, those of secondary spread or systemic manifestations.

Frequent symptoms:

- palpable abdominal mass
- systemic symptoms.

Less frequent symptoms:

- haematuria
- pain
- associated anomalies (15% of patients).

Tumours may be very large; 5% are bilateral and 20% are metastatic at presentation. Differentiation is variable and the tumour may contain muscle, cartilage and epithelial elements if well differentiated.

Differential diagnosis:

- polycystic kidney
- hydronephrosis
- neuroblastoma.

Treatment

Treatment should be carried out according to a precise protocol and will include:

- nephrectomy, or partial nephrectomy
- combination chemotherapy.

It may also include:

- radiotherapy.

Prognosis

The 5-year survival rate is currently 80%.

Renal – adenocarcinoma

This is the most common adult renal malignancy. It is also known as hypernephroma, Grawitz tumour and clear cell carcinoma.

Clinical features

The clinical presentation of renal adenocarcinoma is very variable but it can present with the 'classic triad':

- flank pain
- abdominal mass
- haematuria.

However, it may also present with:

- anorexia and weight loss
- anaemia
- hypertension
- fever
- other paraneoplastic syndromes
- symptoms from metastases.

The tumour spreads by direct invasion through the renal capsule, venous invasion to the renal vein and vena cava, and haematogenous spread to bone and lungs.

Investigation

IVU can show calyceal distortion and a soft tissue mass. Ultrasound differentiates the tumour from a cyst.

Staging

Contrast CT scanning of the abdomen and chest is used to stage the disease and guide treatment planning. It identifies the degree of local spread, such as renal vein or caval involvement, and metastatic disease.

Treatment

Treatment is surgical, by radical nephrectomy, and is considered worthwhile even with major venous invasion or in patients with limited metastatic disease who have symptoms from the primary tumour. Rare spontaneous regression of metastases occurs. There is little effective treatment for metastases but immunotherapy (after surgical debulking of the primary tumour) and progestogens are occasionally used. T1 tumours (confined to the kidney and ≤7 cm) are now commonly treated with laparoscopic radical nephrectomy. Partial nephrectomy may be indicated for small tumours in patients in whom nephron sparing is required, such as solitary kidney.

Prognosis

Although the average survival rate at 5 years is 40%, individual prognosis is very unpredictable, with occasional long-term survival with extensive disease.

Urothelial tumours

Malignant tumours of the lining transitional cell epithelium (urothelium) can occur in the urinary tract at any point from renal calyces to the tip of the urethra. The tumour type is most often transitional cell carcinoma and the bladder is the site that is most frequently involved (90%). In some parts of the world where schistosomiasis is endemic, squamous cell carcinoma of the bladder is common but this tumour type is infrequently seen elsewhere. The most important presenting feature is painless frank haematuria, which should always be investigated urgently.

Causes

Exposure to many chemical carcinogens has been implicated. An occupational history should be taken in all patients with urothelial tumours. The most important agents are:

- azo dyes
- tobacco smoke
- chemicals used in rubber manufacture.

Pathology and staging

Transitional cell carcinoma is more common in men and incidence increases with age. Most tumours are superficial and papillary but they may be papillary or solid, single or multiple, and superficial or deeply invasive. Superficial tumours are mostly well differentiated but muscle-invasive tumours tend to be of a higher grade. Spread is by direct invasion and via lymphatics and the bloodstream. Transitional carcinoma in situ is an important variant that can progress rapidly to invasive disease.

Staging of the local bladder tumour is based on the invasive level (Figure 191):

Ta: tumour is superficial, involving epithelium only
T1: invasion into subepithelial connective tissue, the lamina propria
T2: invasion of muscle (T2a inner half, T2b outer half)

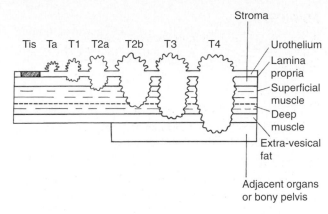

Figure 191 Staging of bladder cancer. Tis, carcinoma in situ.

T3: invasion beyond muscle into perivesical tissue
T4: fixed mass or invading adjacent organ
Tis: carcinoma in situ (CIS), which appears as a flat red patch of high-grade non-invasive tumour, is a special case that, if extensive, progresses rapidly.

Clinical features

Although patients may occasionally present with symptoms due to invasive or metastatic disease, by far the most frequent presenting symptom is painless haematuria, which is either:

- frank – reported by patient
- microscopic – detected by doctor.

Urothelial tumours can also present with recurrent urinary infection or irritative bladder symptoms (dysuria and frequency).

Investigation of haematuria

Investigation of frank haematuria should be urgent and requires upper tract imaging with IVU and ultrasound, and cystourethroscopy. Urothelial tumours may be seen as filling defects on IVU. Exfoliative urine cytology can be useful, especially for upper tract tumours and CIS of the bladder; however, false negatives are common. Bladder tumours are diagnosed, staged and treated by cystoscopy and endoscopic resection.

Treatment

Appropriate treatment depends on the clinical stage and histological grade of the tumour. In the bladder, superficial (Ta or T1) tumours can be managed by endoscopic resection. Follow-up by prolonged endoscopic surveillance is required. Intravesical chemotherapy is used for multiple recurrent superficial lesions. Invasive (T2–T3) bladder tumours require either radiotherapy or radical cystourethrectomy, or both. Intravesical BCG (bacille Calmette-Guérin) provokes a response that can be effective in treating bladder CIS.

In the upper tracts, nephroureterectomy has been traditionally used for unilateral disease because tumours are often multifocal on one side. More conservative surgery is now considered for unifocal disease and for bilateral disease.

Prognosis

Prognosis is dependent on the stage and grade of tumour, with the most superficial tumours resulting in a 90% survival rate at 5 years; this halves to 45% for muscle invasive disease.

Prostate: carcinoma

The incidence of adenocarcinoma of the prostate is increasing worldwide but there is great geographical and racial variation. In the UK, it is now the third most frequent malignant tumour to present in men, and subclinical disease is present in the majority of elderly men. No convincing aetiological factors have been established although there may be a weak familial tendency and environmental factors may be important.

Clinical features

Until recently, almost one-half of patients presented with locally advanced (T3–T4) or metastatic disease. The most frequent metastatic site is the axial skeleton, especially the pelvis and lumbar spine.

Common symptoms are:

- bladder outflow obstruction
- retention of urine.

Less frequent symptoms include:

- bone pain
- ureteric obstruction
- anaemia.

Early stage disease is increasingly being found as a result of 'Well Man' testing, informal screening with prostate-specific antigen (PSA) and an increasing willingness for men to present with mild symptoms.

Diagnosis

Histology The histological diagnosis is established by transrectal ultrasound (TRUS)-guided needle biopsy and sometimes within the specimen by transurethral resection of the prostate.

Markers The serum tumour marker PSA may be elevated or sclerotic metastases may be seen in bone on plain radiograph.

Grade and stage Tumour grade (differentiation) and stage have a bearing on prognosis and both are important in deciding the best treatment. The Gleason grading system is most useful and scores the two main histological patterns to give a sum score between 2 and 10. Poorly differentiated tumours have a higher grade and poorer prognosis. Staging of a local tumour (Figure 192) is most often carried out by digital rectal examination:

T0: no evidence of primary tumour
T1: tumour not detectable by palpation but detected by needle biopsy or TURP (T1a <5% TURP specimen, T1b >5% TURP specimen, T1c detected on needle biopsy)
T2: clinically detectable, not breaching capsule (T2a, less than half of one lobe; T2b, over half of one lobe; T2c, both lobes)

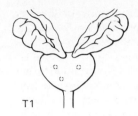
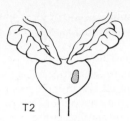
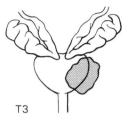
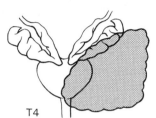

Figure 192 Staging of prostate cancer.

T3: beyond capsule, invading bladder neck or seminal vesicle, not fixed
T4: fixed or invading other local structures.

Metastatic staging is usually established by radioisotopic bone scanning because metastasis to bone is the most common clinically important site.

Treatment

Opinion on the best treatment for prostate cancer is divided but it depends on symptoms, the age and general health of the patient and on the tumour stage.

Clinically localised tumour in a younger patient:

- radical radiotherapy to prostate (external beam or brachytherapy – radioactive seeds placed into prostate)
- radical prostatectomy
- 'active surveillance'–observation of the prostate cancer patient with regular PSA screening, prostate examination and, sometimes, repeat biopsy.

The aim is to cure and the first two treatments are both controversial.

Symptomatic advanced disease at any age Four out of five prostatic cancers are 'androgen dependent' and advanced disease will regress well for a time if the source of circulating testosterone is removed by orchiectomy or the secretion or action of testosterone is blocked by drugs. The main treatments at present are:

- orchiectomy (subcapsular or total): classic treatment – now used much less frequently
- LHRH (luteinising hormone-releasing hormone) analogues (stop testosterone release)
- antiandrogens (block testosterone action).

LHRH analogues cause a transient increase in testosterone before suppressing testosterone production, and are usually used together with an antiandrogen for the first few weeks to avoid temporary stimulation of the tumour (tumour 'flare'). Estrogens have been widely used but are now obsolete because of their cardiovascular side effects.

Asymptomatic locally advanced or metastatic disease Some advocate the use of radiotherapy with adjuvant hormonal therapy in locally advanced disease. Alternatively, hormonal treatment may be given immediately or 'deferred' until the symptoms emerge. The timing is controversial as many elderly men with advanced disease die of other causes without ever becoming symptomatic.

Hormone-relapsed disease Secondary hormone treatment is usually ineffective and treatment is aimed at palliation of symptoms. Recurrent prostatic obstruction can be treated by repeat transurethral resection.

Focal bone pain is palliated by:

* external beam radiotherapy.

Diffuse pain is palliated by:

* hemibody radiotherapy
* bone-seeking isotope therapy.

Opiate analgesia may be required.

Prognosis
Prognosis is very variable but can be predicted by stage. With metastatic disease at presentation, 50% of patients die within 2 years. When there is no metastatic disease at presentation, 50% will die within 4 years.

Testicular carcinoma
Incidence and aetiology
Testicular cancer is one of the most common cancers in young men, with a peak incidence in the third decade. There is some racial variation, with Caucasians having a higher risk of disease. Risk is also higher in testicular maldescent but the aetiology is unknown.

Clinical features
Usually:

* painless lump.

Less often:

* tender inflamed swelling
* history of trauma
* symptoms from metastasis.

Diagnosis
Any lump in the testis is considered a testicular tumour until proven otherwise and should be explored through a groin incision; unless another diagnosis is evident, the testis should be removed. Preoperative ultrasound is helpful in excluding benign testicular pathology and confirming that the abnormality actually lies within the testis itself.

Tumour markers Blood samples for the measurement of tumour markers are taken immediately before and serially after surgery. The following markers are screened for:

* AFP (α-fetoprotein)
* β-hCG (human chorionic gonadotrophin)
* LDH (lactate dehydrogenase).

Pathology
The pathology is very variable. Germ cell tumours of various types predominate. The previous distinction between seminoma and teratoma has now been superseded by classifications that consider the variable amounts of differentiation present. Testicular lymphoma is relatively rare and is seen in an older age group, peaking in the sixth decade.

CIS CIS is sometimes seen in testicular biopsies for infertility and, if present, there is a 50% risk of invasive cancer developing within 5 years.

Spread Spread is by local invasion to adjacent structures and by lymphatic invasion to para-aortic lymph nodes.

Nodal staging Nodal staging is important for treatment and is determined by CT scanning. The Royal Marsden Hospital staging system is widely used:

Stage I: disease is confined to the testis
Stage II: infradiaphragmatic nodes involved
Stage III: supradiaphragmatic nodes involved
Stage IV: extralymphatic disease.

Treatment
Treatment depends on the pathology and the stage but follows detailed national protocols:

* low-stage disease with negative test results for markers:
  - orchiectomy and surveillance, radiotherapy or prophylactic chemotherapy
* nodal disease, persistent tumour markers or relapse on surveillance:
  - combination chemotherapy
* persistent nodes:
  - salvage node dissection
  - repeat chemotherapy.

Prognosis
Prognosis is extremely good for early-treated disease. The prognosis is much worse if nodal disease persists after combination chemotherapy.

Penile carcinoma
Penile carcinoma is uncommon and only affects uncircumcised men. The tumour is a squamous cell carcinoma that most often affects the inner aspect of the foreskin and the glans. Spread is by local direct infiltration and by the lymphatics to the inguinal and then iliac nodes. Inguinal nodes are palpable in 50% of patients at presentation but this is often the result of secondary infection and only one-third of nodes are actually involved by the tumour.

Staging
The TNM classification is most commonly used:

Tis: carcinoma in situ
Ta: superficial disease
T1:   invasion of subepithelial connective tissue
T2:   invasion of corpus cavernosum or spongiosum
T3:   invasion of urethra or prostate
T4:   invasion of other structures.

Treatment

Treatment depends on the stage and grade. Superficial, well or moderately differentiated lesions can be treated with penis-preserving strategies, such as local excision and radiotherapy. High-grade lesions and lesions of T2 and above are treated with radical penectomy, with or without inguinal lymph node dissection. There may also be a place for other adjuvant treatment.

Prognosis

The 5-year survival rate is as high as 80% for well-differentiated lesions, falling to 30% for poorly differentiated lesions.

Self-assessment: questions

Many diseases of the urinary system are common in practice and a thorough revision of the common urinary malignancies, urinary infection and stones is essential examination preparation.

Extended matching items questions (EMI)

EMI 1

Theme: Therapeutic alternatives in urology

A. bicalutamide (an oral antiandrogen)

B. external beam radiotherapy

C. alfuzosin (an alpha-adrenergic blocker)

D. orchiectomy (bilateral)

E. transurethral resection

F. radical nephrectomy

G. extra-corporeal shock-wave lithotripsy (ESWL)

H. orchiectomy

I. nephroureterectomy

J. endoscopic insertion of bilateral ureteric stents

K. finasteride (a 5α-reductase inhibitor)

L. trimethoprim

M. percutaneous nephrostomy

N. goserelin (an LHRH analogue depot)

O. cystectomy and urinary diversion

P. opiate analgesia

Q. diclofenac

R. endoscopic insertion of ureteric stent

For each of the brief case histories below, choose the one or more appropriate therapeutic options from the list above. Each option may be used once, more than once or not at all.

1. A 53-year-old woman with a new diagnosis of high-grade muscle-invasive [T2NxM0 (muscle invasion, nodes not assessed, no metastases)] transitional cell carcinoma of the bladder.

2. An 82-year-old man with severe back pain due to metastatic prostate cancer; hormone therapy started 3 years ago.

3. A 45-year-old man with haematuria from a unilateral transitional cell carcinoma of the renal pelvis.

4. A 68-year-old man with bothersome nocturia, reduced urine flow (maximum flow rate of 9 ml/s, post-void bladder residual of 160 ml) and a clinically enlarged benign prostate.

5. A 73-year-old man with a new diagnosis of locally advanced non-metastatic prostate cancer, with troublesome voiding symptoms, bilateral hydronephrosis and a serum creatinine level of 300 μmol/l.

6. A 42-year-old woman with haematuria and loin pain from a 7 cm solid tumour in the parenchyma of the left kidney, with CT scan evidence of tumour extending into the left renal vein, and a normal chest radiograph.

7. A 26-year-old woman with severe left loin pain radiating to the groin. IVU shows prompt excretion from normal kidney on the right but, on the left, delayed function, hydronephrosis and a 2 cm calculus at the pelviureteric junction.

Constructed response questions (CRQs)

CRQ 1

A man aged 62 years presents with a single episode of painless total haematuria. He has no other voiding symptoms but admits that he had a mild ache in the left loin a few weeks before.

a. How should he be investigated and why?

Before investigations begin he presents to casualty with a 5-h history of severe pain in the left flank, which started abruptly and now radiates to the left groin. He has vomited, is sweating and pale and finds it difficult to lie still to be examined. Urine testing shows microscopic haematuria.

b. What is now the most likely diagnosis and how can it be confirmed? What important differential diagnosis must be excluded?

Imaging shows a 9 mm radiopaque calculus at the pelviureteric junction, with complete obstruction of the left kidney.

c. Outline the steps in clinical management.

CRQ 2

A man of 44 years presents with a 3-year history of increasing frequency of micturition. For the past year he has needed to wake about five times each night to pass urine. He admits that the stream of urine has become weaker and prolonged. About 6 years ago he was involved in a fight and was kicked in the perineum. Examination shows a mild phimosis. Rectal examination reveals a normal prostate. Urinary flow rate is 4 ml/s maximum and it takes 90 s for him to pass 200 ml.

a. What is the most likely diagnosis?

b. What other investigations should he have?

c. How might he be treated initially?

d. Should he have a circumcision and, if so, why?

CRQ 3

A man of 76 years presents with increasing difficulty in passing urine over the past 3 months. He has had a 'bad back' for years but, over the last month, the pain has become much worse and he has had difficulty sleeping, despite taking regular paracetamol and codeine. Examination reveals some tenderness to percussion over the lower lumbar spine, and the prostate is irregular, fixed and stony hard. A PSA screen carried out by his GP is 580 µg/l and a plain radiograph of the lumbar spine shows osteosclerotic deposits.

a. What is the likely diagnosis and how can it be confirmed?
b. If the diagnosis is confirmed, what is the disease stage?
c. What is the prognosis?
d. What initial treatment options are there and what is the likelihood of remission?

His back pain resolves 2 weeks later and this improvement is maintained although he complains of some 'hot flushes'. The PSA level falls to 10 µg/l within 3 months of starting treatment but, by the end of the year, has increased to 150 µg/l. Approximately 15 months after the initial treatment the back pain has returned, with new pain in the left hip that cannot be controlled by simple analgesics.

e. What treatment options remain?

Objective structured clinical examination questions (OSCEs)

OSCE 1

This 83-year-old man has started wetting his bed at night and has anorexia and weight loss. You have his blood biochemistry results and the report of an abdominal ultrasound examination. Look at the results and then explain to the patient what treatment you recommend.

Blood biochemistry: Na, 135 mmol/l; K, 3.8 mmol/l; urea, 42 mmol/l; creatinine, 280 µmol/l. Ultrasound report: liver, gallbladder, spleen unremarkable. There is gross bilateral hydronephrosis and hydroureter. There is marked cortical thinning in both kidneys. The bladder is hugely distended, although the patient has just voided, and the bladder volume is estimated as 3500 ml.

OSCE 2

This 42-year-old smoker has attended for a 'Well Man' visit. He has no urinary symptoms. You have the report of his urinalysis. Explain the urinalysis result to the patient, including a description of the recommended investigations that he will need.

Urinalysis: protein negative, nitrites negative, leucocytes negative, blood positive +++, glucose negative.

Multiple choice questions

1. A man aged 60 years, who denies having other symptoms, reports a single episode of frank painless total haematuria:

a. if culture shows urine infection, bladder tumour is very unlikely
b. cystoscopy is indicated even if urine cytology shows no abnormalities
c. the most likely serious cause is renal adenocarcinoma
d. there is a 20% chance that cystoscopy and IVU will reveal a bladder tumour
e. cystoscopy is indicated if the IVU is reported to show a normal bladder outline

2. With regard to prostate cancer:

a. it is present in most men over 80 years of age
b. a serum PSA greater than 100 µg/l suggests skeletal metastases
c. a serum PSA of 15 µg/l is diagnostic of prostate cancer
d. early disease can often be cured by bilateral orchiectomy
e. abnormal uptake on bone scan can be disregarded if radiographs of the same area are quite normal

3. A man aged 74 years presents with a history of passing no urine for 12 h. He denies having previous urinary symptoms but, on direct questioning, admits that he has needed to get out of bed two or three times each night to pass urine for several years. He is now very restless and uncomfortable, with a constant urge to pass urine:

a. catheterisation should be deferred until renal function has been assessed by urgent blood biochemistry
b. the bladder should be decompressed slowly to avoid causing heavy haematuria
c. the retention may have been precipitated by antidepressant medication
d. the most likely cause is benign prostatic enlargement
e. blood should be taken for a PSA assay within 24 h

4. With regard to transitional cell carcinoma:

a. most patients have advanced disease at first presentation, requiring radical treatment
b. it is more common in cigarette smokers
c. the bladder is affected more frequently than the ureters
d. even if there is no evidence of recurrence after 10 years, follow-up is still justified
e. carcinoma in situ involving the whole bladder usually runs a long benign course

5. A boy of 13 years presents with a 4-h history of pain, swelling and redness of one side of the scrotum:

a. he is likely to have epididymitis
b. he should have early surgical exploration to exclude testicular torsion

   c. a diagnosis of testicular lymphoma should be considered

   d. if the affected testis is infarcted, the unaffected side should be left alone

   e. a twisted appendix testis may be responsible

6. Ureteric obstruction:

   a. is most often caused by calculus

   b. cannot be caused by calculus if the plain KUB radiograph is normal

   c. may be asymptomatic

   d. usually causes an increase in blood urea

   e. should always be relieved when complicating advanced pelvic malignancy

7. An overweight 45-year-old mother of four has used pads to control leakage of urine for 5 years. She has a 'smoker's cough'. She is now finding it difficult to afford the pads and asks for treatment:

   a. most women with incontinence of urine do not seek medical help

   b. her incontinence is almost certainly the result of weakness of the pelvic floor

   c. she may be helped by drug treatment

   d. if she passes urine in small volumes, frequently and urgently, bladder overactivity may be present

   e. if she has genuine stress incontinence she should have surgery without delay

8. A 23-year-old woman has had repeated episodes of frequency and dysuria, occurring every few weeks for 18 months. She left her parents' home shortly before the attacks began and now lives with her boyfriend:

   a. she probably has an underlying urinary tract abnormality

   b. urine should be collected for culture before commencing treatment at each attack

   c. the social history is irrelevant

   d. a vulval disinfectant will not help reduce the number of attacks

   e. she should be advised to decrease her fluid intake and empty her bladder before intercourse

Self-assessment: answers

EMI answers

EMI 1

1. O, B or both. Radiotherapy can be used either as an alternative or as an adjunct to radical surgery, with curative intent in this situation.

2. P, then B. Adequate analgesia should be provided and palliative external beam radiotherapy to the painful sites offered. Hormone therapy should be continued.

3. I. Transitional cell carcinoma is often multifocal on the affected side – the kidney, renal pelvis and ureter down to the bladder should be removed together.

4. C, K (or both), E. Mild bladder outflow symptoms may be helped by alpha-adrenergic blockers or 5α-reductase inhibitors, and it is reasonable to offer these medical alternatives first and offer transurethral resection only if symptoms or post-void residual remain a problem.

5. J or M, D or A and N. Temporary decompression of the obstructed upper tracts should be performed urgently and, if stent insertion is not possible, percutaneous nephrostomy can be used. There is a good expectation of remission with hormonal manipulation: bilateral orchiectomy or the use of an LHRH analogue (with an antiandrogen for 2 weeks to avoid a tumour 'flare') should be offered as alternatives.

6. F. Even with early invasion of the renal vein and vena cava, radical nephrectomy is indicated and may be curative.

7. Q, R or M, then G. Non-steroidal anti-inflammatory agents such as diclofenac provide effective analgesia. The obstructed kidney should be drained promptly, and a stent is useful in helping the stone fragments to clear after ESWL.

CRQ answers

CRQ 1

a. Despite the history of loin pain, the most likely important diagnosis to exclude is urothelial neoplasm of the bladder. Investigation should include urine culture, cystoscopy and upper tract imaging with intravenous urogram, and renal tract ultrasound.

b. The most likely diagnosis is ureteric colic caused by calculus. Although a plain abdominal film and ultrasound may be useful, an intravenous urogram or non-contrast CT give the most useful information in the acute phase. In a man of this age, the most important differential diagnosis is of a leaking abdominal aortic aneurysm.

c. Pain should be relieved using non-steroidal anti-inflammatory agents, such as diclofenac, and antiemetics. A stone of this size is unlikely to pass spontaneously. The obstructed kidney should be decompressed as an emergency, either by percutaneous nephrostomy or by passing a ureteric catheter to the level of the stone and flushing the stone back into the kidney. A ureteric stent should be left in place. The stone can then be electively fragmented by ESWL or removed by percutaneous nephrolithotomy if ESWL is not available. Once the acute episode is over, the patient should be investigated to exclude a treatable cause for stone.

CRQ 2

a. Symptomatic benign prostatic hyperplasia is only occasionally seen at this age, with functional bladder neck obstruction being rather more frequent. This history and findings are, however, most suggestive of obstruction caused by traumatic urethral stricture.

b. A midstream urine specimen should be collected for culture because obstruction is often complicated by infection. The probable diagnosis is best confirmed by flexible (fibre-optic) cystoscopy, although the actual length and position of any urethral stricture may be better defined by contrast urethrography. Urinary tract ultrasound may be indicated if there is evidence of incomplete bladder emptying, and plain abdominal radiography will exclude bladder calculus.

c. Urethral strictures can be managed initially by dilatation with urethral sounds, but endoscopic incision of the stricture (optical urethrotomy) has better long-term results. Open urethroplasty is also a more definitive treatment in selected patients.

d. No; circumcision should be avoided if possible, because long or recurrent strictures may require urethroplasty and the preputial skin may be needed to form a urethral patch.

CRQ 3

a. The likely diagnosis of advanced metastatic prostate cancer should be confirmed without delay. The troublesome bladder outflow symptoms may be improved temporarily by transurethral prostatic resection, which would also provide a tissue diagnosis. Alternatively, the histology could be confirmed by a needle biopsy of the prostate, which can be performed under local anaesthetic and transrectal ultrasound guidance.

b. If the histology is confirmed, the stage of the disease is T4M1.

c. For men with metastatic disease at presentation, the 2-year survival rate is 50% (half die within 2 years).

d. This patient has symptoms from metastases and, therefore, after full discussion with the patient, hormonal treatment ('androgen deprivation') should be initiated by either orchiectomy or with LHRH analogues or antiandrogens. A very useful response is seen in 80% of patients and the remission lasts for about 18 months on average.

e. Palliative radiotherapy can provide very effective temporary relief of symptoms from bone pain. This can be administered by external beam to the affected sites or, if the painful lesions are widespread, by either external beam hemibody irradiation or intravenous administration of a radioactive bone-seeking strontium isotope. Analgesics should be increased, using non-steroidal anti-inflammatory agents and opiates if needed, until the radiotherapy has been allowed to work. Secondary hormonal treatments are of no significant benefit.

OSCE answers

OSCE 1

He has overflow incontinence secondary to bladder outflow obstruction, complicated by obstructive renal failure. You should explain the need for prompt urethral catheterisation, both to relieve the renal obstruction and to treat the incontinence. You should explain the need for close (probably inpatient) monitoring of fluid balance as an obligatory diuresis is likely to occur, which may require fluid replacement. You should consider explaining that the bladder is unlikely to recover and that long-term catheterisation or intermittent self-catheterisation may be needed.

OSCE 2

He has asymptomatic microscopic haematuria. The urinalysis is otherwise negative, so urinary infection is unlikely. You should advise that blood pressure and blood biochemistry be checked. You should explain that, although a serious cause is unlikely to be found, further investigation is recommended and will include upper tract imaging (ultrasound, intravenous urogram) and cystoscopy. There is an association between cigarette smoking and bladder cancer and you should, of course, recommend that he stops smoking.

Multiple choice answers

1. a. **False.** In total, 40% of patients with bladder tumours have a proven urinary infection.

   b. **True.** False negatives are common with urine cytology.

   c. **False.** The most likely serious cause is transitional cell carcinoma of the bladder.

   d. **True.**

   e. **True.** Many bladder tumours are not seen on IVU.

2. a. **True.** However, most men have an asymptomatic microscopic focus.

   b. **True.** About 80% will have a positive bone scan.

   c. **False.** A PSA of 15 µg/l could also be caused by benign conditions. In this situation, prostate cancer should be diagnosed on histology.

   d. **False.** Orchiectomy and other types of hormonal manipulation can produce useful remission of advanced disease but are never curative. Such treatments are not indicated for early asymptomatic disease.

   e. **False.** Although bony secondaries are usually sclerotic, this combination is also diagnostic of metastases.

3. a. **False.** This presentation is of acute retention, and early relief by catheterisation takes priority over investigation.

   b. **False.** Although bleeding can occur from the bladder after decompression by catheterisation, this is more common after chronic retention and, furthermore, is not prevented by slow decompression.

   c. **True.** Any drug with anticholinergic action can precipitate retention.

   d. **True.**

   e. **False.** The PSA level may be spuriously elevated soon after retention or catheterisation.

4. a. **False.** Superficial disease is most common and is amenable to local endoscopic treatment.

   b. **True.** Smoking is thought to produce a urinary carcinogen in susceptible individuals.

   c. **True.** About 95% of transitional cell carcinoma occur in the bladder and the pelvicalyceal system is affected more frequently than the ureter or urethra.

   d. **True.** However, this depends on histology. Superficial well-differentiated transitional cell carcinoma with no recurrence at 5 years can safely be discharged. Other stages require lifelong endoscopic follow-up because recurrence is not unusual, even after 10 years.

   e. **False.** Carcinoma in situ tends to progress to muscle-invasive disease, especially if extensive.

5. a. **False.** Infective causes are unlikely.

   b. **True.** This is a classic presentation and should be dealt with as an emergency to avoid loss of the testis.

   c. **False.** Testicular neoplasms are rare at this age and lymphoma is seen in a much older age group.

   d. **False.** If the affected testis is infarcted, the 'unaffected' side may also be vulnerable to torsion and should be sutured to prevent this.

   e. **True.** This is often only diagnosed at operation, but removing the infarcted appendix testis (a müllerian duct remnant) speeds recovery.

6. a. **True.** About 90% of cases are caused by stone.
   b. **False.** Not all urinary stones are radiopaque.
   c. **True.** Especially when of gradual onset.
   d. **False.** If the other kidney is normal and unobstructed, as is usually the case, blood biochemistry is unchanged.
   e. **False.** Each individual patient should be considered carefully, but it is often considered wrong to relieve a painless terminal complication and then expose the patient to a painful death from other causes.

7. a. **True.** Unfortunately.
   b. **False.** About one-half of women with urinary incontinence have detrusor overactivity. Cystometry is essential to diagnose the mechanism of incontinence before considering surgery.
   c. **True.** If she has an overactive bladder she may benefit from anticholinergic drug treatment.
   d. **True.**

   e. **False.** Weight reduction, stopping smoking and physiotherapy will cure many such women and should always be tried before surgery.

8. a. **False.** Investigation of women in this age group rarely shows any abnormality.
   b. True. It is important to obtain a urine sample to determine the responsible organism and its antibiotic sensitivity before starting treatment, although a 'best guess' antibiotic should be commenced while awaiting the result.
   c. False. Sexual activity is often implicated in the initiation of urinary infection in women.
   d. True. Alteration of the natural vulval flora will often make the situation worse.
   e. False. She should increase her fluid intake. The bladder is better emptied after intercourse to 'flush out' any vulval organisms that may have been introduced.

Plastic surgery

Chapter overview

Injuries to the skin and subcutaneous tissues are among the commonest injuries encountered in primary and secondary health care. Considerable morbidity can result from failure to accurately assess the extent of injury or to initiate appropriate treatment. Understanding the different types of soft tissue damage will help to raise awareness of the patterns of injury and will improve diagnostic accuracy.

An extensive burn injury can be life threatening. Careful assessment of burn depth and airway involvement, together with a knowledge of fluid resuscitation and care of burn wounds, is essential if these patients are to have a successful outcome.

Skin cancers are the most common of all cancers. Recognition of the most frequent types will ensure early diagnosis and treatment. The number of skin cancers is increasing and failure to recognise the characteristic early clinical features of malignant melanoma, for example, can result in a curable condition becoming life threatening. Reconstructive plastic surgery is an important component in the overall management of patients with breast and oral cancer. The principles of reconstructive surgery are outlined in this chapter.

14.1 Soft tissue trauma

Learning objectives

You should:

- understand the different types of soft tissue injury encountered in clinical practice
- be able to assess a soft tissue injury
- know the principles of management
- recognise the importance of the soft tissues in complex limb injuries.

Soft tissue trauma is one of the most frequent causes of attendance at an A&E department. Penetrating lacerations may be life threatening if major vessels are injured (e.g. in the neck). Crush injuries may result in considerable mor-

bidity and delayed healing. Recognition of the different categories of soft tissue injury is important because it reduces the risk of missing injuries to deep structures and it enables appropriate primary management to be instigated. The five main types of soft tissue injury are:

- laceration
- crush injury
- degloving injury
- avulsion injury
- haematoma.

Laceration Stab wounds are typical laceration wounds. The incision-like injury is usually caused by a sharp implement (knife or broken bottle). These wounds are often deep and penetrating with little surrounding bruising. Associated fractures are rare, but vascular or nerve injuries are common, especially in the head and neck. Tendons in the hand are frequently injured. Skin loss is rare.

Crush injury Crush injuries are caused by a blunt force and are characterised by diffuse soft tissue damage. Bone and joint injuries occur more frequently than lacerations,. The force behind the injury causes vessel and nerve compression. Bruising is often extensive. Complete division of neurovascular structures is uncommon. Skin devitalisation is seen more often than in a laceration injury.

Degloving injury In degloving injuries, external forces shear the skin off the underlying tissues, usually in a tissue plane between the subcutaneous fat and deep fascia. This injury is most frequent in the limbs. Severe degloving injuries are classically associated with roller type machinery or a vehicle tyre running over a limb. Less severe, though more common, degloving injuries are seen in elderly patients who strike their legs against a low object such as a table or a bus platform. The skin is degloved between the fixed obstacle and the moving limb. In elderly patients with thin fragile skin, healing can be delayed and morbidity prolonged if the injury is not correctly recognised. These injuries can result in skin necrosis.

Avulsion injury This implies tissue loss after injury and is a characteristic of human and animal bite wounds. Prominent parts of the face or limbs are often affected. Bite wounds are particularly prone to infection because of the large number of organisms in the mouth; they must be meticulously cleaned and debrided before repair. Broad-spectrum antibiotic treatment (flucloxacillin and metronidazole) is essential. These wounds present a formidable reconstructive challenge because of their complexity and location, frequently in cosmetically sensitive areas of the face. Occasionally, avulsed segments (particularly digits) can be reimplanted either as a free graft or by using micro-vascular techniques.

Haematoma These are caused by a blunt force, which results in subcutaneous haemorrhage while the skin overlying the bleeding site remains intact. An expanding haematoma can devascularise the overlying skin and cause necrosis. Applying pressure dressings exacerbates the problem by further reducing the blood supply to the skin. Early diagnosis together with decompression and ligation or cautery of the injured vessels is the treatment of choice. Otherwise, skin necrosis will develop and a skin graft will be required.

Principles of management

Soft tissue trauma alone

Diagnosis
An accurate description of the nature of the injury is almost as important as the clinical examination of the wound. Many injuries, particularly if they are extensive, will be a combination of the various types of soft tissue injury listed above.

Complications
The most important complications following soft tissue trauma are:

- vessel, tendon and nerve injury
- foreign body inclusion
- skin loss and necrosis
- secondary infection.

Treatment
The key steps in treatment are:

1. careful assessment
2. thorough debridement
3. meticulous wound inspection under local or general anaesthetic to assess the extent of damage and to remove foreign bodies, e.g. glass fragments
4. primary repair of all severed structures unless the wound is grossly infected; skin graft as necessary
5. reassessment of tissue viability immediately and at 48 h
6. antibiotic cover for all avulsion injuries and contaminated wounds.

Soft tissue injury in complex limb trauma

Failure to recognise injury to the skin and subcutaneous tissues close to a fracture may compromise the outcome of an otherwise good fracture reduction and fixation. Without adequate management of the soft tissue injury, the wound will break down, exposing the fracture site and leading to osteomyelitis and non-union. Lower limb complex fractures are particularly at risk when associated with a major degloving injury to the limb. Important preventative measures are:

1. careful assessment of the wound, checking for soft tissue viability
2. thorough debridement of non-viable soft tissue at the time of fracture reduction and fixation

3. covering of the fracture site with viable soft tissue within 5 days of the injury. A local or 'free' microvascular flap may be required.

Although these injuries are most commonly seen in the lower limb, the same principles apply in complex upper limb and hand injuries.

14.2 Burns and skin grafts

> **Learning objectives**
>
> You should:
> - understand the pathophysiology of burns including inhalation injury
> - know the diagnostic features of different depths of burn wounds
> - be able to construct a fluid resuscitation regime for burn patients
> - understand the different methods of managing a burn wound.

The epidemiology of burns in the developed world has changed significantly over the last 50 years. Legislation (e.g. outlawing inflammable nightwear for children) has reduced many types of burn injury. The most common burn injuries that remain are:

- scalds in children
- burns in elderly patients
- burns related to medical illness (e.g. following an epileptic fit)
- burns in alcoholics and drug addicts
- burns in major disaster victims (e.g. Piper Alpha oil platform, Bradford football stadium, etc.).

Most burns are small [<2% body surface area (BSA)] and can be dealt with in a casualty department. Burns of >10% BSA in children (>15% in adults) should be admitted for fluid resuscitation. Patients with suspected smoke inhalation should also be admitted.

Pathophysiology

Burn injury results in a large amount of fluid 'leakage' from the circulation into the tissues at the site of the injury. When the size of the burn exceeds 20–30% (BSA), the process becomes generalised. When this oedema is combined with ongoing evaporative loss from the moist burn surface, the plasma volume is significantly decreased, which leads to intravascular hypovolaemia. If this is not corrected, it precipitates organ system failure, especially renal failure. In the case of inhalational injury, oedema of the airways causes acute respiratory obstruction with stridor, etc., requiring urgent intervention with intubation or even tracheostomy.

Types of burn injury

Scald A burn caused by wet heat, usually boiling water or steam.

Flame A direct effect of burning gases on the skin. High temperatures damage skin proteins and cause deep burns with skin staining. Smoke inhalation injury is frequent.

Chemical Caused by direct skin contact with chemicals (usually strong acid or alkali).

Electrical Often causes a deep burn. The severity of damage depends on the tissue resistance (high in skin and bone), voltage and current. The electrical energy is transformed into heat energy. Low-voltage domestic burns often look small but are deep. High-voltage injuries can be fatal, causing cardiac arrhythmias and muscle spasm, which prevents the victim releasing himself from the current source.

Friction Occurs when the body comes into contact with a rapidly moving surface (e.g. a tyre or belt drive). Often these wounds are deep and expose underlying fat or muscle.

Contact Caused by direct conduction of heat from a hot surface to the skin, particularly when protective mechanisms are not functioning (e.g. an epileptic patient who falls into a fire following a seizure).

Inhalation Lung and airway damage follows smoke inhalation. Several factors contribute, including the effects of heat, hypoxia and toxic products in the smoke, as well as secondary changes caused by pulmonary oedema and infection.

Burn depth

There are three categories of burn depth:

- superficial
- deep dermal
- full thickness.

Superficial burns Damage is confined to the epidermis and the superficial dermal layers. Spontaneous healing occurs in 10–14 days as the epidermis regenerates from undamaged epidermal appendages in the dermis (hair follicles and sweat glands).

Deep dermal burns Damage includes deeper layers of dermis. Only a few epidermal appendages remain. Although spontaneous healing occurs, it is often delayed for 3–4 weeks and may result in a hypertrophic scar.

Full-thickness burns The epidermis and dermis are totally destroyed and spontaneous epithelialisation cannot occur. A very small full-thickness burn will eventually heal as the wound contracts by epithelialisation from adjacent tissue.

Clinical features

Correct assessment of the burn depth and extent is the key to successful treatment:

Assessment of depth:

- superficial
  - moist blistered surface
  - sensitive to pinprick
- deep dermal
  - blistering
  - bright red
  - reduced pain sensitivity
  - cream-coloured wound base

Table 18 'Rule of nine' method for estimating burn surface area

Area of body	Percentage of body surface rea
Head/neck	9
Upper limb (each)	9
Front of trunk	18
Back of trunk	18
Lower limb (each)	18
Perineum	1

- full thickness
  - no blistering
  - dry, grey/white leathery appearance
  - absent pain sensation.

Many burns are a combination of categories, e.g. a predominantly deep dermal injury is usually surrounded by a zone of superficial burn injury.

Assessment of extent There are three commonly used methods for assessing the extent of a burn injury:

- *the rule of nine*: this is the most common method of estimating burn surface area (see Table 18). It is less accurate in young children because the head represents a proportionately larger surface area of the body than in adults
- *Lund and Browder charts*: these provide a more detailed mapping system of a burn, again as a percentage BSA. Different charts are available for children and adults
- *palm of hand*: the area of a patient's palm is equal to 1% of the BSA and can be used to estimate the extent of the burn.

Burn management

There are two phases to burn wound management:

- early
- subsequent/late.

Early management

Burns may be part of a multiple systemic injury to a patient; the initial assessment should follow the advanced trauma life support (ATLS) principles (see p. ••). There are two important components to the early management of burn injuries:

- fluid resuscitation
- wound management
  - *open method*
  - *closed method.*

Fluid resuscitation

Fluid resuscitation by an intravenous route is required for burns of >15% BSA in adults and >10% BSA in children. Fluid resuscitation requirements are based on the Parkland formula (see Figure 195).

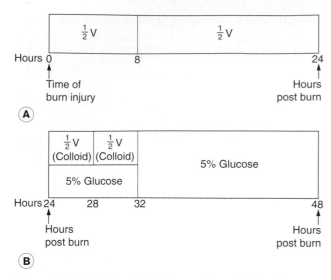

Fourteen

Figure 193 Parkland formula for fluid resuscitation. (A) First 24 h post burn. (B) Second 24 h post burn.

For adults In the first 24 h post burn the fluid requirement (V) is calculated from the following formula: 4 ml × weight of patient (kg) × % BSA burned. Use Ringer's lactate solution and give 50% of the required volume in the first 8 h postburn, with the remaining 50% being given over the next 16 h. (Figure 193A).

The fluid required (V) over the next 24 h is calculated from the following formula: 0.5 ml × weight of patient (kg) × % BSA burned. Use a combination of fresh frozen plasma (or colloid substitute) and 5% glucose solution. This volume is given between 24 h and 32 h post burn. Throughout the 24-h period the volume of 5% glucose solution given to the patient (Figure 193B) is adjusted to maintain a urine output of 60–80 ml/h for a 70-kg adult.

Additional baseline fluid maintenance therapy must be provided for patients who are unable to take oral fluids.

For children: Use the Parkland regime and calculate the additional fluids (use 4% glucose in ¼ or ⅕ normal saline) required for maintenance therapy according to the weight of the child:

- 100 ml/kg up to 10 kg
- 500 ml/kg between 10 and 20 kg
- 20 ml/kg for each kg over 20 kg.

Paediatric expertise must be sought, especially if presentation has been delayed. Under these circumstances, electrolyte balance can be difficult to manage. As a general rule, half the calculated volume is given in the first 8 h with the remainder given over the next 16 h.

These calculations only form a *basis* for resuscitation. The adequacy of resuscitation is monitored using the hourly urine output and haematocrit [packed cell volume (PCV)] as a guide and the infusion rate is adjusted accordingly.

Burn wound care

The main aim is to reduce the risk of infection until spontaneous healing occurs or the wound is ready for split skin grafting.

Open treatment A dry eschar forms over burn wounds during the first few days after injury and acts as a biological barrier. This is particularly useful in burn wounds that are difficult to dress (e.g. face, perineum, buttocks). The crust or eschar slowly separates from the wound margins after 7–10 days. In superficial burns, separation is complete by 14–21 days leaving a freshly epithelialised surface beneath. In deep burns, a granulating surface is left that requires skin grafting. Large burn wounds are treated by exposure. Patients are nursed in a warm room with clean filtered air (this forms the design basis for modern burns units).

Closed treatment After cleaning the burn wound, a dressing is applied. Silver sulfadiazine has antibacterial properties and is particularly useful for burn wounds. If there is a lot of exudate, dressings are changed daily. The wound should be inspected at 5 days to re-evaluate the extent of the injury.

Hand burns can be treated by coating the affected areas with silver sulfadiazine and then applying a plastic bag around the hand and securing the bag at the wrist. Using this treatment, the patient can still use the affected hand to hold utensils, etc.

Subsequent/late management

After resuscitation has been completed, the burn should be reassessed. Unless the burn is superficial or a very small deep dermal/full-thickness injury, skin grafting will probably be required.

Tangential excision

This technique, which is carried out 5–10 days after the injury, involves serial shaving of the burn wound until bleeding occurs from the wound surface:

- immediate bleeding indicates a superficial burn; these wounds are simply dressed until healing occurs
- a white pattern dermis on shaving indicates a deep dermal burn; these wounds are resurfaced with a split skin graft
- subcutaneous fat on shaving indicates a full-thickness burn; these wounds are also resurfaced with a split skin graft.

Key points in major burn management

Analgesia Use intravenous morphine or pethidine in sufficient amounts to relieve pain. Do *not* use subcutaneous or intramuscular routes of administration as drugs will be poorly absorbed initially; later, as resuscitation takes effect, massive absorption of opiates may cause collapse.

Escharotomy Use releasing incisions for deep circumferential burns to limbs. Otherwise, as the tissues swell, dead skin that cannot expand will act as a tourniquet causing distal ischaemia.

Blood transfusion Avoid in the first 24 h after injury unless there is associated trauma. Transfusion exacerbates the haemoconcentration (and peripheral sludging) that follows plasma loss after a burn injury.

Admission to hospital This should occur if:

- intravenous fluids are required
- burns are likely to need early grafting (e.g. eyelids, hands, etc.)
- burns affect difficult areas that are likely to need specialised nursing (e.g. perineum)
- non-accidental injury is suspected (e.g. in children).

Fluid resuscitation Fluid needs should be calculated *from the time of injury* and not from the time of hospital admission. Do not forget daily maintenance requirements.

Inhalation injury

This serious injury is usually associated with burns that occur in a confined space (e.g. in a house fire).

Clinical features

These include:

- burns to face and mouth
- black carbonaceous sputum
- ulcerated and oedematous oral mucosa
- wheezing and stridor.

Investigations

The degree of injury should be investigated by:

- measuring carboxyhaemoglobin levels
- measuring arterial blood gases and monitoring arterial saturation
- obtaining a chest radiograph
- bronchoscopy (flexible).

A carboxyhaemoglobin level of >15%, 3 h after injury, or a P_aO_2 <10 kPa when a patient is provided with 50% oxygen suggests inhalation injury.

Treatment

In the treatment of inhalation injuries:

- provide humidified oxygen via a face mask
- if stridor develops, intubate the patient
- use aggressive physiotherapy
- nurse in the head-up position
- bronchodilators may help but steroids probably will not
- ventilate patients whose P_aO_2 falls below 10 kPa
- consider therapeutic bronchoscopy to clear the airways
- use specific antibiotics after sputum culture.

Prognosis

The outcome after a severe inhalation injury is poor. Patients can die of bronchopneumonia and/or respiratory failure.

Late complications of burn injury

Hypertrophic scarring

Superficial burns heal with virtually no scarring. Many deep dermal and all full-thickness burns will scar and some will become hypertrophic (thickened, red and uncomfortable), especially in children.

Treatment Hypertrophic scarring can be reduced by:

- topical silicone gel
- compression garments: a specially manufactured lycra garment that compresses the scar during maturation (up to 18 months)
- steroid injection: used mainly in small raised scars.

Contractures

These develop where a scar extends longitudinally across a joint crease. They are particularly common in children, who should undergo follow-up until growth is complete. Surgical release may be necessary, with resulting defects being repaired with skin grafts of flaps.

Unstable scar

Breakdown of a scar or graft can occur over bony prominences. Overgrafting or resurfacing with a more robust skin flap may be needed.

Alopecia

Deep scalp burns can cause alopecia. Scalp flaps, which are sometimes combined with tissue expansion, can usefully cover these areas with hair-bearing tissue.

Marjolin's ulcer

Squamous cell carcinoma can develop on an old scar (often from a burn). These develop many years after the original injury, often in elderly patients. Treatment is by excision and skin grafting.

14.3 Skin tumours

> ### Learning objectives
>
> You should:
> - know the clinical features of the common types of skin malignancy
> - have a detailed knowledge of the early features of malignant melanoma
> - know the prognostic indices of malignant melanoma
> - know how to treat and prevent malignant melanoma.

Skin cancer is the most common cancer affecting mankind. The incidence of skin cancer is increasing throughout the developing world and the number of cases of malignant melanoma is doubling every 10 years in the UK at present. There are three common types of skin cancer:

- basal cell carcinoma
- squamous cell carcinoma
- malignant melanoma.

Basal cell carcinoma

This is the most common type of skin cancer. It predominates in the elderly, especially on exposed parts of the body, particularly the face. These tumours generally grow extremely slowly over many years and only rarely metastasise.

Clinical features

Four types of basal cell carcinoma are recognised:

- cystic
- ulcerative
- multifocal, superficial
- sclerosing or morphoeic.

Most basal cell cancers occur on the head and neck; they are much less common on the limbs. They are especially common in fair-skinned people of northern European extraction who are exposed to long periods of sunlight. Basal cell carcinomas usually grow very slowly. Multiple lesions are sometimes found, representing a 'field change' in the skin. Occasionally, basal cell cancers are pigmented and a malignant melanoma must be considered in the differential diagnosis.

Diagnosis

The diagnosis is based on the long history and the appearance of the lesion. Cystic tumours are well circumscribed, have a pearly smooth-domed appearance and small capillaries can be seen tracing across their surface. Ulcerative tumours are the classic basal cell cancer, with an ulcerated centre surrounded by a rolled margin. Multifocal and sclerosing tumours have ill-defined margins and great care is required to ensure that they are completely excised.

Treatment

Surgery As these lesions rarely metastasise, the main aim of surgery is to *ensure adequate local removal*. Careful sharp dissection is required with a gentle 'no touch' and 'non-crush' technique to prevent contamination and seeding of the surgical field. This is particularly important in ulcerated or fungating lesions.

The *margin of excision* varies with the type of lesion being excised. It is always helpful to draw a line around the outline of the lesion with a second line to demarcate the extent of the excision. Usually, a margin of 2–3 mm is adequate for a cystic basal cell carcinoma. In multifocal or sclerosing tumours, great care must be taken to identify the interface between tumour and normal tissue. Under these circumstances, magnification is often helpful. A wider margin of 5–6 mm or more (if the lesion is recurrent) should be measured out prior to excision. If there is any doubt about the adequacy of excision, especially in large deeply invasive recurrent basal cell cancers, frozen section examination at the time of operation is very helpful. An alternative is to use micrographic surgery, a complex dermatological technique, which is useful in recurrent tumours where the margins are distinct. Magnifying loupes should be used when excising these tumours.

Overall, surgical treatment is usually preferred to other treatments because:

- it is a single-stage treatment
- it has a high cure rate
- it provides an opportunity to confirm the tissue diagnosis and adequacy of excision by histological examination.

Radiotherapy Radiotherapy is an effective treatment for basal cell cancers. It is particularly useful for advanced tumours when underlying bone is involved. Radiotherapy is contraindicated in cancers that develop on limbs or for treating recurrence after previous radiotherapy. It should also be avoided in the treatment of lesions of the inner canthus, eyelids, tip of the nose and alar region, base of the ala nasi, external ear and auditory canal.

Topical cytotoxic therapy A preparation of 5-fluorouracil (5-FU) is available as a cream that can be applied topically to basal cell cancers (and to squamous cell cancers). It is applied once or twice per day for 3–4 weeks. Topical 5-FU is usually only effective in very early flat lesions. There is a high recurrence rate.

Imiquimod cream This can be used to effectively treat early superficial basal cell cancers. It is applied once per day for 5 days each week for a total of 6 weeks. The cream should be rubbed in and left for 8 h before being carefully washed off with mild soap and water.

Photodynamic therapy (PDT) This treatment, which uses light to activate topical or systemically delivered cytotoxic agents, is currently being evaluated in the treatment of superficial basal cell and squamous cell carcinomas. Its long-term effectiveness compared with existing treatment options is still unknown.

Squamous cell carcinoma

These cancers are also common in areas of the body that are exposed to sunlight for prolonged periods.

Clinical features

Squamous cell cancers are usually distributed on the head and neck. They occur on the limbs more often than basal cell cancers. These tumours grow more rapidly than basal cell cancers and can metastasise via the lymphatics to regional lymph nodes and via the bloodstream to distant sites, particularly lung and bone. They have an ulcerated surface and irregular margins. The lesions are often friable and bleed easily. Regional lymph nodes should always be examined, especially in large long-standing lesions. Early results of treatment with PDT are promising.

Treatment

Surgical excision or radiotherapy is chosen based on the principles outlined for basal cell cancers.

Bowen's disease

This is a slow-growing, low-grade variant of a squamous carcinoma that develops intraepidermally. The lesion is well circumscribed, slightly raised and often pink/brown in colour with a scaly consistency. Multiple lesions occur on the limbs. Growth is very slow over many years but may progress to a frankly invasive squamous cell carcinoma. Imiquimod cream can also be used to treat Bowen's disease.

Keratoacanthoma

This lesion is *not* a squamous cell carcinoma but is often mistaken for one; it can be very difficult to differentiate between the two on appearance alone. The history is of a rapidly growing exophytic lesion that characteristically has a large central keratin plug. The growth is self-limiting and the lesion slowly regresses leaving virtually no scar. This rapid growth and aggressive appearance causes great alarm to the patient. The diagnosis is usually made on the length of the history.

Treatment

Observation The suspected keratoacanthoma should be observed for a period of *up to 6–8 weeks only*. If there is no sign of spontaneous regression, excision is indicated.

Surgery Excision may be needed followed by skin flap closure or grafting. It is essential that these lesions are sent for histological analysis.

Malignant melanoma

Malignant melanoma accounts for 11% of all skin cancers in the UK. Both the incidence and the death rates have risen significantly over recent years and this trend continues. Malignant melanoma is one of the few cancers to affect young adults; 22% of all melanomas occur in individuals under 40 years of age. The cancer is more common in women and the anatomical distribution differs between the sexes; melanomas are more common on the trunk in men and on the lower limb in women.

Several factors affect a given individual's risk of developing a melanoma:

- excessive exposure to the sun
- skin type
- change in an existing mole
- presence of a large number of naevi
- previous melanoma
- presence of a giant hairy naevus.

Up to 10% of melanomas are thought to be associated with inherited characteristics (dysplastic naevus syndrome). These moles are usually large (>1 cm diameter) with irregular margins and often a variation in pigment density. There is a clear association between sunburn and melanoma.

There are four clinical types of melanoma:

- superficial spreading (50%)
- nodular (20–25%)
- lentigo maligna melanoma (15%)
- acral lentiginous (10%).

Malignant melanoma spreads via the regional lymphatics and bloodstream. Satellite lesions may be found in the skin. Liver, lung, brain and bone are the most frequent sites for metastases.

The prognosis is most accurately related to the thickness of the tumour (Breslow thickness; see Table 19).

Table 19 Breslow thickness and survival rates in patients with melanoma

Thickness of melanoma (mm)	5-year survival rate (%)
Less than 1.5	93
1.5–3.49	67
More than 3.5	37

Treatment

There is no consistently successful treatment for advanced melanoma. Long-term survival is poor for thick lesions. An adequate surgical excision is the mainstay of treatment. For thick lesions, survival appears to remain the same irrespective of the margins of excision. The main thrust of management of this dangerous tumour is *prevention* and *early diagnosis*.

Prevention

Sunlight is the main aetiological risk factor linked with malignant melanoma. Studies have shown that the risk is significantly increased in:

- sunburn during childhood
- fair-skinned people who burn easily, tan poorly and who are exposed excessively to the sun.

These at-risk groups should avoid prolonged exposure to the sun (particularly between 11AM and 3PM). Sun beds and sun lamps should be avoided. Covering the skin with light clothing is effective; broad-brimmed hats afford similar protection for the head and neck. Sunscreens are also helpful, filtering out ultraviolet radiation in the ultraviolet-B range (the cause of blistering and burning). Sunscreens are graded (by factor numbers) according to their ability to filter ultraviolet radiation, e.g. by using a factor 6 sunscreen, a person can spend six times as long in the sun before getting burned. Ideally, nothing less than factor 15 should be used. Sunscreens must be used liberally and reapplied every 2 h if exposure to the sun continues.

Early diagnosis

Early signs of malignancy in a pigmented lesion include a change in size, alteration in pigment (particularly if the mole becomes unevenly pigmented), itching and notching of the margin. Later signs include bleeding and ulceration. Studies have shown that the diagnosis can be aided with the use of a dermatoscope or a siascope, which in the hands of an experienced observer can improve detection of the early signs of malignancy.

Treatment

Surgery Complete excision is essential. Controversy exists with regard to the optimum margin of excision. As a guide, a margin of 1 cm for each mm in Breslow thickness is appropriate. Incisional biopsies are to be condemned, as is an incomplete excision. Prophylactic lymph node dissection does not improve the prognosis.

Sentinel lymph gland biopsy Currently, the potential benefit of sentinal lymph node mapping and biopsy is being assessed in patients with malignant melanoma. This technique uses a radioactive marker and a blue dye marker to identify lymph glands draining a melanoma. The markers are injected into the vicinity of the cancer and the lymphatic drainage can then be tracked to the first or 'sentinal' lymph gland that drains the melanoma. These glands are removed for histological examination. If any melanoma cells are identified, the remaining lymph glands in the entire lymph gland 'basin' that drain the melanoma are removed.

This technique is still controversial and it remains to be seen if it will improve survival in these patients. It should be considered in melanomas of >1 mm Breslow thickness.

Chemotherapy and radiotherapy Various combinations of chemotherapeutic agents have been tried without notable success and trials are continuing. Radiotherapy provides useful palliation, particularly for symptomatic bone metastases. The early results of immunotherapy have been encouraging.

Prognosis

The outcome is closely related to the thickness of the melanoma at the time of excision and is summarised in Table 19.

14.4 Reconstruction following cancer surgery (Breast and oral cancer)

Learning objectives

You should:
- know about the reconstructive options for patients undergoing surgery for breast or intraoral malignancy.

Reconstruction following cancer surgery plays an important role in the overall management and rehabilitation of cancer patients, especially those with breast or oral cancer.

Breast cancer

Once a decision to carry out a mastectomy has been made, reconstruction should be discussed with the patient. Radiotherapy, smoking and poor general health are all factors that may predispose to a poor outcome after this extensive surgery. Reconstruction can be carried out using:

- prostheses (saline or silicone)
- the patients' own tissue (autogenous reconstruction), e.g. using a flap of skin and fat based on the transverse rectus abdominus muscle (TRAM flap) from the lower abdomen
- a combination of these techniques (e.g. latissimus dorsi flap plus prosthesis).

Reconstruction can be carried out at the time of mastectomy (immediate) or at a later date (delayed).

The advantages and disadvantages of each option must be discussed fully with each patient, taking into account their tumour oncology and any personal risk factors. For example, a prosthesis used alone to reconstruct a breast where the overlying skin has been irradiated is likely to be associated with a high complication rate, especially skin breakdown with extrusion of the implant. A flap of 'healthy' living tissue (e.g. a latissimus dorsi myocutaneous flap) combined with a prosthesis would be a much safer option for this patient.

Oral cancer

Reconstruction is required following resection of large tumours of the oral cavity, which often involves removal of part of the mandible. 'Free' tissue transfer (i.e. tissue taken from other parts of the body and revascularised using microvascular surgical techniques) is an essential part of the rehabilitation of these patients in allowing these large defects to be replaced with skin and bone grafts. Examples include:

- radial forearm flap – for small mandibular defects
- fibular flap – for larger mandibular defects
- anterior thigh flap – for large soft tissue only defects in the floor of the mouth.

Self-assessment: questions

Extended matching items questions (EMIs)

EMI 1

Theme: Burns and skin grafts

1. Marjolin's ulcer, left shin	A. tangential excision and grafting
2. deep circumferential burn, right upper arm	B. local steroid injection
3. superficial burn, right hand	C. escharotomy
4. deep dermal burn left thigh	D. wide excision and skin grafting
5. hypertrophic scar, right forearm	E. silver sulfadiazine dressings

Match each of the items in the left-hand column with a single item in the right-hand column.

EMI 2

Theme: Skin cancers

1. cystic basal cell cancer, right inner canthus	A. radiotherapy
2. sclerosing basal cell cancer, left forearm	B. local excision with 1-cm margin
3. superficial spreading melanoma less than 1 mm thick	C. local excision with 3-cm margin; consider sentinel node biopsy
4. histologically proven recurrent basal cell carcinoma involving zygoma in patient unfit for surgery	D. local excision with 3-mm margin
5. nodular melanoma estimated to be 3 mm thick	E. local excision with 6-mm margin

Match each of the items in the left-hand column with a single item in the right-hand column.

EMI 3

Theme: Skin malignancy

1. malignant melanoma
2. squamous cell carcinoma
3. basal cell carcinoma
4. Marjolin's ulcer
5. Bowen's disease

The following clinical statements relate to which of the above diagnoses? Each statement may be used once, more than once or not at all.

A. Tends to be more radiosensitive than other forms of skin cancer

B. Occurs in chronic scars

C. Often, but not exclusively, arises in a pre-existing mole

D. Typically grows on the limbs of elderly patients and can metastasise to the regional lymph nodes

E. Arises superficially in the skin and may be sensitive to imiquimod cream

F. Responds well to chemotherapy in the advanced stages of the disease

EMI 4

Theme: Soft tissue injuries

1. animal and human bite wounds
2. lower limb compound fractures
3. lacerations to the hands/digits caused by a knife or broken glass
4. haematomas of the limbs
5. degloving injuries
6. crush injuries

Match each of the following clinical facts to one of the soft tissue injuries above. Each clinical fact may be used once, more than once or not at all.

A. Require viable soft tissue cover by 5 days post injury.

B. Frequently result in damage to tendons and nerves.

C. Should be drained, the limb elevated and compression bandaging avoided where possible.

D. Are heavily contaminated wounds (including gram negative organisms) and require thorough cleaning and broad-spectrum antibiotic cover.

E. The specific mechanism of injury may result in extensive undermining of the soft tissues with resulting necrosis.

Constructed response questions (CRQs)

CRQ 1

A 19-year-old man was assaulted with a broken bottle as he came out of a pub. The injury to the left cheek was in the form of an inverted 'C' (see Figure 194). The ambulance crew reported that there had been excessive bleeding from the wound.

a. What type of soft tissue injury is this likely to be?

b. List five important steps in the management of this injury.

Look at the site of the injury.

c. List four important structures that could have been damaged.

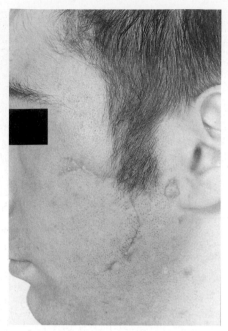

Figure 194

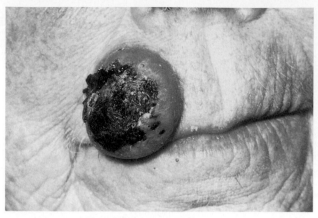

Figure 195

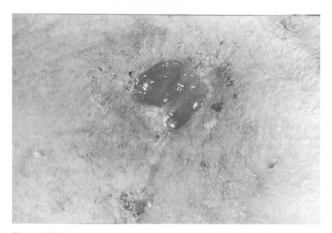

Figure 196

d. What long-term complications can develop as a result of this injury. List two of them.

CRQ 2

A 37-year-old woman is brought into the A&E department after being rescued from a house fire. On admission she is very distressed and appears to be wheezing. Her weight is 70 kg and the burns are mainly confined to her trunk, face, right upper limb (including the hand) and right thigh, affecting 30% of the body surface area in total excluding areas of erythema. The burn to the right arm was noted to be full thickness extending around the whole limb. The burn injury occurred at 9.30PM and the patient was admitted to hospital at 11.30PM. Fluid resuscitation commenced at 12.30AM, 3 h post burn.

a. List four important points in the *early* management of this patient.

b. What analgesia would you use?

c. Describe: (i) the route of delivery that you would choose and (ii) why?

d. Using the Parkland formula: (i) calculate the fluid replacement that the patient will require and (ii) outline the initial fluid replacement regime.

e. What type of fluid would you use?

Two hours after admission you are asked to assess the patient's progress.

f. Describe two indices that would be most useful in assessing the adequacy of fluid replacement in this patient.

The patient is particularly concerned about the burn injury to her right hand.

g. Outline four key points in the management of the burn injury to the right hand.

Objective structured clinical examination questions (OSCEs)

OSCE 1

Look at the accompanying photograph (Figure 195). This large crusted lesion has grown rapidly to its present size over a 3- to 4-week period. It is not painful. On examination it is raised and well circumscribed. There is no history of bleeding. Answer the following questions:

a. What is the most likely diagnosis?

b. What is the key differential diagnosis?

c. What else should your clinical examination include?

d. How would you treat this patient?

OSCE 2

Look at the accompanying clinical photograph (Figure 196) and read the following history that relates to this patient.

A 75-year-old retired soldier who has spent much of his time abroad in the tropics attends your surgery for a routine hypertension check. While you record his blood pressure you notice an ulcerating lesion on his arm, measuring approximately 6 cm in diameter and arising in an old scar from a war injury. The margin is irregular and

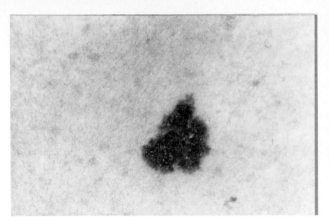

Figure 197

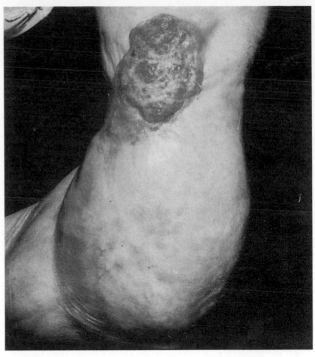

Figure 198

friable (the patient usually keeps it covered with a dry dressing). There is also evidence of long-standing sun damage to the surrounding skin with multiple keratoses.

Taking the history and clinical photograph together, answer the following questions:

a. What is the most likely diagnosis?

b. What else should you examine?

c. What investigations would be appropriate?

d. How would you manage this patient?

OSCE 3

Examine the accompanying photograph (Figure 197) and read the following history that relates to this patient.

A 32-year-old woman gives a history of a long-standing mole on her leg. Over the last 6 months it has become darker in colour and has begun to itch. She regularly holidays abroad in Spain. On examination she has an irregular pigmented lesion measuring 1.5 cm in diameter on her leg.

Answer the following questions:

a. What is the diagnosis?

b. What other areas of the body should you examine?

c. What investigations would be appropriate?

d. What is the correct treatment?

e. The pathology report indicates that the lesion is 2.5 mm thick. What is the prognosis?

f. What key advice would you give regarding the prevention of further similar lesions?

OSCE 4

Look at this clinical photograph (Figure 198) and read the following history that relates to this patient.

A 70-year-old woman attends surgery with a long-standing lesion (several years) on her upper arm that has been steadily increasing in size. It is not causing any symptoms but she is concerned because it is not 'going away'. On examination she has a well-circumscribed lesion measuring 1.5 cm on her upper arm. It is circular in outline, ulcerated and has a raised margin.

Answer the following questions:

a. What is the likely diagnosis?

b. Name two treatment options.

c. Is this lesion likely to metastasise?

Multiple choice questions

1. Inhalation burn injury:

   a. is often associated with burns on the face

   b. can be difficult to diagnose in the early stages

   c. can be rapidly fatal

   d. may need to be treated by early endotracheal intubation

   e. is suggested by a carboxyhaemoglobin level of 5%

Self-assessment: answers

EMI answers

EMI 1

Theme: Burns and skin grafts

1. D. A Marjolin's ulcer is a squamous cell carcinoma that develops in an old scar, often many years after the original injury. It requires a wide local excision and usually skin grafting to cover the remaining defect.

2. C. An escharotomy is often necessary for this type of injury. This 'releasing incision' will prevent the deep circumferential burn wound from acting as a tourniquet, causing distal ischaemia as the limb swells and becomes oedematous in response to the injury.

3. E. Silver sulfadiazine has antibacterial properties and is particularly useful in burn wounds. Burns to the hand can be treated by coating the affected areas with silver sulfadiazine and then securing the hand in a plastic bag enabling some useful function to be maintained as the injuries heal.

4. A. Tangential excision, carried out 5–10 days after the burn injury, involves serial shaving of the burn wound until bleeding occurs from the wound surface. In this way, the depth of the burn wound is carefully gauged and only a minimal amount of viable tissue is removed before simple dressings or skin grafts are applied, depending upon the depth of the wound.

5. B. Hypertrophic scars are the sequel to some but not all deep dermal and full-thickness burns. They are more common in children. Steroid injection is one option in the management of these wounds. It is more effective in small raised scars.

EMI 2

Theme: Skin cancers

1. D. A small but clear margin (3 mm) is adequate for a cystic basal cell tumour, especially in a cosmetically sensitive area on the face. Radiotherapy is contraindicated in this area as it may produce scarring or radiation dermatitis.

2. E. A sclerosing basal cell cancer does not have as clearly a defined edge and requires a wider margin of excision to ensure complete clearance and to prevent local recurrence.

3. B. As a general rule, a margin of 1 cm for each mm in Breslow thickness is appropriate. This superficial spreading type melanoma is thin and a 1-cm margin should be sufficient.

4. A. Fixation to underlying tissues such as bone is an indication for treatment with radiotherapy.

5. C. This nodular melanoma is estimated to be 3 mm thick. As a consequence it will require a wide excision providing a margin of at least 3 cm.

EMI 3

Theme: Skin malignancy

1. C. Although many melanomas do arise in pre-existing moles (melanotic naevi), patients do not always recollect a pigmented lesion at the site of a melanoma. A significant risk factor for melanoma is the presence of large numbers of benign melanocytic naevi as well as the existence of large numbers of atypical or dysplastic naevi.

2. D. These tumours tend to be commoner in the elderly, typically on the limbs, but can occur on the face and scalp, especially in older bald men with evidence of sun damage to the scalp.

3. A. These are best treated surgically although radiotherapy is useful in recurrent lesions particularly when there is bony involvement. Radiotherapy should be avoided on the limbs.

4. B. Typically, they appear more than 10 years following the burn injury.

5. E. Imiquimod is likely to be most effective in early superficial Bowen's disease lesions. It is also effective for superficial basal cell carcinomas. The histology should always be confirmed by biopsy before commencing the cream.

EMI 4

Theme: Soft tissue injuries

1. D. Animal and human bite wounds tend to be heavily contaminated with aerobic as well as anaerobic organisms. Thorough cleaning (and debridement) of these wounds is essential, together with broad-spectrum antibiotic cover and tetanus prophylaxis.

2. A. Thorough debridement of non-viable tissue, wound irrigation and coverage of the fracture site with viable tissue by 5 days post injury significantly reduces the risk of osteomyelitis or non-union.

3. B. It is a useful guideline to assume that these injuries cut through everything until they reach the bone; assume that underlying tendons and nerves have been cut until proven otherwise.

4. C. These injuries cause pressure to the overlying skin and, in turn, reduce its blood supply. Simply applying a tight constricting bandage will further compromise the already precarious

blood supply to the involved skin. Drainage of the haematoma and elevation of the limb are the steps that are necessary to preserve the blood supply to the overlying skin.

5. E. It is essential to ascertain the exact mechanism of injury. Frequently, there is an extensive undermining of the soft tissues in this type of injury, which will lead to an extensive tissue loss from necrosis if the mechanism of the injury is not recognised. Take an accurate history.

CRQ answers

CRQ 1

a. This is a laceration injury caused by a sharp glass.

b. Check vital signs.

Establish intravenous infusion.

Check full blood count, blood group and save serum if appropriate.

Plan to explore under general anaesthetic.

Apply local compression to wound to control haemorrhage.

This patient has lost a significant amount of blood. Pulse and blood pressure should be checked to ensure that he is not in shock. An intravenous infusion should be established. The wound needs to be carefully explored in view of its extent, site and a chance that a major vascular structure may have been damaged in the depths of the wound. Exploration should be carried out under general anaesthetic. Local pressure with a bandage should control the haemorrhage until definite exploration can be carried out.

c. Facial nerve branches.

Parotid duct.

Superficial temporal artery and vein.

Maxillary artery.

Infraorbital nerve.

All of these responses will score points. These are the key anatomical structures that are related to this wound.

d. Facial muscle weakness following nerve injury.

Hypertrophic scarring causing disfigurement.

A salivary fistula from the parotid gland.

Any of these responses will score marks. These are the most serious complications that could follow this injury.

CRQ 2

a. Check blood gases.

Chest radiograph.

Analgesia.

Intravenous access.

Escharotomy for right arm circumferential wound.

Catheterise patient.

Any of these responses will score points. This patient has a significant burn requiring fluid replacement and may

have a smoke inhalation injury. The initial management plan must address these problems. In addition, she has a circumferential burn to the right arm and may require an escharotomy to prevent a 'tourniquet effect' from the burn, which might endanger the blood supply to the limb.

b. Morphine or pethidine.

Burn wounds are painful and require strong opioid analgesics to provide effective pain relief.

c. (i) Intravenous.

(ii) Provides controlled delivery.

Intravenous morphine or pethidine would be the analgesics of choice. This route of administration is preferred because subcutaneous or intramuscular absorption in burn patients can be erratic leading to under- or overdosage.

d. A 30% burn in a 70-kg patient, resuscitation commencing 3 h postburn.

For the first 24 h:

Fluid requirements are calculated using the Parkland formula: 4 ml × weight (kg) × % body surface area burned.

In this patient: $4 \times 70 \times 30 = 8400$ ml.

Half of this is given in the first 8 h postburn, i.e. 4200 ml over the first 8 h, *but* 3 h have already elapsed since the burn injury so this volume of fluid (4200 ml) has to be given over the next 5 h. Therefore, infuse at a rate of 840 ml/h (4200/5).

At the end of 5 h, the rate of infusion is adjusted to deliver 4200 ml over the next 16 h. Infuse at a rate of 263 ml/h (4200/16). The rate of fluid administered should be adjusted according to the hourly urine output and haematocrit (PCV), which should be checked every 4 h.

For the second 24 h:

Over the next 24 h, fresh frozen plasma and 5% glucose should be used for fluid resuscitation. This is calculated as follows: 0.5 ml × weight (kg) × % body surface area burned.

In this patient: $0.5 \times 70 \times 30 = 1050$ ml.

This is delivered over 8 h so infuse at a rate of 130 ml/h (1050/8). At the same time infuse 5% glucose at a rate to maintain urine output at 60–80 ml/h.

e. Ringer's lactate solution (for first 24 h).

f. Packed cell volume.

Hourly urine output.

g. Clean hand.

Apply silver sulfadiazine.

Cover with plastic bag.

Tangential excision and skin graft.

After the initial management further definitive treatment will be required because this is a full-thickness burn. Tangential excision and skin grafting will be required 5–7 days after the burn.

OSCE answers

OSCE 1

a. Keratoacanthoma. The history and clinical appearance are typical of this condition.

b. Squamous cell carcinoma.

c. Regional lymph nodes. The neck should be carefully examined paying particular attention to the submandibular, submental and parotid groups of lymph nodes.

d. Conservatively. If your diagnosis is correct, a spontaneous resolution can be expected. An expectant policy should only be pursued for 4–6 weeks. Thereafter, if there is no evidence of resolution, the lesion should be excised. At this site, a complex flap reconstruction will have to be carried out to minimise distortion of the lip.

OSCE 2

a. Either a squamous or a basal cell carcinoma. These tumours can sometimes be difficult to distinguish.

b. The regional lymph glands in the axilla.

c. A chest radiograph. This is quite a large tumour and metastatic spread is a possibility.

d. Excision and grafting. This lesion needs to be excised. Because of its size and site, a skin graft will be needed to repair the resulting defect. A diagnostic biopsy would be useful prior to formal excision.

OSCE 3

a. Malignant melanoma. This patient presents with early symptoms of itching and colour change. 'Notching' of the outline of the mole is also evident.

b. Surrounding skin.

Regional lymph nodes.

Liver.

The surrounding skin should be examined to ensure that there are no satellite nodules in the skin or subcutaneous tissues. The regional draining lymph nodes in the popliteal fossa and groin should also be examined, as should the liver for signs of hepatomegaly.

c. Chest radiograph

Liver function tests

Ultrasound scan of the liver (if there is evidence of hepatomegaly).

d. Complete excision of the lesion. This is the key treatment. Partial biopsy should not be carried out.

As this lesion is quite small, it should be possible to close the resulting defect without skin grafting.

e. The 5-year survival rate is 67%.

f. Avoid prolonged exposure to sunlight. This patient is at a slightly higher risk than the general population of developing a further melanoma. She should be advised to avoid getting burned in the sun, to use a high factor sunscreen (factor 15 or over) and to reapply her sunscreen every few hours when out of doors, particularly in the middle of the day. Any remaining moles can be photographed as a baseline to enable future changes to be identified.

OSCE 4

a. Basal cell carcinoma.

b. Surgical excision.

Radiotherapy.

The advantage of surgery is that histological analysis can be performed and the completeness of excision confirmed. Basal cell cancers are, however, sensitive to radiotherapy.

c. No. Only in exceptional circumstances do basal cell carcinomas metastasise to regional lymph nodes.

Multiple choice answers

1. a. **True.** Particularly if soot staining is noted around the mouth and lips.

   b. **True.** The history is important. Inhalation injury should be suspected after a burn that has occurred in a confined space. Always look for signs of burning to the face or evidence of difficulty with breathing.

   c. **True.** As oedema increases in the airway, respiration becomes progressively more difficult.

   d. **True.** Intervention and ventilation may be necessary in a severe inhalation injury.

   e. **False.** Although the carboxyhaemoglobin level is important, other investigations and signs and symptoms must be taken into account. A carboxyhaemoglobin level of 15% or greater suggests a significant inhalation injury.

Neurosurgery

Chapter overview

Neurosurgery deals with disease and injury of the brain and spinal cord. The most common conditions are traumatic injury, spontaneous haemorrhage and a variety of benign and malignant tumours. Traumatic and degenerative conditions of the spinal column are dealt with in section 3 on Orthopaedic surgery.

The key aims of neurosurgical practice are to localise, identify and treat pathology, and to protect the brain or spinal cord from further damage to maximise the chances of survival or recovery of function. Assessment of neurosurgical conditions usually follows a standard approach: taking a clinical history, examination of the patient (with particular regard to the nervous system) and specific investigations such as cross-sectional imaging. This approach is modified in the initial assessment of a serious head injury, when the first priority is to identify and treat immediately life-threatening complications, even in the absence of a full history.

All neurosurgeons work within multiprofessional teams of doctors, nurses, allied health professionals such as therapists, and clinical psychologists, but they also work particularly closely with other doctors such as neuroradiologists and neuroanaesthetists, who contribute special skills to the diagnosis and treatment of a patient's condition.

15.1 Head injury

Learning objectives

You should:
- understand the pathological basis of head injury care
- know the priorities when assessing and managing a seriously brain-injured patient
- understand the principles of surgical and non-surgical treatment (including rehabilitation) in head injury.

Epidemiology and causes

Head injury is common. In the UK, of the one million people who attend hospital annually for head injury, 100 000 are admitted and 10 000 of these are transferred to neurosurgical units.

There are three categories depending on the seriousness of the injury:

- mild head injury not requiring hospital admission
- moderate head injury requiring hospital admission
- severe head injury requiring transfer to a neurosurgical unit.

Most moderate and severe head injuries result from road accidents (50%), falls (30%) and assaults (10%). Many minor head injuries result from accidents in sport and play.

Pathology of traumatic brain damage

There are two types of brain damage that occur after head injury:

- primary brain damage occurring at the time of injury
- secondary brain damage as a result of later events.

A good result after a serious head injury often depends upon preventing secondary brain damage by prompt recognition and treatment of complications.

Primary brain damage: 'impact injury'

There is a wide spectrum of severity in primary brain damage, from mild concussion to instant death. Mechanical deceleration forces act on the brain at the moment of impact, transferring energy and disrupting neurones and the cerebral microcirculation.

The severity of primary brain damage is assessed by measuring the conscious level. There may be focal neurological signs, depending on the exact pattern of damage throughout the brain.

The management of primary brain damage is to prevent complications while any recovery takes place by:

- maintaining cerebral perfusion and oxygenation
- preventing or treating raised intracranial pressure (ICP).

Secondary brain damage: 'second insult'

Secondary brain damage occurs any time after injury when events reduce cerebral blood supply (and oxygen supply) to the injured neurones. The main causes are:

- extracranial
  - hypoxia and hypercarbia (e.g. blocked airway, inadequate ventilation)
  - shock (e.g. blood loss from other injuries)

- intracranial
  - intracranial haematoma
  - epileptic seizures (if prolonged or repeated)
  - meningitis/brain abscess (after a penetrating injury).

All of these complications cause brain swelling and a rise in ICP, which aggravates existing damage to the neurones. Neurotoxic molecules such as free radicals and neurotransmitters do further damage.

Raised intracranial pressure

There is little spare room within the skull and the cranial contents are not easily compressed. A small increase in intracranial volume can be accommodated with little rise in ICP but, if the volume goes on increasing (e.g. because of haematoma or brain swelling), the ICP rises steeply (Figure 199). This, in turn, decreases cerebral blood flow and oxygen supply. Whether the resulting damage to neurones is reversible or not depends on the severity and duration of the high ICP, so prompt diagnosis and correction are vital.

Clinical assessment of the head-injured patient

History

Some history may be available from the patient or a witness. The ambulance crew are an invaluable source of information about the time and circumstances of injury (e.g. pattern of vehicle damage, height of fall, type of weapon) and whether the patient has improved or deteriorated since the injury. It is extremely important to know how much neurological function the patient had immediately following the injury and to use this as a baseline for the Glasgow Coma Scale (see below).

Priorities in assessment and treatment

Standard protocols are used in the initial assessment of every seriously injured patient, to identify and treat life-threatening problems. The priorities are:

A. airway (with cervical spine control)
B. breathing (with high-flow oxygen)
C. circulation (with haemorrhage control)
D. dysfunction (of the nervous system)
E. exposure and identification of injuries.

Assessing conscious level

The Glasgow Coma Scale (Table 20) is used throughout the world. Conscious level is based on three independent variables:

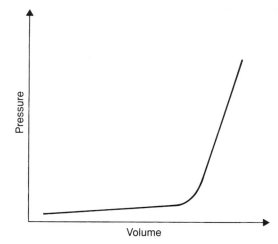

Figure 199 Intracranial pressure—volume relationship.

Table 20 Glasgow Coma Scale and score

Response	Extent of response	Point scale
Eye opening response	Spontaneous	4
	To speech	3
	To pain	2
	No response	1
Best motor response	Obeys commands	6
	Localises painful stimuli	5
	Withdraws from painful stimuli	4
	Spastic flexion	3
	Extension	2
	No response	1
Best verbal response	Orientated	5
	Confused	4
	Inappropriate words	3
	Incomprehensible sounds	2
	No response	1
Minimum score		3
Maximum score		15

- eye opening response
- best motor response in the upper limbs
- best verbal response.

The 'score' for each of the three variables (see Table 20) can be added together to yield a coma score of between 3 and 15. Measurements of conscious level should be made as soon as possible after injury, repeated often and charted to monitor the trend. Changes in conscious level are the most sensitive index of a patient's progress. A falling score warns of continuing neurological damage.

Focal neurological signs

Focal neurological signs reflect damage to specific areas of the brain. The most common are:

- asymmetry of pupil size or response to light stimulus
- asymmetry of motor response between left and right limbs.

A dilated pupil indicates damage on the same side of the brain. Unilateral limb weakness (hemiparesis) indicates damage on the opposite side of the brain. Receptive or expressive dysphasia indicates damage to the speech centres in the fronto-temporal area of the dominant cerebral hemisphere (usually the left).

Radiological assessment

This takes second place to the recognition and correction of life-threatening injuries and complications. Only stable patients should be sent to the computed tomography (CT) suite or radiology department.

Computed tomographic scan

Unlike skull films, CT scanning can provide direct evidence of structural intracranial damage – haematomas, contusions, brain swelling, skull fracture or penetrating injury – and is increasingly used as the only imaging technique in a patient with a head injury that is not clearly minor. Its disadvantages (cost, higher radiation dose and the potential delay and risk involved in sending the patient to the CT suite) are more than outweighed by the value of the information that a CT scan can provide.

CT scanning should be done in a head-injured patient with any of the following features:

- a deteriorating conscious level
- not speaking or not eye opening to speech (Glasgow Coma Scale score 12/15 or worse)
- confusion or drowsiness (Glasgow Coma Scale score 13–14/15), which does not improve within 4 h
- severe headache, vomiting, altered behaviour or a fit, even when fully conscious
- focal neurological signs
- clinical or radiological evidence of a skull fracture.

Skull films

Figure 200 shows the classification of skull fractures. The indications for skull films need to be considered in the context of CT scanning. If an emergency CT scan is planned, there is no need for skull films. If a CT scan is not planned or is not available, skull films are indicated in the following circumstances:

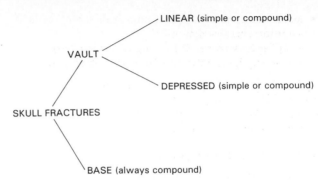

Figure 200 Classification of skull fractures.

- if the patient has any impairment of conscious level (Glasgow Coma Scale score 14 or less)
- if the patient is alert, orientated and obeying commands (Glasgow Coma Scale score 15) but:
  - *the mechanism of injury was not trivial (e.g. road accident, fall from a height or assault with a weapon)*
  - *consciousness has been lost at any stage*
  - *the patient has a loss of memory or has vomited*
  - *the history is inadequate.*

Early management and transfer

Careful monitoring of a patient's vital signs is important. Shock is almost never caused by the head injury, but blood loss elsewhere may have been overlooked and should be sought and treated.

Unexpected neurological deterioration

Common reasons for unexpected deterioration are hypoxia, hypercarbia, shock or a fit. It is essential to check that:

- the airway is clear
- the patient is breathing adequately and has high-flow oxygen
- the patient is not shocked.

If the patient has had a fit, the airway should be protected until the fit stops. Anticonvulsants are given only if the fit is prolonged or repeated. Intravenous or rectal diazepam will abort a fit. Intravenous phenytoin (given slowly to prevent cardiotoxicity) prevents further fits.

If these complications are all excluded, or if focal neurological signs develop, the deterioration is probably caused by a critical degree of brain compression by an intracranial haematoma. The patient should be intubated and ventilated and urgently referred to a neurosurgical unit. Mannitol, an osmotic diuretic, can be given to control raised ICP (after neurosurgical consultation). Corticosteroids have no place in the management of acute head injury.

Referral to a neurosurgeon

Late referral to neurosurgery still causes avoidable death and disability, as complications such as haematoma are missed and treatment is delayed. The patient should be referred for neurosurgical assessment and possible intervention if a CT scan in the general hospital shows a recent intracranial lesion or if a scan cannot be done there soon enough despite the criteria being met. The patient should also be referred if any of these features are present:

- persisting coma (Glasgow Coma Scale score 8 or less) after initial resuscitation
- confusion that persists for more than 4 h
- deterioration in conscious level after admission
- focal neurological signs
- a seizure without full recovery
- depressed skull fracture
- definite or suspected penetrating injury
- a cerebrospinal fluid (CSF) leak or other sign of a skull base fracture.

The decision to transfer

Image transfer systems allow the neurosurgeon to assess the patient and the CT scan before a decision is made whether or not to transfer the patient to the neurosurgical unit. Transfer is necessary when the neurosurgeon has to (or may have to) operate. Increasingly, patients are being transferred to neurosurgical intensive care facilities in order to access the specialist care that is available there, whether or not operation is needed.

Safe transfer to the neurosurgeon

Transfer can be a time of great danger. The patient must be resuscitated and stabilised before the journey begins, monitored during transfer and accompanied by an escort able to deal with any problems en route (e.g. airway obstruction, respiratory arrest, fits). A doctor must accompany every patient with a serious head injury during transfer.

Neurosurgical management

The role of the neurosurgeon is to deal with complications of head injury that threaten life or the quality of survival. These include intracranial haematomas, contusions, brain swelling and penetrating brain injuries.

Haematomas and contusions

There are three types of post-traumatic intracranial haematoma. All are diagnosed by CT scan:

- extradural
- subdural
- intracerebral.

An *extradural haematoma* forms when a skull fracture tears a dural blood vessel. Usually, conscious level is altered from the start because of associated primary brain damage but some patients have a 'lucid interval' before the conscious level starts to fall – sometimes dramatically. The expanding haematoma compresses and distorts the brain, raises ICP and impairs cerebral perfusion. As the conscious level falls, focal signs develop: a dilating pupil on the same side as the haematoma and weakness of the contralateral limbs. Without timely surgery, signs of brainstem compression or 'coning' develop (rising blood pressure, falling pulse rate and slowing respiration). If the haematoma is not promptly removed, the patient dies or suffers permanent brain damage. With early surgical intervention, over 90% of patients will survive and most recover well.

A *subdural haematoma* results from a tear of a vein draining blood from the brain surface to a venous sinus. Conscious level is almost always abnormal from the time of injury because of associated primary brain damage. A large subdu-

ral haematoma causes a clinical picture similar to that of an extradural haematoma and treatment is equally urgent.

Intracerebral haematomas and cerebral contusions are most common in the frontal and temporal lobes. They vary in size and clinical importance. Large intracerebral haematomas and contusions cause the same signs of progressive brain compression as extradural and subdural haematomas, and surgical evacuation is essential.

A large haematoma or area of contused brain ('burst lobe') is evacuated through a craniotomy – a hole cut in the overlying skull and hinged back as a flap. Small haematomas and contusions can be left alone if the patient is well but, if in doubt, the ICP can be measured by implanting an intracranial pressure transducer for a few days and measuring the ICP.

Diffuse brain swelling

The treatment is mainly supportive and pharmacological:

- control blood gases by ventilation (avoid hypoxia, hypercarbia)
- reduce brain water with diuretics (e.g. mannitol)
- reduce cerebral metabolic rate using drugs (e.g. the anaesthetic agent propofol).

Neuroprotective drugs may become available soon that can inactivate toxic molecules, block unnecessary depolarisation by neurotransmitters or protect key intracellular processes.

Penetrating injuries

Three clinical types of penetrating injury can be distinguished:

- compound depressed fracture of skull vault
- fracture of skull base
- penetration of the cranial cavity by a missile or sharp object.

Compound depressed fractures usually result from a direct blow from a blunt object. The main complications are epilepsy and intracranial infection. Epilepsy is more likely if there is underlying dural laceration or cortical contusion. Treatment of the injury includes surgical wound toilet, elevation of bone fragments and repair of any underlying dural tears under antibiotic cover.

Skull base fractures form a pathway for endogenous pathogens like pneumococci to enter the brain and cause infection. A CSF leak may develop from the nose or ear. Anti-pneumococcal antibiotics are usually given until the leak stops. Some patients need surgical repair of the leak.

Brain penetration by a sharp weapon or a missile such as a bullet or bomb fragment is uncommon in the UK but common in many other countries. Basic surgical principles are applied: surgical wound toilet, removal of devitalised tissue and broad-spectrum antibiotic therapy.

Outcome, recovery and disability

After a severe head injury:

- one-third of patients make a good recovery
- one-third survive with disabilities
- one-third die.

The prognosis depends on the initial injury (primary brain damage), the amount of any secondary brain damage and the age of the patient; very young and elderly patients fare worse.

The biology of recovery

Most patients with a mild head injury recover quickly. Recovery after severe brain damage is slow and can continue over months or years, especially in younger people. Injured neurones have limited potential for repair but can sometimes reform synapses with other neurones to re-establish functional circuits. Recovery is best seen in parts of the brain concerned with learning and memory because these neurones are normally in a constantly dynamic state. Other recovery mechanisms include the activation of dormant circuits and the creation of new ones. There is growing interest in how stem cells can differentiate and multiply to replace lost cells, the role of glial cells in repairing the injured brain and how pharmacology and molecular biology might be used to stimulate or modify these recovery processes.

Disabilities

Common disabilities include:

- physical
  - *headache and facial pain*
  - *limb weakness*
  - *poor hand function*
  - *impaired balance/vision/hearing*
  - *seizures*
- mental
  - *personality change*
  - *depression*
  - *loss of short-term memory*
  - *poor concentration*
  - *learning problems*
  - *communication problems (expressive or receptive).*

The Glasgow Outcome Scale (Table 21) measures outcome in broad categories but a more detailed assessment by physiotherapists, occupational therapists, speech therapists, clinical psychologists, etc. can identify specific

Table 21 Glasgow Outcome Scale

Outcome	Characteristics
Good recovery	Normal social/family life; can return to work; may have minor deficits
Moderate disability	Independent but disabled; can feed/wash/dress; can use public transport; may be able to work
Severe disability	Dependent for some daily activities
Persistent vegetative state	Non-functioning cerebral cortex; some preserved function in deep hemisphere centres and brainstem
Death	

physical and mental deficits needing correction. Good motivation and a supportive family are invaluable. Neurological rehabilitation is complex and some patients need the intensive multidisciplinary approach of special rehabilitation units.

15.2 Subarachnoid haemorrhage

Learning objectives

You should:
- know the important causes of intracranial haemorrhage
- understand the principles of investigation, diagnosis and treatment of ruptured cerebral aneurysms and other vascular anomalies.

Classification of cerebrovascular disease

Cerebrovascular accidents (CVAs) are common and, like all degenerative diseases, occur more often in middle or old age. Prevention is better than any attempt to repair the damage caused. Cigarette smoking, poorly controlled hypertension, a fat-rich diet, obesity and too little exercise all increase the risk of a CVA. Arterial occlusion (by thrombosis or embolism) causes 80% of CVAs and usually affects vessels that are chronically narrowed by atheroma. Haemorrhage from rupture of a vessel weakened by atheroma or a congenital anomaly causes the remaining 20%. The treatment of most CVAs is medical rather than surgical but, in some cases, the neurosurgeon can intervene to remove an intracranial haematoma or prevent a further bleed, especially after a subarachnoid haemorrhage.

Subarachnoid haemorrhage

Aetiology and pathogenesis

Subarachnoid haemorrhage (SAH) means bleeding into the subarachnoid space and, therefore, into the CSF. Bleeding can spread into the ventricles or the brain, the clinical effects of which can outweigh those of the SAH itself.

The amount of escaped blood varies but even small volumes cause profound symptoms. At first, the CSF is uniformly bloodstained but, after some days, it becomes yellowish (xanthochromic) as the blood starts to break down. These breakdown products can cause spasm of the cerebral microcirculation and aggravate the clinical picture.

Although head injury commonly causes SAH, by convention, the term refers only to cases in which the subarachnoid bleeding results from other causes including:

- cerebral aneurysm — 80%
- arteriovenous malformation (AVM)
- cavernous angiomas (cavernomas)
- dural fistulae
- vascular tumours } 10%
- no identifiable cause ('cryptogenic') — 10%.

Aneurysms form when smooth muscle in the arterial wall is weakened or congenitally deficient – often where vessels branch. Most occur at well-defined sites on or near the circle of Willis and are more common in patients with hypertension and cigarette smokers. About 10% are multiple. The hydrostatic pressure within the lumen gradually bulges and thins the arterial wall out to form a blister-like saccular or 'berry' aneurysm. Rupture can occur once the aneurysm is >7 mm in diameter, although sometimes an aneurysm can be >2.5 cm before bleeding occurs, causing an SAH. Once ruptured, an aneurysm is liable to rebleed unless treated.

An AVM is a congenital tangle of abnormal blood vessels in the brain containing fistulous connections between arteries and veins. The veins become dilated, tortuous and friable as blood at arterial pressure is shunted into them. Dural fistulae are closely related to AVMs. They are partly formed from vessels in the dura.

Clinical features

The onset of SAH is dramatic. Headache is severe and sudden, often described by the patient as an 'explosion' of pain, usually occipital at first but radiating quickly over the top of the head to the frontal area. Most patients also have neck pain, nausea, photophobia and vomiting, caused by escaped blood irritating the meninges. Some have an epileptic fit at the time of the bleed. In 50% of patients, the conscious level is affected and the extent depends on the severity of the bleed. SAH is an important cause of sudden death.

Neck stiffness is the most consistent finding on physical examination. Some patients are febrile. Focal neurological signs such as hemiparesis or pupillary asymmetry indicate that the bleeding has caused a focal haematoma in the brain; retinal or subhyaloid haemorrhages may be evident. The most severe cases show signs of brainstem compression: bradycardia, rising hypertension and irregular respiration.

Differential diagnosis

Sometimes a patient is found collapsed, unable to give a history and with altered consciousness, headache and neck stiffness. Apart from SAH, the two main alternative diagnoses are meningitis and other types of CVA. In other types of CVA (e.g. cerebral infarction), profound focal neurological deficits dominate the clinical picture. Acute bacterial meningitis usually has a less dramatic onset than SAH, but other diagnostic clues (high fever, skin rash) are not always present.

Diagnosis

The diagnosis is confirmed by:

CT brain scan If this is carried out within 72 h it will confirm the bleed and also show complications (brain swelling, hydrocephalus).

Lumbar puncture A lumbar puncture is essential if CT is not available or if the scan is normal despite a good clinical history. Uniformly bloodstained or xanthochromic CSF confirms the diagnosis. Lumbar puncture carries risks if ICP is raised but must be done if bacterial meningitis is a possible diagnosis.

Cerebral angiography This is used to show the detailed anatomy of the cerebral vessels and any abnormality (e.g. an aneurysm) causing the SAH. Direct catheter angiography is the most sensitive method, but newer techniques such as CT angiography are almost as sensitive with less risk of complications.

Complications of SAH

These are common and include:

- recurrent SAH
- cerebral ischaemia
- hydrocephalus
- systemic complications.

Recurrent SAH Ruptured aneurysms and AVMs tend to rebleed. The risk is highest initially and falls over the following weeks. A recurrent bleed can kill the patient or add to existing neurological deficits.

Cerebral ischaemia Cerebral autoregulation malfunctions after SAH and cerebral perfusion can also fall if the patient is dehydrated from vomiting or poor fluid intake. Breakdown products of subarachnoid blood can cause cerebral vasospasm and ischaemia, with infarction in severe cases. Vasospasm can be confirmed using transcranial Doppler ultrasound. The calcium channel-blocking drug nimodipine gives some protection against vasospasm.

Hydrocephalus Blood in the subarachnoid space and ventricles can impede the normal CSF flow, causing hydrocephalus and a rise in ICP. The CSF must then be diverted by an external drain or an internal shunt.

Systemic complications SAH can cause subendocardial ischaemia, which can progress to myocardial infarction. Cardiac ischaemia and disturbance in the electrical rhythm is a cause of sudden death after SAH. Sodium loss in the renal tubule often lowers the serum sodium concentration severely, with a reduction in consciousness and risk of seizures. This is treated by sodium supplements, not fluid deprivation.

Other clinical effects of aneurysms and arteriovenous malformations

A giant aneurysm (>2 cm diameter) can act like a brain tumour and cause symptoms of raised ICP or focal deficits. Acute expansion of some aneurysms can cause a painful third nerve palsy (diplopia, dilated pupil and severe retro-orbital pain). Urgent treatment is needed to avert aneurysm rupture.

An AVM can cause epilepsy by directly damaging adjacent brain tissue or by causing ischaemia. AVMs can 'steal' blood from the brain and cause progressive neurological symptoms such as hemiparesis or intellectual disturbance.

Treatment of aneurysms

The main risk is that a ruptured aneurysm will rebleed, and the aim is to seal the aneurysm before this can happen. There are two treatment options.

Surgery Until recent years this was the usual treatment, using a special metal clip to isolate the aneurysm from the parent artery. Most neurosurgeons operate within a few days of the bleed. There is a balance of risks, which depends on:

- age and general condition of the patient
- neurological status (conscious level, focal deficits)
- any complications (e.g. vasospasm)
- likelihood of technical difficulty.

Interventional radiology This has overtaken surgery in recent years. A fine catheter is guided through the arterial tree into the aneurysm and used to position soft metallic detachable coils, which induce thrombosis. There is evidence that this is safer than surgery and just as effective.

Some patients are treated conservatively because they are unfit, have neurological damage or refuse treatment.

Treatment of arteriovenous malformations

Patients with AVMs tend to be younger and fitter than those with aneurysms, but the lesions are often more difficult to deal with because of their size or position or because of a complex arterial supply and venous drainage. Conservative management is more common than with aneurysms, especially if the AVM has not bled. The three options for active treatment are:

- surgery
- interventional radiology
- high-intensity ionising radiation (radiosurgery).

The aim of treatment is to destroy the lesion completely; anything less leaves the patient liable to further bleeds. The likelihood of achieving a complete surgical removal must be set against the risk of causing harm by damaging brain tissue. Interventional radiology can obliterate even large AVMs by embolisation, either as a definitive procedure or as preparation for surgical removal; however, it is not without risk. In radiosurgery, a highly focused beam of ionising radiation is directed onto the AVM, damaging its vessels and causing a slow obliteration over the next 2–3 years.

Prognosis and outcome

SAH is an important cause of sudden death. Many survivors have significant neurological or neuropsychological disabilities. The pattern of damage resembles that seen after a head injury and rehabilitation has the same aim – to identify and treat specific problems and restore as much brain function as possible.

15.3 Brain tumours

Learning objectives

You should:
- understand the classification of brain tumours
- be able to recognise the natural history and clinical presentation
- know how to investigate a suspected brain tumour
- understand the principles of surgical and non-surgical treatment of brain tumours.

Classification

There are three types of tumour found in the brain:

- primary and benign (e.g. meningioma)
- primary and malignant (e.g. most gliomas)
- secondary and malignant (e.g. metastatic bronchial carcinoma).

Malignant primary brain tumours infiltrate the brain but almost never spread (metastasise) outside the CNS. *Primary tumours* can be further subdivided as follows:

- glioma: usually malignant
- meningioma: benign
- pituitary tumours: benign
- schwannoma (neuroma): benign
- developmental tumours: usually malignant.

Secondary tumours are malignant.

Clinical features

Most brain tumours are more common in the middle-aged or elderly. There are three types of clinical presentation:

- raised intracranial pressure (ICP)
- focal damage to affected areas of the brain
- epileptic fits.

The speed of onset of symptoms depends on the tumour type and rate of growth.

Raised intracranial pressure Many patients with a brain tumour gradually develop a constant, pounding, generalised headache that steadily worsens, peaking in the early morning and waking the patient from sleep. Nausea and vomiting are common. Confusion, drowsiness and coma develop if the raised ICP is not relieved.

Focal brain symptoms The pattern of focal brain damage depends on the location of the tumour:

- frontal lobe: personality change, contralateral hemiparesis
- occipital lobe: contralateral homonymous hemianopia
- dominant temporal lobe: receptive dysphasia and short-term memory loss
- cerebellum: ataxia and incoordination.

Epileptic fits A first epileptic fit may be the catalyst that makes a patient seek help. Symptoms of raised ICP or focal brain damage extending back over weeks or months often then emerge. Three types of fit occur:

- generalised (grand mal) convulsions
- focal seizures of limbs or face
- complex partial seizures.

Generalised fits involve tonic–clonic jerking movements of all limbs, loss of consciousness and incontinence of urine and can threaten the airway. During focal seizures, the patient remains conscious and the fit can be followed by temporary paralysis of the affected limbs (Todd's palsy). Complex partial seizures are often caused by tumours deep within the cerebral hemispheres.

Diagnosis

CT scan A CT scan enhanced by intravenous contrast is useful in emergency diagnosis. It will show tumour size, position, contour and internal structure, as well as peritumoral oedema, distortion of adjacent brain tissue and evidence of raised ICP.

Magnetic resonance imaging (MRI) This is the investigation of choice where available. Its superior resolution and multiplanar capability are useful in surgical planning and some physico-chemical information may be obtained by MR spectroscopy.

Surgical biopsy The clinical features or scan appearances are not always diagnostic. If not, a surgical biopsy of the tumour allows the most appropriate treatment to be planned. Computer-guided techniques (stereotactic biopsy) allow precise positioning of the biopsy needle even into a very small tumour.

Treatment

There are four main treatment options, which can be combined for maximum effect:

- surgery
- radiotherapy
- chemotherapy (cytotoxic or endocrine)
- steroids (dexamethasone).

The potential benefits of treatment must always be balanced against the possible risks.

Surgery Surgery can cure a benign tumour and is the treatment of choice for meningiomas, acoustic schwannomas and pituitary tumours. Cure rates can exceed 90% but the surgery needed for some large tumours can be technically challenging and risky.

Surgery can palliate symptoms from an incurable tumour by improving the quality of life and extending survival. Severe headache can be relieved by excising the bulk of a large infiltrating tumour or by draining a large fluid-filled tumour cavity. Operative damage may be reduced by using the rapidly evolving technique of 'computer-aided neuro-navigation' to make resection as complete and precise as possible without unnecessary sacrifice of brain tissue or undue risk to major vessels and other structures.

Radiotherapy Radiotherapy provides useful palliation. Its effectiveness can be increased by:

- surgical debulking of the tumour (cytoreductive therapy)
- single-dose stereotactic radiosurgery (the 'Gamma Knife').

Ionising radiation can damage normal tissue in the brain and elsewhere (radionecrosis). Doses are given in multiple fractions over several weeks to minimise the systemic upset – important for the quality of life in patients with limited life expectancy. Special care is needed in the developing brain and radiotherapy is seldom used for brain tumours in children less than 3 years of age.

Cytotoxic chemotherapy These agents can be used to complement surgery and radiotherapy. They may be given topically at the time of surgery or systemically at a later date. Many chemotherapeutic drugs do not penetrate well into CNS tumours, thus lowering their effectiveness.

Endocrine therapy Some brain tumours (e.g. meningiomas) express receptors for hormones such as estrogen on their cell surfaces. However, endocrine manipulation does not affect their recurrence. Endocrine-secreting pituitary tumours, especially prolactinomas, may respond very well to hormone antagonists (e.g. cabergoline).

Steroids Glucocorticoids such as dexamethasone reduce brain swelling around a tumour, which often contributes to symptoms, and can give remarkable relief of headache, drowsiness and focal neurological deficits within a day or two.

Specific types of brain tumour

Glioma

These are the most common primary CNS tumours. They occur throughout the brain and spinal cord in all age groups. The main histological types are:

- astrocytoma (80%)
- oligodendroglioma
- ependymoma.

Gliomas cause gradually worsening symptoms of raised ICP, focal neurological damage or fits. They show a wide spectrum of biological and clinical behaviour. Low-grade tumours have few mitoses and grow slowly for years. High-grade tumours show rapid growth, killing the patient within months. Low-grade gliomas contain areas of more active growth, which eventually dominate the tumour and change its behaviour. The treatment and prognosis are guided by the grade of tumour, determined by biopsy.

Gliomas infiltrate adjacent brain tissue early on. Even when the CT scan shows a well-defined tumour, glioma cells will already have migrated some distance and will cause recurrence even after apparently successful treatment. For this reason, the treatment of gliomas is palliative and not curative. Surgery aims to debulk large tumours or drain a cyst; radiotherapy and chemotherapy are used to shrink the tumour. Genetic profiling of gliomas may soon be available as a clinical tool to predict responsiveness to radiotherapy and distinctive chemotherapeutic agents. Steroids are useful for short-term alleviation of the symptoms of raised ICP.

Apart from the benign pilocytic astrocytoma of childhood, most tumours recur after an interval that is dependent upon the histological grade. Further treatment is usually ineffective and attention turns to symptomatic relief (headache, nausea, etc.) using palliative care.

Meningioma

These are benign, slow-growing, usually solitary tumours that arise from the arachnoidal layer of the meninges inside the skull base, on the falx or tentorium, or overlying the convexity of the brain. Usually, a meningioma is a solid mass; less often, it occurs as a sheet of tumour spreading over the dura (an 'en plaque' meningioma).

Meningiomas occur mainly after the age of 40 and more often in women. Symptoms of raised ICP and focal brain damage develop slowly, often so gradually that they are attributed to normal ageing. Tumours in eloquent areas like the motor cortex are usually diagnosed earlier. An epileptic fit can precipitate diagnosis.

A CT scan shows a well-defined mass enhancing evenly with intravenous contrast. MR scanning can define invasion or occlusion of nearby venous sinuses, and gives a multiplanar relationship to other intracranial structures. Surgery is the treatment of choice. Even large meningiomas do not infiltrate surrounding brain tissue and a cure is theoretically possible. Difficult access or the involvement of major vessels or cranial nerves can make surgery risky. After surgery, 10% of meningiomas recur, although the exact rate varies with completeness of excision. Radiotherapy, particularly single-dose (radiosurgery) techniques, may reduce the growth rate of residual tumour.

The prognosis for most patients is good: 90% cure and 10% risk of significant complications.

Pituitary adenomas

These are solitary, benign, slow-growing tumours of the glandular tissue of the anterior pituitary lobe. Large adenomas (macroadenomas) grow out of the pituitary fossa and compress the optic chiasm, causing progressive visual field loss (typically a bitemporal hemianopia). A few become big enough to compress the brain itself and cause frontal lobe symptoms or hydrocephalus. Although they do not secrete hormones, macroadenomas compress and damage the normal pituitary tissue and cause chronic hypopituitarism or acute haemorrhagic infarction and swelling of the pituitary gland (pituitary apoplexy). They can sometimes invade and destroy the bone of the pituitary fossa and skull base.

Microadenomas are confined to the gland and over-produce one of the anterior pituitary hormones, causing acromegaly (growth hormone), Cushing syndrome (adrenocorticotropic hormone; ACTH) or infertility and galactorrhoea (prolactin).

Whatever the tumour size, the diagnosis is confirmed by MR or CT scan. Three treatment options may be used individually or in combination:

* surgical excision (usually by the trans-sphenoidal route)
* radiotherapy
* hormone antagonist drugs (e.g. cabergoline).

The prognosis is usually excellent, although a few pituitary adenomas will recur. Some patients will need long-term endocrine replacement therapy.

Secondary brain tumours

Cancers often metastasise to the brain via the bloodstream. Lung and breast are the most frequent primary sites, with relatively few metastasising from the gastrointestinal tract. Others arise from malignant melanoma, lymphoma, testicular tumours and head and neck cancers (which reach the brain by eroding through the skull).

The clinical history is short and distinctive: headache, altered mental state and focal neurological features that worsen rapidly over a few days. Sometimes the underlying primary tumour is already known. Diagnosis is by CT or MR scan, which typically shows multiple small lesions in the white matter that often cause a considerable space-occupying effect because of surrounding oedema. If a single tumour is seen, the diagnosis may need biopsy confirmation.

Surgical decompression can be useful for a single metastasis at an accessible site (e.g. cerebellar hemisphere, frontal lobe) and stereotactic localisation can help locate the tumour with minimal disruption of brain tissue. In most cases, treatment is by radiotherapy or chemotherapy, supported by steroids. Death ensues within a few months and good quality palliative care is important.

15.4 Spinal tumours

Learning objectives

You should:
* know the types of tumour that develop in or around the spinal cord
* be able to recognise their natural history and clinical features
* know how to diagnose a spinal tumour
* understand the principles of treatment.

Classification

Tumours can arise within:

* the spinal cord
* the nerve roots, which emerge from the cord
* the bone of the vertebral column.

There are several types of spinal tumour:

* primary tumours:
  – intramedullary (within cord): glioma
  – extramedullary (outside cord): meningioma, neurofibroma
* secondary tumours (extradural):
  – carcinoma
  – lymphoma
  – malignant melanoma
  – multiple myeloma.

Clinical features

Spinal tumours compress and damage the spinal cord and/or nerve roots, according to the site and nature of the tumour:

* cord compression causes myelopathy below that segmental level (upper motor neuron lesion)
* root compression causes radiculopathy in the distribution of that root (lower motor neuron lesion).

A spinal tumour usually causes a developing myelopathy. Control of the lower limbs (and upper limbs too, if the tumour compresses the cervical spinal cord) is progressively lost. Tone and reflexes are increased in the affected limbs with extensor plantar responses, reflecting damage to the upper motor neurons of the spinal cord. If the myelopathy is untreated, muscle power decreases to the point of paralysis: paraplegia (the lower limbs) or tetraplegia (all four limbs). Sensation is disturbed and ultimately lost below the segmental level of cord compression. Proprioception (dorsal column sensation) is affected before deep pain and temperature (spino-thalamic) sensation. Sphincter control and sexual function are impaired and then lost.

Less often, a spinal tumour causes a developing radiculopathy, with progressive pain, weakness and sensory disturbance in the distribution of that nerve root. The pain often has a burning 'dysaesthetic' quality. Lower motor neuron damage is evident in the distribution of the affected root, with reduced power, muscle bulk, sensation and reflexes.

These symptoms and signs can develop over days, weeks or months. Some patients with a spinal tumour show features of both a myelopathy and a radiculopathy.

Diagnosis

The differential diagnosis of a suspected cord or root compression includes:

- other causes of compression:
  - spinal trauma
  - disc prolapse
  - spondylosis (bony degeneration)
  - syringomyelia (cyst within cord)
  - haematoma (spontaneous or traumatic)
  - abscess
- non-compressive disease:
  - demyelination
  - infection
  - inflammation
  - infarction
  - degenerative cord syndromes.

Further investigations are always necessary to establish whether there is cord or root compression and the likely cause. The most useful investigations are:

- MR imaging: delineates tumour in great detail
- CT scan: shows relationship of tumour to cord and spinal column
- plain radiograph films: bony infiltration or collapse
- myelography: 'filling defect' or block of flow to contrast.

Treatment and prognosis

The main methods of treatment are surgery and radiotherapy (the choice depends on the type of tumour), with steroids as an adjunct. Chemotherapy is often more useful with spinal tumours than with brain tumours. The benefits and risks of any treatment must be individualised for each patient.

Survival depends on the tumour type. The prognosis for neurological improvement depends on the severity and duration of spinal cord or nerve root compression before treatment. Cord compression recovers less well than root compression.

Specific types of spinal tumour

Intramedullary tumours

Spinal gliomas behave like brain gliomas, growing with variable speed but infiltrating and surrounding the spinal cord early on. They can extend over many segments of the cord and even into the brainstem. They cause progressive myelopathy affecting the lower limbs and sphincters and (in a cervical glioma) the upper limbs as well. Pain is rare, but patients steadily lose power, sensation, coordination and sphincter control.

Other spinal tumours, motor neuron disease, vasculopathies and multiple sclerosis are the main differential diagnoses. MR imaging is the investigation of choice. Open biopsy guides management by differentiating slow-growing from fast-growing tumours.

Treatment is palliative. Surgical decompression is useful for low-grade tumours containing cysts or those with a good plane of cleavage from normal tissue. Radiotherapy can be used alone or in combination with surgery. Steroids have a useful palliative effect. Death is from damage to respiratory centres in the cervical cord or brainstem.

Extramedullary tumours

Meningiomas and neurofibromas (schwannomas) are benign, slow-growing tumours that arise on a nerve root. They cause a radiculopathy in the distribution of that nerve root and, if large enough, compress the spinal cord and cause a myelopathy. Meningiomas and schwannomas never infiltrate the cord or metastasise but can reach a large size and erode adjacent vertebrae. Although usually solitary, multiple neurofibromas arise on the spinal nerves in the hereditary condition of neurofibromatosis (von Recklinghausen syndrome) and can become large enough to extend out of the spine into the neck, chest, or abdomen.

Symptoms develop slowly. The diagnosis is often delayed until an important function like hand coordination is affected. Plain films, myelography and CT scanning are all useful but the best investigation is MR imaging. Surgical excision of the tumour is usually curative but there is a risk of increasing the neurological deficit in large tumours that compress the cord.

Extradural tumours

Secondary tumour deposits reach the extradural space via the bloodstream or by direct extension from a vertebral focus. Most originate in carcinomas (lung, breast, prostate, kidney), malignant melanoma, lymphoma and multiple myeloma. They grow quickly, destroying bone and infiltrating paraspinal soft tissues. The features of spinal cord compression develop rapidly and can progress to a complete paraplegia within a few days. Investigation and treatment are urgent.

Plain films show bone destruction, and myelography shows a partial or complete block to contrast flow at the tumour site. CT and MR scanning are of value in showing the extent of tumour spread within and outside the spine. A percutaneous biopsy under radiographic control can yield tissue for histology.

There is an urgent need to shrink the tumour and decompress the cord. If bladder control is already lost, the window of opportunity for rescue is only 24 h. Surgery, radiotherapy, chemotherapy and steroids are used alone or in combination.

Survival depends on the tumour type. Recovery of cord function depends upon the duration and extent of cord compression. Often the diagnosis is made too late to restore function.

Self-assessment: questions

Extended matching items questions (EMIs)

EMI 1

Theme: Head injury

1. hypercarbia	A. major pelvic fracture
2. inadequate cerebral perfusion	B. severe diffuse axonal injury
3. lucid interval after head injury	C. skull base fracture
4. CSF rhinorrhoea	D. extradural haematoma
5. deep coma immediately after accident	E. blocked airway

Match each of the items in the left-hand column with a single item in the right-hand column.

EMI 2

Theme: Brain and spinal tumours

1. progressive loss of temporal visual fields	A. thoracic neurofibroma
2. multiple cerebral lesions on cerebral CT scan	B. fronto-parietal meningioma
3. focal motor seizures worsening over several months	C. frontal lobe tumour
4. change of personality with impaired cognition	D. secondary carcinoma
5. increasingly stiff legs for last few months	E. pituitary tumour

Match each of the items in the left-hand column with a single item in the right-hand column.

Constructed response questions

CRQ 1

A 10-year-old boy, previously well except for mild asthma, falls off his bicycle and strikes his head on a kerbstone. He does not lose consciousness but vomits shortly afterwards and returns home. About an hour later, significant headache develops but the child is neurologically normal. He vomits again and becomes a little restless and breathless.

a. The child lives in the country, in a remote part of your practice where you are working as a GP. You are contacted by the boy's parents. What would be the most appropriate response?

Before they have time to act on your advice, the child has a grand mal fit at home. An ambulance is called and the child is sent to the local hospital. On arrival he is shaking on the left side. His right pupil is larger than the left but responds to light.

b. What other important neurological signs should the casualty officer seek?

The ambulance crew tell you that he is not as alert as he was at the scene of the accident.

c. What is the most likely cause of this child's presentation?

Within an hour of admission he becomes comatose.

d. What investigations should be arranged?

This examination shows evidence of a significant intracranial injury.

e. What would be the most appropriate management?

CRQ 2

A 55-year-old company executive collapses on the floor of his office and is at first unresponsive. Within a minute or two he starts to wake up and complains of severe headache and nausea. He regains full consciousness and is taken to hospital, where a history of recent overwork and much foreign business travel is elicited. His blood pressure is 190/105 mmHg, there is mild neck stiffness and a temperature of 37.5°C is recorded.

a. From the history and clinical signs as presented, what do you think is the most likely clinical diagnosis?

The patient has recovered sufficiently for you to obtain a full history.

b. What questions would you ask the patient?

At the time of the collapse, your patient was chairing an important meeting. He is accompanied to the hospital by several of his colleagues who witnessed the collapse.

c. What question would you ask any witness?

The patient is cooperative enough to enable you to complete a full physical examination.

d. What additional neurological signs would you seek?

The patient is understandably anxious and asks if he will require any tests.

e. What would be the most appropriate line of investigation?

CRQ 3

A 64-year-old housewife with a long history of hypertension and mild depression has complained of frontal headaches over about 2 months, which she feels are getting worse. Two paracetamol tablets no longer clear the headache, which wakes her now most days. She visits her GP for advice. She denies any other symptoms. A neurological examination shows slightly brisker reflexes on the right side, but general examination is normal. It is not possible to obtain a good view of her optic fundi.

a. What is the most appropriate management at present?

A week later her husband telephones the GP. He is worried because she has become 'odd' in the last few days, forgetting meals and once talking about her dead sister as if she was still alive. He thinks she is perhaps becoming depressed again and asks the GP to see her. It is found that her right hand is a little weak but she seems unconcerned about this and her headache.

b. What is the most likely diagnosis at this stage?

The GP phones the local hospital and speaks to a consultant physician who agrees to admit her for tests later that week. However, that night he is called to see her as she has fallen out of bed and become very drowsy. He finds her lying on the bedroom floor, eye opening to speech and mumbling incoherently. Her right side is weak and there is twitching of the right side of the face. The left pupil is larger than the right but both react to light. Her blood pressure is 200/130 mmHg. There is no external evidence of injury.

c. Describe the features of emergency treatment at this stage.

Multiple choice questions

1. In the clinical management of head injury:
   a. the first priority in the management of an unconscious head injury is the assessment of pupil and limb responses
   b. a patient with a skull fracture who is fully conscious can safely be sent home from the A&E department
   c. a patient in a coma after a head injury should be intubated and ventilated before transfer to a neurosurgical unit
   d. a patient who has had an epileptic fit after a head injury should be given 10 mg of diazepam as quickly as possible
   e. clinical signs of shock are unlikely to be caused by the head injury itself

2. A deteriorating level of consciousness in the A&E department an hour after serious head injury:
   a. is almost certainly caused by an expanding intracranial haematoma
   b. may reflect rising intracranial pressure
   c. should routinely be treated with mannitol and steroids
   d. is not significant unless the patient also develops focal neurological signs
   e. automatically requires immediate transfer to the nearest CT scanner

3. The clinical features of a large left-sided acute extradural haematoma are likely to include:
   a. left hemiparesis
   b. dilated left pupil
   c. left-sided skull fracture
   d. deteriorating conscious level
   e. tachycardia

4. Which of the following statements about head injury are true?
   a. about one million patients are admitted to hospital in the UK each year because of head injury
   b. fractures of the skull base are usually diagnosed on clinical rather than radiological grounds
   c. outcome from an acute intracranial haematoma is not related to the patient's preoperative conscious level
   d. the risk of post-traumatic epilepsy is increased by a depressed fracture with a dural tear and cortical contusion
   e. cognitive deficits are common in survivors of severe head injury

5. Which of the following statements about cerebrovascular accidents are true?
   a. they never occur in patients in their 20s
   b. they are more common in women than in men
   c. high blood pressure is an important risk factor
   d. haemorrhages are more common than infarcts
   e. damage to the brain can never recover

6. Clinical features of a diffuse subarachnoid haemorrhage include:
   a. a severe occipito-frontal headache
   b. neck stiffness
   c. constricted pupils
   d. sudden onset of symptoms
   e. repeated vomiting

7. Cerebral berry aneurysms:
   a. are usually present at the time of birth
   b. occur mainly where arteries bifurcate
   c. are usually multiple

    d. can only be treated by a surgical operation

    e. can become large enough to compress nearby cranial nerves

8. Common complications of aneurysmal subarachnoid haemorrhage include:

    a. a further haemorrhage

    b. congestive cardiac failure

    c. salt-losing nephropathy

    d. communicating hydrocephalus

    e. cortical blindness

9. Presenting features of a glioma of the left temporal lobe may include:

    a. progressive headache

    b. weakness of the left hand

    c. focal seizures of the right hand

    d. expressive dysphasia

    e. jaundice from liver secondaries

10. Intracranial meningiomas:

    a. are usually multiple tumours

    b. infiltrate the surrounding brain at an early stage

    c. can present with an epileptic fit

    d. are very radiosensitive

    e. can usually be cured by surgical excision

11. Which of the following statements about secondary brain tumours are true?

    a. the history is usually short and rapidly progressive

    b. the most common primary sites are lung, stomach and colon

    c. the CT scan often shows a great deal of oedema

    d. surgery is never useful in their treatment

    e. steroids may give dramatic symptomatic relief

12. Radiotherapy for brain tumours:

    a. can cause brain damage unless the dose is carefully controlled

    b. is the ideal treatment for brain tumours in children under 3 years of age

    c. has its greatest effects with rapidly dividing tumours

    d. causes side effects that are well tolerated by most patients

    e. is ineffective in pituitary tumours

13. The clinical features of a myelopathy that has been rapidly progressive over 1 week are likely to include:

    a. preservation of proprioceptive sensation

    b. increased knee and ankle reflexes

    c. sciatic pain

    d. marked wasting of muscles of the lower limbs

    e. loss of bladder control

14. Spinal cord compression from an extradural secondary tumour at the level of the fourth thoracic vertebra:

    a. causes progressive weakness of all four limbs

    b. is often associated with destructive changes in the adjacent bone

    c. can lead to loss of bladder control within a few days

    d. always requires surgical decompression

    e. can be the first presentation of a bronchogenic carcinoma

15. A neurofibroma arising from the left eleventh thoracic nerve root:

    a. is likely to cause symptoms that progress slowly

    b. may cause a band of pain around the left loin

    c. can cause vertebral erosion that is visible on plain films

    d. causes an extradural block to contrast flow on myelography

    e. has a 10% chance of infiltrating the surrounding spinal cord tissue by the time of diagnosis

Self-assessment: answers

EMI answers

EMI 1

Theme: Head injury

1. E. A blocked airway or inadequate ventilation are potent causes of hypercarbia and hypoxia. These are among the commonest causes of secondary brain damage (secondary insult), following on from primary brain damage at the time of injury. Hypercarbia causes brain swelling and a rise in intracranial pressure by causing cerebral vasodilatation.

2. A. A major pelvic fracture can cause 2–3 l of blood loss. If this volume is not promptly replaced, the resulting cardiovascular shock can lead to inadequate cerebral perfusion, another significant cause of secondary brain damage.

3. D. A 'lucid interval' before the conscious level starts to fall is characteristic of an extradural haematoma. Following injury, a haematoma develops after a skull fracture tears a dural artery. Eventually, the expanding haematoma compresses and distorts the brain leading to impaired consciousness.

4. C. A leak of CSF either from the nose or ear is pathognomonic of a skull base fracture.

5. B. Deep coma immediately after an accident is the hallmark of a diffuse severe brain injury. It is important to record the neurological status immediately following injury and to use this as a baseline for the Glasgow Coma Score.

EMI 2

Theme: Brain and spinal tumours

1. E. As they slowly increase in size, pituitary tumours grow 'out' of the pituitary fossa and compress the optic chiasm that lies immediately above the pituitary fossa. This causes progressive damage to the visual fields. Initially, it is the central nerve fibres in the optic chiasm that are damaged, producing a bitemporal hemianopia.

2. D. Secondary tumours metastasise to the brain via the bloodstream. A CT scan will typically show multiple, often quite small, lesions that can be surrounded with oedema.

3. B. Meningiomas are slow growing and typically produce symptoms over a period of months or even years. Focal motor seizures that affect the limbs or face are in keeping with a slowly developing tumour that is affecting the motor cortex in the posterior part of the frontal lobe.

4. C. The pattern of brain damage depends on the site of the tumour. Frontal lobe tumours are characterised by alterations in personality. The initial changes are often subtle and can be mistaken for degenerative neurological disease leading to a delay in diagnosis.

5. A. A spinal tumour usually causes a progressive myelopathy (an upper motor neuron lesion) below the spinal segmental level where the tumour is growing. In this case, a thoracic neurofibroma will cause upper motor neuron signs in the lower limbs; the upper limbs will not be affected. Initially, the tone and reflexes will be increased in the lower limbs and this will be expressed by the patient as an increasing stiffness in the legs.

CRQ answers

CRQ 1

a. Urgent referral to the nearest A&E department.

This boy initially seemed fine after an apparently minor head injury but his increasing headache and persistent vomiting are warnings that all is not well. These clinical features should always be taken seriously in a child who has had a head injury and justify prompt referral to an A&E department.

b. Assess his conscious level using the Glasgow Coma Score.

Look for focal neurological signs in his limbs.

The boy deteriorated before arrival at hospital and may have had a focal epileptic seizure. Evaluation of any neurological injury is based on an assessment of the conscious level using the Glasgow Coma Scale and the presence of any focal neurological signs. The most important are asymmetry of pupil size or response to light stimulus, or asymmetry of the motor response between the left and right limbs.

c. Right-sided extradural haematoma.

The clinical findings at hospital – left-sided focal fits and an abnormal right pupil – strongly suggest a right-sided cerebral hemisphere expanding lesion. An apparently 'minor' precipitating injury followed by a lucid interval before a neurological deterioration are the hallmarks of an extradural haematoma.

d. CT scan of the brain.

A CT scan provides direct evidence of structural intracranial damage – haematomas, contusions and brain damage. In addition, any skull fracture will be identified. If an emergency CT scan is planned, as in this case, skull radiographs will be unnecessary and will simply delay the child's management.

e. This child requires urgent consultation with a view to transfer to the nearest neurosurgical unit. The child's clinical condition is likely to deteriorate further, possibly with dramatic speed, and he must be referred at once.

CRQ 2

a. Subarachnoid haemorrhage.

The features of this man's sudden illness all strongly suggest an intracranial bleed, most likely a subarachnoid haemorrhage. The key features are the loss of consciousness, headache and neck stiffness, together with the low-grade fever.

b. Where did the headache start?

Has the headache moved (radiated)?

Does he feel sick or photophobic?

Any of these answers will score marks. A sudden-onset, severe headache, which begins in the occipital area and spreads quickly over the top of the head to the frontal area, is characteristic of a subarachnoid haemorrhage. Nausea, vomiting and photophobia are all signs of cerebral 'irritability' and should be looked for in any patient with a suspected subarachnoid haemorrhage.

c. Did the patient have a fit?

This important piece of information may also point toward an intracerebral event.

d. Focal neurological signs.

Retinal or subhyaloid haemorrhage.

Focal neurological signs such as hemiparesis or pupillary asymmetry indicate that the bleed has caused a focal haematoma in the brain. Retinal haemorrhages may develop because blood in the subarachnoid space surrounding the optic nerves compresses the central retinal vein and raises the pressure in the retinal veins causing haemorrhage

e. CT scan of the brain.

Lumbar puncture.

The key investigation is a CT scan, which would almost certainly show free blood after a subarachnoid haemorrhage. A lumbar puncture several hours after the bleed is almost as sensitive but carries a small risk of complications (if the intracranial pressure is raised by the bleed). When a subarachnoid haemorrhage has been diagnosed by CT scan, a lumbar puncture becomes redundant. It is best reserved for those few cases in which the CT scan is equivocal.

CRQ 3

a. The headache has some features of raised intracranial pressure and the focal neurological signs (unilateral brisk reflexes) in this woman should alert the GP to the possibility of an intracranial mass lesion. The GP should refer the patient urgently to a physician or (if available) a neurologist or neurosurgeon, with a view to investigation by CT scanning. Simply reassuring the patient or

prescribing strong analgesics without referring the patient is not appropriate.

b. The new symptoms reported by the patient's husband the following week suggest a progressive change in personality and behaviour. Although depression can cause such symptoms, their association with brisk right-sided reflexes and right-hand weakness points strongly to a focal lesion in the brain, most likely in the left frontal lobe. The gradual and progressive tempo of the illness suggests a tumour rather than a stroke, but urgent hospital investigation is needed.

c. The next day the illness has worsened dramatically. Although her husband describes a fall, the circumstances of this make it more likely to be the result of, rather than the cause of, her deterioration. She may have been having focal seizures of the right-sided limbs but, unless these lead to repeated or prolonged generalised convulsions, intravenous diazepam is not indicated. Although she is hypertensive (and has a history of this), this may be a response to raised intracranial pressure, and antihypertensive medication may be dangerous and is contraindicated. She should go to hospital by ambulance after basic resuscitation.

Multiple choice answers

1. a. **False.** The management of any seriously injured patient begins with the identification and correction of life-threatening problems of the airway, breathing and circulation.

   b. **False.** A patient with a skull fracture should always be admitted for observation or referred for a CT scan, even if neurologically well, as a fracture is a powerful risk factor for an intracranial haematoma.

   c. **True.** An unconscious patient should be intubated and ventilated before being transferred out of the resuscitation room.

   d. **False.** Diazepam is a respiratory depressant and should only be given to a patient whose fit lasts for more than a minute or two and then only in small increments with facilities available for respiratory support.

   e. **True.** Shock is almost never caused by the head injury itself but by blood loss from extracranial injuries, which initially may be unrecognised.

2. a. **False.** A falling level of consciousness after head injury is a sensitive warning of continuing brain injury and must always be taken seriously. It can be caused by intracranial complications or by systemic injuries and complications that reduce cerebral perfusion and oxygenation.

   b. **True.** A rise in intracranial pressure is paralleled by a fall in conscious level, in response to brain compression and reduced cerebral perfusion.

   c. **False.** Mannitol lowers raised intracranial pressure for less than an hour. Steroids carry no benefit (and possibly some detriment) in the management of acute head injury.

    d. **False.** It is dangerous to wait for focal neurological signs before acting.

    e. **False.** The patient should not be transferred to the CT scanner or neurosurgical unit until life-threatening problems have been excluded or corrected.

3. a. **False.** A right hemiparesis develops.

    b. **True.** The pupil of the left eye dilates because of compression of the oculomotor nerve.

    c. **True.** An extradural haematoma is almost always caused by an overlying skull fracture that lacerates a dural vessel.

    d. **True.**

    e. **False.** If the haematoma is not evacuated, brainstem compression causes a slowing of the pulse rate.

4. a. **False.** Most of the one million head-injured individuals who attend hospital in the UK each year do not need admission, but it is important to identify the 10% who do. This group are at risk of complications and prompt intervention is needed to minimise the harmful effects of these complications.

    b. **True.** Meningitis can result from neglect of the clinical signs of a radiologically invisible fracture of the skull base.

    c. **False.** The worse a patient's conscious level has become before removal of the intracranial haematoma, the worse the outcome is likely to be.

    d. **True.** A depressed skull vault fracture carries a risk not only of infection but also of epilepsy, especially if the underlying dura and brain are damaged.

    e. **True.** Survivors of severe head injury often have cognitive deficits, which can be marked.

5. a. **False.** Cerebrovascular accidents can occur in all age groups, although they are more common in the middle-aged and elderly.

    b. **True.** Cases in women outnumber those in men by about 6:4.

    c. **True.** Uncontrolled hypertension is a key risk factor, along with cigarette smoking, hyperlipidaemia, obesity, stress and diabetes.

    d. **False.** Infarcts are much more common (80%) than haemorrhages (20%).

    e. **False.** Infarcts and haemorrhages both cause neuronal death in an area of the brain. Damage to surrounding neurones can recover with time and supportive therapy, leading to recovery of function.

6. a. **True.** The usual history of a subarachnoid haemorrhage involves the sudden onset of a severe generalised headache.

    b. **True.** The neck is usually stiff.

    c. **False.** Focal neurological signs can be present or absent, but the pupils are normal or dilated in this condition.

    d. **True.**

    e. **True.** The features of meningeal irritation (nausea, photophobia, repeated vomiting) usually accompany a subarachnoid haemorrhage.

7. a. **False.** The muscle abnormality is congenital, but the aneurysm itself almost always develops only in adult life.

    b. **True.** A cerebral aneurysm arises where an artery branches. Pressure from blood in the vessel causes the wall to balloon out where the smooth muscle layer is weak.

    c. **False.** Most are single but 10% are multiple.

    d. **False.** Options for management now include endovascular obliteration by radiological techniques as well as surgical treatment.

    e. **True.** The most common nerve to be affected is the oculomotor nerve, causing a dilated unreactive pupil on the same side as the aneurysm.

8. a. **True.** The main fear with a ruptured aneurysm is that it will rupture again. This risk is especially high in the early weeks after the initial bleed.

    b. **False.** A cardiac dysrhythmia is the most common cardiac complication.

    c. **True.** The salt-losing nephropathy can cause severe hyponatraemia.

    d. **True.** The hydrocephalus is usually of the communicating type, caused by clogging of the arachnoid villi by blood.

    e. **False.** Vasospasm induced by blood breakdown products in the subarachnoid space causes ischaemia, but the occipital cortex is rarely sufficiently affected to cause blindness.

9. a. **True.** The space-occupying effect of a glioma and its surrounding oedema steadily raises intracranial pressure and makes headache worse.

    b. **False.** A left-sided cerebral lesion will produce right-sided neurological signs.

    c. **True.**

    d. **True.** Focal damage is likely to affect the speech centre (causing expressive dysphasia).

    e. **False.** No matter how aggressive its behaviour within the brain, a glioma will not metastasise to other parts of the body.

10. a. **False.** A meningioma is usually solitary.

    b. **False.** Meningiomas do not infiltrate the surrounding brain.

    c. **True.** It grows steadily and the symptoms of raised intracranial pressure and focal brain damage are at first underestimated by the patient, often until a dramatic event, such as a fit, takes place.

d. **False.** Radiotherapy has little effect on such a slow-growing tumour.

e. **True.** Even a large meningioma can usually be cured by surgical excision.

11. a. **True.** They grow quickly and cause symptoms quickly but this is often because of marked cerebral oedema rather than the size of the metastases themselves.

b. **False.** Most cerebral metastases arise from carcinoma of the lung or breast – few are from gastrointestinal tumours.

c. **True.**

d. **False.** Palliative surgery can help to relieve troublesome pressure symptoms from a large and apparently solitary metastasis, even when the long-term outlook is poor.

e. **True.** The patient's headache and other symptoms of raised intracranial pressure resolve rapidly with steroids.

12. a. **True.** The risk of radiation damage to normal tissue limits the dose that can be given.

b. **False.** The risk is especially high in the developing brain, and radiotherapy is only justified in children under 3 years of age if it is a life-saving measure and no other treatment is effective.

c. **True.** Radiotherapy is especially useful for fast-growing tumours.

d. **True.** Systemic side effects on bone marrow, skin, hair and gut are usually well tolerated at the doses used.

e. **False.** Even a pituitary tumour which grows slowly will shrink or cease growth after treatment.

13. a. **False.** Proprioception tends to be affected before deep pain sensation.

b. **True.** This reflects signs of an upper motor neuron lesion below the level of cord compression.

c. **False.** Radicular pain (e.g. sciatica) is not a feature of myelopathy.

d. **False.** There is no wasting of muscles until the myelopathy has caused disuse atrophy.

e. **True.** This is also a sign of an upper motor neuron lesion below the segmental level of cord compression.

14. a. **False.** The myelopathy caused by a tumour in this position causes motor and sensory loss in the lower limbs but not the upper limbs.

b. **True.** Such tumours destroy bone extensively.

c. **True.** Loss of sphincter control under these circumstances can be rapid.

d. **False.** The extensive adjacent bone involvement often limits the value of surgery, especially in an elderly or frail patient. Radiotherapy and/or chemotherapy (with steroids) often provides equally effective palliation.

e. **True.** The likeliest primary tumour is a carcinoma, hitherto undiagnosed.

15. a. **True.** A neurofibroma grows slowly.

b. **True.** It arises on a spinal root in its intervertebral foramen and causes slowly worsening features of a radiculopathy in the distribution of that root, which in this case would include a sensory disturbance in the left loin.

c. **True.** As it enlarges, erosion of the adjacent vertebra occurs and can be seen on plain films.

d. **False.** They are intradural tumours, and the appearance of a filling defect on a myelogram distinguishes them from extradural tumours.

e. **False.** Neurofibromas displace nervous tissue rather than infiltrating it and, even when very large, they remain well demarcated.

Transplantation

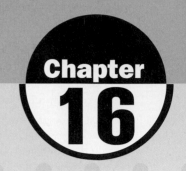

Chapter overview

Whole organ transplantation has revolutionised the management of patients with end-stage organ failure, the majority of whom, before the advent of transplantation, would have ultimately died of their illnesses. Transplant surgery has evolved rapidly over the last 40 years. Success in kidney transplantation has been followed by liver, heart, lung and, more recently, pancreas transplantation. This chapter outlines the general principles which govern rejection and immunosuppression that are common to all organ transplants and describes the indications, methods and outcomes of most common organ transplants.

16.1 General principles

Learning objectives

You should:
- understand the mechanisms and types of organ rejection
- know the effects and side effects of the major immunosuppressive drugs.

Although the technical barriers to whole organ transplantation were overcome at the beginning of the twentieth century, successful whole organ transplantation was impracticable until the phenomenon of rejection was understood and reliable methods of immunosuppression had been developed. The modern era of transplantation really began in the 1960s with the first successful series of kidney transplants.

Currently, the most frequently performed transplants are:

- kidney
- liver
- heart
- lung.

Various terms and definitions are used in transplant technology. *Allotransplantation* means transplantation from a non-identical donor to a recipient of the same species (i.e. an allograft). Almost all human transplants are in this category. *Xenotransplantation*, transplanting between members of different species, is rare. *Grafts* that are implanted into a recipient are termed *orthotopic* if they occupy their normal anatomical site (e.g. liver transplants) or *heterotopic* if they occupy an ectopic site (e.g. renal transplants).

Rejection and immunosuppression

Early transplants inevitably failed because of a complex rejection process, which involves cellular immunity (T- and B-cell lymphocytes) and humoral immunity (circulating antibody) mechanisms.

The host response to the donor graft depends upon the tissue matching. The two most important compatibility systems are:

- ABO blood group
- HLA (human leucocyte antigen) class I and class II systems.

On the rare occasions when donor and recipient are identical twins, tissue matching will be perfect and there will be no antigenic difference and no rejection.

ABO blood group compatibility is essential. Placing a blood group B graft into a blood group O recipient, for example, will lead to immediate rejection because of circulating (humoral) anti-group B antibodies in the recipient.

The HLA class I and class II antigen systems are extremely complex. Although close matching between donor and recipient confers a survival advantage of the graft in the recipient, such matching is not always possible because of the wide number of antigen permutations. It may be impossible to set up the perfect match between donor and recipient. Instead, it is necessary to settle for the best available match between a given donor and recipient.

The therapeutic goal of *immunosuppression* is to override any response of the immune system to tissue histoincompatibility while at the same time preserving the remaining functions of the recipient's immune system to protect against infection.

Three patterns of rejection are recognised:

- hyperacute
- acute
- chronic.

Hyperacute rejection This is uncommon and occurs within minutes to hours after transplantation. The transplanted organ becomes swollen and tender and there is severe vascular damage, with thrombosis and endothelial damage. There is an abrupt cessation of graft function. This injury is mediated by circulating recipient antibodies and is usually caused by a major ABO or HLA system incompatibility.

Acute rejection This occurs more often and develops within a few weeks/months of transplantation and is of rapid onset. The graft becomes tender and swollen and there is a deterioration in function. The rejection process is mediated by a combination of cellular and humoral (antibody) mechanisms. Biopsy of the graft will reveal a mixed cellular infiltrate (lymphocytes, monocytes and plasma cells) together with evidence of antibody-mediated vascular endothelial damage.

Chronic rejection This begins months/years after transplantation. It is characterised by a progressive deterioration in function of the transplanted organ, with a mononuclear cellular infiltration on graft biopsy.

Methods of immunosuppression

Drug therapy is the cornerstone of immunosuppression. The main targets of immunosuppressive drugs are the CD4 T lymphocytes, which play a critical role in orchestrating the rejection response. The principal agents used are given in Table 22. A wide variety of combinations of these agents are used to combat rejection. Therapy is begun immediately following transplantation and continues indefinitely, usually with a combination of a steroid, a calcineurin inhibitor and an antiproliferative agent.

Many of the improvements in the long-term survival of organ transplants of all types have been attributed to the introduction of new immunosuppressive drugs such as tacrolimus and mycophenolate mofetil (see Table 22), coupled with the ability to prevent or overcome opportunistic infection [e.g. cytomegalovirus (CMV) infection] by using more effective antiviral treatments.

Anti-lymphocyte globulin (ALG) and anti-thymocyte globulin (ATG) are useful adjuncts that allow other immunosuppressants to be used at lower doses that are less toxic.

16.2 Types of organ transplantation

Learning objectives

You should:
- know the indications for the most common types of organ transplantation
- have an understanding of the outcome in these groups of transplant patients.

Renal transplantation

This is the most frequently carried out and successful organ transplant procedure. Most major medical centres in the UK have an established renal transplant programme and, nationwide, 3000 transplants are performed each year.

The main indication for transplantation is irreversible renal failure. The three most frequent causes are:

- chronic glomerulonephritis
- chronic pyelonephritis
- diabetic nephropathy.

Most patients who are on a transplant waiting list will require peritoneal dialysis or haemodialysis until a suitable kidney becomes available.

Donor sources

Kidneys for transplantation come from two sources:

- brain-dead donors (cadaveric transplants)
- living donors.

Most donor kidneys come from patients who have recently died in hospital, following either a stroke or a major head injury. Donors are accepted provided that there is no evidence of active infection, extracerebral malignancy, hepatitis A, B or C infection, tuberculosis or HIV infection.

Once brainstem death is confirmed and consent obtained, the kidneys are harvested as part of a multiple organ donation involving liver, kidneys, heart and lungs.

Table 22 Immunosuppressive drugs used in transplantation

Drug	Action	Side effects
Calcineurin inhibitors[a] Tacrolimus, ciclosporin A	Inhibit immunoactive leucocytes (CD4 T lymphocytes)	Nephrotoxic
Antiproliferative drugs[b] Mycophenolate mofetil, azathioprine	Inhibit RNA and DNA synthesis	Bone marrow suppression
Steroids	Inhibit inflammation	Growth retardation, hypertension, increased infection risk
Anti-lymphocyte globulin	Reduces lymphocyte numbers	
Anti-thymocyte globulin	Reduces thymocyte numbers	

[a]These drugs inhibit calcineurin, which is essential for the growth of T lymphocytes.
[b]These drugs prevent proliferation of T lymphocytes.

Immediately the circulation is arrested, the intra-abdominal organs are perfused with a cold preservation fluid to minimise the period of warm ischaemic time and thus prevent organ degeneration. Most kidneys can be preserved for up to 24 h.

Live donation is usually reserved for related donors who wish to help a family member with renal disease. Transplantation between unrelated individuals is less common and is fraught with ethical problems. Because of the limited number of cadaveric donors available to provide kidneys, increasing use is being made of living related and unrelated donation.

Transplant surgery

The kidney is transplanted into a heterotopic site in either the left or the right iliac fossa. An extraperitoneal pouch is prepared to receive the kidney and the renal vessels are anastomosed to the adjacent external iliac artery and vein.

The ureter is usually implanted into the recipient's bladder. Implantation into the colon or an isolated small bowel loop (an ileal conduit) is rarely used.

Outcome and prognosis

Rejection episodes are uncommon with the newer regimens of immunosuppression, outlined on p. 325. Although recipients cope well with common viral illnesses, they are prone to opportunistic infection with *Pneumocystis* spp. or CMV. Cancer (usually lymphoma or skin cancer) is also more common in transplant recipients.

Current long-term graft survival rates average 80% for cadaveric transplants and 90–95% for living related grafts.

Liver transplantation

The first successful liver transplants were carried out in the late 1960s. Before 1980, the 1-year survival rate was less than 40%. The introduction of ciclosporin and, more recently, tacrolimus has revolutionised liver transplantation and, in the USA alone, more than 5000 transplants are performed every year, with the 1-year survival rate approaching 90%.

The main indications for transplantation in adults are:

- cirrhosis secondary to viral hepatitis
- biliary cirrhosis
- fulminant liver failure.

    Transplantation is performed less often for:

- hepatocellular cancer
- alcoholic cirrhosis.

    In children, congenital biliary atresias are the most widespread indication for liver transplantation.

Donor sources

Whole organ livers are obtained from brain-dead donors. Because technical difficulties are encountered when transplanting a large liver into a small recipient (e.g. from an adult to a child), several alternative types of transplant have been developed. These are:

- reduced-size transplants: using part of the left lobe of the liver only as a graft; this is especially useful in children
- split-liver transplants: dividing the liver into two anatomical halves, corresponding to the left and right lobes, to enable two transplants from one donor.

Living related transplants are occasionally undertaken, again using part of the left lobe. This form of transplantation is usually undertaken between mother and child.

Transplant surgery

The operative procedure is complex. Essentially, the organ is transplanted orthotopically after the recipient liver has been removed. During this procedure, the venous return to the heart is diverted away from the liver bed by an extracorporeal veno-venous bypass.

Outcome and prognosis

Haemorrhage and biliary complications, including obstructive jaundice, are the most common early postoperative complications. Opportunistic infections related to immunosuppression are also frequent.

Despite these setbacks, patients can expect a 1-year survival rate of up to 90%.

Cardiac transplantation

Successful cardiac transplantation was established between 1970 and 1980. Currently, about 3000 transplants are performed annually worldwide.

The main indication for cardiac transplantation is end-stage cardiac failure, which is most commonly caused by:

- viral cardiomyopathy
- ischaemic heart disease.

    Less common indications include:

- valvular heart disease
- congenital heart disease.

    There are few contraindications to transplantation other than the presence of active infection (especially HIV or hepatitis) or major liver or renal dysfunction.

Donor sources

Donor hearts are invariably obtained as part of a multiple organ retrieval from a brain-dead donor. In contrast to kidney and liver transplants, a freshly harvested cold perfused heart has a short survival time of only 4–6 h. Because of this, recipient preparation and organ retrieval, which often take place at different centres, have to be carefully coordinated to minimise any delays.

Transplant surgery

Cardiopulmonary bypass is established and the recipient's heart excised before performing an orthotopic heart transplant.

Outcome and prognosis

Despite a technically successful transplant some patients will die in the early postoperative period because of the severity of their pre-existing cardiac illness. Sepsis precipitated by immunosuppression is another important cause of mortality. Deaths caused by rejection are less common.

About 80% of all transplant patients will survive for at least 1 year after operation.

Pulmonary transplantation

Successful lung transplantation has only been achieved since the late 1980s. Today, in the USA alone, over 1000 lung transplants are performed each year. The main indications for transplantation are:

- chronic fibrotic lung disease
- chronic obstructive airways disease
- chronic pulmonary sepsis
- pulmonary hypertension.

Transplant surgery

There are three types of operation:

- combined heart and lung transplants
- single lung transplants
- bilateral lung transplants.

The choice of operation depends upon the extent of pulmonary disease and any coexistent cardiac disease.

Outcome and prognosis

Rejection and/or infection are the main causes of graft failure. Lung transplantation is less successful than heart, liver or renal transplantation; approximately 60% of patients will survive for 1 year after surgery.

Pancreas transplantation

Pancreas transplantation is undertaken to prevent the complications of type 1 diabetes mellitus, usually nephropathy, retinopathy or atherosclerosis, and to avoid the requirement for exogenous insulin administration. Because these patients will require immunosuppression, pancreas transplantation is usually only offered to diabetic patients who are receiving immunosuppression already (e.g. a diabetic renal transplant patient) or diabetic patients in renal failure who will undergo a combined pancreas–kidney transplant.

Donor sources

The donor pancreas is usually obtained as part of a multiple organ retrieval from a brain-dead donor who has no history of alcohol abuse or glucose intolerance.

Transplant surgery

Usually, the entire pancreas and duodenum is transplanted into the recipient. The pancreatic exocrine secretion is drained into either the recipient's urinary bladder or the small intestine. The allograft is positioned in the recipient's lower abdomen with vascular attachments to the recipient iliac artery and vein.

Outcome and prognosis

Success rates have slowly improved in the last decade and up to 80% of patients will remain insulin independent after transplantation.

Small bowel transplantation

Small bowel transplantation has lagged behind other forms of organ transplantation because of frequent graft rejection followed by sepsis and multiorgan failure. Potent new immunosupressive agents such as tacrolimus have now made intestinal transplantation a viable option in patients with intestinal failure. The main indication for transplantation is intestinal failure in patients who have had massive small bowel resection and who can no longer be treated by total parenteral nutrition (TPN), either as a result of liver failure caused by prolonged TPN or because the routes of venous access have become exhausted.

Transplant surgery

There are two types of operation:

- isolated small bowel transplantation
- combined liver and small bowel transplantation.

The choice is determined by the presence or absence of any coexisting irreversible liver disease, which may have been caused by TPN.

Outcome and prognosis

About 50% of patients will survive for 5 years after a small bowel transplant.

Sixteen

Self-assessment: questions

Multiple choice questions

1. With regard to transplantation in general:
   a. currently, most human transplants are xenotransplants
   b. a renal transplant is an example of an orthotopic transplant
   c. allotransplantation means transplantation from a non-identical donor to a recipient of the same species
   d. heterotopic transplants are rarely performed
   e. currently, renal transplants are the most commonly performed transplant operation

2. With regard to transplant rejection:
   a. a blood group A graft placed in a blood group O recipient will not be rejected if there is a good HLA system match between donor and recipient
   b. close HLA class I and II matching is essential if rejection is to be prevented
   c. an acute pattern of rejection usually develops within weeks/months of transplantation
   d. hyperacute rejection is characterised by severe vascular damage, with thrombosis and endothelial destruction
   e. cellular and humoral mechanisms are responsible for the phenomenon of acute rejection

3. With regard to renal transplantation:
   a. most kidneys can be preserved for up to 24 h between harvesting and transplantation
   b. a 60% survival rate can be expected following cadaveric transplantation
   c. the kidney is usually transplanted into a heterotopic site in either the left or right iliac fossa
   d. renal transplant patients are prone to infection with *Pneumocystis* spp. or cytomegalovirus
   e. diabetic nephropathy can recur in a healthy kidney following transplantation

4. With regard to liver transplantation:
   a. biliary atresia is a common indication for transplantation in adults
   b. multiple transplants can be provided from a single donor liver
   c. liver transplantation is an example of an orthotopic transplant
   d. up to 70% of all transplant patients can expect to live for 1 year after transplantation
   e. liver transplantation is contraindicated in patients with hepatocellular carcinoma

5. With regard to cardiac and pulmonary transplantation:
   a. a freshly harvested cold perfused heart will survive for up to 12 h before transplantation
   b. acute rejection is the most frequent cause of death following cardiac transplantation
   c. cardiopulmonary bypass is an essential step prior to performing an orthotopic cardiac transplant
   d. ischaemic heart disease accounts for 40% of all patients requiring cardiac transplantation
   e. coronary artery disease can develop in a healthy transplanted heart

Self-assessment: answers

Multiple choice answers

1. a. **False.** Xenotransplantation means transplanting between members of different species. Most human transplants are allotransplants, i.e. transplanting between members of the same species.

    b. **False.** Grafts are termed orthotopic if they are transplanted into their 'normal' anatomical site. Renal transplants are usually heterotopic, occupying an ectopic site usually in the right or left iliac fossa.

    c. **True.** Most human transplants are allografts.

    d. **False.** Renal transplants, the most common of all human transplants, are heterotopic.

    e. **True.** Approximately 3000 renal transplants are performed every year in the UK. The usual limiting factor is the availability of suitable donor kidneys.

2. a. **False.** The ABO blood group is one of the key compatibility systems in tissue matching. A blood group A graft will be immediately rejected by a blood group O recipient because of circulating anti-blood group A antibodies in the recipient. This will occur even if there is a good donor/recipient match in the HLA system.

    b. **False.** The HLA class I and class II antigen systems are extremely complex and perfect matching is rarely achieved between donor and recipient because of the wide number of antigenic permutations. However, this does not prevent transplantation. Immunosuppressive agents such as ciclosporin are used to override the recipient immune response to the graft.

    c. **True.** Hyperacute rejection occurs within minutes of transplantation. An acute rejection response occurs within several months of transplantation.

    d. **True.** The transplanted organ becomes acutely swollen and tender and ceases to function. Vascular thrombosis and endothelial damage are the key microscopic features.

    e. **True.** Only hyperacute rejection is mediated predominantly by circulating humoral antibodies.

3. a. **True.** There is a functional deterioration if transplantation is delayed beyond this time.

    b. **False.** Graft survival rates following transplantation average 80%.

    c. **True.** A renal transplant is the most common type of heterotopic transplant.

    d. **True.** Opportunistic infections are more frequent in patients following renal or other types of transplant. This is related to suppression of the patient's own immune system by the immunosuppressive agents used to prevent rejection.

    e. **True.** Diabetic nephropathy and some forms of glomerulonephritis can recur in a transplanted kidney. Occasionally, repeat transplantation is required.

4. a. **False.** This is the major indication for transplantation in childhood. Most adult transplants are undertaken for cirrhosis secondary to viral hepatitis or for fulminant liver failure.

    b. **True.** A split liver transplant, dividing the liver into two anatomical halves corresponding to the left and right lobes of the liver, enables two transplants from one donor.

    c. **True.** The liver is transplanted into its normal anatomical site, i.e. it is an orthotopic transplant.

    d. **True.** The immunosuppressive agent ciclosporin has revolutionised the outcome of liver transplantation. Currently, 70% of transplanted patients will survive for 1 year.

5. a. **False.** A heart has a short survival period after harvesting, usually 4–6 h. For this reason, recipient preparation and donor harvesting, which often take place at different centres, need to be carefully coordinated.

    b. **False.** Most early deaths are caused by the severity of the patient's pre-existing cardiac illness. These patients will die despite a technically successful transplant.

    c. **True.** Cardiopulmonary bypass enables systemic perfusion to continue during the transplant procedure.

    d. **True.** Ischaemic heart disease and viral myocarditis together account for 80–90% of all transplant patients.

    e. **True.** 'Transplant' coronary artery disease does occur. It is probably a form of chronic rejection rather than a complication of developing atheromatous disease.

Ophthalmology

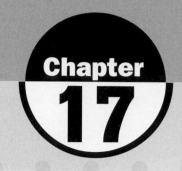

Chapter 17

Chapter overview

This chapter outlines core material related to ophthalmology. First, a description of how to take an ophthalmic history and measure a patient's visual acuity is provided. The importance of history taking is highlighted and the specific ophthalmic complaints of red eye and visual disturbance are discussed in more depth. Second, a systematic description of the common conditions encountered by an ophthalmologist is given. Further detail on how to examine specific parts of the eye is provided in the discussion of each clinical condition. The clinical features, basic management and potential complications of common conditions are outlined. It is important to have an understanding of ocular anatomy to appreciate the symptoms and signs being discussed. Some basic ocular anatomy is provided throughout the chapter, however, the emphasis is on clinical presentation. As well as common conditions affecting specific ocular structures, there are sections on the optics of the eye, glaucoma, ocular injuries and neuro-ophthalmology. The self-assessment section helps to clarify some of the key concepts in the chapter and provides additional clinical examples and photographs.

History and examination

17.1 History

Learning objectives

You should:
- be able to take a directed ophthalmic history
- be able to measure a patients visual acuity
- be able to note the history and examination findings.

Asking a patient open questions about their symptoms will help to identify the predominant complaint or suggest a likely diagnosis. It is then useful to clarify specific aspects of the presenting complaint with some closed questions. These include:

- whether this is the first episode or a recurrent condition
- whether one or both eyes are affected
- the duration of symptoms
- whether the symptoms are intermittent or constant

- whether anything relieves or aggravates the symptoms
- whether the problem is getting better, staying the same or worsening
- whether there are any associated systemic or neurological symptoms (e.g. headache or nausea).

In addition, it is useful to explore some aspects of certain symptoms further. This will help to create a differential diagnosis. For example:

Red eyes:

- both eyes affected suggests infective or allergic conjunctivitis
- purulent discharge may suggest bacterial conjunctivitis
- itch may suggest allergy
- photophobia suggests inflammation of the anterior segment (e.g. iritis or keratitis)
- a red eye with reduced visual acuity suggests more serious pathology (e.g. acute closed-angle glaucoma, iritis, corneal ulcer).

Visual disturbance:

- both eyes affected suggests a postchiasmal neurological lesion
- one eye affected suggests pathology of the globe or optic nerve
- acute visual loss in a quiet white eye with temporal headache and scalp tenderness suggests temporal arteritis

- acute visual loss with a red eye and systemic upset such as vomiting may suggest acute closed-angle glaucoma
- gradual painless visual loss suggests either cataract or age-related macular degeneration.

After taking the ocular history it is important to explore the general medical history, drug history, family history and social history. It is also important to determine the patients perspective on the problem, in particular, how their daily life is affected. This helps greatly when considering surgical intervention, e.g. cataract surgery.

17.2 Examination

Before starting the examination it is important to take a few moments to observe the patient for clues that may help to identify the diagnosis.

The complete systematic examination should include:

- visual acuity
- external eye
- anterior segment
- pupil responses
- ocular motility
- field of vision
- ophthalmoscopy.

Visual acuity

Vision is most commonly assessed using a standard Snellen chart (Figure 201A). Each eye is tested in turn, with the

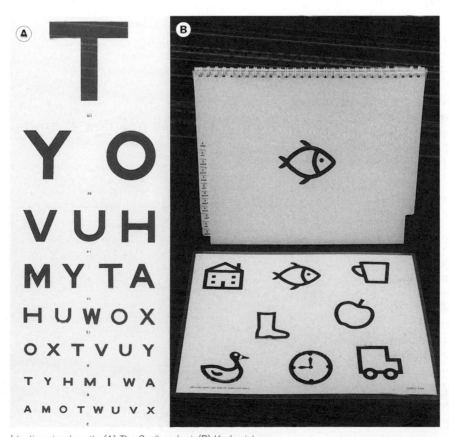

Figure 201 Methods of testing visual acuity. (A) The Snellen chart. (B) Kay's pictures.

right eye tested first as routine. If the patient wears glasses they should be worn for the test and if the patient is unable to read the chart they should be asked to look through a pin-hole aperture as this 'neutralises' any refractive error. The chart should be placed 6 m from the patient, who is asked to read the chart from the top with one eye covered by an occluder. If the patient is only able to see the top letter, the acuity is documented as 6/60 (a person with normal vision should be able to see the top letter from 60 m away). If the chart can be read down to the bottom, the acuity is documented as 6/6, i.e. 'normal' vision. If the patient is unable to see the chart at all, vision should be recorded progressively as the ability to count fingers (CFs), perceive hand movements (HMs), perceive light (PL) or not perceive light (NPL).

Near vision should also be tested. This can be carried out using a standard reading book although, if this is not available, any text will do.

In younger children, visual acuity assessment can be challenging. A variety of methods are employed depending on the child's age. For children of less than 18 months, preferential looking tests using simple patterns are used. For children older than 18 months, matching tests using shapes, pictures (see Figure 201B) or letters (Sheridan–Gardiner test) can be employed.

The rest of the ocular examination will be considered during the relevant sections of this chapter.

The history and examination should be noted clearly in the patients notes. Typically, right occular findings are written or drawn diagrammatically on the left-hand side of the page, i.e. as if you are looking at the patient. This should be followed by the differential diagnoses and management plan.

The eyelids and lacrimal system

17.3 Infection and inflammation

> **Learning objectives**
>
> You should:
> - know the cause of lid infection and inflammation
> - recognise lid malposition and know the possible causes
> - be able to identify a basal cell carcinoma of the lid
> - know the causes of a watery eye.

The eyelashes and eyelid meibomian glands are common sites of staphylococcal infection.

Hordeolum (stye)

Clinical features
There is an acute, red, tender swelling of the lid margin, which 'points' at the lash line.

Management
Topical broad-spectrum antibiotics and steam bathing will help during the acute infection. Styes usually discharge spontaneously and resolve within 1–2 months.

Chalazion
If the opening of a meibomian gland on the lid margin becomes blocked, the gland will swell creating a chalazion.

Clinical features
A red, localised, occasionally tender swelling occurs within the lid. Chalazia are often associated with blepharitis (see below).

Management
The majority of acute chalazia will settle spontaneously over a 1- to 3-month period, often leaving a small, residual, firm, painless nodule. If a large or painful chalazion persists, incision and drainage will often hasten resolution. Topical antibiotics are often prescribed although their therapeutic benefit is unproven.

Blepharitis
Blepharitis is chronic inflammation of the lid margins and associated meibomian glands. It is a common cause of irritable red eyes.

Clinical features
The lid margins are red and swollen. There may be crusting around the lashes in severe disease. This is a chronic disease in which the eyes are persistently gritty and sore. Patients are more likely to develop chalazia.

Management
The lids should be cleaned using cotton buds dipped in a dilute solution of baby shampoo. This removes crusts and clears meibomian gland orifices. Artificial tear supplements may be required.

17.4 Lid position abnormalities

Ptosis
Drooping of the upper eyelid is known as ptosis and may be congenital or acquired. Causes include:

- neurogenic
  - third cranial nerve palsy
  - Horner's syndrome (see Figure 202)
- myogenic
  - weakness of the levator muscle (e.g. 'senile ptosis')
- neuromyogenic
  - myasthenia gravis

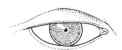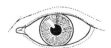

Figure 202 Right Horner's syndrome.

- mechanical
  - cysts or swelling of the upper lid.

Clinical features

The upper lid usually overlies the cornea by 1 mm. In ptosis, this position is lower than normal. The extraocular movements and pupils should be examined for any associated features.

Management

If an underlying cause such as myasthenia gravis is identified this should be treated appropriately, otherwise, treatment is surgical. In congenital ptosis, surgical correction is required promptly if the visual axis is occluded to prevent the development of amblyopia.

Lower lid entropion

Clinical features

In entropion, which is usually a condition of the elderly, the eyelid turns in and the lashes abrade the cornea. The lashes rub on the cornea and conjunctiva causing redness, pain and the feeling that there is something in the eye. Instillation of fluorescein will often reveal small corneal abrasions.

Management

Treatment is surgical by placing everting sutures.

Lower lid ectropion

Clinical features

In ectropion, the lower lid turns out and the exposed tarsal conjunctiva becomes red and thickened (Figure 203). The eye may water because tears cannot drain into the everted lower lacrimal punctum or it may feel gritty because of exposure.

Management

The symptoms of grittiness and exposure may improve with the use of artificial tears. Otherwise, treatment is surgical, although this is often not required.

17.5 Tumours

Basal cell carcinoma

Basal cell carcinomas (BCCs) account for 95% of eyelid tumours. Characteristically, BCCs rarely metastasise although they do invade locally. The remaining 5% of eyelid tumours comprise squamous cell carcinoma, sebaceous gland carcinoma and malignant melanoma.

Clinical features

BCCs are usually raised painless lesions with a pearly telangiectatic margin and an ulcerated centre. They are commonly found on the lower lid margin.

Management

Treatment is by surgical excision.

17.6 Abnormal lacrimal flow

Lacrimal outflow obstruction (watery eyes)

Tears drain from the conjunctival sac through the lacrimal puncta and canaliculi into the lacrimal sac in the medial wall of the orbit. From here, they drain down the nasolacrimal duct to its opening in the nose beneath the inferior turbinate (Figure 204). Obstruction at any point along this pathway results in epiphora (watering of the eye). This may be congenital or acquired.

Congenital nasolacrimal duct obstruction

Membranous obstruction of the lower end of the nasolacrimal duct may be present if incomplete canalisation occurs. In the vast majority of children (>90%), the mem-

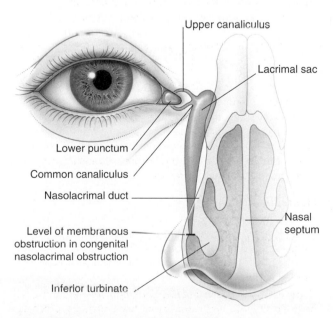

Figure 204 The lacrimal drainage system.

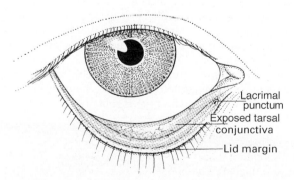

Figure 203 Lower lid ectropion.

branous obstruction opens spontaneously during the first year of life and the symptoms resolve completely.

Clinical features

There is painless watering of the eye, which may be worse in cold winds. The eyelids appear healthy with no eyelid position abnormality and a normal tear film.

Management

The obstruction is bypassed by creating a direct communication between the lacrimal sac and the nasal mucosa. This is known as a dacryocystorhinostomy (DCR).

Dacryocystitis

Dacryocystitis is an infection of the lacrimal sac, often secondary to nasolacrimal duct obstruction.

Clinical features

Acute dacryocystitis This is an extremely painful, tender, red swelling at the medial canthus. Pus builds up in the lacrimal sac and, without treatment, may discharge through the skin.

Chronic dacryocystitis Chronic infection causes a painless swelling of the sac. Mucopurulent material accumulates in the sac and can be expressed through the lacrimal puncta by pressure on the swelling.

Management

Dacryocystitis requires systemic antibiotics. Once the infection has settled, a DCR is necessary to avoid recurrent attacks.

Complications

Lacrimal sac infections can lead to episodes of preseptal and orbital cellulitis.

Keratoconjunctivitis sicca (dry eyes)

The tears lubricate the ocular surface and contain antibacterial substances that protect against infection. Keratoconjunctivitis sicca is an extremely common cause of ocular discomfort, especially in the elderly.

The underlying pathology is atrophy and fibrosis of the lacrimal gland caused by:

- senile changes in the lacrimal gland
- connective tissue diseases, e.g. Sjogren syndrome, which is characterised by keratoconjunctivitis sicca, dry mouth and autoimmune diseases such as rheumatoid arthritis.

Clinical features

The patient complains of dry, gritty eyes. Paradoxically, the eyes may water from reflex secretion because of the surface irritation. By placing small strips of filter paper into the lower fornix, an assessment of tear production can be made. This is known as Schirmer's test.

Management

Artificial tear drops and lubricating ointments may provide symptomatic relief. The rate of drainage can be reduced

by blocking the lacrimal puntal openings on the eyelid margins.

The conjunctiva, cornea and sclera

17.7 The conjunctiva

Learning objectives

You should:
- be aware of the major causes of conjunctivitis
- be able to recognise a dendritic ulcer and know the importance of appropriate management
- be able to differentiate between episcleritis and scleritis.

The conjunctiva is a clear mucous membrane that covers the globe and the inner surface of the eyelids. The most common conditions of the conjuctiva include infective and allergic conjunctivitis.

Infection

Bacterial conjunctivitis

Clinical features

Patients may give a history of acute-onset, red, gritty eyes with a purulent discharge that characteristically causes the eyelids to be stuck together on wakening. The redness is diffuse and most prominent deep in the conjunctival fornices rather than around the cornea. Vision is usually unaffected.

Management

The most common causative pathogens are staphylococci, streptococci and *Haemophilus influenzae*. Treatment is with broad-spectrum topical antibiotic drops or ointment, such as chloramphenicol.

Adenoviral conjunctivitis

Clinical features

Although bilateral, this infection is often asymmetrical. The eyes are red with a watery discharge. The redness is diffuse but most prominent deep in the fornices rather than around the cornea. Superficial punctate corneal lesions can often be seen, particularly if stained with fluorescein. These lesions are largely responsible for the symptoms of grittiness and photophobia. Occasionally, they can reduce visual acuity. The preauricular lymph nodes are also often enlarged and tender.

Management

Antiviral agents are ineffective and, consequently, treatment is symptomatic. The condition is highly contagious and the patient should be advised on hygiene techniques to reduce spreading the infection, e.g. not sharing a face towel with another family member.

Complications

The keratitis can become chronic. If this occurs, mild topical steroid drops can help resolve the corneal lesions, improving symptoms.

Chlamydia conjunctivitis

Conjunctivitis caused by *Chlamydia trachomatis* can be divided into two distinct groups: endemic trachoma and sexually transmitted conjunctivitis.

Endemic trachoma This infection is common in developing countries in areas of poor sanitation. Scarring of the tarsal plate and in-turning of the lashes results in opacification of the cornea. It affects several million people worldwide and is one of the leading causes of preventable blindness.

Sexually transmitted conjunctivitis This condition tends to affect young adults. A bilateral conjunctivitis develops approximately 2 weeks after sexual exposure. The eyes become red with follicular changes in the fornices and palpebral conjunctiva. The discharge tends to be mucopurulent and stringy with non-tender enlargement of the preauricular lymph nodes. This condition is not sight threatening.

Management

If the diagnosis is suspected clinically, topical chlortetracycline is initially prescribed and appropriate swabs taken. Once the diagnosis is confirmed, referral to genito-urinary medicine (GUM) is necessary to enable further investigations to be performed to confirm the GU infection. Treatment with systemic doxycycline or azithromycin is recommended, as well as initiation of contact tracing.

Neonatal conjunctivitis (ophthalmia neonatorum)

This is a conjunctivitis occurring in the first month of life. It is a notifiable disease. The usual source of infection is the mother's genital tract or the environment, and the most common causative organisms are *Chlamydia* and staphylococci. Gonococcal infections are very rare but may cause severe conjunctivitis with keratitis. Herpes simplex can also cause neonatal conjunctivitis with keratitis.

Clinical features

The clinical features are dependent on the aetiology. *Chlamydia* may cause a mucopurulent discharge up to several weeks after birth. Gonococcus tends to present earlier with a more purulent discharge.

Management

Bacterial infections resolve quickly with topical broad-spectrum antibiotics. Chlamydial infection should be treated with systemic erythromycin rather than tetracycline as this binds to calcium, thus staining growing teeth. If a sexually transmitted disease is confirmed, the mother should be referred to GUM.

Complications

Chlamydial neonatal conjunctivitis may rarely lead to pneumonitis.

Allergic conjunctivitis

Hay fever conjunctivitis

Hay fever conjunctivitis is a very common self-limiting acute conjunctivitis caused by a type I immediate hypersensitivity reaction to pollens.

Clinical features

The eyes become red and itchy with a watery discharge. There may be marked oedema and swelling of the conjunctiva (chemosis). This condition tends to be seasonal and patients often have a history of asthma or eczema (atopy).

Management

Avoiding the precipitating antigen may reduce episodes. Topical antihistamine drops may be used prophylactically as well as during an attack to improve symptoms. Under ophthalmological supervision, topical steroids may be prescribed.

Vernal keratoconjunctivitis (spring catarrh)

Vernal keratoconjunctivitis (VKC) is an allergic condition that is normally only seen in children. It is caused by the release of inflammatory mediators from conjunctival mast cells and basophils in response to environmental antigens.

Clinical features

The most prominent symptoms of VKC include itch and photophobia. Reduced visual acuity is often noted as a result of corneal abnormalities and associated poor tear film. There tends to be a mucopurulent discharge with exacerbations occurring in the spring. Boys are more commonly affected than girls. There is a tendency towards spontaneous remission in adolescence but this is not always the case. There is an association with atopy.

Management

The most important element of management is antigen avoidance. The most common antigenic precipitant is the house dust mite. Measures that can be used to reduce exposure include careful vacuuming and dusting of the child's bedroom and consideration of a wooden rather than a carpeted floor, the use of 'sealed' pillowcases and duvet covers, and placing soft toys in the freezer to kill the mites. Combining reduction of antigen load with anti-inflammatory medication is more likely to achieve symptomatic improvement.

Complications

Corneal scarring is the most common sight-threatening complication. Glaucoma and cataract may develop secondary to steroid treatment.

Seventeen

17.8 The cornea

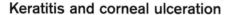

The cornea is the major refracting structure of the eye and its clarity is essential for good vision. The cornea is made up of three structural layers:

1. The surface of the cornea is a combination of the tear film and a multilayered epithelial membrane that is continuous with the conjunctiva at the limbus.
2. The middle layer of the cornea is the stroma, which consists of collagen fibres combined in such a way that they allow the passage of light. The stroma is continuous with the sclera.
3. Lining the inner aspect of the stroma is a layer of endothelium. The endothelium actively pumps water out of the stroma, maintaining the overall clarity of the cornea.

Keratitis and corneal ulceration

Keratitis is any inflammatory or infective process affecting the cornea.

Bacterial keratitis

The combination of normal lid anatomy, healthy tear film, intact corneal epithelium and a normal immune system protects the cornea from infection. If corneal infection develops it is usually associated with a predisposing factor such as:

*   lid abnormality (entropion, ectropion, lid retraction)
*   keratoconjunctivitis sicca
*   trauma (corneal abrasion)
*   contact lens wear
*   corneal paraesthesia
*   immunocompromised host
*   keratitis
*   corneal ulceration.

Clinical features

The clinical features vary according to the causative pathogen. The condition is usually unilateral. The patient presents with a red eye associated with a discharge. There is intense pain and photophobia with reduced vision, particularly if the ulcer is in the centre of the cornea. An opacified area of the cornea represents the stromal focus of infection. An overlying corneal epithelial defect may be easily seen if stained with fluorescein. Often, there is a secondary anterior uveitis with inflammatory cells circulating in the anterior chamber. These cells may settle in the inferior aspect of the anterior chamber creating a white fluid level known as a 'hypopyon'.

Management

The patient is usually admitted for round-the-clock intensive topical antibiotic treatment. Any predisposing abnormalities should be reversed, such as augmenting the tear

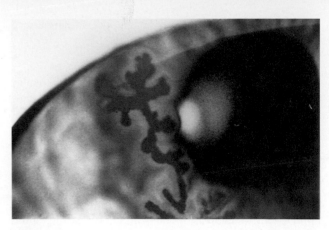

Figure 205 Dendritic ulcer.

film with copious artificial tears or surgically correcting an entropion.

Complications:

*   corneal perforation
*   corneal scarring
*   loss of the eye.

Herpes simplex (dendritic ulcer)

Clinical features

This condition is classically unilateral with recurrences always occurring on the same side. Photophobia, pain and blurred vision are common symptoms. The eye appears diffusely red with a watery discharge. The virus characteristically produces a branching, dendritic epithelial defect (Figure 205) that stains with fluorescein. The virus remains latent in the trigeminal ganglion and may become reactivated. With successive attacks, scarring of the cornea can occur.

Management

Topical aciclovir will normally help ulcers to heal within 1–2 weeks. Topical steroids must *not* be prescribed. Steroids will reduce the local effect of the immune system making the eye more comfortable but will stop the ulcer healing; this often results in the ulcer becoming larger and deeper. Because of this risk, patients with an acute red eye must *not* be given topical steroids except under the supervision of an ophthalmologist.

Complications:

*   corneal scarring and loss of vision
*   corneal paraesthesia with secondary bacterial ulceration.

17.9 The sclera and episclera

The sclera is the tough white collagenous wall of the eye. It is continuous with the cornea at the limbus. The episclera is an overlying layer of blood vessels, nerves and connective tissue.

Episcleritis

Clinical features

The patient complains of mild irritation, usually in one eye. The affected eye displays sectoral injection in the interpalpebral area.

Management

This condition usually resolves spontaneously within a few weeks. Resolution may be hastened by instilling a mild topical steroid or non-steroidal anti-inflammatory under ophthalmic supervision.

Scleritis

Pathologically, scleritis represents a form of immune complex deposition. Most cases are idiopathic. Systemic associations include any type III hypersensitivity vasculitic disease. Rheumatoid arthritis is the most common systemic association.

Clinical features

The most characteristic feature is severe ocular pain, which serves to differentiate scleritis from episcleritis. The globe is exquisitely tender and appears either diffusely red or injected in a sectorial fashion (Figure 206).

Management

Investigations for an underlying connective tissue disease are performed. The mainstay of treatment is the use of topical and systemic steroids although other immunosuppressive drugs are sometimes used.

Complications

If scleritis affects the posterior globe, swelling of the retina can occur resulting in loss of vision. Rarely, the sclera can become dramatically thin: this is known as 'scleromalacia perforans'.

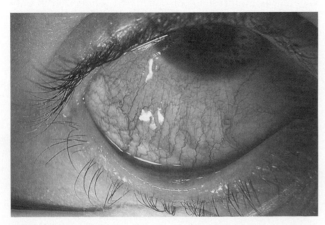

Figure 206 Scleritis.

The optics of the eye

17.10 Disorders of refraction

Learning objectives

You should:
- understand the different types of refractive error
- understand the anatomical reasons for refractive error
- understand the principles involved in correcting refractive error
- be able to recognise cataracts and understand the principles of cataract surgery.

The main structure in the eye that focuses light is the cornea. The lens provides additional focusing power, which can be adjusted for new objects (accommodation) (Figure 207). If, on entering a 'relaxed' non-accommodating eye, parallel light from a distant object focuses directly onto the retina, the eye is considered to be physiologically normal or emmetropic. If the light comes to a focus short of the retina, the eye is considered to be short-sighted or myopic, and if the light focuses behind the retina, it is considered to be long-sighted or hypermetropic.

Myopia (short sight)

In myopia the globe is bigger and, therefore, the eye is relatively longer than normal from front to back. As a consequence, the image of a distant object is brought to focus in front of the retina and a blurred image is formed at the retina. Distance vision is therefore reduced but can be corrected by using a concave (diverging) spectacle lens. Individuals with myopia have good near vision, hence

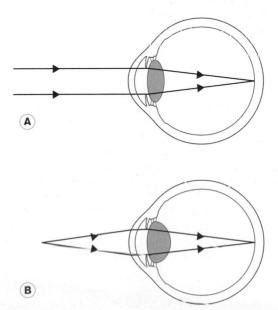

Figure 207 (A) Normal eye: emmetropia. (B) Accommodation: the lens becomes thicker and more curved, increasing its power and allowing the eye to focus on a near object.

Seventeen

337

the term short sight (see Figure 208). These individuals are more prone to spontaneous and traumatic retinal detachment.

Hypermetropia (long sight)

In hypermetropia the globe is smaller and the eye is relatively shorter than normal from front to back. As a consequence, the image of a distant object is theoretically brought to a focus behind the plane of the retina and a blurred image is formed on the retina. A convex (converging) lens will correct this (Figure 209). Because the eye is smaller, the structures in the anterior part of the eye tend to be 'anatomically crowded', which increases the chance of developing closed-angle glaucoma, especially if the pupil is dilated.

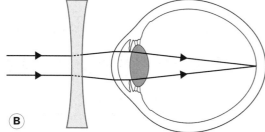

Figure 208 (A) Myopia. (B) Corrective lens for myopia.

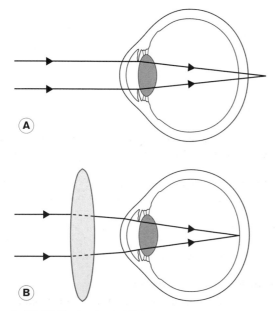

Figure 209 (A) Hypermetropia. (B) Corrective lens for hypermetropia.

Astigmatism

Regular astigmatism

The refractive power of the cornea is dependent upon its curvature. In astigmatism, the corneal curvature is not uniform, making it impossible to bring an image into sharp focus on the retina. An astigmatic cornea can be considered to be more the shape of a rugby ball than a football (normal), being more curved in one axis than another. An astigmatic spectacle lens can neutralise the differences in corneal curvature enabling a single sharp image to be focused on the retina.

Presbyopia

Accommodation for near work is dependent upon the plasticity of the lens and the power of the ciliary muscle. With increasing age, the lens becomes more rigid and it cannot assume the more rounded and thicker shape associated with higher focusing power. The ciliary muscle also weakens and the combination of these effects leads to a reduced ability to increase the focusing power of the eye for near vision. By the fifth decade most individuals will begin to hold reading material progressively further away. This is a normal process termed presbyopia. Reading glasses are required to focus on a near object.

Treatment of refractive disorders

There are a number of methods used in treating refractive errors:

- spectacle correction is the traditional method of improving vision
- contact lenses are preferred by some patients; the previously popular hard lenses have been replaced with rigid lenses (gas permeable) or soft lenses
- refractive surgery: several methods are available to alter the intrinsic refractive power of the eye; remodelling the cornea with an excimer laser has become increasingly popular.

17.11 Disorders of the lens

Cataract

Cataract is the presence of opacity in the lens. It is only considered clinically relevant if the patient has symptoms from the opacity. This is the most common cause of treatable visual impairment worldwide. Opacification of the lens commonly forms in three distinct portions. An opacity in the central portion of the lens is termed nuclear sclerosis; this is the most common form of age-related lens opacity. Cataract in the periphery of the lens has a radial spoke-like pattern and is called cortical cataract. An opacity at the posterior aspect of the lens is called a posterior subcapsular cataract; this type of cataract can be particularly visually disabling causing early loss of reading vision and glare in bright lights.

Most cataracts are the consequence of ageing. A minority of cataracts develop secondary to:

- ocular trauma
- ocular disease, e.g. uveitis

- metabolic disorders: diabetes is the most common with galactosaemia and hypercalcaemia being very rare
- drug use: notably prolonged use of systemic steroids
- congenital and hereditary disorders.

Clinical features
Patients with cataract can have a variety of symptoms such as:

- no symptoms (an incidental finding), which is very common
- reduced visual acuity leading to difficulty with
  - *reading the newspaper*
  - *reading prices of items in shops*
  - *watching the television*
  - *reading signs*
- glare
  - *in low sunlight*
  - *from car headlights*
- monocular diplopia.

The lens opacity can be noted on ophthalmoscopy as a disturbance of the red reflex. If the lens opacity is very advanced the pupil can appear white on macroscopic examination. This is known as 'leucocoria'.

Management
The only definitive means of dealing with cataract is surgical removal of the opacified lens. Surgery should be considered when the vision is reduced to the point where the patient is having problems with activities of daily living. Most operations are performed under local anaesthetic by infiltrating anaesthetic around the globe. The pupil is widely dilated to allow access to the lens. Cataract extraction is the most common operation performed worldwide.

Phaco-emulsification cataract surgery A small incision is made close to the limbus of the eye and a round tear in the anterior capsule of the lens is made. The lens is fragmented and sucked out of the eye by a sharp, oscillating, hollow tip known as a phaco-emulsification probe. A small, often foldable, lens is inserted via the incision and placed within the capsule bag upon the posterior capsule (see Figure 210). The incision wound is normally self-sealing and does not require any sutures. This technique allows rapid patient visual rehabilitation.

Postoperative care Topical steroids and antibiotics are prescribed routinely for a short period after cataract surgery to prevent infection and reduce inflammation.

Complications of cataract surgery
Cataract extraction surgery is generally a successful procedure. Complications include:

- opacification of the posterior capsule that holds the lens: this is more common in younger patients and can lead to blurred vision. It can be easily treated using a laser to disrupt and clear the opacified capsule
- intraocular infection (endophthalmitis)
- retinal detachment
- corneal decompensation.

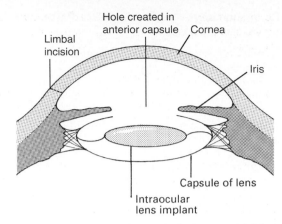

Figure 210 Intraocular lens implant inside the lens capsule at the end of an operation.

All infants should be screened routinely at birth for the presence of lens opacities by observing the red reflex of each eye with a direct ophthalmoscope. Screening is important to allow early treatment and reduce the chance of developing amblyopia. In a child with a dense lens opacity the diagnosis can be made more easily as the pupil appears white (leucocoria).

The uveal tract

17.12 Uveitis

> **Learning objectives**
> You should:
> - know the anatomy of the uveal tract
> - be able to differentiate uveitis from other causes of a red eye
> - understand the principles of uveitis management.

The uveal tract: structure and function
The uveal tract consists of three components from anterior to posterior:

- iris
- ciliary body
- choroid.

The iris is a diaphragm that contains a central opening (the pupil) that controls the amount of light entering the eye.

The ciliary body secretes aqueous humour and contains the ciliary muscle, which controls the focusing power of the lens.

The choroid is the highly vascular and deeply pigmented middle layer of the eye, which is sandwiched between the inner retina and outer sclera.

Classification of uveitis
Inflammatory conditions of the uveal tract are referred to as 'uveitis'. Depending on the component of the uveal tract

that is predominantly involved, uveitis can be classified into four main groups:

- *anterior uveitis*: the iris is predominantly involved, commonly known as 'iritis'
- *intermediate uveitis*: the ciliary body is predominantly involved
- *posterior uveitis*: the choroid is predominantly involved, commonly known as 'choroiditis'
- *pan-uveitis*: the whole uveal tract is inflamed.

Anterior uveitis (iritis)

Anterior uveitis is the most common of the four manifestations of uveitis. The other forms are fortunately rare as they can often have severe effects on visual function.

Clinical features

Anterior uveitis is usually unilateral. The patient has a photophobic, painful, watering, red eye with moderately reduced visual acuity. The presence of a sticky discharge or symptoms of itch and grittiness are not characteristic and instead would suggest a conjunctivitis.

Examination of the eye reveals diffuse redness that is most prominent around the limbus (junction of the cornea and sclera). This is also known as ciliary or circumcorneal injection. The pupil is usually small but may also be irregular because of adhesions between the anterior lens surface and the pupil margin (posterior synechia) (Figure 211).

Slit lamp examination is helpful in making the diagnosis as this reveals flare (proteinaceous exudates) and cells (immune cells) in the anterior chamber, which have leaked from the dilated iris blood vessels. In the majority of cases of unilateral acute anterior uveitis no cause can be identified and they are therefore considered idiopathic.

An underlying systemic association is more commonly found if the condition is bilateral, chronic or both. Systemic associations include:

- ankylosing spondylitis
- inflammatory bowel disease (both Crohn's disease and ulcerative colitis)
- sarcoidosis
- Reiter syndrome
- Behçet syndrome

- psoriatic arthropathy
- juvenile idiopathic arthritis
- tuberculosis
- syphilis.

Management

Intensive topical steroid drops reduce the inflammation. Cycloplegic drops such as cyclopentolate and atropine aid in relieving the prominent symptom of photophobia. Dilating the pupil also breaks pre-existing posterior synechiae and reduces the formation of new adhesions.

The retina

17.13 The retina: structure and function

Learning objectives

You should:
- know the basic structure and function of the retina
- recognise the symptoms of retinal detachment
- recognise the features and impact of age-related macular degeneration
- be able to differentiate between retinal vein and retinal artery occlusion
- recognise the features and understand the management of diabetic retinopathy.

Tiny light-sensitive cells (photoreceptors) at the back of the eye collect information about the visual world. There are two types of photoreceptor. *Rod photoreceptors* are very sensitive to dim light but cannot assess the colour (frequency) of the light. *Cone photoreceptors* are sensitive to bright light and, because there are three different types of cones, they are capable of assessing the frequency of light.

Each light photoreceptor transmits its information down nerves to the brain. The optic nerve is a collection of all of these nerves. All of the photoreceptors together make up a thin light-sensitive layer at the back of the eye known as the retina. The retina is divided into three separate anatomical and functional areas:

1. The peripheral retina is the area beyond the temporal arcade blood vessels. This area is dominated by rod photoreceptors. Functionally, it has low visual acuity (as the photoreceptors are relatively widely spaced) and poor colour vision but it functions well in dim light and is very sensitive to movement. This part of the retina serves the peripheral visual field.

2. The macula is the area of the retina within the temporal arcade blood vessels. This part of the retina is functionally dominated by the cone photoreceptors and, therefore, has good colour vision. The photoreceptors are more tightly packed together and, consequently, this area has better

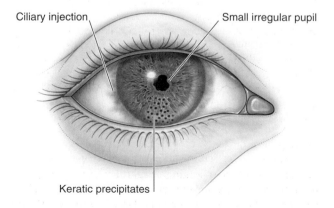

Ciliary injection — Small irregular pupil — Keratic precipitates

Figure 211 Anterior uveitis.

visual acuity than the periphery. The posterior pole serves the central 20–30° of vision.

3. The fovea is the central part of the macula. Cone photoreceptors are very densely packed in this area providing sharp central visual acuity for fixating and identifying fine-detailed objects.

17.14 Retinal detachment

There are several mechanisms by which the retina can detach from the back of the eye, including:

- fluid from the vitreous flowing through a retinal hole or tear. This is known as a 'rhegmatogenous' detachment and is the most common mechanism (Figure 212)
- severe proliferative diabetic retinopathy, which may lead to contracting scar tissue pulling the retina off the back of the eye causing a 'tractional' detachment (see section 17.18 on Diabetic retinopathy).

Predisposing factors for rhegmatogenous detachment include:

- myopia
- cataract surgery
- blunt trauma
- YAG laser posterior capsulotomy
- inherited peripheral retinal degeneration
- posterior vitreous detachment.

Clinical features of rhegmatogenous retinal detachment

Most patients present complaining of peripheral flashing lights and 'floaters'. The patient also describes a 'black curtain' or 'shadow'.

On examination, the patient may have reduced visual acuity, a field defect or relative afferent pupillary defect. On ophthalmoscopy (see Box 1), an anteriorly placed, slightly pale area of retina may be seen ballooning forwards.

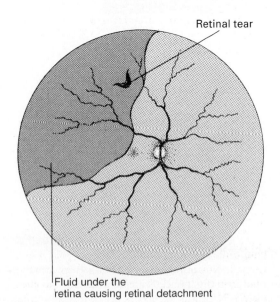

Retinal tear

Fluid under the retina causing retinal detachment

Figure 212 Retinal detachment.

> **Box 1:** Ophthalmoscopy
>
> - Sit patient in dark room; preferably, pupils should be dilated with drops, e.g. 1% tropicamide
> - With ophthalmoscope set at zero, observe red reflex in both eyes from 1 m
> - Dial lens to +10 (usually black numbers) and move to within 10 cm of the patient's eyes
> - The ophthalmoscope should now be focused on the front of the eye
> - Dial lens down towards zero until the retina comes into focus
> - Note any anterior segment abnormalities, e.g. cataract, as you focus towards the back
> - Once the retina is in focus, observe the optic disc, blood vessels, macula and periphery

Management

Treatment is surgical; visual recovery is uncertain. Untreated retinal detachment results in a blind eye.

Posterior vitreous detachment

The vitreous is a gel that fills the posterior segment of the globe. In young people, the vitreous is attached to the retina, but with age it peels away leading to a 'posterior vitreous detachment'. Patients often complain of floaters and peripheral flashing lights during the vitreous detachment. These symptoms normally settle after a few months. In the process of detaching, the vitreous can occasionally pull a small hole or tear in the retina, which may progress to a retinal detachment.

17.15 Age-related macular degeneration

This degenerative change of the macula is the commonest cause of reduced vision in the elderly. Age-related macular degeneration (ARMD) can be classified into two types: 'dry' (Figure 213) and 'wet' (or disciform) degeneration (Figure 214).

Clinical features

The patient usually complains of a gradual deterioration in vision. Ophthalmoscopy demonstrates pigmentary mottling in the macular region around areas of pale atrophic-looking retina. Well-demarcated yellow deposits known as hard drusen may be seen in association with these changes (see Figure 213). The condition is bilateral although it may be asymmetrical. In wet ARMD, haemorrhage or a grey subretinal neovascular membrane may be seen. These patients may complain of distortion, i.e. straight lines appear bent.

Management

Treatment is generally supportive rather than curative. With the use of good lighting, magnifiers and bigger print, the patient can maximise their functional reading vision. Newer treatments for certain types of wet ARMD called photodynamic therapy and anti VEGF intravitreal

Seventeen

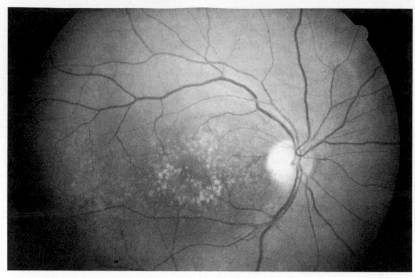

Figure 213 Dry ARMD. There is evidence of drusen and pigmentary disturbance at the macula.

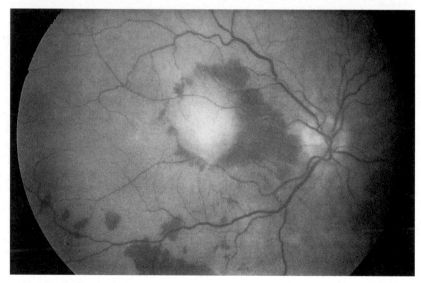

Figure 214 Disciform ARMD. There is evidence of a pale raised lesion in the macular area with haemorrhage around the lesion. Some of this haemorrhage has spread inferiorly.

injections may reduce progression in a few cases. The patient may be eligible for partial sight or blind registration. The advantage of such registration is that the patient may receive financial, practical, social and educational benefits from local social services and visual impairment societies. The current definition of 'blind' in the UK is 'a person who is so blind that they are unable to perform work for which vision is required'. This generally equates to having vision of equal to or less than 3/60 or having a significant visual field defect such as a hemianopia or grossly constricted fields because of glaucoma.

17.16   Retinal artery occlusion

Arterial occlusion causes sudden profound uniocular visual loss (usually to counting fingers or less).

Risk factors for an arterial occlusion include:

- carotid artery disease
- smoking
- hypertension
- diabetes (this is a risk factor for *all* arterial disease; it is treatable and must be excluded in all cases of central retinal artery occlusion)
- hypercholesterolaemia
- cardiac arrhythmia
- heart valve disease
- giant cell arteritis.

The commonest cause is an embolus from an atheromatous plaque in the internal carotid artery. If the visual disturbance lasts for less than 24 h, it is known as 'amaurosis fugax'. An embolus is assumed to have passed through the retinal circulation with no irreversible consequences. This is the eye equivalent of a cerebral transient ischaemic attack.

Clinical features

Central retinal artery occlusion causes complete painless uniocular loss of vision. A branch arterial occlusion leads to loss of function in one part of the retina, usually resulting in an 'altitudinal' field defect in which the upper or lower half of the visual field is lost.

Visual acuity is normally profoundly reduced to counting fingers or less. A dense relative afferent pupillary defect is present. Fundoscopy reveals a swollen pale retina, characteristically with a 'cherry-red spot' at the centre of the macula. An embolus may be seen lying within an arteriole.

Management

If the patient presents within 6–12 h of onset of the visual disturbance, efforts should be made to dislodge the embolus. Techniques include massage of the globe, lowering of intraocular pressure with intravenous diamox and 'rebreathing' into a paper bag to precipitate vascular dilatation (by increasing systemic carbon dioxide levels).

A standard systemic examination and investigation protocol should be performed to exclude an underlying reversible cause of emboli. Systemic examination should specifically exclude an irregular pulse, hypertension, a carotid bruit and any heart murmurs. Hyperviscosity states should be excluded and the cholesterol level checked. A carotid ultrasound examination is recommended to exclude significant stenosis.

Medical or surgical management should be instigated to reduce future cardiovascular morbidity. Interventions include low-dose aspirin, lipid-lowering agents and hypertension treatment and, in cases with significant carotid stenosis, carotid endarterectomy is considered. Patients should stop smoking.

17.17 Retinal vein occlusion

Visual loss in retinal vein occlusions is not usually as profound as in retinal artery occlusions. Branch retinal vein occlusions are more common than central vein occlusions.

Risk factors for a vein occlusion include:

- increasing age
- hypertension
- diabetes
- hyperviscosity syndromes.

Clinical features

In a central retinal vein occlusion (Figure 215) the patient complains of a sudden generalised loss of vision. Only part of the visual field will be affected in those with a branch vein occlusion.

The characteristic fundal appearance of vein occlusions includes:

- flame-shaped haemorrhages
- dilated tortuous veins
- cotton-wool spots
- macular oedema
- iris new vessel growth.

Management

It is important to consider the problem on two levels. First, any systemic risk factors that may have precipitated the vein occlusion need to be identified and treated. Second, the ocular consequences have to be considered. The two main causes of loss of vision are macular oedema and the development of a painful red eye with raised intraocular pressure (rubeotic glaucoma). Laser treatment is sometimes helpful.

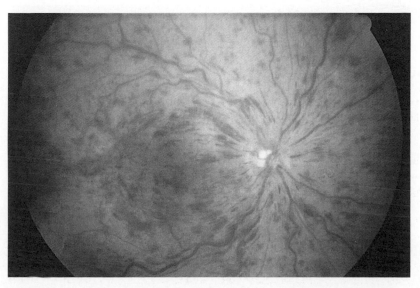

Figure 215 Central retinal vein occlusion. Note the flame-shaped retinal haemorrhages and the dilated tortuous veins.

Seventeen

17.18 Diabetic retinopathy

Diabetic retinopathy is the most common cause of blindness in the working population. Individuals with diabetes must have annual systemic examinations and ophthalmoscopy to enable medical treatment to be optimised and laser treatment to be performed early to prevent visual loss.

Pathophysiology

The loss of normal glycaemic control leads to damage of the cells that line blood vessels. This leads to:

- dilatation of local blood vessels, which leak protein and lipid-rich fluid causing hard exudate deposition and retinal oedema, defining diabetic maculopathy
- the release of angiogenic growth factors resulting in new vessel growth, defining proliferative diabetic retinopathy.

The retinal changes can be assessed on ophthalmoscopy by identifying specific clinical signs. These signs help classify the stages of diabetic retinopathy (Box 2).

Non-proliferative diabetic retinopathy

Non-proliferative diabetic retinopathy (NPDR) represents a spectrum of clinical signs depending on the level of retinal ischaemia (Figure 216). The vision is typically normal.

Box 2: Classification of diabetic retinopathy

- Non-proliferate diabetic retinopathy
- Proliferative diabetic retinopathy
- Diabetic maculopathy

Mild to severe NPDR clinical signs include:

- microaneurysms
- dot haemorrhages
- hard exudates
- cotton wool spots
- extensive deep blot haemorrhages
- venous beading.

Increasing severity of signs secondary to ischaemia

Proliferative diabetic retinopathy

The hallmark of proliferative disease is the presence of new vessels growing on the retina. It may be complicated by:

- vitreous haemorrhage as a result of bleeding from fragile new vessels: this presents as acute, painless, profound loss of vision and, on ophthalmoscopy, the red reflex is absent
- tractional retinal detachment, because of contraction of the supporting connective tissue
- rubeotic glaucoma, caused by growth of new vessels at other sites within the eye, such as the drainage angle.

If vitreous haemorrhage, tractional retinal detachment or rubeotic glaucoma develop, visual acuity is reduced (new vessels alone are usually associated with normal vision).

Diabetic maculopathy

Macular oedema and hard exudates may coexist with other signs of non-proliferative or proliferative diabetic retinopathy. Visual acuity may be reduced.

Management of diabetic retinopathy

NPDR does not generally require laser treatment; however, patients still require regular fundal examination and

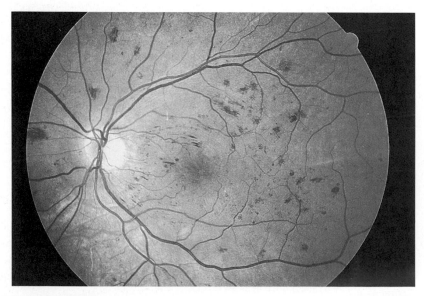

Figure 216 Non-proliferative diabetic retinopathy.

systemic examination for cardiovascular risk factors such as hypertension and hypercholesterolaemia. Control of associated cardiovascular risk factors will reduce the chance of retinopathy progression and visual loss. The more advanced the retinopathy, the more regular the examinations should be.

If the retinopathy progresses to the proliferative stage, argon laser ablation of the peripheral retina is indicated. Laser treatment reduces the amount of ischaemic tissue present and, therefore, reduces the overall oxygen demand.

Oedematous maculopathy requires direct but gentle laser treatment.

Vitrectomy involves removal of the vitreous. This is useful for cases of vitreous haemorrhage or tractional retinal detachment.

Strabismus

Each eye has six extraocular muscles (the medial, lateral, inferior and superior rectus muscles, and the inferior and superior obliques). The movements of each eye are finely coordinated with those of the opposite eye, so that both eyes normally function as one unit when fixating an object of interest in different fields of gaze. When the eyes become misaligned so that the visual axis of one eye is not directed to the same fixation point as the other, a squint, or strabismus, is present.

Classification of squints:

- concomitant
  - convergent (esotropia) (Figure 217A)
  - divergent (exotropia) (Figure 217B)
  - vertical (hyper/hypotropia) (Figure 217C)
- incomitant
  - cranial nerve palsies
  - dysthyroid eye disease
  - myasthenia gravis
  - trauma.

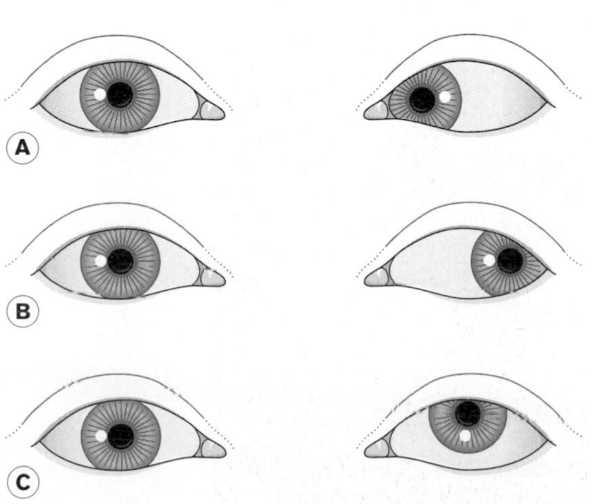

A concomitant squint is one that stays the same size no matter which direction the patient looks in and the patient has a full range of eye movements. An incomitant squint varies in size depending on the direction of gaze and there is evidence of weakness or tightness of one or more of the extraocular muscles. This distinction is important as it has implications regarding the underlying aetiology, which is important in terms of investigation and management.

17.19 Concomitant squints

> ### Learning objectives
>
> You should:
> - be able to perform a cover test and examine the extraocular movements
> - know the difference between concomitant and incomitant squint
> - know the possible causes of incomitant squint.

Convergent squint (esotropia)

Clinical features

There is a strong association between hypermetropia (long-sightedness) and childhood esotropia.

This type of squint usually becomes evident from about the age of 18 months to 3 years, when the child's near reflex (i.e. the ability to converge and focus on a near object) is developing, so that the eyes tend to over-converge when trying to focus on a near object.

One eye turns inwards (Figure 217A), which is confirmed by the cover test (see Box 3). This eye commonly becomes amblyopic without treatment. The eye movements are full.

> **Box 3:** Cover test and examination of extraocular movements
>
> ### Cover test
>
> - Ask the patient to fix on an interesting target held 60–90 cm away, e.g. small, detailed picture. Look for any obvious misalignment
> - Cover the left eye and observe the right eye for movement. Then, cover the right eye and observe the left eye (see Figure 218)
>
> ### Extraocular movements
>
> - Request the patient to fixate and follow a pen torch
> - Ask the patient to report any double vision during the test
> - Move the pen torch from the centre (primary position) into the other eight positions of gaze, returning to the primary position each time (see Figure 219)

Figure 217 Squints. (A) Left esotropia. (B) Left exotropia. (C) Left hypertropia.

The squint may start as intermittent but becomes constant with time. There are usually no symptoms (such as double vision) as the patient develops suppression of the squinting eye.

Management

In this age group, any child with a squint should be tested for glasses (refracted) and correction given to see if this improves or alters the angle of squint. If there is any amblyopia, this should be treated by patching the better eye. Patching the better eye forces visual stimulation of the amblyopic eye, assisting normal visual development. In patients whose vision is not corrected with spectacles, surgery is usually required.

Divergent squint (exotropia)

Divergent squints are much more rare in children than convergent ones. The age of onset of this type of squint is

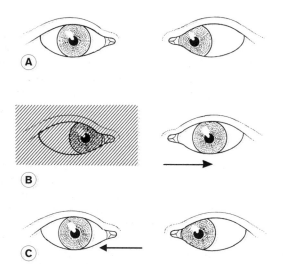

Figure 218 The cover test. (A) Patient fixating on the target; the left eye appears convergent. (B) The right eye is covered and the left eye moves out to take up fixation on the target, confirming a left convergent squint. (C) The cover is removed and the left eye becomes convergent again.

from the very young infant to 5–6 years of age. The aetiology is unknown.

17.20 Incomitant squints

Motor nerve palsies

The motor nerves to the extraocular muscles may be affected by a variety of disease processes such as:

- microvascular disease (in association with hypertension, diabetes or atherosclerosis)
- demyelination
- intracranial aneurysms
- infection (e.g. herpes zoster, meningitis)
- trauma
- intracranial neoplasms.

Clinical features

The features depend on the affected nerve.

Third nerve palsy All muscles except the lateral rectus and superior oblique are innervated by the third (oculomotor) nerve. Features of a third nerve palsy include:

- divergent hypotropic eye
- dilated unreactive pupil
- ptosis (droopy upper lid).

In many patients the condition is partial, either by sparing the pupil or lid or by leaving some movements partially or fully intact. A painful third nerve palsy must be considered as a neurosurgical emergency as it may be caused by enlargement of a posterior communicating artery aneurysm, which may be at risk of bleeding with catastrophic consequences.

Fourth nerve palsy The fourth, or trochlear, nerve innervates the superior oblique muscle. The affected eye cannot look downwards fully while adducted (turned inwards). Patients notice diplopia in which the images are on top of each other (vertical diplopia) and tilted at an

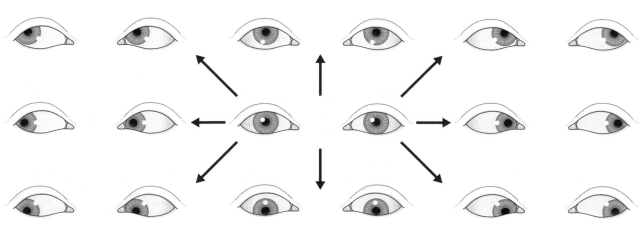

Figure 219 The nine positions of gaze.

angle to each other (torsional diplopia). To compensate for this, patients commonly tilt their heads away from the affected side (Figure 220).

Sixth nerve palsy Sixth (abducent) nerve palsy is the most common cranial nerve palsy. It causes an isolated lateral rectus weakness, which presents as double vision in which the images are side by side. The diplopia is maximal (i.e. the images are most widely separated) on looking towards the affected side and when looking in the distance (Figure 221).

Management

Patients should be investigated for an underlying cause. The majority of nerve palsies improve spontaneously over a few months. An orthoptist can monitor the improvement of a palsy by examining the patient and recording the movements. During this time, the patient should be treated symptomatically to relieve any diplopia. This is done by patching one eye to occlude the second image or by sticking a plastic prism on to the glasses in front of one eye to allow the eyes to function together. In the long term, those that do not improve may require surgery.

Dysthyroid eye disease

Thyroid gland dysfunction can be associated with a disturbance of eye movements.

Clinical features

Patients often present with vertical or horizontal diplopia. In addition, they usually have other features of dysthyroid eye disease, such as ocular discomfort and redness, lid retraction, lid lag and proptosis (Figure 222). The abnormality of muscle function is not a weakness but a restriction caused by contraction of the affected muscles.

Management

Patients with characteristic eye findings who have not previously been diagnosed as dysthyroid should have their thyroid function tested (thyroxine, triiodothyronine and thyroid-stimulating hormone). Computed tomography (CT) or magnetic resonance imaging (MRI) demonstrates thickened rectus muscles. Any underlying thyroid disorder should be treated. However, this probably does not influence the clinical course of the eye disease. The condition runs an active course during which there may be

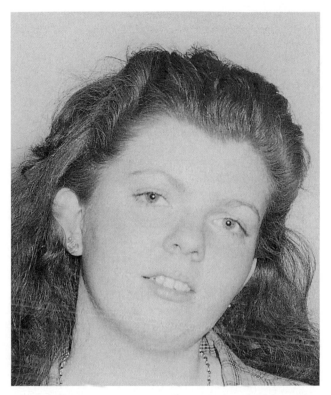

Figure 220 Right fourth nerve palsy. Patient tilts their head away from the affected side.

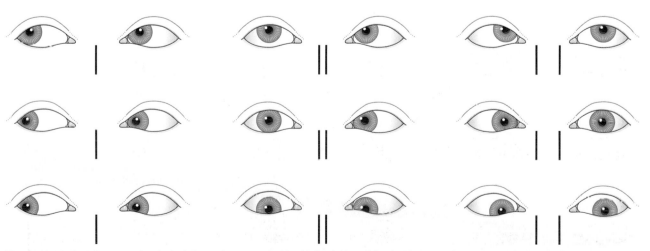

Figure 221 Left sixth nerve palsy. A single image is seen on looking to the right, and the double images become progressively further apart when looking left.

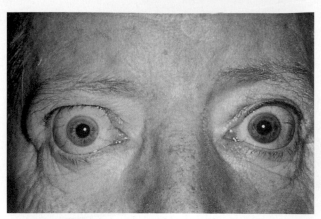

Figure 222 Dysthyroid ophthalmopath. Both upper and lower lids are retracted. Both eyes show proptosis.

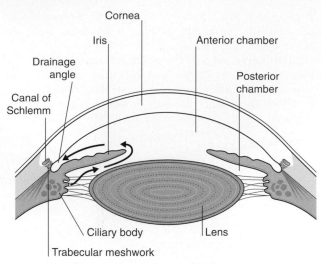

Figure 223 Aqueous production, flow and drainage.

continuing changes in the eye position, and during this time the patient should be kept comfortable with prisms or patches. After some months or years, it eventually stabilises and, at this point, the resultant ocular motility defects can be treated definitively by operating to weaken (or recess) the restricted extraocular muscles.

Complications:
• chronic diplopia
• exposure keratitis
• irreversible loss of vision.

Myasthenia gravis

Myasthenia gravis is an autoimmune condition in which neuromuscular transmission is affected by autoantibodies to acetylcholine receptors.

Clinical features

The most common ocular sign is ptosis although the patient may complain of diplopia, which may vary throughout the day and is characteristically worse at night. There is no pattern to the motility disturbance and it may simulate any nerve palsy.

Management

Treatment is with pyridostigmine. Patients suspected of having myasthenia should have a therapeutic trial of pyridostigmine.

Glaucoma

17.21 The glaucomas

Learning objectives

You should:
• understand the classification of glaucoma
• recognise the features of primary open-angle and acute closed-angle glaucoma.

Introduction

The glaucomas are a group of conditions with the common pathological end point of optic nerve neuropathy commonly associated with raised intraocular pressure. The optic neuropathy can be observed clinically as optic disc cupping. The neuropathy leads to peripheral visual field loss and, if untreated, to blindness.

Intraocular pressure is dependent on the balance between the rate of production and drainage of aqueous humour (outflow). Aqueous fluid is produced by the ciliary body. It flows from the posterior chamber into the anterior chamber via the narrow gap between the lens and the iris (see Figure 223). The fluid then drains mainly through the trabecular meshwork situated in the angle between the iris and the cornea into the canal of Schlemm and subconjunctival venous circulation. Intraocular pressure within the normal population is less than 21 mmHg.

17.22 Primary open-angle glaucoma

Primary open-angle glaucoma (POAG) is a bilateral condition that is usually seen in those over 40 years of age. It has a familial tendency with 10% of first-degree relatives developing the condition.

Clinical features

The onset is insidious and the patient is asymptomatic until very late in the disease. Patients with POAG may be identified at the asymptomatic stage by finding raised intraocular pressure (>21 mmHg) and optic disc cupping with associated visual field defects (Figure 224). The visual field loss characteristically occurs initially as an arcuate pattern (see Figure 225). The condition is therefore suitable for screening in the community. All patients attending an optometrist who have a family history of POAG or who are over the age of 40 have these tests performed.

Medical management

Medical management is normally first line and takes the form of a variety of topically applied intraocular pressure-lowering drops:

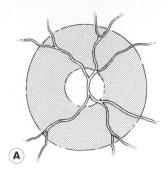

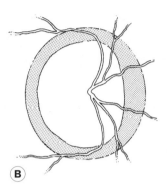

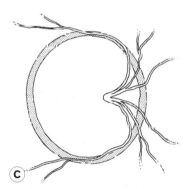

Figure 224 Optic disc. (A) Normal optic disc with small central cup. (B) Early glaucomatous cupping with extension of the cup vertically. (C) Advanced glaucomatous cupping.

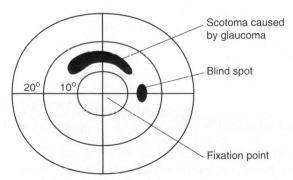

Figure 225 Pattern of field loss in early open-angle glaucoma caused by arcuate scotoma (or nerve fibre bundle defect).

- prostaglandin analogues (e.g. latanoprost); increase aqueous drainage
- beta blockers (e.g. timolol); reduce aqueous production at the ciliary body. Beta blockers should not be prescribed, even topically, to patients with reversible airways disease or heart block as they are absorbed systemically and may aggravate these conditions
- sympathomimetics (e.g. brimonidine); reduce aqueous production
- para-sympathomimetics (e.g. pilocarpine); reduce aqueous production and increase outflow via the trabecular meshwork. They cause miosis and often induce 'brow ache'. The miosis may lead to reduced visual acuity in patients with cataract. The drops need to be administered up to four times per day, which may reduce compliance in some patients
- carbonic anhydrase inhibitors (e.g. dorzolamide drops topically and acetazolamide systemically); act at the ciliary body to reduce aqueous production.

Surgical treatment

A surgical trabeculectomy is an operation that creates a fistula between the anterior chamber and the subconjunctival venous plexus, bypassing the trabecular meshwork. This creates a new channel for aqueous drainage, which leads to reduced intraocular pressure. Trabeculectomy has a high success rate but may be complicated by intraocular infection, intraocular haemorrhage and premature cataract formation.

Ocular hypertension

In some patients, the intraocular pressure is greater than 21 mmHg but there is no evidence of optic disc cupping or typical visual field loss. This is termed 'ocular hypertension' (OHT). The patient does not require any treatment although they should be reviewed regularly as they are at an increased risk of developing glaucoma.

Low-tension glaucoma

A group of patients show evidence of optic disc cupping and typical visual field loss despite having consistently normal intraocular pressures (<21 mmHg). After an intracranial cause of visual field loss has been excluded, a diagnosis of low-tension glaucoma (LTG) is made. This condition is very common and accounts for approximately 40% of patients suffering from glaucoma.

17.23 Acute closed-angle glaucoma

Pathophysiology

Acute closed-angle glaucoma (ACAG) develops when the normal flow of aqueous fluid between the lens and the iris at the pupil meets resistance. The resistance is known as 'pupil block' and is maximal when the pupil is mid-dilated. The aqueous fluid becomes trapped in the posterior chamber causing the iris to bow anteriorly (see Figure 226). The peripheral iris obscures the trabecular meshwork in the drainage angle causing an acute, marked reduction in

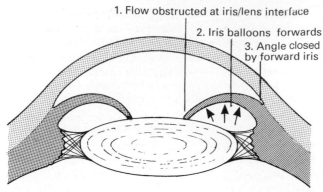

Figure 226 Sequence of events in acute closed-angle glaucoma.

1. Flow obstructed at iris/lens interface
2. Iris balloons forwards
3. Angle closed by forward iris

aqueous outflow. The intraocular pressure rises rapidly leading to pain and loss of vision. ACAG is more common in people with relatively small eyes with anatomically crowded anterior segment structures. Most patients with relatively small eyes are hypermetropic. The condition is also more common in elderly females, occurring in the evening and winter months when the pupil is more likely to be mid-dilated. The instillation of dilating drops may also precipitate an attack.

Clinical features

The patient presents with an extremely painful red eye, which may be associated with nausea and vomiting. The eye is diffusely red, there is no discharge, the cornea is cloudy and the pupil is mid-dilated and fixed. There is usually profound visual loss.

Before the acute episode, the patient may give a history of intermittent episodes of ocular pain and seeing haloes round lights, especially in the evenings.

The diagnosis is made on the basis of a typical history in association with a shallow anterior chamber, extremely high intraocular pressure and a pupil that is mid-dilated and fixed. Digital pressure (i.e. simply pressing on the eye) reveals a brick-hard eye.

Management

The intraocular pressure should be lowered as quickly as possible using intravenous carbonic anhydrase inhibitors and topical hypotensive agents (see medical management of POAG). Intensive topical pilocarpine will miose the pupil, breaking the pupil block and opening the drainage angle to increase aqueous outflow.

After the acute attack has been reversed, a laser peripheral iridotomy should be performed to prevent a further episode of ACAG. Because the fellow eye is similarly anatomically predisposed to an attack of ACAG, both eyes should be treated. A peripheral iridotomy is a small hole in the peripheral iris that allows aqueous fluid to flow directly from the posterior chamber into the anterior chamber, bypassing the pupil and any associated 'pupil block'. This results in equal pressure in the posterior and anterior chambers, reducing iris bowing and thus preventing a further episode of angle closure. Pressure control is not always achieved and medical treatment or tubeculectomy may be required (see POAG).

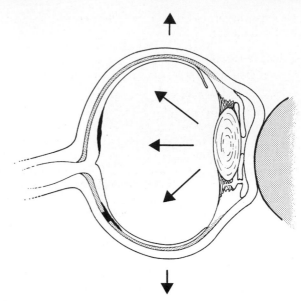

Figure 227 When the eye is struck, it is deformed and intraocular structures are damaged.

Ocular injuries

Introduction

Injuries to the eye are an important cause of ocular morbidity and visual impairment. The majority occur in young men. The common causes are sport and leisure activities, accidents in the workplace or home, assaults and road traffic accidents.

Prevention of injuries

The treatment of eye injuries is expensive and, in many cases, disappointing. The best method of reducing this burden is prevention. Although effective protective eyewear is available for most high-risk activities, such as sports and work, unfortunately, it is infrequently worn properly.

17.24 Blunt injuries

> **Learning objectives**
>
> You should:
> - appreciate the importance of injury prevention
> - recognise the features of blunt injuries
> - recognise the features of penetrating injuries
> - be able to initiate immediate treatment for chemical burns.

Blunt injuries are the most common type of eye injury. They are caused by a direct blow to the eye and surrounding tissues by an object such as a fist or a ball.

If the eye is struck, the globe flattens antero-posteriorly and becomes stretched equatorially (Figure 227); thus, intraocular structures are damaged by a combination of contusional and tearing forces. No penetration takes place although, in severe cases, rupture of the periorbital skin or eyeball may occur.

Clinical features

Common features of blunt ocular trauma include:

- periorbital haematoma (black eye)
- blow-out fracture (or orbital floor fracture). Significant blunt trauma leads to a rapid rise in intraorbital pressure. The contents of the orbit decompress into the sinuses surrounding the orbit causing a fracture of the floor of the orbit in which the orbital rim remains intact (Figure 228). This often leads to double vision and the appearance of a sunken orbit (enophthalmos). It is often also associated with infraorbital paraesthesia
- subconjunctival haemorrhage (diffuse bleeding under the conjunctiva)
- corneal abrasion: an acutely painful injury that can be detected by instilling fluorescein drops into the conjunctival sac. The abraded area will stain bright green when viewed with a blue light
- hyphaema (blood in the anterior chamber; see Figure 229). This indicates that the eye has suffered a significant injury with damage to the intraocular

structures. The eye is usually acutely painful, especially if the intraocular pressure is elevated, which is a common effect of blood in the eye
- sight-threatening complications such as retinal holes, choroidal tears and rupture of the globe.

Management

Black eyes and subconjunctival haemorrhages settle spontaneously over a few days without any treatment. Corneal abrasions are treated with antibiotic ointment and firm padding. Blow-out fractures only require surgical intervention if double vision persists or the appearance is cosmetically unacceptable. In cases of intraocular damage, full examination of the eye may not be possible until bleeding has settled and the eye is comfortable, which may not be until 3–4 weeks after the injury. Examination should include an evaluation of the peripheral retina for tears and an assessment of the drainage angle.

Early complications:
- raised intraocular pressure
- uveitis
- rebleeding of hyphaemas.

Long-term complications:
- premature cataract
- glaucoma
- retinal detachment.

17.25 Small flying particle injuries

Low-velocity foreign material tends to lodge on the cornea as a corneal foreign body (CFB) or under the lid as a subtarsal foreign body (STFB). High-velocity particles penetrate the globe to become intraocular foreign bodies (IOFB). Any injury that may have been caused by a high-velocity small particle (e.g. hammering injuries) should be treated as a potentially penetrating IOFB until proven otherwise, i.e. a radiograph of the eye should be performed or an experienced ophthalmologist's opinion sought before discounting this diagnosis.

Clinical features

Superficial foreign bodies cause a significant amount of pain, watering, redness and photophobia. Paradoxically, intraocular foreign material may be less painful and the symptoms are frequently minor.

CFBs can usually be seen on close inspection of the cornea, and staining with fluorescein helps to demarcate the area. STFBs can be seen when the upper eyelid is everted (Figure 230). IOFBs may be difficult to see on examination.

Management

CFBs can be removed with a small cotton tip or a sharp needle (under magnification after the administration of topical anaesthetic). A STFB can be swept off the inside of the lid with a cotton tip after everting the lid. If there is any epithelial damage from the superficial foreign body, topical antibiotic agents should be prescribed.

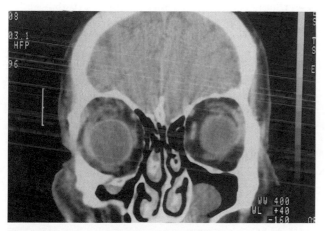

Figure 228 A 'blow-out' fracture of the right orbit, shown on CT scan. The orbit is expanded and there is evidence of a prolapse of tissue into the maxillary antrum through the orbital floor (the tear-drop sign).

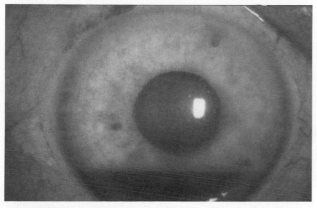

Figure 229 Hyphaema.

Seventeen

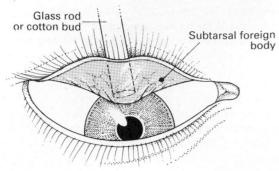

Figure 230 Everting the upper lid. Ask the patient to look downwards and evert the lid over a glass rod or cotton bud by pulling on the lashes.

IOFBs require surgical removal. This may involve loss of the lens, iris or vitreous humour if they are damaged by the injury.

Complications

The damaged epithelium of the cornea may not heal satisfactorily after a CFB or a STFB leading to a recurrent corneal erosion, a painful condition caused by recurrent breakdown of a tiny area of the epithelial surface.

The long-term effects of an IOFB depend on the degree of intraocular damage and the type and size of material that penetrated the eye. Organic material may rapidly lead to suppuration of the intraocular contents, and metallic foreign bodies oxidise and combine with intraocular proteins (siderosis) if not removed in the early period.

17.26 Large sharp objects

Injuries caused by large sharp objects may penetrate the eye.

Clinical features

The clinical features depend on the extent of the injury, ranging from superficial damage to the lids and eye to full ocular penetration with globe disruption.

Ocular penetrations may manifest as an irregular pupil, because the iris plugs the wound to prevent the loss of intraocular contents, or the eye may be softer than normal (Figure 231). Vision is usually reduced.

One should always be suspicious that full-thickness lid lacerations may involve the underlying sclera and retina.

Management

Lid lacerations, like any facial injuries, require careful skin closure. However, as the lacrimal drainage apparatus is situated at the medial aspect of the lid, injuries in this area may require specialist evaluation and treatment.

A primary repair for globe penetration should be performed urgently. Multiple surgical procedures may subsequently be required for the optimum result.

Complications

- corneal scarring
- cataract
- endophthalmitis

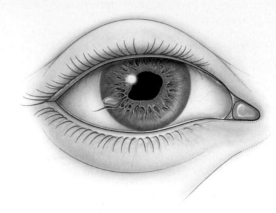

Figure 231 Penetrating injury. A corneal laceration is seen, with the iris plugging the wound causing an irregular pupil.

- sympathetic ophthalmia
- astigmatism.

Sympathetic ophthalmia is a very rare granulomatous inflammation that affects both eyes after a penetrating injury to one eye. The injured (exciting) eye sets up this response in itself as well as in the other (sympathising) eye. This usually occurs within 3 months of the injury. Removal of the injured eye before the sympathetic response starts prevents the onset of the condition; however, once established, removal of the exciting eye does not help. The response to steroids and immunosuppressants is usually favourable. Removal of an injured eye should, therefore, not be considered purely on the grounds of the risk of sympathetic ophthalmia but be based on the visual potential of the eye.

17.27 Chemical burns

Burns caused by acids or alkalis are a medical emergency. Alkalis denature proteins and their burns tend to be more extensive and penetrating than acid burns.

Clinical features

Patients with chemical burns to the eye are in severe pain. There may be lid swelling, oedema of the conjunctiva, corneal and conjunctival epithelial loss, uveitis, raised intraocular pressure, corneal melting, cataract and peripheral retinal damage.

Management

Any patient with a history of a chemical being splashed into the eyes must be treated with immediate copious irrigation (at least 1 l) of the affected eyes with water or normal saline. Any particulate material (e.g. lime) should be looked for and removed from the fornices or subtarsal areas urgently. There should be no delay in obtaining a careful history or in examining the eyes.

Once thorough irrigation has been completed (20–30 min), the extent of damage may be evaluated. pH paper can be applied to the tear film to assess if all of the acid or alkali has been removed. If the pH is not around neutral, irrigation should be recommended until all of the chemical has been washed away.

Corneal and conjunctival epithelium may be totally lost. In addition, the blood vessels may be destroyed, leading to areas of scleral ischaemia, and the cornea may be rendered opaque.

Complications

Complications are more commonly seen in alkali injuries:

- severe corneal and conjunctival scarring
- raised intraocular pressure
- cataract
- necrosis of sclera
- ultimate perforation of the eye with loss of useful vision.

Acids may cause corneal and conjunctival injury but without the other complications listed above.

Neuro-ophthalmology

17.28 Prechiasmal pathway

Learning objectives

You should:
- know the anatomy of the visual pathway
- be able to examine the pupils
- be able to examine a patient's visual fields to confrontation
- recognise features of pre- and postchiasmal lesions.

Optic nerve

The optic nerve is part of the central nervous system and, as such, can be involved in neurological diseases as well as diseases of the eye (e.g. glaucoma). In this section, the following conditions of the optic nerve will be considered:

- optic neuritis
- anterior ischaemic optic neuropathy
- papilloedema
- optic atrophy.

Optic neuritis

This is inflammation of the optic nerve, which usually occurs in adults aged from 15 to 50 as a result of demyelination or viral infections. Many cases are idiopathic.

When the optic nerve head is involved it is termed papillitis and when the nerve behind the globe is affected it is called retrobulbar neuritis. These conditions have the same aetiology, management and implications; they simply involve slightly different areas of the optic nerve.

Clinical features

The main clinical features are:

- usually one eye affected
- reduction in vision over a few days with loss of colour vision (may be mild or severe, but the patient finds that bright red appears as a desaturated red or pink)
- pain when moving the eye, especially upwards
- gradual recovery of visual function begins 1–4 weeks after the onset
- further blurring of vision with exertion or heat exposure (Uhthoff's phenomenon).

The only sign of optic neuritis may be an afferent pupillary defect (see below) in association with poor visual acuity. Patients with papillitis also have swelling of the optic nerve head. Field of vision testing demonstrates a central scotoma in the affected eye. The visual evoked response demonstrates increased latency.

Management

Management is simply observation while awaiting the spontaneous recovery of vision.

Complications

In a small proportion of patients, vision does not recover; in particular, the colour perception remains abnormal.

Anterior ischaemic optic neuropathy

Anterior ischaemic optic neuropathy (AION) represents an infarction of the optic nerve head, usually affecting patients over the age of 60. It is caused by vascular disease. Two types of AION are recognised:

- arteritic (most commonly due to giant cell arteritis)
- atherosclerotic.

Clinical features

The clinical features of each type of AION are similar:

- rapid, painless loss of vision in the affected eye but may affect the upper or lower field only (altitudinal field defect; Figure 232)
- vision usually significantly impaired (counting fingers or less)
- disc swelling, with haemorrhages around the posterior pole
- no visual recovery.

It is important to differentiate between arteritic and atherosclerotic causes, as this has important implications regarding management.

Arteritic Diagnosis of the arteritic variety is made on the basis of the patient suffering from a systemic disorder consisting of general malaise, headaches, muscle

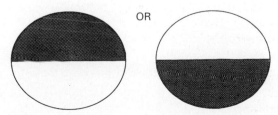

Figure 232 Altitudinal field defect; loss of upper or lower field.

tenderness and jaw claudication in the presence of an elevated erythrocyte sedimentation rate (usually >100) or elevated plasma viscosity. A temporal artery biopsy is indicated to establish the diagnosis unequivocally.

Atherosclerotic Those with the atherosclerotic type may have symptoms of generalised arteriopathic disease, such as angina or intermittent claudication.

Management

Arteritic Systemic steroids are used in those with giant cell arteritis. High doses of systemic steroids for those with features of giant cell arteritis must be commenced immediately to preserve the vision in the other eye, which is also at risk of developing visual loss. Steroid treatment may be required for many years. There is a 65% chance of the other eye being affected within 10 days.

Atherosclerotic No effective treatment is available for atherosclerotic cases. Associated risk factors such as hypertension, diabetes and hypercholesterolaemia should, however, be identified and treated.

Complications:

- the other eye becomes affected (almost invariably in those with temporal arteritis without treatment, and in approximately 30% of others)
- generalised complications of vascular disease.

Papilloedema

This term refers to swelling of the optic nerve head caused by increased intracranial pressure. Intracranial space-occupying lesions and idiopathic intracranial hypertension (pseudotumour cerebri) are the most common causes.

Clinical features

The main clinical features are:

- symptoms of raised intracranial pressure (headaches, nausea and vomiting)
- ophthalmoscopy reveals elevation of the optic disc, blurring of the disc margins, dilatation of the retinal veins and haemorrhages around the disc
- field of vision testing may show an enlarged blind spot
- visual acuity is usually unaffected.

Intracranial imaging with CT or MRI should reveal any intracranial mass. If this is negative, a lumbar puncture should be performed to measure the intracranial pressure.

Management

Management involves treating the cause of the raised intracranial pressure.

Optic atrophy

This is not a diagnosis but a clinical sign that may result from a number of different disease processes that affect the optic nerve:

- optic neuritis
- ischaemic optic neuropathy

- chronic papilloedema
- optic nerve tumours
- optic nerve trauma
- ocular disease (e.g. glaucoma, retinal artery occlusion).

Clinical features

Reduction in visual acuity or field of vision is a usual clinical finding. The presenting complaint usually depends on the underlying cause.

Management

Management involves treating the underlying cause.

Optic chiasm

The optic chiasm is the area of the visual pathway where the optic nerves partially cross. The chiasm is situated just above the pituitary gland and enlarging adenomas of the pituitary are a common cause of compression of the chiasm.

With respect to age, the common causes of chiasmal compression include:

- <40 years of age: craniopharyngioma
- 40–60 years of age: pituitary tumour
- >60 years of age: meningioma.

Clinical features

Patients with pituitary adenomas classically present with:

- headache
- hormonal disturbance
- bitemporal hemianopia (Figure 233).

CT scan of the chiasmal region will usually reveal the underlying pathology.

Management

Neurosurgical decompression is required.

17.29 Postchiasmal pathway

The retrochiasmal pathway includes the optic tract, lateral geniculate body, optic radiation and the occipital cortex. These postchiasmal optic pathways may be involved in:

- cerebrovascular accidents
- tumours
- infections (meningitis, cerebral abscesses).

These lesions cause defects in the visual field of both eyes and may also be responsible for other neurological deficits. The field defects depend on the area of the pathway that is affected, but postchiasmal lesions are always homonymous (i.e. affect the same side of the visual field in each eye) (Figure 233).

Clinical features

The presentation may be part of a more generalised neurological disorder, e.g. a cerebrovascular accident or raised intracranial pressure. Visual fields should be tested to identify the site of the lesion (Figure 233; see Box 4). Intracranial imaging using MRI identifies the site and nature of the lesion.

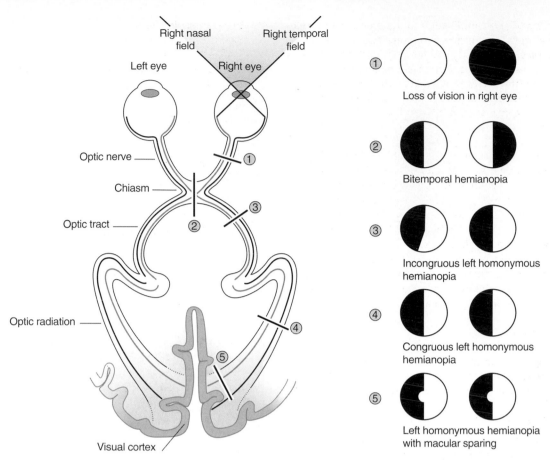

Figure 233 Field of vision defects in relation to the anatomical pathway.

Box 4: Examination of visual fields

When assessing a patient's field of vision, the examiner should compare their own field of vision with that of the patients, i.e. 'to confrontation'

- Observe the patient for clues regarding any field defect, e.g. hemiparesis, head turn
- Initially present your hands either side of the midline and ask the patient how many hands they can see (see Figure 234). This will detect any gross hemianopia
- Ask the patient to cover their right eye and you cover your left eye
- Imagine the visual field split into four quadrants with the centre on the patient's pupil
- Present one or two fingers in the centre of each quadrant and ask the patient how many fingers they can see
- Repeat for the other eye

NB This form of examination is useful for identifying gross neurological visual field defects such as hemi- and quadrantanopias. It is less appropriate for assessing subtle prechiasmal visual field defects such as in glaucoma, for which more sophisticated field analysis is usually employed.

Management

Visual field anomalies are usually irreversible although, if caused by pressure, they may improve after neurosurgical intervention.

17.30 The pupils

Abnormalities of the pupils may reflect neurological disease. The afferent limb of the pupillary light reflex is via the retina, optic nerve, chiasm and optic tract. This passes to the third nerve nucleus and synapses there to form the efferent part of the reflex that runs in the third nerve to constrict the pupil (Figure 235). Adie's pupil and third nerve palsies are defects of the efferent or outflow aspect of the pupil reflex.

The pupil is innervated by sympathetic (dilatation) and parasympathetic stimuli (constriction). Horner syndrome is an anomaly of the sympathetic innervation of the pupil (see Box 5).

Horner's syndrome

If the sympathetic nerve supply to the face is damaged, the patient develops Horner's syndrome (Figure 236). This can be caused by:

- neck trauma
- Pancoast's tumour (apical lung carcinoma)

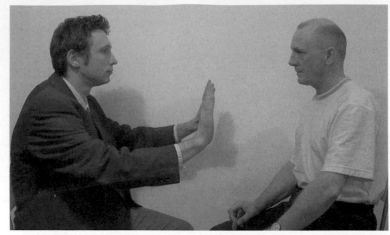

Figure 234 Assessing a patient's field of vision. Sit opposite the patient with your eyes at the same level. Present targets equidistant in the middle of a quadrant, avoiding the horizontal and vertical meridia.

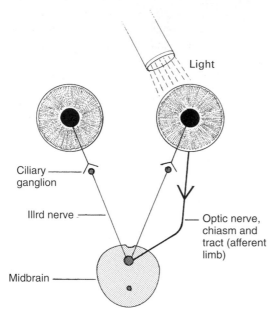

Figure 235 The pupillary light reflex.

> ### Box 5: Examination of the pupils
>
> - Observe pupil size and shape. Note any anisocoria (unequal pupil size), abnormality of lid position or ocular alignment
> - Instruct patient to fixate on a distant target (to prevent accommodative miosis).
> - Using a bright torch, examine the direct light response of one eye
> - Repeat the previous step, looking at the opposite eye to confirm the presence of the consensual response
> - Briskly move the torch from one eye to the other, resting on each eye for a second or two. This is the swinging flashlight test (see Figure 236)
> - To test pupil response to accommodation, ask the patient to look into the distance and then fix on an object that you are holding 30 cm away from their nose. Both pupils should constrict

- congenital anomalies
- idiopathic (probably vascular).

Clinical features

The characteristic features of Horner's syndrome are:

- small pupil (miosis)
- slight ptosis
- reduced sweating of the skin on the ipsilateral side of the face.

Management

No specific treatment is possible. Investigation for any underlying cause should be carried out.

Adie's pupil

In Adie's pupil, the affected pupil is dilated. It usually affects young women and a viral infection of the ciliary ganglion is the probable cause.

Clinical features

Characteristics of the affected pupil include:

- dilated
- absent response (either directly or consensually) to light
- slow response to accommodation and tends to remain miosed for a prolonged period after accommodating
- full eye movements.

Management

Reassurance is essential. Although the accommodative response is present, it is commonly reduced and the patient may require assistance, such as glasses for reading.

Third nerve palsy

The pupil is dilated and does not react to light or accommodation, either directly or consensually (see section 17.20 on Strabismus).

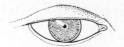

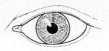

Figure 237 Right Horner's syndrome.

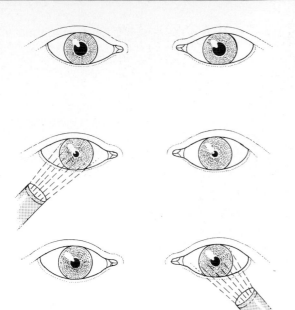

Figure 236 An afferent pupillary defect as demonstrated using the swinging flashlight test. The consensual response of the left pupil is stronger than the direct response. There is, therefore, paradoxical dilatation of the pupil whilst shining the light at the abnormal eye.

Afferent defect

If the consensual pupillary response is stronger than the direct response, this suggests an anomaly of the afferent pathway, i.e. retina or optic nerve (the afferent limb of the pupil response).

Clinical features

The vision is usually reduced in the affected eye. The direct pupillary response to light is diminished. This may be obvious but swinging the light stimulus briskly to and fro between each eye and watching for any change in the response can pick up more subtle defects. The affected pupil will appear to dilate when the light is shone directly into it as the consensual response is so much stronger (Figure 236).

Management

Management depends on the cause of the problem.

Seventeen

Self-assessment: questions

History and examination

Extended matching items questions (EMIs)

EMI 1

Theme: History

A. left-sided cerebrovascular accident of the postchiasmal visual pathway

B. left retinal detachment

C. acute closed-angle glaucoma affecting the right eye

D. dense cataract of the left eye

E. primary open-angle glaucoma of the left eye

F. right-sided cerebrovascular accident of the postchiasmal visual pathway

G. primary open-angle glaucoma of the right eye

H. giant cell arteritis causing a left anterior ischaemic optic neuropathy

I. space-occupying lesion of the right occipital lobe

J. chiasmal compression from a pituitary tumour

Choose the most likely diagnosis from above for each of the histories given below.

1. Painless sudden-onset flashing lights with a dark shadow in the peripheral visual field of the left eye in a 25-year-old short-sighted man.

2. Painless acute-onset right-sided visual field loss affecting both eyes in a 65-year-old man with a past medical history of hypertension and hypercholesterolaemia.

3. Acute-onset complete loss of vision in the left eye of a 82-year-old woman with associated temporal headache, shoulder pain and weight loss.

EMI 2

Theme: History

A. subconjunctival haemorrhage

B. bilateral anterior uveitis

C. acute closed-angle glaucoma of the right eye

D. anterior uveitis of the right eye

E. acute closed-angle glaucoma of the left eye

F. rubeotic glaucoma of the right eye

G. primary open-angle glaucoma of the right eye

H. chemical conjunctivitis

I. bacterial conjunctivitis

J. allergic conjunctivitis

Choose the most likely diagnosis from above for each of the histories given below.

1. A 63-year-old woman with a painful, firm, red left eye and reduced visual acuity with cloudy cornea. The pupil is mid-dilated and unreactive. She is long-sighted with a history of similar episodes, which normally resolve spontaneously.

2. A 6-year-old boy with an 18-month history of intermittently bilateral itchy red eyes. The symptoms are worse in spring and summer. He has a past medical history of asthma and eczema.

3. A 27-year old man with a 1-week history of a photophobic, watering, red right eye. He has previously had similar episodes, which, after having seen an ophthalmologist, settled with topical steroids. He has a past medical history of ankylosing spondylitis.

The eyelids and lacrimal system

Extended matching items questions (EMIs)

EMI 1

A. entropion

B. ectropion

C. senile ptosis

D. Horner's syndrome

E. blepharitis

F. Sjogren syndrome

G. keratoconjunctivitis sicca

H. ptosis secondary to a third nerve palsy

I. ptosis secondary to myasthenia gravis

J. congenital ptosis

For each of the symptoms and signs listed below, select the most appropriate diagnosis from the list above:

1. An out-turning eyelid causing drying to the surface of the eye.

2. An in-turning eyelid causing abrasions to the corneal surface from abrading eyelashes.

3. A droopy upper lid, noted since birth.

EMI 2

A. malignant melanoma

B. hordeolum

C. basal cell carcinoma

D. chalazion

E. blepharitis

F. Sjogren syndrome

G. dacryocystitis

H. squamous cell carcinoma

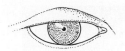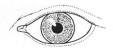

Figure 238

I. lacrimal gland swelling

J. Horner's syndrome

For each of the symptoms and signs listed below, select the most appropriate diagnosis from the list above.

1. Painless, pink, raised, pearly-edged telangiectatic lump on the medial aspect of the lower eyelid with a central ulcerated area.

2. A very tender, red, hot, raised lump on the skin just nasal to the medial canthus associated with a watering eye.

3. Red swollen lid margins with blocked meibomian orifices, associated with a poor tear film and acne rosacea.

Objective structured clinical examination questions (OSCEs)

OSCE 1

A 48-year-old woman visits her GP complaining that the appearance of her eyes has changed over the past month.

a. Look at Figure 238 and describe the appearance of her eyes.

b. List some causes of ptosis.

c. In your opinion, what is the most likely aetiology of this patient's ptosis.

The conjunctiva, cornea and sclera

Extended matching items questions (EMIs)

FMI 1

A. bacterial conjunctivitis

B. adenoviral conjunctivitis

C. scleritis

D. uveitis

E. neonatal conjunctivitis

F. herpes simplex keratitis

G. marginal keratitis

H. trachoma

I. allergic conjunctivitis

J. episcleritis

For each of the symptoms and signs listed below, select the most appropriate diagnosis from the list above.

1. Unilateral photophobic red eye with a watery discharge. Central corneal dendritic-shaped epithelial defect.

2. Bilateral, gritty, watering eyes with diffuse conjunctival injection and punctate corneal epithelial

erosions and associated preauricular and submandibular lymphadenopathy. The patient also has a sore throat and flu-like illness.

3. Chronic bilateral sticky red eyes with a mucopurulent discharge. In-turning eyelashes and corneal scarring. This is the second most common cause of preventable and treatable visual loss in the world.

Constructed response questions (CRQs)

CRQ 1

A young mother brings a 14-day-old girl to the clinic with a sticky red eye. The eyelids are swollen and closed.

a. What is the diagnosis?

b. What organisms may cause this infection?

c. How is the diagnosis confirmed?

d. How should the problem be managed?

CRQ 2

A 30-year-old management executive has had an acute red eye for 4 days. The patient normally wears soft contact lenses and thinks that he may have hurt the eye putting the lenses in. The lids are stuck together in the mornings because of a green discharge and, for the last 24 h, the pain has become severe and vision reduced. On examination, the eye is extremely red and there is a central corneal epithelial defect. There is a white opacity under the epithelial defect and a hypopyon.

a. What is the likely diagnosis?

b. What factors predispose to infection?

c. How should this patient be managed?

d. What complications may occur?

Objective structured clinical examination questions (OSCEs)

OSCE 1

A 21-year-old student returns from a holiday in Ibiza 2 weeks before important examinations. She complains of a photophobic red right eye for 1 week. The patient complains that her vision is very blurred in the right eye. This is the fourth similar episode in the past 3 years. A watery discharge is present. She has had a cold sore on her lip for the past 10 days. The visual acuity in the right eye is reduced to 6/60. Figure 239 shows the appearance of the right cornea.

a. What is the common stain used to highlight diseases of the surface of the cornea?

b. Describe the findings.

c. What is the likely diagnosis?

d. Describe the appropriate management for the problem.

e. What topical medication is contraindicated during an active infection?

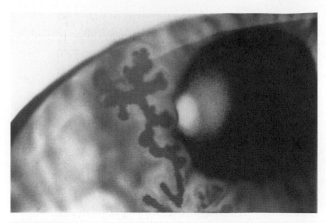

Figure 239

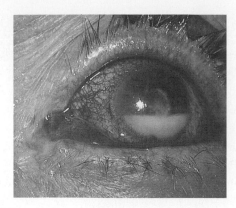

Figure 240

The optics of the eye

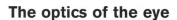

Constructed response questions (CRQs)

CRQ 1

A 67-year-old man is referred to the eye clinic because his optometrist has noted reduced visual acuities in both eyes of 6/12 uncorrected. The vision does not improve with a new prescription or a pin-hole.

a. What is the most likely diagnosis?

b. Discuss other possible diagnoses (information from other sections is required to answer this question).

c. What kind of symptoms is the patient likely to complain of?

After a full examination, a diagnosis of cataracts in both eyes is made.

d. Briefly describe the operation of phaco-emulsification cataract extraction and lens implantation.

The patient does not complain of any significant visual symptoms despite the reduced visual acuities.

e. Should this man proceed with cataract extraction?

CRQ 2

A 36-year-old woman complains of increasingly blurred vision when reading the newspaper. The television still appears clear and she has no problems reading street signs. Using a pin-hole she can read small print clearly. Her mother recently suffered an attack of closed-angle glaucoma.

a. What refractive problems might this patient be suffering from?

b. Is she likely to have relatively small or relatively large eyes?

c. What type of spectacle correction would improve her symptoms?

d. In 30 years' time, what further problems might she complain of?

Objective structured clinical examination questions (OSCEs)

OSCE 1

A 69-year-old woman presents to A&E complaining of a painful red right eye with profoundly reduced visual acuity. She had undergone uncomplicated cataract extraction in the symptomatic eye 5 days previously.

a. List some of the postoperative complications of cataract surgery.

Figure 240 shows the appearance of the eye on presentation.

b. Describe the main abnormality seen in the anterior chamber.

The red reflex is absent and the visual acuity is only perception of light.

c. In your opinion, what complication has this patient developed?

d. How should her management proceed?

The uveal tract

Constructed response questions (CRQs)

CRQ 1

A 35-year-old man presents with a red right eye. He complains of having had reduced vision with associated photophobia for the last 24 h. There is no history of trauma and no stickiness or discharge. He has a past medical history of ankylosing spondylitis. Examination reveals a red eye with ciliary injection. The pupil is miosed. There is no corneal staining with fluorescein.

a. What is the most likely diagnosis?

b. What is the treatment?

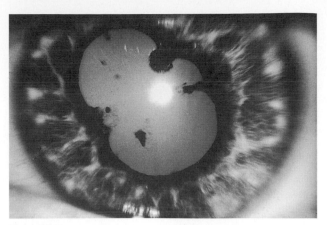

Figure 241

c. Discuss the differential diagnosis (information from other sections is required to answer this question).

Objective structured clinical examination questions (OSCEs)

OSCE 1

A 23-year-old man presents with a 2-day history of a red photophobic right eye. There is a watery discharge. His vision is 6/12. Figure 241 shows his symptomatic eye.

a. Describe the findings seen in the photograph.

b. What is the likely diagnosis?

c. What are the common systemic associations of this condition?

d. Describe the appropriate management of this condition.

The retina

Constructed response questions (CRQs)

CRQ 1

A 29-year-old insulin-dependent diabetic patient presents with sudden, painless complete loss of vision in her right eye. She has never been seen in the eye department before.

a. What are the possible causes of the visual loss?

b. What are the important clinical signs to look for on examination?

c. What treatment is she likely to need?

Objective structured clinical examination questions (OSCEs)

OSCE 1

A 42-year-old woman presents with sudden painless loss of vision in one eye.

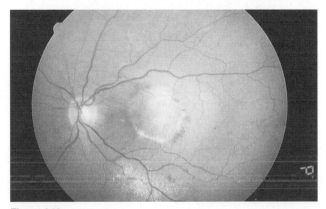

Figure 242

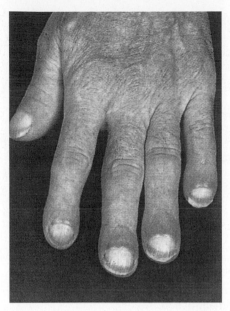

Figure 243

a. Describe the clinical findings in Figure 242.

b. What are the recognised systemic associations of this finding?

c. How might these systemic associations have led to her presentation?

d. Describe some investigations that would help in identifying an underlying cause.

OSCE 2

A 92-year-old man presents to his GP complaining of difficulty watching television and recognising faces in the street. His visual acuities measure 3/60 in both eyes corrected.

a. Describe the fundal appearances of the patient's left eye as seen in Figure 243.

b. What is the most likely diagnosis?

c. State the legal definition of 'blind' in the UK.

d. What can be done to help this patient?

Strabismus

Extended matching items questions (EMIs)

EMI 1

Theme: Strabismus

A. Weakness of down gaze in adduction of the right eye with a head tilt to the left. The patient complains of double vision with tilting of the images.

B. Intermittent double vision that is worse towards the end of the day, associated with variable bilateral ptosis.

C. Vertical double vision associated with a right ptosis and a 'down and out' eye position on the same side.

D. Weakness of all eye movements of the left eye except abduction and depression.

E. A manifest convergent squint with weakness of right abduction.

F. Weakness of all eye movements of the right eye except abduction and depression.

G. Constant double vision with marked restriction of up gaze. The eyes appear prominent. There is bilateral lower lid retraction.

H. Weakness of down gaze in adduction of the left eye with a head tilt to the right. The patient complains of double vision with tilting of the images.

I. Vertical double vision associated with a left ptosis and a 'down and out' eye position on the same side.

J. A manifest convergent squint with weakness of left abduction.

Match the diagnoses below with the most appropriate clinical descriptions from above.

1. Myasthenia gravis.
2. Right fourth cranial nerve palsy.
3. Right sixth nerve palsy.

Constructed response questions (CRQs)

CRQ 1

A 68-year-old woman presents to her GP complaining of horizontal double vision. The double vision is worse for distance and on looking to the left but does not bother her for near vision. She is otherwise asymptomatic. She has a past medical history of obesity and a family history of cerebrovascular accidents.

a. What cranial nerve palsy is most likely to be responsible for this patient's double vision?

b. What are the possible aetiologies of the cranial nerve palsy?

c. What investigations would it be appropriate to perform in the surgery?

The patient is referred to the eye department for further management.

d. What important signs must the ophthalmologist examine for to clinically exclude a space-occupying lesion?

e. What are the management options for improving the symptoms of double vision?

Objective structured clinical examination questions (OSCEs)

OSCE 1

A 54-year-old woman is referred to the eye clinic. She has a past medical history of hyperthyroidism and thyroid eye disease.

a. Describe the clinical signs seen in Figures 244 and 245.

Her eyes are currently comfortable with no redness or symptoms of grittiness and burning.

b. What problems may this patient complain of?

c. Outline the general management of thyroid eye disease.

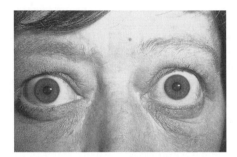

Figure 244

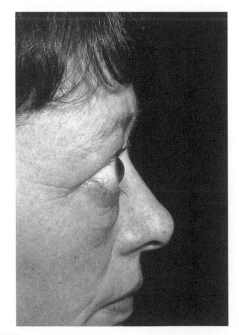

Figure 245

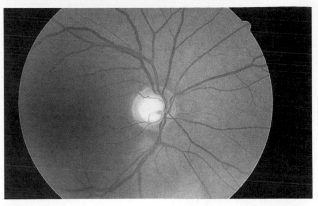

Figure 246

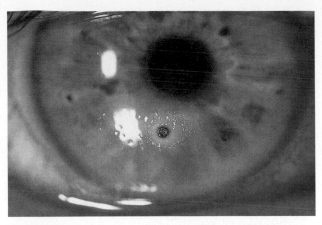

Figure 247

Glaucoma

Objective structured clinical examination questions (OSCEs)

OSCE 1

A 71-year-old man who suffers from asthma is referred to the eye clinic because at a recent routine optometry appointment an 'abnormal' optic disc was noticed in the right eye. The patient is asymptomatic.

a. Describe the abnormalities in the patient's right optic disc that can be seen in Figure 246.

b. What condition might the patient have?

c. What other tests might the optometrist perform to help make a diagnosis?

d. What field defect might the patient display?

e. What group of intraocular pressure-lowering drugs are contraindicated in this patient?

f. Name two other classes of topical intraocular pressure-lowering drugs that would be suitable alternatives.

Ocular injuries

Objective structured clinical examination questions (OSCEs)

OSCE 1

A 54-year-old builder presents to A&E complaining of a gritty, red, photophobic, watering right eye.

a. Describe the findings as shown in Figure 247.

b. What questions should the examining doctor ask regarding the mechanism of the injury?

c. What management is recommended?

d. What physical signs might suggest an intraocular foreign body injury?

e. What investigation in A&E would help confirm a metallic intraocular foreign body injury?

Multiple choice questions

1. In the management of alkali burns of the eye, which of the options below describes the best immediate management?

   a. neutralisation of the alkali with acid

   b. immediate irrigation with normal saline before an examination of the eye

   c. irrigation with saline following a complete history and examination of the eye

   d. treatment with chloramphenicol ointment and a pressure patch

   e. referral to an ophthalmology department for irrigation

Neuro-ophthalmology

Extended matching items questions (EMIs)

EMI 1

Theme: Neuro

A. chiasmal compression from a pituitary tumour

B. oculofacial sympathetic palsy on the right side

C. right anterior ischaemic optic neuropathy

D. parasympathetic palsy of the right eye

E. right occipital lobe stroke

F. right temporal lobe space-occupying lesion

G. recent-onset optic neuritis of the left eye

H. bilateral papilloedema

I. traumatic left optic neuropathy

J. right parietal lobe stroke

For each of the visual field defects described below, choose the pathology from above that would be the most likely cause.

1. Complete, irreversible loss of vision in the right eye.

2. A complete left homonymous hemianopia.

3. Bitemporal hemianopia.

EMI 2

Theme: Neuro pupils

A. chiasmal compression from a pituitary tumour
B. oculofacial sympathetic palsy on the right side
C. anterior ischaemic optic neuropathy of the right eye
D. parasympathetic palsy of the right eye
E. right occipital lobe stroke
F. left temporal lobe space-occupying lesion
G. recent-onset optic neuritis of the left eye
H. bilateral papilloedema, left eye worse than right
I. bilateral papilloedema, right eye worse than left
J. right parietal lobe stroke

Match the pathology above with the most appropriate clinical signs from below.

1. Reduced direct pupillary light response in the left eye.
2. Unequal-sized pupils with the right being larger than the left.
3. Reduced direct pupillary light response in the right eye.

Objective structured clinical examination questions (OSCEs)

OSCE 1

A 70-year-old man is referred to the eye clinic because at a recent routine optometry appointment an abnormal visual field was plotted.

a. Describe the visual field defect seen in Figure 248.
b. What pathology might explain this type of visual field loss?

His wife comments that over the past few years his facial appearance has slowly changed. Photographs from 5 years ago confirm that his jaw is more prominent and his features generally coarser.

c. What is the relevance of the change in his facial features?

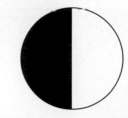
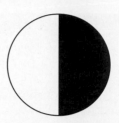

Figure 248

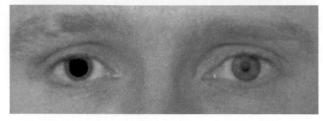

Figure 249

d. If the visual field loss crossed the vertical midline would this alter the differential diagnosis?
e. How should his management proceed?

OSCE 2

A 23-year-old woman presents complaining of recent-onset marked inequality of pupil size and slightly blurred vision of the right eye, especially for near vision.

a. Describe the findings seen in Figure 249.

On examination, the right pupil does not constrict to light whereas the left pupil reacts normally.

b. State a possible differential diagnosis for this appearance.
c. Describe the steps involved in examining the pupil responses.

The pupil constricts slowly to an accommodative target and remains miosed after the target has been taken away.

d. What is the diagnosis?
e. What advice should the patient be given?

Self-assessment: answers

History and examination

EMI answers

EMI 1

Theme: History

1. B   The symptoms described are characteristic of retinal detachment, with short-sightedness being a risk factor for the development of a spontaneous 'rhegmatogenous' detachment. Cataract and glaucoma tend to affect older patients, are of gradual onset and do not characteristically cause symptoms of flashing lights.

2. A   As both eyes are affected, the pathology is likely to be postchiasmal. The past medical history of hypertension and hypercholesterolaemia raises the possibility of a cerebrovascular accident, which, if affecting the visual pathway on the left side of the brain, would lead to the symptoms on the contralateral side.

3. H   Complete uniocular sudden-onset loss of vision suggests optic nerve pathology. In an elderly woman with an associated temporal headache, giant cell arteritis is a possible diagnosis and must be excluded.

EMI 2

Theme: History

1. E   The symptoms described are consistent with closed-angle glaucoma. The history of similar previous episodes which resolved suggests that she has a chronic intermittent form of the condition. Long-sightedness is a risk factor for the development of closed-angle glaucoma.

2. J   Recurrent red itchy eyes, particularly if seasonal and seen in an atopic individual, are highly suggestive of allergy.

3. D   The symptoms are consistent with anterior uveitis, which is often unilateral and idiopathic but may be associated with ankylosing spondylitis and inflammatory bowel disease. The condition is usually recurrent and should be managed by an ophthalmologist, only settling with topical steroids.

The eyelids and lacrimal system

EMI answers

EMI 1

1. B   An ectropion is where the lower eyelid turns out leading to corneal exposure and drying. The patient often complains of a gritty eye.

2. A   An entropion is where the lower eyelid turns in causing abrasions to the surface of the eye.

3. J   A ptosis is of the lower-positioned upper lid. If it is noted from birth it is, by definition, a congenital ptosis.

EMI 2

1. C   This is the classic appearance of a basal cell carcinoma, a common non-metastasising but locally invasive skin tumour.

2. G   If the nasolacrimal duct becomes blocked, stagnant fluid collects within the sac. During an episode of dacryocystitis, the stagnant fluid becomes infected. As the sac is found just nasal to the medial canthus, this area becomes red, swollen and tender. Because the nasolacrimal duct is blocked, the eye is always watery.

3. E   This is the classic appearance of blepharitis, a common condition of the lid margins.

OSCE answers

OSCE 1

a. Right ptosis and miosis.

b. Neurogenic: third cranial nerve palsy or Horner syndrome.

   Myogenic: congenital dystrophic levator muscle or age-related levator disinsertion.

   Neuromyogenic: myasthenia gravis.

   Mechanical: cysts or tumours of the upper lid.

c. The patient has sudden-onset mild ptosis with associated miosis. Clinically, this appears to be a right-sided oculofacial sympathetic palsy or Horner syndrome.

The conjunctiva, cornea and sclera

EMI answers

EMI 1

1. F   Herpes simplex virus characteristically causes a unilateral infection, unlike most other infective conjunctivitis conditions, which tend to be bilateral. Photophobia rather than itch is the predominant symptom and, therefore, infective keratitis is more likely than an allergic conjunctivitis. The characteristic corneal epithelial defect is dendritic shaped.

2. B   Adenoviral conjunctivitis and keratitis is characteristically bilateral. Local lymph nodes are often swollen and the patient may have a systemic illness with a sore throat and flu-like

illness. Most other infective causes of conjunctivitis do not cause a systemic illness.

3. H Trachoma is a bilateral condition seen in children and adults in developing countries in areas of poor sanitation. The infective organism is *Chlamydia trachomatis*. It characteristically causes a bilateral conjunctivitis, which, with time, becomes scarring causing the eyelids to turn inwards. The rubbing of the eyelashes on the cornea leads to abrasions, infection and scarring of the cornea with associated loss of vision. Trachoma is second only to cataract in the world's leading causes of visual loss.

CRQ answers

CRQ 1

a. The child is only 14 days old. Any conjunctivitis occurring within the first month of life is, by definition, a 'neonatal' conjunctivitis (ophthalmia neonatum).

b. It is usually caused by infective agents from either the mother's birth canal or the environment. These infective agents include *Chlamydia*, gonococci, herpes simplex and staphylococci.

c. Conjunctival swabs.

d. Appropriate topical antibiotics are prescribed based on the aetiology suggested by the history and clinical examination. Once the results of microbiology investigations are available, treatment can be altered and tailored to the sensitivities of the causative organism. If *Chlamydia* is confirmed, systemic treatment with erythromycin is required and the child should be seen by a paediatrician because of the risk of pneumonitis. If *Chlamydia* or any other sexually transmitted organism is identified, the mother must be referred to the genito-urinary clinic for investigation, treatment and contact tracing.

CRQ 2

a. The likely diagnosis is bacterial keratitis because there is a purulent discharge, an epithelial defect with associated opacified cornea and a hypopyon.

b. The major predisposing factor is soft contact lens wear, which may cause a corneal abrasion and introduce infection. Other potentially predisposing factors include: lid abnormalities (entropion, ectropion, lid retraction); dry eye; trauma (corneal abrasion); corneal paraesthesia; and immunocompromised host.

c. The patient should be admitted for intensive treatment with antibiotic drops. Conjunctival swabs and scrapings of the ulcer should be examined microscopically and cultured for organisms.

d. The complications that may occur include corneal scarring with loss of vision and corneal perforation with endophthalmitis and loss of the eye.

OSCE answers

OSCE 1

a. Fluorescein drops help to identify any epithelial defects.

b. Dendritic-shaped epithelial defect in the centre of the cornea.

c. Herpes simplex keratitis.

d. Topical aciclovir ointment to treat active herpes simplex infection.

e. Topical steroids are contraindicated during active herpes simplex infection as they prolong the course and have the potentially serious ocular side effects of increasing intraocular pressure and cataract development.

The optics of the eye

CRQ answers

CRQ 1

a. The most common cause of gradual deterioration of vision in this age group is cataract.

b. Other possible causes for these symptoms in a man of this age include age-related macular degeneration and primary open-angle glaucoma that has advanced to a late stage.

c. He may complain of difficulty reading the newspaper and price tags in shops, watching television, navigating in the home and outside and recognising faces, and of glare in bright lights.

d. The pupil is fully dilated. Local anaesthetic is infiltrated around the globe. A small incision is made close to the limbus of the eye and a round tear in the anterior capsule of the eye lens is made. The lens is fragmented and sucked out of the eye by a phaco-emulsification probe. A new lens is placed within the capsule bag upon the posterior capsule. The incision wound is normally self-sealing and does not require any sutures.

e. If the patient does not have any visually impairing symptoms then the cataract extraction is not necessary. The cataract itself will not harm the eye and does not need removal for its own sake with the associated risks of surgical intervention.

CRQ 2

a. Hypermetropia and early presbyopia. She is having difficulty seeing at short distance but can see clearly at long distance; she is therefore long-sighted (hypermetropic). She may have presented at this age because she is losing the ability to accommodate (presbyopia), which is 'unmasking' her hypermetropia. She also appears to have a family history of hypermetropia.

b. Hypermetropia is associated with relatively small eyes with anatomically crowded anterior segment structures.

c. Spectacles with convex (plus) lenses to converge the light to focus on the back of her eye.

d. Theoretically, she has an increased risk of developing acute closed-angle glaucoma as hypermetropia is a risk factor for this condition. She may also develop any of the other common visually impairing age-related eye conditions such as cataract or age-related macular degeneration.

OSCE answers

OSCE 1

a. Anterior uveitis, intraocular infection (endophthalmitis), cystoid macular oedema, opacification of the posterior capsule, retinal detachment and corneal decompensation.

b. A pale fluid level is seen in the anterior chamber. This represents a collection of inflammatory cells known as a hypopyon.

c. An intraocular infection known as endophthalmitis.

d. She should be referred to the ophthalmology team as an emergency.

The uveal tract

CRQ answers

CRQ 1

a. The symptoms of photophobia with reduced visual acuity, in the absence of itch or a discharge, are highly suggestive of an anterior uveitis (iritis). Identifying a well-recognised systemic association such as ankylosing spondylitis raises the suspicion of this being anterior uveitis.

b. Topical steroids, cycloplegics, analgesia and dark glasses

c. The differential diagnoses of a red eye are conjunctivitis (infective or allergic), corneal abrasion/foreign body injury, subconjunctival haemorrhage, episcleritis, scleritis, corneal ulceration (infective or inflammatory), uveitis and acute-angle

closure glaucoma. Table 23 lists the principal differences in these diagnoses.

OSCE answers

OSCE 1

a. This is a photograph of the anterior segment of an eye demonstrating an abnormality of the iris. Adhesions are seen between the iris and the lens. These are known as posterior synechiae. They are likely to be associated with inflammatory cells and flare in the anterior chamber.

b. Anterior uveitis.

c. Some of the common systemic associations of this condition are ankylosing spondylitis, inflammatory bowel disease (both Crohn's disease and ulcerative colitis), sarcoidosis, Reiter syndrome, Behçet syndrome, psoriatic arthropathy, juvenile idiopathic arthritis, tuberculosis and syphilis.

d. Topical steroids, dilating drops (cyclopentolate or atropine), analgesia and dark glasses.

The retina

CRQ answers

CRQ 1

a. Vitreous haemorrhage is the most likely cause of the visual loss, as it tends to be an acute loss with no pain. Maculopathy and tractional retinal detachment both tend to cause a more slowly progressive visual disturbance. Rubeotic glaucoma is characteristically painful.

b. Visual acuity reduction, abnormal pupil reflexes, corneal clarity, new vessel growth on the iris, intraocular pressure, the red reflex and fundoscopy. A vitreous haemorrhage will often result in very poor vision, such as hand movements, and an absent red reflex.

c. Vitrectomy and argon laser pan-retinal photocoagulation.

Table 23 Differential diagnoses of red eye

	Vision	Pain	Discharge	Area	Fluorescein staining	Pupil	Laterality
Conjunctivitis	Normal	Gritty	Sticky	Generalised	No	Normal	Both
Subconjunctival haemorrhage	Normal	No	No	Diffuse	No	Normal	One
Episcleritis	Normal	No	No	Interpalpebral	No	Normal	One
Corneal ulcer	Reduced	Yes	Yes/no	Limbal	Yes	Normal	One
Scleritis	Reduced	Yes	No	Variable	No	Normal	One/both
Uveitis	Reduced	Yes	No	Limbal	No	Small	One
Acute closed-angle glaucoma	Reduced	Yes	No	Diffuse	No	Mid-dilated	One (second eye at risk)

OSCE answers

OSCE 1

a. Finger clubbing.

b. Neoplasia, chronic obstructive airways disease, bronchiectasis, chronic hypoxia, endocarditis (among many).

c. Neoplasia: metastasis to the choroid.

 Endocarditis: retinal arteriole embolus from a heart-valve vegetation.

d. Full blood count, plasma viscosity/erythrocyte sedimentation rate/C-reactive protein, chest radiograph, carotid ultrasound scan, blood gases, blood culture, echocardiogram.

OSCE 2

a. The central part of the macula appears pale with well-demarcated but irregular borders. There is *no* associated haemorrhage or exudates.

b. The appearances are in keeping with age-related macular degeneration.

c. The patient should be added to the blind register if they are so blind that they are unable to do work for which vision is essential. In most circumstances, this equates to a visual acuity of lower than 3/60 corrected in the better eye, a visual field of less than 10° or a hemianopia. If a patient has a hemianopia it is at the discretion of the examining consultant ophthalmologist as to whether the patient should be added to the blind register; this is often based on the level of visual acuity.

d. Ensure that he is wearing his best spectacle correction. Issue low visual aids for near and distance vision. If he fulfils the criteria for registration, add to the blind register to allow access to social services and help from the local visual impairment society.

Strabismus

EMI answers

EMI 1

Theme: Strabismus

1. B The presentation of myasthenia gravis can be highly variable. The signs characteristically worsen towards the end of the day because of fatigue. Ptosis is a characteristic finding.

2. A The superior oblique muscle is supplied by the fourth cranial nerve. Weakness of this muscle causes torsional (tilting) double vision and a head tilt away from the side of the lesion.

3. E The lateral rectus muscle is supplied by the sixth cranial nerve. Weakness of this muscle may present as a convergent squint and weakness of abduction of the affected eye.

CRQ answers

CRQ 1

a. A left sixth nerve palsy with consequent abducting weakness of the left eye. This characteristically causes horizontal double vision, which worsens when the affected eye moves into the direction of action of the weakened muscle. The abducting weakness does not affect the patient when converging for near work.

b. In order of likelihood:

  • microvascular ischaemia of the nerve secondary to risk factors associated with cardiovascular morbidity

  • space-occupying lesion

  • raised intracranial pressure causing a 'false localising sign'

  • mid-brain stroke

  • demyelination

  • vasculitis.

c. Investigations aimed at identifying cardiovascular disease risk factors, including:

  • blood pressure level

  • urinalysis to exclude glycosuria and haematuria

  • cholesterol level

  • fasting blood glucose level

  • plasma viscosity to exclude a vasculitis such as giant cell arteritis.

d. Associated cranial nerve palsies and swollen optic discs, suggesting a space-occupying lesion and raised intracranial pressure.

e. Occluding the vision from one eye either by patching or fogging a lens in the patient's spectacles. Alternatively, if the angle of squint is not too large, a prism may be applied to a spectacle lens, which will maintain binocularity.

OSCE answers

OSCE 1

a. Bilateral proptosis and lid retraction with the right eye appearing worse than the left.

b. Problems may include corneal exposure leading to gritty uncomfortable eyes with mild blurring of vision, restrictive myopathy leading to double vision and tender eye movements and proptosis and 'puffy' periorbital tissues leading to concerns regarding cosmesis.

c. If an underlying thyroid gland dysfunction is present then this should be treated. Most patients can be managed conservatively with symptomatic treatment. Sometimes, if double vision occurs, prisms or extraocular surgery are required.

Glaucoma

OSCE answers

OSCE 1

a. Optic disc cupping with an uneven neuroretinal rim.

b. These signs are characteristic of glaucomatous optic nerve neuropathy. The patient may have primary open-angle glaucoma. An open-angle form is most likely as the patient is asymptomatic with no pain or redness.

c. Visual field examination using automated perimetry: if visual field loss consistent with the optic disc appearance is confirmed, the presence of glaucoma is more likely.

   Intraocular pressure check: if the intraocular pressure is raised (>21 mmHg), glaucoma is more likely. Even if the pressure is within the normal range, low-tension glaucoma may still be present.

d. Arcuate visual field defects.

e. Beta blockers.

f. Suitable second-line agents include:
   - carbonic anhydrase inhibitors (dorzolamide)
   - parasympathomimetics (pilocarpine)
   - sympathomimetics (brimonidine)
   - prostaglandin analogues (latanoprost).

Ocular injuries

OSCE answers

OSCE 1

a. A central dark corneal opacity is seen. The conjunctiva is only mildly injected. The pupil is round and the pupil space appears dark with no evidence of lens opacity. There is no evidence of hyphaema in the anterior chamber. The appearances are suggestive of a metallic corneal foreign body that has rusted. There is no evidence of a penetrating injury.

b. It is important to exclude a 'hammer and chisel' type injury in which a small high-velocity foreign body may have penetrated the eye. A penetrating injury is more likely if the patient was not wearing eye protection, which must also be enquired about in the history.

c. Remove the foreign body and rust and prescribe chloramphenicol ointment. If the patient is photophobic, topical cyclopentolate and analgesia may help. A dilated examination is important to exclude an intraocular foreign body.

d. Reduced or normal visual acuity, corneal laceration, flat anterior chamber, irregular-shaped pupil, lens opacity, vitreous haemorrhage and a retinal tear or detachment.

e. An orbital radiograph.

Multiple choice answers

1. b. Prompt action is essential to minimise damage. At least 1 l of natural saline should be administered immediately. This is easier if given through an i.v. giving set. The pH of the tear film should be checked afterwards to ensure that it has returned to 7. Remember, when treating chemical injuries, shoot first, ask questions later.

Neuro-ophthalmology

EMI answers

EMI 1

Theme: Neuro

1. C Anterior ischaemic optic neuropathies tend to cause profound irreversible loss of vision. An episode of optic neuritis may also lead to significant reduction in visual acuity but is usually less marked and improves after 2–3 months.

2. E A left-sided field defect that obeys the vertical meridian must be postchiasmal and on the right side of the visual pathway. Complete hemianopias are usually secondary to pathology of the occipital lobe. Parietal lobe lesions cause inferior quadrantanopias and temporal lobe lesions cause superior quadrantanopias.

3. A Bitemporal hemianopias are characteristically caused by chiasmal lesions, most commonly a result of compression from an expanding pituitary gland mass.

EMI 2

Theme: Neuro pupils

1. G Optic neuritis presents with reduced visual acuity, impaired colour vision (particularly to red) and tender eye movements. Optic nerve function is impaired by the episode of demyelination and, therefore, the direct pupillary light response is reduced.

2. D Inequality in the size of pupils (unless physiological) is caused by an imbalance between the parasympathetic and sympathetic motor nerve supply to the iris muscles and not by optic nerve damage (sensory loss). Loss of the parasympathetic supply to the sphincter muscles leads to dilated pupil because of the unopposed action of the sympathetic-driven dilator muscle. This is seen in Adie's pupil or third nerve palsy.

3. C Loss of the blood supply to the optic nerve, as occurs in anterior ischaemic optic neuropathy, causes irreversible loss of function with an associated reduced direct pupillary light response.

OSCE answers

OSCE 1

a. Bitemporal hemianopia.

b. Chiasmal compression.

c. The patient may have a growth hormone-secreting pituitary adenoma.

d. Chiasmal and postchiasmal visual pathway lesions cause visual field defects that 'obey' the vertical meridian. If a field defect crosses the vertical meridian then it is more likely to be due to a lesion anterior to the chiasm, such as optic nerve or retinal disease.

e. To confirm chiasmal compression, an MRI scan of the suprasellar region should be requested. Opinion should be sought from an endocrinologist regarding the clinical impression of acromegaly.

OSCE 2

a. The patient demonstrates anisocoria: the right pupil is larger than the left. The right pupil measures approximately 8 mm in diameter whereas the left only measures 5 mm. There is no associated ptosis or squint.

b. Adie's pupil: this is the most likely diagnosis as the patient describes a recent change and is symptomatic with blurred near vision. This condition is more common in women in the third and fourth decades of life.

Third nerve palsy.

Physiological anisocoria.

Left sympathetic palsy.

Instillation of a dilating drop such as tropicamide to the right eye.

c. Observation, direct light response, consensual light response, relative afferent defect (swinging light test) and the response to a near accommodative target.

d. Adie's pupil.

e. The patient should be reassured. The palsy is most commonly idiopathic or postviral and does not represent serious disease. The condition may develop in the other eye. Accommodation can be reduced for a period of time and, consequently, near vision may feel blurred.

Ear, nose and throat

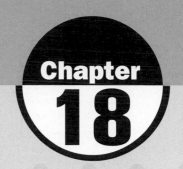

Ear

Chapter part overview

The ear is divided into three parts – the external, middle and inner ear. The external and middle ears function to channel and amplify sound waves into the cochlea of the inner ear, where they are converted into electrical impulses that travel along the cochlear part of the vestibulo-cochlear (eighth) nerve.

Any dysfunction of the external or middle ears causes a conductive loss. Dysfunction of the inner ear causes a sensory loss, whereas dysfunction of the eighth nerve causes a neural loss.

Examination of the tympanic membrane is performed with an otoscope, hearing is tested with a pure tone audiogram and balance function is tested with a caloric test (among others).

Hearing loss may be treated surgically, with a hearing aid if conductive, or by a variety of electronic aids if sensorineural.

Each part of the ear and surrounding structures has disease processes that are particular to it.

18.1 Anatomy and physiology

Learning objectives

You should:
* understand the basic anatomy of the ear – external, middle and inner
* know the two functions of the ear – *hearing* and *balance*
* know the five presenting complaints of ear disease.

The ear is subdivided into three parts (Figure 250):

* external
* middle
* inner.

External ear

The external ear is composed of the auricle and the external auditory canal, and extends to the tympanic membrane. The ear canal skin covers bone medially and cartilage laterally. Epithelial migration of the skin of the ear canal is from medial to lateral. Laterally, the skin contains hair follicles and ceruminous glands. The tympanic membrane has an upper thin part, the pars flaccida, and a lower thicker part, the pars tensa (Figure 251). The malleus handle is embedded in the substance of the tympanic membrane and the long process of the incus may be seen deep to the tympanic membrane postero-superiorly.

Middle ear

The middle ear is connected to the nasopharynx via the eustachian tube and also posteriorly to the mastoid air cells. The ossicular chain comprises three ossicles, the malleus, incus and stapes. They transmit vibration from the tympanic membrane to the inner ear. The stapedius and tensor tympani muscles are attached to the stapes and

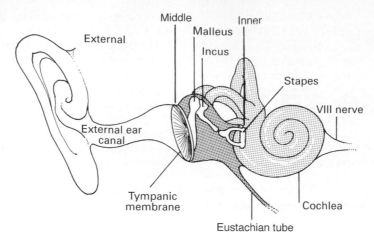

Figure 250 Anatomy of the ear.

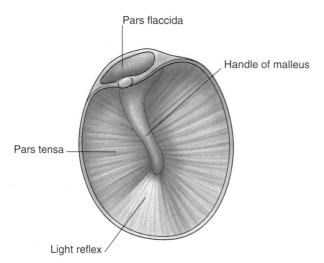

Figure 251 The left tympanic membrane.

malleus respectively. The facial nerve lies in a narrow bony tunnel (fallopian canal) in the temporal bone and may be damaged by disease of the surrounding bone.

Inner ear

The inner ear comprises the cochlea, concerned with hearing, and the semicircular canals, utricle and saccule, concerned with balance. These structures relay neural impulses to the central auditory and central vestibular systems respectively. The central vestibular system also receives and coordinates proprioceptive and visual information.

Common presenting complaints related to the inner ear are:

- hearing loss
- tinnitus
- vertigo
- aural discharge
- otalgia.

18.2 Clinical examination

Learning objectives

You should:
- know how to use an otoscope to examine the tympanic membrane
- know the difference between conductive and sensorineural hearing loss
- understand how tuning fork tests can tell us which type of hearing loss a patient has
- be aware of the basic tests of hearing and balance – *audiometry* and *caloric tests*
- understand the basic functioning of a hearing aid.

Ear examination involves inspection of the surrounding skin as well as inspection of the ear canal and tympanic membrane with a battery-powered otoscope.

Initially the ear is inspected for surgical scars, both postaural and endaural. To straighten the ear canal for otoscopic examination in adults, gently pull the auricle up and back. In children, gently pull the auricle straight back and, if necessary, slightly downwards. The otoscope should be held like a pen. This initially feels awkward but allows easier, more gentle inspection. Remember that in some patients, not all of the tympanic membrane can be seen. In particular, the antero-inferior part of the tympanic membrane may be obscured by a prominent anterior canal wall. The pneumatic attachment to the otoscope can be used to assess the mobility of the tympanic membrane (Seigeloscopy).

A 512-Hz tuning fork is used for the Rinne and Weber hearing tests.

Investigations

Tests of hearing

Assessment of hearing is made initially by noting the patient's response to a normal conversational voice. Hearing loss caused by disease of the external or middle ear is termed conductive hearing loss, that caused by disease of the inner ear is termed sensory hearing loss and that caused by disease of the auditory nerve is termed neural hearing loss. In practice, it is often difficult to distinguish between the last two types of hearing loss and they are commonly referred to as sensorineural or perceptive hearing loss.

Tuning fork tests

The 512-Hz tuning fork is struck on the tester's knee or elbow, and air and bone conduction hearing is tested.

The Rinne test compares air conduction with bone conduction in the test ear. The tuning fork is placed lateral to the ear to test air conduction and on the mastoid process to test bone conduction. In the normal ear, air conduction should be greater than bone conduction. This is called a positive Rinne test. It may also indicate sensorineural hearing loss. If bone conduction is greater than air conduction, a negative Rinne test, conductive hearing loss is present in the test ear.

A false-negative Rinne test occurs in the test ear when this ear has a severe sensorineural hearing loss. This is because bone conduction is heard in the opposite ear when the tuning fork is applied to the mastoid of the ear with the sensorineural loss. The introduction of a blocking sound to the non-test ear (masking) is required.

The Weber test compares bone conduction in both ears. The tuning fork is placed in the midline of the skull. If the sound is heard in midline the test is normal. In an abnormal test, the sound lateralises to the side of conductive hearing loss and away from the side of sensorineural loss.

Audiometric tests

These may be subjective or objective.

Subjective Pure-tone audiometry measures hearing over a range of frequencies in each ear by air and bone conduction. Speech audiometry tests speech reception thresholds and speech discrimination.

Objective Impedance audiometry detects middle ear disease such as otitis media with effusion and can also assess the condition of the ossicular chain. Evoked-response audiometry measures evoked potentials from the brainstem, mid-brain and auditory cortex. These may be used to determine auditory thresholds, and brainstem audiometry is a useful screening test for retrocochlear disease such as acoustic neuroma.

Tests of balance

Maintenance of balance involves integration of information provided by the inner ears, the eyes and the proprioceptive organs. This integration occurs in the central vestibular system. Disruption of the integrity of the vestibular system results in vertigo, which is a hallucination of movement of self or surroundings.

The labyrinths send nerve impulses to the brainstem and their function is analogous to that of a twin-engined aeroplane. Loss of function of one end organ can be compensated for by central mechanisms, but acute loss is characterised by vertigo and nystagmus. Compensation occurs rapidly in the young but, in the elderly, complete compensation may not be achieved.

The integrity of the vestibular apparatus may be tested in various ways. In the Hallpike test, the patient sits on an examination couch in the erect position. The patient's head is then brought briskly to hang over the end of the couch and the eyes are examined for nystagmus. The patient returns to the original position and the test is repeated with the head rotated to the left and again with the head rotated to the right. The fistula test is performed by applying positive pressure to the column of air in the ear canal, either by digital pressure on the tragus or by using a pneumatic otoscope. If a fistula to the inner ear is present, the patient will complain of imbalance or vertigo and nystagmus may be observed.

Caloric stimulation of the inner ear by irrigation of the ear canal with warm (44°C) or cold (30°C) air or water results in nystagmus, which may be measured to assess the integrity of the labyrinth being stimulated.

Imaging

The middle and inner ears, as well as the posterior cranial fossa, may be imaged by conventional computed tomography (CT) scanning and magnetic resonance imaging (MRI).

Aids to hearing

A hearing aid has three components: a microphone, an amplifier and an earphone. Sound is conducted to the ear via an ear mould or, very occasionally, through the skull via a bone vibrator. 'In-the-ear' aids and 'in-canal' aids are available commercially and in-the-ear aids are now being introduced in the UK through the NHS. Larger body-worn aids are sometimes helpful for those who have difficulty manipulating the small controls of conventional hearing aids. Analogue hearing aids have an O/T/M switch. O is for off, M is for microphone and T is for switching the microphone to the telecoil for use with an induction loop system. This allows the direct broadcast of signals to the hearing aid and eliminates background noise. This system is used in many public buildings such as cinemas, theatres and churches. Frequency adjustment may be made using the H (high) and L (low) tone screw. Most hearing aids issued now use a digital system that allows them to be programmed using the patient's audiogram as a guide and can give superior hearing for some users. Their functions are modified using a single small control button.

Even the most sophisticated hearing aid is essentially an amplifier. Patients with conductive hearing loss do well with properly adjusted hearing aids, but patients with poor speech discrimination tend to do less well. Patients fitted with hearing aids should be reviewed routinely to identify problems as they arise. Other devices such as telephone amplifiers, loud doorbells and flashing alarm lights can improve the quality of life of the hard of hearing. Cochlear implants are appropriate only for patients who are profoundly deaf in both ears. Cochlear implantation is now being undertaken in both adults and children.

18.3 Diuseases of the ear

Learning objectives

You should:

- be aware of the treatment of external otitis and foreign bodies in the external ear
- know the symptoms and treatment of acute otitis media and otitis media with effusion
- know that cholesteatoma is the presence of squamous epithelium in the middle ear; how it presents; the complications and the treatment
- know that presbycusis is the high-tone sensorineural hearing loss of old age and be aware of the other main causes of hearing loss
- understand the symptoms and treatment of Menière's disease.

The external ear

Infection

Infection of the external ear is also known as otitis externa, often called swimmer's ear, and is caused by opportunistic bacteria or fungi. This condition is treated by local debridement and ear drops, which usually contain a steroid in combination with an antibacterial or antifungal agent.

Obstruction

Osteomas (solitary benign bony tumours) and exostoses (diffuse, usually multiple, bony swellings) narrow the ear canal. They may not produce symptoms but, if they result in wax impaction and otitis externa, they need to be surgically removed.

Foreign bodies in the ear canal usually occur in toddlers. If not easily removed, referral to an otologist is required and, occasionally, general anaesthesia is needed. More damage may be done to the ear by unskilled attempts at removal than by the presence of the foreign body itself.

Wax impaction can obstruct the ear. The wax may be softened by use of bicarbonate, olive oil or almond oil ear drops. Once soft, wax may be removed by syringing but, if perforation of the tympanic membrane (current or healed) is suspected, a wax curette should be used. Occasionally, wax removal under magnification using the operating microscope is necessary.

The middle ear

Infection

Acute otitis media is most common in young children and is usually caused by *Haemophilus influenzae* infection. It presents with otalgia, hearing loss and, if the tympanic membrane ruptures, discharge. It is usually preceded by an upper respiratory tract infection and antibiotics are usually given. Tympanic membrane perforations follow-

ing this condition usually heal spontaneously. Should the perforation fail to heal spontaneously, surgical repair of the tympanic membrane (myringoplasty) may be undertaken. If the ossicular chain has been damaged, it may be repaired by ossiculoplasty. Myringoplasty has a very high success rate – usually over 90%. Temporalis fascia is the most commonly used graft material. Ossiculoplasty results are much less predictable as the grafts or prostheses used to reconstruct the ossicular chain are subject to infection, migration and extrusion.

Otitis media with effusion is common in children. It is associated with a conductive hearing loss and may present as slow speech development, poor performance at school and disruptive behaviour. Fluid accumulates in the middle ear space as a result of eustachian tube blockage. The fluid is usually sterile. The condition is usually self-limiting but, if persistent, may require myringotomy, possibly with the insertion of a grommet to maintain ventilation. Sometimes, adenoidectomy is also required. Depending on the design, grommets tend to extrude spontaneously after 6–12 months. Occasionally, grommets need to be removed surgically.

Chronic suppurative otitis media is associated with tympanic membrane perforation and aural discharge. There may be associated external otitis. Gram-negative organisms are usually involved. It may respond to medical therapy but, if cholesteatoma is present, surgery is usually required.

Cholesteatoma results from the presence of keratinising squamous epithelium in the middle ear. It presents as a chronic, smelly aural discharge. The epithelium invades the underlying bone and may result in complications such as intracranial infection, labyrinthitis and facial nerve paralysis. Mastoid surgery is required to remove the disease and prevent the development of complications. Such surgery may result in the creation of a mastoid cavity, which will require periodic debridement by the otologist throughout the patient's life. Nowadays, it is sometimes possible to remove cholesteatoma without the creation of a mastoid cavity (intact canal wall procedure).

Hereditary disease

Otosclerosis results in fixation of the stapes footplate with resultant conductive hearing loss. The inner ear is sometimes involved with associated sensory hearing loss. The condition is familial and is transmitted by autosomal dominant inheritance with incomplete penetrance. The incidence is likely to be similar in both sexes but, because of hormonal influences, it presents twice as commonly in females. Treatment is by hearing aid or operation (stapedotomy), which replaces the immobile stapes with a prosthesis. Stapedotomy is generally a very successful operation resulting in elimination of the conductive hearing loss (closure of the air–bone gap on the audiogram). Occasionally, damage to the inner ear occurs, resulting in sensorineural hearing loss, tinnitus and vertigo. These risks need to be explained to the patient. Because of the risks, stapedotomy is not undertaken in an only hearing ear.

Tumours

Tumours of the external, middle and inner ears are uncommon. Glomus tumours involving the middle ear or the base of the skull may present as unilateral pulsatile tinnitus. They are treated by surgery, sometimes preceded by embolisation.

Trauma

Minor trauma results from foreign bodies being inserted into the ear canal in an attempt to remove wax. This usually results in further wax impaction.

The inner ear

Hearing loss of old age

Presbycusis is the hearing loss of old age. Higher frequencies of hearing tend to be affected first and patients have difficulty hearing female voices in background noise. There is associated deterioration of the central auditory system. A hearing aid is usually helpful but requires quiet surroundings to function best.

Noise-induced hearing loss

Noise-induced hearing loss may result from industrial or recreational noise exposure. Initially, the hearing loss is often reversible but, with repeated exposure, permanent damage occurs. The loss is often greatest initially at 4 and 6 kHz. Avoidance of hazardous noise exposure is best but, if this is not possible, adequate hearing protection should be worn.

Trauma

Trauma to the temporal bone may result in conductive, sensory or mixed hearing loss with or without facial paralysis. The inner ear is well protected in the petrous temporal bone and fractures of this bone usually result from considerable force, often associated with loss of consciousness.

Drugs

Ototoxic drugs, e.g. aminoglycosides, may affect the auditory, vestibular or both parts of the inner ear. Most ototoxic drugs induce permanent changes in the inner ear, but a few drugs such as aspirin and quinine result in reversible damage.

Sudden hearing loss

Sudden sensorineural hearing loss results from viral or vascular damage to the inner ear. Hearing loss may be temporary, but in some patients it is permanent and profound.

Tumour

Acoustic neuroma, more properly termed vestibular schwannoma, commonly presents with unilateral tinnitus and hearing loss. Imbalance is common but true vertigo is unusual. Any unexplained, progressive unilateral or asymmetrical sensorineural hearing loss should be investigated for possible acoustic neuroma. An MRI scan of the posterior fossa and internal auditory meatus is the definitive investigation. Ideally, acoustic neuromas are detected when small and are treated surgically by removal with minimal morbidity. The approach to the tumour may be neurosurgical, otological or combined. In elderly unfit patients with minimal symptoms, slowly growing tumours may best be left untreated. Serial MRI scans allow tumour growth to be assessed over time.

Ménière's disease

Ménière's disease is characterised by fluctuating sensory hearing loss, tinnitus and vertigo. There is often an associated feeling of fullness in the affected ear. The aetiology is unknown. The disease is usually unilateral but, with time, the other ear may become affected. There is no clear evidence that the natural course of the condition is affected by medical therapy. Various operations are described for severe, intractable disease. Destructive operations, such as labyrinthectomy and division of the vestibular nerve, are effective in controlling symptoms. Labyrinthectomy, by definition, destroys the hearing function of the inner ear and is only undertaken when the affected ear has very poor hearing. Non-destructive procedures include decompression and shunting of the endolymphatic sac, but the efficacy of such procedures remains in doubt.

Vertigo

Vestibular neuronitis presents as acute vertigo with no associated hearing loss or tinnitus. It is self-limiting over a period of days or weeks.

Benign positional vertigo results from semicircular canal dysfunction and is characterised by episodic vertigo consequent upon adopting a given head position. It may occur after head injury and is usually self-limiting after some months.

18.4 Miscellaneous conditions

Learning objectives

You should:
- be aware of Bell's palsy and know that it is a diagnosis of exclusion
- be aware of Ramsay–Hunt syndrome and its clinical presentation
- know what tinnitus means and that unilateral tinnitus requires investigation
- understand that pain in the ear may be referred from elsewhere.

Diseases of the facial nerve

Bell's palsy is an isolated, idiopathic lower motor neuron paralysis of the facial nerve, which is suspected to be caused by herpes virus infection. The eye becomes vulnerable if it does not close completely and tear production may be diminished. The patient should be advised about the need for eye protection. In total, 90% of patients with an incomplete facial palsy will recover full function, but a complete palsy may not recover entirely. Treatment with oral steroids and aciclovir may be effective although the evidence base for this is currently lacking. Patients who have recurrent palsies and those who do not recover function should be investigated further, often requiring an MRI scan of the posterior cranial fossa. Other diseases that may result in lower motor neuron facial paralysis, such as cholesteatoma, acoustic neuroma and parotid malignancy, must be excluded.

Ramsay–Hunt syndrome results from herpes zoster involvement of the inner ear. It is characterised by hearing loss, vertigo and facial nerve palsy. Recovery of the facial nerve palsy may be incomplete. Systemic antiherpetic therapy may be helpful in relieving symptoms.

Trauma to the facial nerve may occur at any point along its course. A stab of the cheek may result in peripheral division of the nerve, whereas fractures of the temporal bone may damage it more proximally. Early surgical repair with grafting, if indicated, offers the best chance of recovery in a facial nerve that has been divided.

Tinnitus

Tinnitus, commonly described as buzzing or hissing noises in the ears or head, is common and usually associated with hearing loss. Resolution of the hearing loss may improve the tinnitus because of the masking effect of previously unheard sounds. Bilateral tinnitus is rarely of serious significance and patients should be reassured. Unilateral tinnitus requires further investigation. Background noise or a masker often helps to suppress the tinnitus. Anxiety and depression should be treated appropriately.

Referred otalgia

Pain felt in the ear in the absence of any ear disease is very common. Although the teeth and temporo-mandibular joints are common sources, disease of the tongue and throat must be excluded. Occasionally, pain is referred from the thyroid (de Quervain's thyroiditis) or trachea.

The nose and paranasal sinuses

Chapter part overview

The nose functions to allow the passage of air to the lungs and to the olfactory mucosa for smell. It warms, cleans and humidifies the air as it passes. The paired paranasal sinuses (frontal, maxillary, anterior and posterior ethmoid, and sphenoid) surround the nose, with all but the sphenoid and posterior ethmoid sinuses draining to the middle meatus, the key area in the treatment of sinus disease.

Nasal obstruction, discharge, sneezing, loss of sense of smell and facial pain are common symptoms of sinonasal disease. These problems are often associated with anatomical abnormalities, such as deviation of the nasal septum, or with mucosal inflammation, such as is found with allergic rhinitis.

Epistaxis (nose bleed) is usually trivial and easily controlled but can be life threatening, especially in older patients.

18.5 Anatomy and physiology

Learning objectives

You should:
- understand the basic anatomy and functions of the nose – *smell* and *breathing*
- know the names of the paranasal sinuses and where they drain.

The nose

The external nose (Figure 252)

The upper one-third of the external nose is bony and covered by mobile thin skin. The lower two-thirds is cartilaginous and covered by tightly adherent skin that contains multiple sebaceous glands.

The nasal cavities

These pass in an antero-posterior (not superior) direction in the skull for 6–7 cm in the adult. They are divided by a bony and cartilaginous nasal septum (Figure 253), which is rarely absolutely in the mid-line. The major features of the lateral nasal wall (Figure 254) are the superior, middle and inferior turbinates, which contain erectile tissue. The cavities are lined by respiratory epithelium, which is thick over the turbinates and thinner over the septum. The nose has a rich blood supply from both the external and internal carotid arterial systems. Some nasal venous drainage passes intracranially to the cavernous sinuses.

Function

Besides being the olfactory organ, the nose warms and humidifies the inspired air. Particulate matter is trapped anteriorly at the nasal vestibule by the nasal vibrissae. Smaller particles adhere to the mucus blanket that lines the nasal mucosa and are transported posteriorly by muco-

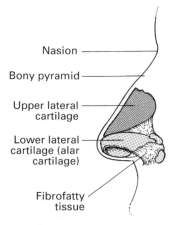

Nasion

Bony pyramid

Upper lateral cartilage

Lower lateral cartilage (alar cartilage)

Fibrofatty tissue

Figure 252 The external nose.

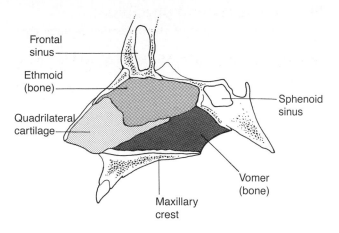

Figure 253 The nasal septum.

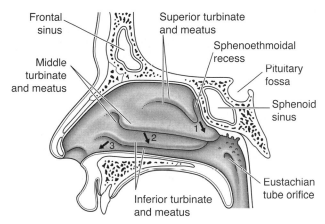

Figure 254 Structure of the lateral wall of the nasal cavity, showing the superior (1), middle (2), and inferior (3) meatuses.

ciliary activity and swallowed. The olfactory epithelium is located high in the nasal cavity below the cribriform plates. Nasal obstruction from any cause results in reduced air flow and reduced sense of smell. Nasal obstruction may also result in loss of vocal resonance. Excess nasal patency also alters voice quality.

Paranasal sinuses

These are paired structures (Figure 255) comprising:

- anterior group: frontal, maxillary and anterior ethmoid sinuses; these all drain to the middle meatus below the middle turbinate
- posterior group: posterior ethmoid and sphenoid sinuses; these drain to the sphenoethmoidal recess.

Not all paranasal sinuses are present at birth. They tend to enlarge rapidly in late childhood and at puberty as the facial bones grow anteriorly and inferiorly from the skull base. In humans, the paranasal sinuses have no known function.

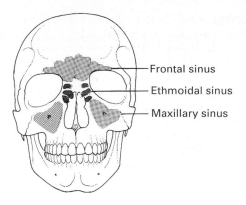

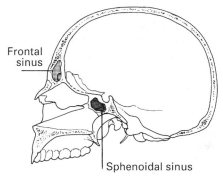

Figure 255 The paranasal sinuses.

18.6 Clinical examination

Learning objectives

You should:

- know the common presenting features of nasal disease
- be aware of the methods that are available to examine the nose
- know how to differentiate a polyp from a turbinate
- be aware of the two methods of testing for allergy – *skin prick testing* and *RAST*.

Clinical features

Obstruction

This is the most common problem and may be unilateral or bilateral. The cause may be structural or related to mucosal swelling. Common causes of nasal obstruction include deviation of the nasal septum, mucosal inflammation (rhinitis), nasal polyps and, more rarely, neoplasia.

Discharge

This may be clear or coloured, unilateral or bilateral, anterior or posterior (catarrh). Unilateral bloodstained nasal discharge suggests the presence of a foreign body in a toddler or a neoplasm in the elderly.

Sneezing

This results from nasal mucosal irritation and is a common feature of allergic rhinitis.

Pain

Facial discomfort and pain may be secondary to sinus obstruction and inflammation.

Anosmia

Anosmia (lack of sense of smell) is commonly secondary to nasal obstruction. In the absence of nasal obstruction, alteration of smell may result from disease in the anterior cranial fossa.

Cosmesis

Cosmetic nasal deformities are common and include humps, sagging of the nasal dorsum and deviation of the nose. Complaints about nasal size are also common. Nasal appearance is often racially determined and complaint thresholds vary from culture to culture. Some patients present with complaints about nasal function when their main concern is cosmetic.

Investigations

The exterior and interior of the nose must be carefully examined in all patients with nasal complaints. The external nose should be examined for deviation, scars and skin abnormalities. Standard anterior rhinoscopy using a nasal speculum allows a very limited assessment of the nasal cavities and this examination is best undertaken nowadays with a rigid or flexible endoscope, which allows an assessment of the nasopharynx.

In children, the internal nose can be inspected by tilting the nasal tip with the examiner's thumb: instruments tend to frighten children.

The anterior end of the inferior turbinate is often mistaken for a nasal polyp; gentle probing will elicit discomfort from a turbinate but not from a polyp.

Gentle stimulation of a locally anaesthetised nasal septal mucosa will often allow identification of a bleeding spot in Little's area.

Physical examination may be supplemented by imaging including CT and MRI scanning. Allergy testing by skin prick or RAST (radioallergosorbent test) is helpful in patients suspected of having allergic rhinitis. Mucociliary clearance testing and rhinomanometry are becoming more routinely used.

18.7 Infection and inflammation

> **Learning objectives**
>
> You should:
> - know the symptoms and signs of acute and chronic sinusitis and be aware of the appropriate treatment
> - be aware of the causes and presentation of atrophic rhinitis
> - know the causes and presentation of allergic rhinitis
> - be aware of the treatment of allergic and vasomotor rhinitis.

Rhinitis

The most frequent cause of rhinitis is the common cold resulting from viral infection. This condition is characterised by nasal obstruction, nasal discharge and sneezing. It is usually self-limiting within 4–5 days but may be complicated by secondary bacterial infection. It is most common in young children who have not yet developed immunity to the causative viral agents. Symptoms tend to be more severe and longer lasting in smokers, who have impaired mucociliary function.

Sinusitis

Acute sinusitis may be a complication of the common cold as ventilation of the paranasal sinuses may be impaired by swollen mucosa and thick secretions. Steam inhalations and local or systemic decongestants produce symptomatic relief. Secondary bacterial infection may be treated with broad-spectrum antibiotics. Occasionally, maxillary sinusitis is associated with infection of the apices of the premolar and molar teeth, which protrude into the sinus cavity. Such infections are commonly caused by anaerobic organisms. Typically, acute sinusitis of rhinogenic origin is associated with pain located over the affected sinus, nasal obstruction and sometimes purulent nasal discharge. Medical treatment is by decongestants, analgesics and antibiotics. Occasionally, surgical intervention is required to drain the maxillary or frontal sinuses if pain is severe or complications such as orbital cellulitis or intracranial spread of infection threaten.

If acute sinusitis does not resolve adequately, *chronic* sinusitis may develop with further damage to the mucosal lining of the involved sinuses. Medical treatment to improve sinus drainage and reduce infection may help, but surgical intervention is sometimes necessary. Nowadays this is commonly accomplished by functional endoscopic sinus surgery (FESS) rather than by older operations, which were designed to remove damaged mucosa and to provide large drainage channels from the sinuses to the nasal cavity.

Nasal vestibulitis

Inflammation of the nasal vestibules may be secondary to infected anterior nasal discharge or may result from infection of the hair follicles, usually by *Staphylococcus aureus*. In children, vestibulitis is sometimes associated with a foreign body or, more rarely, with unilateral choanal atresia. Careful examination of the nose is required. Pus should be sent for culture and sensitivity testing, followed by appropriate antibiotic treatment. Diabetic and immunosuppressed patients are more prone to recurrent infection of the hair follicles in the nasal vestibules (furunculosis).

Atrophic rhinitis

This rare condition appears to be associated with poor hygiene and malnutrition. It is characterised by nasal crusting and often by foetor (ozaena). Medical treatment involves removal of the crusts and application of nasal douches and drops. Surgical treatment to reduce the size of the nasal cavities is sometimes needed.

Allergic and non-specific (vasomotor) rhinitis

Allergic rhinitis may be either seasonal or perennial. In the UK, common seasonal allergens include tree and grass pollen in spring and summer respectively. Mould spores may cause allergies in the autumn. In the USA, ragweed pollen is a potent source of allergic symptoms in the late summer.

Perennial allergic rhinitis commonly results from exposure to animal dander, feathers and the house dust mite. Some patients develop nasal symptoms resulting from ingested allergens such as eggs, milk products and various nuts. Allergic rhinitis is common, affecting up to one in five of the population. It results from a type I hypersensitivity reaction in which an immunoglobulin (Ig)E and allergen complex binds to mast cells. These cells degranulate releasing inflammatory mediators including histamine.

The nasal mucosa may also react to non-specific stimuli, such as changes in temperature and humidity, and to stress and hormonal changes, such as those occurring at puberty and during pregnancy. This type of non-allergic rhinitis is known as *non-specific* or *vasomotor* rhinitis and is mediated by the autonomic innervation of the nasal mucosa.

In both allergic and non-specific rhinitis, nasal obstruction, clear nasal discharge and bouts of sneezing occur. The mainstay of treatment for allergic rhinitis is the regular use of a topical nasal steroid spray; for vasomotor rhinitis, an ipratropium spray is used. These may be used long term but, after symptom control is established, a minimum maintenance dose of the spray should be employed. In allergic rhinitis, topical and systemic antihistamine therapy may help, as may topical sodium cromoglycate. Surgery, in the form of turbinate reduction, may help nasal obstruction but does not benefit other manifestations of allergic and vasomotor rhinitis.

Prolonged use of topical nasal decongestants may itself result in nasal inflammation, producing a condition known as rhinitis medicamentosa. This is treated by stopping the use of the topical decongestant and substituting a steroid nasal spray. Compliance is better if one nostril is treated at a time. Systemic decongestants may also help.

18.8 Nasal septum

Learning objectives
You should:
- be aware of the management of septal haematoma and nasal fracture
- know the term for the procedure to straighten the nasal septum – *septoplasty*
- be aware of the symptoms and causes of septal perforation.

Trauma

Injuries to the nose may result in damage to nasal soft tissues, cartilage and bone. Patients presenting with nasal injuries should be assessed for associated damage to the head, neck and facial bones. If a nasal septal haematoma is present, it should be drained, the nose packed to prevent reaccumulation of blood and systemic antibiotics given. If the nasal bones are fractured the nose should be re-examined after a few days, when the bruising and swelling has settled, to assess any residual cosmetic deformity. This should be corrected by nasal manipulation within 10–14 days of the injury, otherwise the bones will heal and the deformity will require formal correction by rhinoplasty. Septal deviations resulting from injury may require surgical correction. Untreated, a septal haematoma may form an abscess with the risk of intracranial spread of infection. Later, resorption of the septal cartilage may cause a saddle nose deformity.

Deviation

This may result from differential nasal growth or from trauma. It may involve bone or cartilage of the septum or both. Cartilaginous septal deviations may result in deviation of the external nose. Asymptomatic septal deformities require no treatment but, if there is compromise of function or cosmesis, surgical correction by submucosal resection of the septum, septoplasty or septorhinoplasty is indicated.

Perforation

Perforations are commonly asymptomatic and are seen as an incidental finding. If symptomatic, they may produce bleeding, crusting and whistling. They usually result from trauma, often surgical, but may be caused by nose picking and cocaine abuse. Rare infections such as tuberculosis or syphilis may result in septal perforation.

If asymptomatic, perforations require no treatment. Small to medium-sized perforations can be closed surgically or, more simply, by the placement of a silastic obturator. Large septal perforations may not be amenable to any form of therapy.

18.9 Epistaxis

Learning objectives
You should:
- know the usual site of bleeding within the nose – *Little's area*
- understand the reasons why posterior epistaxis may result in life-threatening haemorrhage
- be aware of the various ways that epistaxis can be controlled
- be aware of the investigations and management that are appropriate for a patient with severe epistaxis.

Nose bleeds usually result from disruption of blood vessels in the anterior portion of the septum (Little's area). This area is the site of a rich vascular anastomosis and is relatively easily traumatised. Bleeding is readily controlled by sitting the patient up with the head slightly forward and pinching the tip of the nose. Blood loss from such bleeding is usually not severe. Cautery of the bleeding area can be carried out under local anaesthesia using silver nitrate sticks or electrocautery.

Potentially more serious nose bleeding results from rupture of larger unsupported posteriorly placed vessels. This type of nose bleed tends to occur in elderly patients who are hypertensive and have arterial disease. Blood loss may be extremely rapid and the patient must be assessed clinically for shock. Blood loss in this situation is often underestimated as the patient swallows a great deal of blood. Measurement of pulse and blood pressure is essential and intravenous infusion and blood transfusion are often necessary. The exact site of a posterior nose bleed is often difficult to determine even with adequate illumination and suction. If a bleeding point can be identified with a nasal endoscope, it may be cauterised under endoscopic control. Most such bleeding is controlled by anteriorly placed nasal packing but, occasionally, postnasal packing is required. The latter usually requires general anaesthesia. Compressive balloons are available to control bleeding and, in an emergency, a Foley catheter may be used as a posterior pack. If anterior packing is to be in place for more than 48 h, systemic antibiotics should be given. The presence of a posterior pack mandates the use of antibiotics.

Underlying causes of severe or continuous bleeding should be sought. Coagulation disorders and patients on anticoagulant therapy may present with severe nose bleeds. Associated conditions such as hypertension need to be controlled. If conservative measures do not control the bleeding, arterial ligation may be necessary. Vessels commonly ligated are the anterior ethmoid and maxillary arteries or, occasionally, the external carotid artery. The sphenopalatine artery may also be ligated endoscopically.

18.10 Nasal obstruction

Learning objectives

You should:
- understand the term choanal atresia and its management
- know what a polyp is and where it comes from
- understand why a unilateral polyp requires further investigation
- be aware of the significance of a unilateral nasal discharge in a child – *foreign body*
- know what a rhinolith is.

Choanal atresia

Choanal atresia results from failure of breakdown of the bucco-nasal membrane. If bilateral, it presents as an acute respiratory obstruction in the neonate, as neonates are obligate nasal breathers. Unilateral cases present later in infancy or childhood with unilateral purulent nasal discharge and obstruction.

Diagnosis

Diagnosis is confirmed by the failure to pass a soft catheter through the nostril. Atresia can be definitively imaged by CT scanning, which helps to differentiate bony from membranous atresia.

Management

Bilateral atresia in neonates requires establishment of an oral airway as an emergency followed by urgent surgical correction of the atresia. Surgery may be delayed in unilateral cases.

Polyps

Nasal polyps are made up of redundant oedematous mucosa and usually arise from the ethmoid sinuses. Most commonly they are bilateral and present in the middle meatus causing nasal obstruction. Occasionally, they arise from the maxillary sinus, in which case they pass posteriorly and are known as antrochoanal polyps. They are often associated with non-allergic asthma and aspirin intolerance but do not occur in children except in association with cystic fibrosis. Typically, polyps have the appearance of skinned green grapes and are insensitive to probing, unlike inferior turbinates for which they are often mistaken.

Unilateral nasal polyps should be regarded with suspicion. In infants, a polypoid nasal mass may be a congenital abnormality such as a meningoencephalocoele. In adults, unilateral polyps may result from neoplastic growth.

Large polyps require surgical removal, possibly with surgery to the associated sinus. Small polyps may be managed by the use of local steroid sprays.

Foreign bodies

These are usually seen in toddlers and occasionally in mentally disturbed patients. Inert foreign bodies such as small pebbles or metal ball bearings may produce few symptoms. Other materials such as foam, wool or vegetable matter result in a brisk inflammatory reaction, which produces a purulent, often blood stained, nasal discharge. This can result in vestibulitis of the ipsilateral nasal skin.

Unless the foreign body can be easily and safely removed, referral to a rhinologist is indicated. Inhalation of the foreign body during manipulation is a risk and, in young children, general anaesthesia is sometimes required.

Rhinoliths result from the accumulation of calcium and magnesium salts around a foreign body. They may reach a very large size and produce obstruction and discharge. General anaesthesia is often required for their removal.

The throat

Chapter part overview

The term 'throat' covers the oropharynx, hypopharynx and larynx and, therefore, the functions of swallowing, breathing and voice. Common symptoms in this area are pain in the throat, difficulty swallowing, changes in the voice and airway obstruction.

Pharyngitis and tonsillitis may be viral or bacterial and are usually treated supportively or, occasionally, with antibiotics. Painless difficulty in swallowing may suggest more serious disease. The cause of a change in voice may range from an entirely benign process such as laryngitis to malignant disease in the neck or chest. Hoarseness for more than 3 weeks should therefore be investigated.

Airway obstruction in children may be caused by infection, as in croup or supraglottitis, or result from a congenital disease such as laryngomalacia. In adults, malignancy must be considered.

18.11 Clinical examination

Learning objectives

You should:
- know how to examine the mouth and neck, and be aware of the techniques of examination of the larynx and pharynx
- be aware of the use of endoscopic equipment and MRI and CT scanning in the examination of the head and neck.

Common symptoms are:

- sore throat
- difficulty in swallowing
- changes in the voice
- airway obstruction.

With a good source of illumination, tongue depressors, gauze swabs (to gently draw the tongue forwards) and appropriate mirrors, the entire oral cavity, pharynx and larynx can be examined. Mucosal surfaces should be carefully inspected and, if necessary, palpated. Palpation is particularly important in assessing oral cavity lesions. Fibre-optic telescopes, both rigid and flexible, may be necessary to examine those patients in whom mirrors do not give an adequate view. Examination of the neck includes inspection and palpation in a systematic fashion. The entire neck should be exposed, which may necessitate the removal of high-necked shirts.

Imaging techniques, including plain and contrast radiology, and CT and MRI scanning, are useful adjuncts to physical examination.

18.12 Sore throats

Learning objectives

You should:
- be aware that most sore throats have a viral cause
- know the symptoms of bacterial tonsillitis
- know the indications for and complications of tonsillectomy.

Pharyngitis

Throat infections are usually caused by viruses and are associated with other upper respiratory tract symptoms. Bacterial infection, commonly streptococcal, may be primary or secondary. Infected sore throats should be treated with oral analgesics, plentiful oral fluids and, if severe, bed rest. Antibiotics are given only if bacterial infection is suspected. Other types of infection include *Candida* spp., which may occur in diabetic or immunocompromised patients and is sometimes seen in patients who use steroid inhalers for asthma. It presents as fluffy white patches on the fauces and responds to topical antifungal agents.

Tonsillitis

Bacterial tonsillitis is characterised by:

- sore throat lasting for a week
- dysphagia (difficulty swallowing)
- odynophagia (pain on swallowing)
- fever
- cervical lymphadenopathy
- malaise.

If recurrent attacks significantly interfere with school or work, tonsillectomy should be considered. Tonsillectomy is generally not indicated for less than three or four attacks of tonsillitis per year.

Occasionally a patient may present with a peritonsillar abscess (quinsy). This is usually unilateral and causes the tonsil to be pushed medially. The treatment is usually needle aspiration of the pus and antibiotic therapy although, if the quinsy recurs, tonsillectomy may be indicated.

Complications of tonsillectomy:
- reactionary haemorrhage, occurring in the first 24 h following tonsillectomy
- secondary haemorrhage, usually occurring a week or so after surgery and associated with separation of slough from the tonsillar bed.

18.13 Disorders of swallowing

Learning objectives

You should:
- know the definition of dysphagia (*difficulty in swallowing*) and odynophagia (*pain on swallowing*)
- be aware of the progression of the severity of dysphagia, which ranges from difficulty with solids to semi-solids to liquids
- know the term *globus* for a sensation of a lump in the throat without dysphagia
- be aware that dysphagia may be a presenting feature of carcinoma of the pharynx or oesophagus.

Clinical features

Organic dysphagia may arise acutely from foreign body impaction, but this history may be difficult to elicit from young children. More characteristically, dysphagia presents as a progression of severity, from difficulty in swallowing solids to difficulty with semi-solids to difficulty swallowing liquids. It is usually associated with weight loss. If associated with hoarseness, cervical lymphadenopathy and otalgia cancer should be suspected. Dysphagia associated with aspiration of liquids suggests neuromuscular disease. The sensation of a lump in the throat without dysphagia is termed globus pharyngis. The need to swallow twice, particularly if associated with regurgitation of undigested food following a meal, suggests a pharyngeal pouch.

Diagnosis

A limited examination of the hypopharynx can be undertaken using the laryngeal mirror or fibre-optic endoscope. A barium swallow will usually define a lower lesion.

Classification:

- intrinsic lesions, e.g. neoplasia, diverticulum, stricture, achalasia
- extrinsic lesions, e.g. goitre, mediastinal masses
- generalised disease, e.g. scleroderma, dermatomyositis
- neuromuscular disorders, e.g. myasthenia gravis, motor neuron disease, disseminated sclerosis.

18.14 Change in the voice

Learning objectives

You should:
- be aware of some of the causes of hoarseness – *laryngitis, nodules, polyps, cancer*
- understand why a patient who is hoarse for 3 or more weeks must have their larynx examined
- be aware of the role of the speech therapist.

Dysphonia is an alteration in the quality of the voice. Aphonia is absence of voice. The most common cause is acute laryngitis associated with viral infection, which is self-limiting. The inflammation is exacerbated by smoking, alcohol and voice abuse. If these factors are not corrected, chronic laryngitis may develop.

Voice abuse may lead to nodules (singer's or screamer's nodules) at the junction of the anterior third and posterior two-thirds of the true vocal cord. It may also result in polypoid changes in the vocal cords and frank polyps may form. Speech therapy is essential to correct poor vocal habits. Surgical removal is indicated for lesions that do not resolve with conservative therapy. Hoarseness may result from neoplastic disease of the larynx and a patient with hoarseness that persists for more than 3 weeks should have their larynx examined by indirect laryngoscopy.

The voice quality in unilateral vocal cord palsy is variable depending on the position of the paralysed cord in relation to its mobile partner. If there is a significant gap between the vocal cords on phonation, the voice is weak and breathy. The patient may also have difficulty with aspiration of liquids. In bilateral cord palsy, the voice may be good but the airway is often inadequate. Vocal cord palsy may be idiopathic or result from damage to the laryngeal nerve supply anywhere between the brainstem and the mediastinum.

18.15 Airway obstruction

Learning objectives

You should:
- know the definition of the terms stertor, snoring, stridor and wheeze, and where in the airway they are produced
- be aware of the causes of sleep apnoea
- understand the presentation of supraglottitis and the need for urgent treatment to establish an airway
- be aware that carcinoma of the larynx occasionally presents as an acute airway obstruction.

Stertor is the name given to the sound resulting from obstruction of the airway above the larynx. The sound is characterised by a snuffling, snorting quality. Snoring results from vibration of the tissues of the soft palate and pharynx. Complete or partial airway obstruction during snoring may result from collapse of the hypopharyngeal airway and also from posterior displacement of the base of the tongue. During sleep, the airway may periodically become completely obstructed causing sleep apnoea. In young children, the tonsils may be relatively large and the pharynx relatively small, which is a recognised cause of sleep apnoea; this is an indication for tonsillectomy in the young child. In older children and young adults, infectious mononucleosis may result in marked tonsillar hypertrophy, again with the risk of airway obstruction. Tumours of the tongue base and pharynx rarely become large enough to produce airway obstruction – dysphagia is a more common presenting feature.

Airway obstruction resulting from laryngeal disease may present at any age. Congenital abnormalities of the larynx may result in stridor at birth. Laryngomalacia, a condition in which the laryngeal cartilages are soft and floppy, is a common cause of stridor in the first year of life. Acute supraglottitis (epiglottitis) results from *H. influenzae* infection and presents with airway obstruction and drooling in the young child. The onset is rapid and the child sits in an upright position struggling for breath. This is an acute emergency. The child requires immediate transfer to hospital where the airway is usually established by passage of a nasotracheal tube in a setting where facilities for bronchoscopy and tracheostomy are available.

Bilateral paralysis of the vocal cords is a rarer cause of airway obstruction in all ages. Carcinoma of the larynx occasionally presents as airway obstruction. This is particularly true when the tumour involves the supraglottis or subglottis. Such patients are occasionally misdiagnosed as having asthma. The noisy breathing in this condition is stridor not wheeze!

Head and neck neoplasia

Chapter part overview

Most cancers of the head and neck are squamous cell carcinomas and are often, though not always, linked to excessive consumption of alcohol and tobacco. If presenting in the glottis (the vocal cords), they are often found early as they cause hoarseness and the cure rate is high. Other sites in the larynx present later with poorer results. The usual treatment is radiotherapy or laryngectomy. Tumours of the oral cavity present earlier the more anterior they arise. Posterior tumours may produce few symptoms and present later. Pharyngeal tumours may present with referred pain to the ear or dysphagia. They often present late and have a poor prognosis. The tonsil may be the site for extranodal lymphoma.

Nasopharyngeal carcinoma is commonest amongst the Chinese population and is linked to the Epstein–Barr virus. It may present with a unilateral otitis media with effusion and is treated with radiotherapy.

18.16 Clinical examination

Learning objectives

You should:
- remember that most malignant tumours of the head and neck are squamous cell carcinomas
- know the functions that these tumours may impair – *breathing*, *swallowing* and *speech*
- be aware of the methods used to diagnose these tumours
- be aware of the treatment for these tumours – *surgery*, *radiotherapy* and, occasionally, *chemotherapy*.

Presentation

Most malignant tumours of the mucosal surfaces of the head and neck are squamous cell carcinomas. Adenocarcinomas and lymphomas are less common. Squamous cell carcinomas spread by metastasising locally to the regional cervical lymph nodes. These tumours may disrupt breathing, swallowing and speech, are often painful and may alter the patient's appearance. Most squamous cell carcinomas of the mucosal surfaces of the head and neck in Western countries are associated with tobacco and alcohol abuse. In the Indian subcontinent, betel nut chewing is a predisposing factor. The Epstein–Barr virus has been implicated in the development of nasopharyngeal carcinoma and Burkitt's lymphoma and may possibly predispose to other head and neck cancers too. Exposure to radiation may result in the development of malignancy many years later. Premalignant conditions include leucoplakia (white mucosal patches), erythroplakia (red mucosal patches) and erosive lichen planus.

Diagnosis

In the clinical examination, the oral cavity should be examined in a systematic fashion, with careful inspection of the floor and roof of the mouth. When a laryngeal mirror is used, the tongue is pulled very gently to avoid pressure on the undersurface of the tongue from the lower teeth. A flexible rhinolaryngoscope allows ready examination of the nasopharynx, larynx and hypopharynx.

The regions of the neck are examined in a systematic fashion. To palpate the deep cervical lymph nodes, place the examining fingers deep to the anterior border of the sterno-mastoid muscle: warn the patient that this may be slightly uncomfortable.

The clinical examination is supported by endoscopy and biopsy.

Management

Most squamous cell cancers of the head and neck are treated primarily by surgery, radiation or a combination of both. Chemotherapy is best used in the context of controlled clinical trials. Occasionally, patients present with such advanced disease that no curative treatment is possible. Such patients require physical and psychological support, often best provided in hospice care.

18.17 The larynx

Learning objectives

You should:
- know the definitions of stridor and wheeze
- know the presenting sign of squamous carcinoma of the glottis – *hoarseness*
- be aware of the methods of treatment for laryngeal cancer – *radiotherapy* and/or *laryngectomy*
- be aware of the methods used to rehabilitate speech postoperatively.

It is important to distinguish between stridor, which arises from large airway obstruction, and wheeze, which originates in the smaller airways. Stertor is the term used to denote noisy breathing resulting from partial airway obstruction above the larynx.

Benign tumours

These are best treated with a carbon dioxide laser. Multiple treatments may be required.

Malignant tumours

Squamous cell carcinoma of the larynx most commonly affects the glottis (vocal cords) and presents with hoarseness. Any patient whose hoarseness persists for more than 3 weeks should be examined by indirect laryngoscopy. Early glottic disease has a good prognosis. The true vocal cords have no lymphatic drainage and 95% of patients with squamous cell carcinoma limited to the glottis can, therefore, be cured by radical radiotherapy. Cancers involving the area of the larynx above the vocal cords (supraglottis) and below the vocal cords (subglottis) have a much poorer prognosis as they present later and spread to cervical lymph nodes is more common because of the rich lymphatic drainage from these areas. Patients with very large tumours may present with stridor and dysphagia. Such patients may require urgent tracheostomy prior to definitive therapy.

Management

A few patients with laryngeal carcinoma may be suitable for partial laryngectomy but, in the UK, most laryngeal cancers are treated with radical radiotherapy. Once a radical course of radiotherapy has been completed, further radiotherapy cannot be given because of the risk of damage to normal tissue.

Total laryngectomy is reserved for patients with very large tumours at presentation and those who fail to respond to radiotherapy. Total laryngectomy involves the creation of an end tracheostome, which is brought out to the surface of the skin. The pharyngeal mucosa is reconstituted over a nasogastric tube and healing occurs in non-radiated patients within 7–10 days. Healing takes about twice as long in patients who have previously undergone radiotherapy.

Following total laryngectomy, about one in five patients develops oesophageal speech, which involves vibration of a segment of the reconstituted pharynx and upper oesophagus by swallowed air. Alternative methods include various hand-held battery-powered devices that are held against the neck skin and produce vibration in the pharyngo-oesophageal segment.

18.18 The oral cavity

Learning objectives

You should:
- know that anterior tumours present earlier and with less chance of metastasis than posterior ones
- know the usual presentation of carcinoma of the tongue – *an ulcer on the lateral border*
- be aware of the techniques that are available to reconstruct the oral cavity and oropharynx
- be aware of the use of the laser within the oral cavity.

Most malignancies are squamous cell carcinomas and the prognosis tends to be worse the further back in the mouth the tumour is sited. Neoplasms presenting anteriorly in the oral cavity are readily seen, whereas those more posteriorly placed often grow large, producing relatively few symptoms, and metastasise early to the cervical lymph nodes. As well as tobacco and alcohol exposure, poor dental hygiene and teeth with sharp irregular edges are thought to promote malignant change in the oral epithelium. In the Indian subcontinent, consumption of betel nut quid, which contains tobacco, is an important causative factor.

Squamous carcinomas of the lip are usually treated by surgical excision. They present early and usually have a good prognosis.

Carcinoma of the tongue usually presents as an ulcerated lesion on the lateral border. The ulcer is initially painless but, when superinfection and deeper invasion occur,

pain is experienced either locally or referred to the ipsilateral ear. Tumours arising in the posterior third of the tongue and in the area of the retromolar trigone (posterior to the third molar tooth) often present late with cervical metastases, so the prognosis is poorer.

Management

Small malignancies of the oral cavity do well with either surgery or radiotherapy. Larger tumours do poorly no matter what modality of treatment is employed. With improved reconstructive techniques, large oral cavity defects can be closed providing adequate rehabilitation of speech and swallowing. Free radial forearm flaps and pectoralis major myocutaneous flaps are routinely used in this type of reconstruction. If the mandible is involved by tumour, marginal mandibulectomy may be possible to a limited degree, preserving the integrity of the mandibular arch. If full-thickness bone of the mandible is removed, it can be replaced by bone from the radius in association with a forearm flap.

Carcinoma of the buccal mucosa, often associated with pipe smoking, may be treated by vaporisation using a carbon dioxide laser. An alternative approach uses excision of the mucosa in association with split skin grafting. Metastatic cervical lymph node disease is usually managed by neck dissection, but small nodes may respond to radiotherapy. When surgery is performed, the primary tumour and the neck dissection specimen are removed in continuity.

18.19 The pharynx

Learning objectives

You should:
- know that pharyngeal tumours often present late with cervical node involvement
- be aware that hypopharyngeal tumours may require excision by laryngopharyngectomy and oesophagectomy
- know that non-Hodgkin's lymphoma may present in the tonsil
- be aware of the term angiofibroma and in whom this condition presents – *adolescent boys*
- know that nasopharyngeal carcinoma is common in Chinese populations and how it may present – *cervical lymphadenopathy* and *unilateral otitis media with effusion*.

Oropharynx

The oropharynx and hypopharynx have a rich lymphatic supply and squamous cell cancers in these areas commonly present with cervical lymphadenopathy. Tumours in this area have a large space in which to grow before symptoms are apparent. Referred otalgia may be a presenting complaint. Patients with tumours in this area often have a high alcohol intake and are heavy smokers who often take little care of themselves. The extent of disease is assessed (usually under general anaesthesia) by inspection and palpation. Imaging with MRI and CT is helpful in determining the exact degree of tissue involvement.

Management

Treatment involves surgery, radiotherapy or a combination of both. Following surgery, reconstruction is by local or distant flaps.

Hypopharyngeal tumours may require laryngopharyngectomy with or without oesophagectomy, and reconstruction is by an interposed viscus, such as stomach, colon or jejunum.

The oropharynx is the most common site of presentation of extranodal lymphoma. These are normally non-Hodgkin's lymphomas and they present as mass lesions, usually in the area of the tonsil. Staging studies need to be undertaken. If localised, they respond to radiotherapy.

Nasopharynx

Benign tumours

Angiofibroma of the nasopharynx is a rare tumour, which typically presents in adolescent males with nasal obstruction and epistaxis. Although histologically benign they are often locally aggressive, extending laterally into the infratemporal fossa and occasionally through the skull base to the intracranial cavity.

CT, MRI and angiography are all used to define the extent of tumour.

They are usually removed surgically, sometimes with immediate preoperative embolisation to reduce vascularity. For those lesions that cannot be surgically removed safely, radiation is an alternative treatment.

Malignant tumours

Carcinoma of the nasopharynx has its highest incidence in south-east Asia, particularly in the Chinese population of Hong Kong. The Epstein–Barr virus has been implicated in the development of this tumour. The viral genome is incorporated into the DNA of the normal cell, which may become malignant in response to other environmental agents. Because the tumour has a large space in which to grow undetected, presentation is late and variable.

Clinical features:

- cervical lymphadenopathy
- otitis media with effusion (indicating obstruction of the eustachian tube)
- facial pain and altered facial sensation (indicating fifth nerve involvement)
- Horner syndrome (indicating invasion of the sympathetic chain).

Diagnosis

Diagnosis is made by examination and biopsy. Submucosal lesions can be difficult to detect clinically and may even be missed by biopsy. The extent of the tumour is defined by CT or MRI scanning. Epstein–Barr virus antibody titres may be used to follow the response to treatment and to detect recurrence of disease.

Management

These tumours are treated by radiotherapy. The prognosis is poor, with only about one-third of patients surviving for 5 years.

18.20 The nose and paranasal sinuses

> ### Learning objectives
>
> You should:
> - be aware of the variety of benign and malignant tumours that affect this area
> - know that the maxillary sinus is the sinus most frequently affected by malignancy, usually squamous carcinoma
> - be aware of the presentation of Wegener's granulomatosis
> - understand the significance of a unilateral nasal polyp.

Benign tumours

Benign tumours are:

- osteoma
- papilloma: squamous or transitional cell.

Squamous papillomas are common in the nasal vestibule and are treated with cautery or excision. Inverting papilloma, although histologically benign, behaves aggressively and requires extensive removal of the lateral nasal wall. About 10% of inverting papillomas are associated with squamous cell carcinoma.

Osteomas of the fronto-ethmoid complex often present with symptoms of obstruction of the fronto-nasal duct. They are slow growing but require removal if symptomatic.

Malignant tumours

Malignant tumours include:

- squamous cell carcinoma (most common)
- adenocarcinoma
- transitional cell carcinoma
- anaplastic tumours and lymphoma
- olfactory aesthesioneuroblastoma
- minor salivary gland tumours
- melanoma.

Wegener's granulomatosis is a systemic disease that is associated with necrotising granulation of the nose. Death is usually caused by associated renal disease.

Lethal mid-line granuloma is a T-cell lymphoma and is treated by radiotherapy.

Clinical features

The maxillary sinus is most commonly involved in malignancy. The patient presents with features resulting from the tumour breaching the walls of the antrum. Diplopia indicates orbital involvement; ill-fitting teeth or dentures indicate extension to the oral cavity. Nasal obstruction results from a breach of the medial wall of the antrum.

Eighteen

A bleeding polyp in an elderly patient should be regarded with suspicion.

Diagnosis

The extent of disease is defined by CT scanning and a tissue diagnosis obtained by biopsy.

Management

Treatment involves radical radiotherapy followed by surgery. Functional and cosmetic rehabilitation is usually provided by prostheses. The prognosis is poor with a 66% mortality rate at 5 years.

18.21 The salivary glands

Of all salivary gland neoplasms, 80% occur in the parotid gland and, of these, 80–90% are benign. Generally speaking, however, the smaller the salivary gland the more likely it is that a tumour involving the gland will be malignant. In the submandibular gland, about 50% of tumours are malignant and, in the minor salivary glands, about 90% are malignant.

Benign tumours are:

- pleomorphic adenoma
- monomorphic adenoma
- Warthin's tumour.

Malignant tumours are:

- adenoid cystic carcinoma
- squamous cell carcinoma
- pleomorphic carcinoma.

Tumours of intermediate malignancy are:

- mucoepidermoid tumour
- acinic cell tumour.

Pleomorphic adenoma

This presents as a slowly growing painless lump, usually below and a little behind the earlobe. It should not be mistaken for an upper cervical lymph node. It does not invade the facial nerve but, if present for many years, may undergo malignant change.

Fine needle aspiration cytology may help in establishing a histological diagnosis.

Treatment is by superficial or total parotidectomy, depending on the part of the gland involved, taking care to preserve the facial nerve.

Warthin's tumour

This parotid tumour usually occurs in older men and is often bilateral. Clinically, it feels soft. Histological examination reveals lymphoid tissue.

Malignant tumours

These tend to grow rapidly, invade the facial nerve and are usually painful. Adenoid cystic carcinoma is the most common. This tumour spreads by invasion of the perineural spaces. Local spread is to the cervical lymph nodes and distant spread is commonly to the lungs.

CT and MRI scans show the extent of disease.

Treatment involves parotidectomy with facial nerve excision if necessary.

Self-assessment: questions

Ear

Extended matching items questions (EMIs)

EMI 1

Theme: Diagnosis

A. vestibular neuronitis

B. Bell's palsy

C. otosclerosis

D. Menière's disease

E. otitis media with effusion

F. otitis externa

G. presbycusis

H. tympanosclerosis

I. cholesteatoma

J. glomus tumour

Match the clinical findings below to the most appropriate diagnosis from the list above:

1. A patient presents with a discharging ear and a facial palsy.

2. A patient presents with conductive hearing loss in both ears, although her tympanic membranes look normal.

3. A patient complains of recurrent vertigo, hearing loss and tinnitus.

EMI 2

Theme: Diagnosis

A. unilateral otitis media with effusion

B. aural discharge

C. sensorineural hearing loss

D. impedance audiometry

E. tinnitus

F. pure tone audiometry

G. vertigo

H. caloric testing

I. facial palsy

J. brainstem audiometry

For each of the questions below, choose the single option from above that most accurately answers the question:

1. Nasopharyngeal carcinoma may present with which ear problem?

2. Disorders of the semicircular canals will mainly cause which of the above?

3. Which of the above tests the function of the semicircular canals?

Constructed response questions (CRQs)

CRQ 1

Olivia is a 3-year-old girl who appears to be having problems with her hearing. She also has recurrent episodes of pain in her ears with occasional slight discharge. Her parents are concerned and take her to you, their GP.

a. Which two main diagnoses will you be considering?

b. Apart from her hearing, what other developmental problems might she have because of her ear disease?

c. You treat her conservatively for 3 months, but her problems become more severe. You refer her to the local ENT department. Which two surgical procedures may be considered?

d. When she is 16 years old she returns to your surgery complaining of recurrent discharge from her right ear. She has also failed a hearing test for the Royal Air Force and is concerned as this is her chosen career. Which two diagnoses are most likely, given her history?

e. Name *one* surgical procedure to treat one of your diagnoses from above.

CRQ 2

A 43-year-old schoolteacher complains of tinnitus and mild hearing loss affecting the left ear for several months. She has also noticed slight unsteadiness when getting up to go to the bathroom in the dark. Her ears look normal on examination. Using the 512-Hz tuning fork, the Rinne test is positive on both sides and the Weber test lateralises to the right ear. You are concerned that she may have a vestibular schwannoma (acoustic neuroma).

a. Which type of hearing loss does this patient probably have?

b. Which other physical examinations would you perform?

c. Which audiological tests might be appropriate?

d. Which radiological tests are appropriate?

e. Assuming that she has a vestibular schwannoma, what treatment would you offer and what complications would you discuss?

Objective structured clinical examination questions (OSCEs)

OSCE 1

Look at the photograph shown in Figure 256.

a. What is this device?

b. Look at the controls. What do O, T and M stand for?

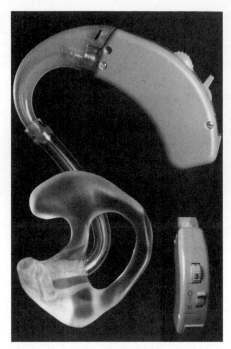

Figure 256

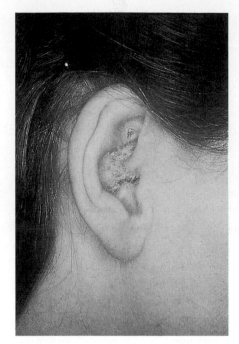

Figure 257 (Reproduced courtesy of Mr RS Dhillon FRCS.)

c. Hearing aids sometimes whistle when fitted incorrectly. What is this whistling noise caused by?

d. What is the name given to the hearing loss suffered by many elderly people?

e. Which frequencies are mainly affected in this type of hearing loss – high, middle or low?

f. Name three other aids that may help a person with hearing loss.

OSCE 2

Look at Figure 257. This shows the ear of a 52-year-old woman who is complaining of right otalgia and facial weakness. She has Ramsay–Hunt syndrome.

a. What abnormalities do you see?

b. What has caused these lesions?

c. What other symptoms may this patient have?

d. What treatment would be appropriate?

e. What long-term problems may the patient have?

Best of 5s questions

1. The usual method of dealing with a patient with cholesteatoma is by:
   a. stapedotomy
   b. issuing a hearing aid
   c. grommet insertion
   d. mastoidectomy
   e. labyrinthectomy

Multiple choice questions

1. Recognised complications of acute otitis media include:

a. tympanic membrane perforation
b. facial nerve paralysis
c. temporal lobe abscess
d. sensorineural hearing loss
e. recurrent tonsillitis

2. Conductive hearing loss is a symptom of:
   a. clinical otosclerosis
   b. Menière's disease
   c. cholesteatoma
   d. Bell's palsy
   e. acoustic neuroma

The nose and paranasal sinuses

Extended matching items questions (EMIs)

EMI 1

Theme: Anatomy

A. sphenoid sinus
B. pituitary fossa
C. middle meatus
D. anterior ethmoid sinus
E. inferior meatus
F. frontal sinus
G. middle turbinate
H. nasal septum
I. Little's area
J. inferior turbinate

Which of the anatomical areas above most accurately fit the descriptions given below:

1. The anterior ethmoid and maxillary sinuses drain into this area.
2. The nasolacrimal duct drains here.
3. This is the usual site for minor epistaxis to start.

EMI 2

Theme: Diagnosis

A. vasomotor rhinitis

B. allergic rhinitis

C. nasal polyp

D. choanal atresia

E. atrophic rhinitis

F. vestibulitis

G. anosmia

H. sinusitis

I. orbital cellulitis

J. rhinolith

Which of the diagnoses above most accurately fit the conditions given below:

1. This condition presents with nasal crusting and a bad smell from the nose.
2. This condition may occur because a foreign body has been left in the nose for a long time.
3. This condition may occur as a complication of acute ethmoiditis.

Constructed response questions (CRQs)

CRQ 1

Jamie is a 25-year-old veterinary surgeon. He has problems with nasal obstruction every summer, which is accompanied by itching of his eyes and palate.

a. What is the correct name for the problem that Jamie has and what is he probably allergic to?

b. Name two tests that could be performed to determine what he is allergic to.

c. Which two groups of drugs might be useful in managing this condition?

d. When his symptoms are particularly bad he sometimes becomes short of breath. What may he be suffering from and what treatment should you give him?

e. Jamie also has a severe allergic reaction when he comes into contact with cats. Because of his job, it is impossible for him to avoid cats. What type of treatment can we offer him that may permanently resolve this problem?

CRQ 2

Jill is a 30-year-old woman with a long history of asthma. She has no history of nasal trauma but has noticed increasing bilateral nasal obstruction and loss of sense of smell. She comes to see you, her GP.

a. Which diagnoses will you consider the most likely?

b. You look in her nose with a torch and see something that looks swollen. How can you differentiate an inferior turbinate from a nasal polyp?

c. She appears to have polyps in both nostrils. How would you treat her initially?

d. After 3 months of treatment, Jill still has a very poor nasal airway. You refer her to the ENT department of your local hospital and it is decided that she needs surgery. Which surgical procedures might be used to deal with her polyps?

e. Jill asks you about the risks of the operation. What would you tell her?

Objective structured clinical examination questions (OSCEs)

OSCE 1

Look at Figure 258. This patient has had an epistaxis.

a. What has this patient had done to stop the bleeding?

b. Name two other methods that are available to try to stop bleeding from the nose.

c. In the elderly population, which two common drugs may make this condition more severe?

d. Elderly patients are more prone to arterial bleeding in the nose than younger people. Apart from drugs, why is this?

e. Name three blood tests that you would perform on this patient and state why they would be relevant to the current problem.

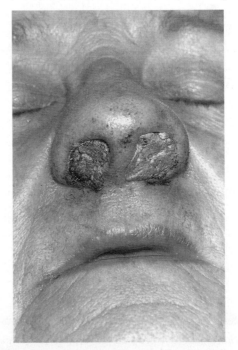

Figure 258

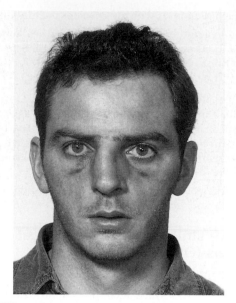

Figure 259

OSCE 2

Look at Figure 259. This patient has recently been struck in the face with an iron bar and has had his nose broken.

a. Which clinical examinations would you perform to rule out other associated injuries?

b. He may need to have his nasal bones manipulated. What would make you decide that this was necessary?

c. For how long after the injury will it be possible to manipulate the nasal bones?

d. If the nasal bones are not manipulated within this period, what treatment may he eventually require?

Best of 5s questions

1. Which class of immunoglobulins is predominantly involved in the immediate reaction seen in allergic rhinitis?

   a. IgA
   b. IgG
   c. IgD
   d. IgE
   e. IgM

Multiple choice questions

1. Causes of recurrent maxillary sinusitis include:

   a. apical dental infections
   b. repeated epistaxes
   c. recurrent bouts of otitis media
   d. deviation of the nasal septum
   e. nasal foreign body

2. Allergic rhinitis:

   a. is caused by a type I hypersensitivity reaction
   b. is best treated by turbinate surgery

c. is commonly complicated by profuse nose bleeds

d. increases the risk of development of nasal carcinoma

e. produces symptoms mainly in elderly people

The throat

Extended matching items questions (EMIs)

EMI 1

Theme: Terminology

A. odynophagia

B. laryngitis

C. hoarseness

D. stridor

E. stertor

F. tonsillitis

G. vocal cord palsy

H. dysphagia

I. laryngomalacia

J. pharyngitis

Which of the diagnoses above most appropriately fit the descriptions given below:

1. Vocal abuse commonly presents with this symptom.

2. This word describes pain on swallowing.

3. This describes the sound made when the laryngeal airway is narrowed.

EMI 2

Theme: Diagnosis

A. post-cricoid web

B. unilateral quinsy

C. laryngeal nodules

D. Epstein–Barr virus

E. pharyngeal pouch

F. Reinke's oedema

G. bilateral abductor palsy of the vocal cords

H. infectious mononucleosis

I. laryngitis

J. adenoid hypertrophy

Which of the answers above match the questions given below:

1. Paterson–Brown Kelly syndrome (Plummer–Vinson syndrome) is associated with which abnormality?

2. This disease may require emergency tonsillectomy to protect the airway.

3. This problem may result in aspiration pneumonia.

Constructed response questions (CRQs)

CRQ 1

Thomas is 6 years old and has been suffering from recurrent sore throats. His mother brings him to your surgery and wonders whether he should have his tonsils removed.

a. Which four questions would you ask her?

b. He has been having episodes of tonsillitis for 3 years. How many attacks per year would he have to suffer before you would consider tonsillectomy?

c. Name two postoperative complications that Thomas might suffer.

d. Name three reasons (other than recurrent tonsillitis) why a patient may require a tonsillectomy.

CRQ 2

Nelly is an 85-year-old female patient with increasing dysphagia of 8 months' duration who feels generally lethargic and has lost 5 kg in weight over the last few months. Clinical examination of the head and neck reveals no abnormalities. Her full blood count shows that she is anaemic, with a haemoglobin of 8.7 g/dl, and the film shows a microcytic picture.

a. Which radiological investigation would you request?

b. Your investigation reveals that she has a post-cricoid web. What will you do next?

c. Will correcting her anaemia with ferrous sulphate therapy cause the web to resolve?

d. In a patient with a post-cricoid web, what would you be concerned about?

e. If this more serious condition had developed, how would you treat her?

Objective structured clinical examination questions (OSCEs)

OSCE 1

Look at Figure 260. Note particularly the swelling lateral to the right tonsil. This tissue is firm, reddened, swollen and painful. A needle mark can be seen in the anterior pillar on the right.

a. What disease process does it show?

b. Give two symptoms that the patient might be complaining of that would make you decide to admit her?

c. What treatment would you give soon after admission?

d. Which factors in her history would help you decide whether she requires a tonsillectomy, and when would you perform it?

e. Following tonsillectomy, how long will you tell her to stay off work and how long will her throat be painful?

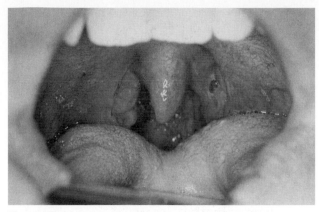

Figure 260

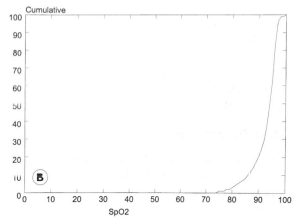

Figure 261

OSCE 2

Look at Figure 261, which shows some of the results of a sleep study performed on a 3-year-old child. The oxygen saturation during 3 h of sleep is shown in (A): the top line of each section is a saturation of 100% and the bottom line a saturation of 70%. The average oxygen saturation curve is shown in (B). His parents tell you that he snores and seems to struggle to breathe at night.

a. What do you notice about the oxygen saturation values shown in A?

b. The average value for oxygen saturation shown in B is approximately 92%. What is the range of normal values?

c. What is the name for the problem that this child is likely to be suffering from?

d. What symptoms may he have because of this problem?

e. What operative procedures may he benefit from?

Best of 5s questions

1. Which of the following symptoms is not usually experienced by a patient with a peritonsillar abscess (quinsy)?
   a. otalgia
   b. dysphagia
   c. hoarseness
   d. trismus
   e. odynophagia

Multiple choice questions

1. Hypopharyngeal diverticulum:
   a. is associated with achalasia of the oesophagus
   b. is a premalignant condition
   c. is uncommon in people over the age of 50 years
   d. tends to regress with time
   e. is associated with iron-deficiency anaemia

2. A 6-month-old baby has had mild inspiratory stridor for the last 2 months. Possible causes include:
   a. subglottic stenosis
   b. acute epiglottitis
   c. croup
   d. tonsillar hypertrophy
   e. laryngomalacia

Head and neck neoplasia

Extended matching items questions (EMIs)

EMI 1

Theme: Management

A. radiotherapy

B. oesophagectomy

C. laryngectomy

D. maxillectomy

E. parotidectomy

F. radical neck dissection

G. glossectomy

H. chemotherapy

I. tracheostomy

J. biopsy

Which of the procedures above most appropriately match the descriptions given below:

1. This procedure is designed to remove a tumour that has spread to the cervical lymph nodes.

2. This procedure is used for excision of the tongue.

3. This operation may be performed as a superficial or total procedure depending on the location of the tumour.

EMI 2

Theme: Disease processes

A. inverting papilloma

B. squamous cell carcinoma

C. adenocarcinoma

D. leucoplakia

E. pleomorphic adenoma

F. Warthin's tumour

G. Wegener's granulomatosis

H. Epstein–Barr virus

I. adenoid cystic carcinoma

J. lymphoma

Which of the disease processes above best match the descriptions given below:

1. This disease often presents with involvement of the kidneys and lungs.

2. This is the commonest tumour found in the parotid gland.

3. This is the commonest malignant tumour of the maxillary sinus.

Constructed response questions (CRQs)

CRQ 1

You are an ENT surgeon seeing a patient whom a GP colleague has referred urgently to you. Colin is a 57-year-old alcoholic who has smoked 100 g of tobacco per week in 'roll ups' for at least 40 years. He has recently been losing weight and complains of a pain in his left ear.

a. You think that he may have cancer. Which two sites are the most likely given his symptoms?

b. Name two procedures that you would want to perform on the day that you see him.

c. Name two investigations that you would book to be done urgently.

d. Unfortunately, Colin continues to lose weight rapidly and starts coughing up blood. What other pathology may he be suffering from?

e. Colin can no longer swallow food or liquid, including his own saliva. He is also in pain. What methods do we have to palliate symptoms in patients such as Colin?

CRQ 2

Rhoda is a 60-year-old woman who has noticed a slowly growing mass in her right cheek, just below and behind her ear. It is painless and she has no evidence of a facial palsy.

a. What is the most likely diagnosis?

b. How could a histological diagnosis be made without performing an open biopsy?

c. Is the facial nerve likely to be involved?

d. What treatment should Rhoda receive?

e. What complications of your treatment should Rhoda understand before you start?

Objective structured clinical examination questions (OSCEs)

OSCE 1

Look at Figure 262.

a. What procedure has this patient undergone?

b. For which two reasons might we perform this procedure?

c. Which two complications of this procedure might your patient suffer?

d. Three weeks after the operation you are called to see the patient at 4AM. He is having great difficulty breathing. What is likely to be wrong, and what would you do about it?

e. Give three symptoms that a patient with laryngeal cancer might present with?

OSCE 2

The patient in Figure 263 has a carcinoma of the hypopharynx and has had treatment with radiotherapy. This is a view of her abdomen.

a. What is the name of the procedure that has been performed?

b. What is the function of this device?

c. What symptoms may this patient have that require such a device?

d. Why might she have such symptoms?

e. Describe briefly how most of these devices are inserted.

Best of 5s questions

1. Which type of cancer is most commonly found in the larynx?

   a. squamous carcinoma
   b. adenocarcinoma
   c. adenoid cystic carcinoma
   d. sarcoma
   e. lymphoma

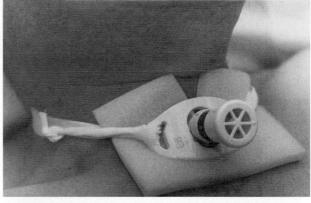

Figure 262

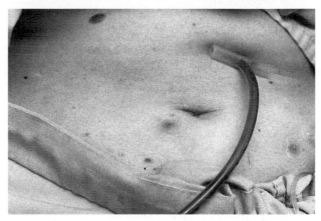

Figure 263

Multiple choice questions

1. Nasopharyngeal carcinoma:

   a. is most common in people from south-east China
   b. presents early with nasal pain
   c. is treated by wide surgical excision
   d. is monitored by measurement of Epstein–Barr virus antibodies
   e. is curable in 90% of patients

2. Carcinoma of the hypopharynx:

   a. is usually an adenocarcinoma histologically
   b. may present with referred otalgia
   c. is best treated by chemotherapy
   d. is often disseminated widely throughout the body at time of presentation
   e. is curable in 90% of patients

Self-assessment: answers

Ear

EMI answers

EMI 1

Theme: Diagnosis

1. I   Discharge from the ear and a facial palsy suggest a cholesteatoma that has eroded the bone overlying the facial nerve and caused the nerve to stop functioning. A Bell's palsy is a viral infection that affects the nerve causing a palsy – it is not associated with an aural discharge.

2. C   Otosclerosis is a condition that affects the bone around the footplate of the stapes in the oval window. There is overgrowth of the bone, which fixes the footplate in position, stopping effective transmission of sound to the cochlea and giving a conductive hearing loss. Otitis media with effusion and tympanosclerosis may also cause a conductive loss, but the tympanic membrane will not look normal.

3. D   This trio of symptoms is classic for Menière's disease, which presents with episodic attacks of vertigo, a low-frequency hearing loss and tinnitus. A vestibular schwannoma (acoustic neuroma) may present in the same way and an MRI scan of the internal auditory canals is usually required to make a diagnosis. Vestibular neuronitis (a presumed viral infection of the vestibular nerve) causes vertigo without other symptoms.

EMI 2

Theme: Diagnosis

1. A   Nasopharyngeal carcinoma may cause obstruction of the lower end of the eustachian tube in the nasopharynx and the consequent development of an effusion. A unilateral effusion (particularly if the patient is of Chinese origin) necessitates examination of the nasopharynx and possible biopsy.

2. G   The semicircular canals are involved with balance. Dysfunction causes vertigo and imbalance.

3. H   A caloric test is performed by putting warm and then cool water, or air, into the ear canals and measuring the nystagmus caused. The different temperatures of the water cause heating and cooling of the fluid in the semicircular canals and, consequently, it flows around them. If they are functioning normally this will cause nystagmus.

CRQ answers

CRQ 1

a. Recurrent acute otitis media or otitis media with effusion (glue ear).

Recurrent acute otitis media is more likely to cause pain in the ears as it involves infection in the middle ear space, but otitis media with effusion may also cause discomfort. Both will cause reduction of hearing.

b. Speech and language delay.

Behavioural problems.

Poor coordination/clumsiness/imbalance.

If hearing is affected, children do not develop language as well as they should because they cannot hear words to repeat them. Behavioural problems often arise because of boredom as the child cannot hear what is going on around them. Imbalance appears to arise because of an effect of the effusion on the vestibular system.

c. Grommet insertion.

Adenoidectomy.

Insertion of a grommet allows the middle ear pressure to return to normal with resolution of the effusion. Adenoidectomy removes the excess tissue that is causing obstruction to the eustachian tubes in the postnasal space. This allows air to pass up the tube and equalise middle ear pressure.

d. Chronic suppurative otitis media (perforated eardrum).

Cholesteatoma.

Long-standing ear disease as a child may predispose to a chronic perforation with consequent discharge and hearing loss. Cholesteatoma arises if the attic area of the tympanic membrane is retracted and squamous epithelium becomes trapped. This causes a smelly discharge and hearing loss (usually due to erosion of the long process of the incus).

e. Myringoplasty.

Mastoidectomy.

Myringoplasty is the term given to repair of the tympanic membrane (usually with temporalis fascia). Mastoidectomy usually involves drilling out the mastoid bone and opening the middle ear and mastoid spaces to the outside. This stops the cholesteatoma spreading intracranially.

CRQ 2

a. A left sensorineural loss.

The presence of unsteadiness suggests a possible peripheral vestibular disorder. The tuning fork tests suggest either a left sensorineural hearing loss or a mild right conductive loss. Given that the patient complains of left-sided hearing loss, it is most likely to be sensorineural.

b. Examination of the trigeminal and facial nerves

Look for nystagmus

Test balance and cerebellar function.

Cranial nerves V and VII should be examined as these may be involved in cerebello-pontine angle lesions such as vestibular schwannoma. Evidence of spontaneous, gaze and positional nystagmus should be looked for. Cerebellar and posterior column function should be tested.

c. Pure tone audiometry

Speech audiometry

Brainstem evoked responses.

Pure tone audiometry is essential to confirm the hearing loss, and speech audiometry may also be useful. Brainstem responses (to see if there is a delay on one side suggestive of a schwannoma) are still occasionally performed but their reliability is limited.

d. MRI of the posterior fossa and internal auditory meatus.

CT of the posterior fossa and internal auditory meatus.

MRI scanning of the posterior fossa and internal auditory meatus is now the standard investigation for suspected cases of vestibular schwannoma. CT scanning will show larger tumours but will miss smaller ones.

e. Craniotomy and removal of tumour.

Complications are of hearing loss, possible facial nerve damage, vertigo and cerebrospinal fluid leak, among others. In a younger patient, removal of the tumour is appropriate but, in elderly or frail patients, annual scanning may be performed to monitor the tumour, which is usually very slow growing. The main complications of removal of a vestibular schwannoma relate to the surrounding nerves, the auditory and facial, with possible deafness and facial palsy; vertigo because of the surgery involving the vestibular nerve; cerebrospinal fluid leak through the craniotomy; and a variety of complications common to all intracranial procedures.

OSCE answers

OSCE 1

a. A hearing aid.

A hearing aid is made up of a microphone, an amplifier and a speaker. The speaker is attached to the ear mould, which should fit snugly into the ear.

b. O for off.

T for telecoil or telephone.

M for microphone.

The T setting is used when an induction loop facility is available. This transmits radio signals from the sound source (such as a microphone in church or the sound track of a film in the cinema) directly to the hearing aid, so reducing the problem of background noise. The M setting allows normal use.

c. Feedback.

If the ear mould is loose and allows sound to escape from the ear canal this may be picked up by the microphone and a feedback loop set up causing whistling.

d. Presbycusis.

Presbycusis is the symmetrical, high-frequency sensorineural hearing loss found in the elderly. The prefix presby- means old (as in presbyopia).

e. High.

The higher frequencies are lost first, possibly because the first turn of the cochlea, which deals with the higher frequencies, is nearest to the stapes and receives most noise trauma over a lifetime.

f. Flashing doorbell.

Flashing/amplified telephone.

Vibrating alarm clock.

Subtitles on television.

Flashing smoke alarm.

Spectacles to allow lip-reading.

Hearing dog for the deaf.

There are many aids that a person with hearing difficulties may find useful. A hearing therapist and the social work department of the local council should be approached for advice.

OSCE 2

a. Vesicles and crusting of the pinna.

Vesicles and crusting of the pinna associated with pain is very typical of Ramsay–Hunt syndrome (herpes zoster oticus).

b. Herpes zoster virus.

The lesions and the facial palsy are caused by the herpes zoster virus.

c. Hearing loss and vertigo.

She may suffer from a variety of cranial nerve disorders secondary to a neuritis caused by the virus. Facial palsy, hearing loss and vertigo result from involvement of cranial nerves VII and VIII. Involvement of nerve IX leads to vesicular eruptions on the palate; involvement of nerve X leads to vocal cord palsy.

d. Analgesia.

Bed rest if vertigo is severe.

Antiviral therapy such as aciclovir.

Systemic antiviral therapy, such as aciclovir, may shorten the attack, although whether it is useful in promoting recovery of facial nerve function is less certain.

e. Facial palsy.

Hearing loss.

Neuralgia.

In contrast to Bell's palsy, in which 90% of patients recover facial function, only about 60% do so after Ramsay–Hunt syndrome. Post-herpetic neuralgia may be troublesome and the hearing may not recover.

Best of 5s answers

1. d. **Mastoidectomy.** Stapedotomy is performed if the footplate of the stapes is fixed in otosclerosis, grommet insertion is appropriate with a middle ear effusion and labyrinthectomy is occasionally performed for unrelieved vertigo. Mastoidectomy involves drilling out the diseased bone and squamous epithelium from the mastoid to make the ear safe.

Multiple choice answers

1. a. **True.** Rupture of the tympanic membrane in acute otitis media is often associated with bloodstained purulent discharge and relief of pain.

   b. **True.** Facial nerve paralysis may occur when the bony covering of the nerve in its passage through the middle ear is thin or absent.

   c. **True.** Possible but extremely rare. Intracranial complications are much more likely to occur when cholesteatoma is present.

   d. **False.** Conductive hearing loss is a feature of acute otitis media. Sensorineural hearing loss implies involvement of the labyrinth.

   e. **False.** Acute otitis media results from infection ascending from the nasopharynx. Recurrent tonsillitis may occur in association with acute otitis media but is not a complication.

2. a. **True.** Progressive conductive hearing loss is the cardinal feature of clinical otosclerosis.

   b. **False.** Menière's disease is characterised by a fluctuating, progressive sensory hearing loss.

   c. **True.** Cholesteatoma damages and frequently destroys parts of the ossicular chain. Hearing may be preserved by transmission of sound through the cholesteatoma. The conductive hearing loss may, therefore, be greater following surgery to eradicate cholesteatoma.

   d. **False.** Bell's palsy is not associated with hearing loss.

   e. **False.** Acoustic neuroma is characterised by a neural (retrocochlear) hearing loss that is unilateral. The patient often notices tinnitus before hearing loss.

The nose and paranasal sinuses

EMI answers

EMI 1

Theme: Anatomy

1. C   The middle meatus is the area under the middle turbinate. The frontal, maxillary and most of the ethmoid sinuses drain into it. The sphenoid sinuses drain into the sphenoethmoidal recess at the back of the nose.

2. E   The nasolacrimal duct is the only structure to drain into the inferior meatus.

3. I   Little's area is the name given to the anterior part of the nasal septum. A number of veins and small arteries are found in the mucosa, which may bleed as it is an area that is frequently traumatised by picking the nose. Older patients may have arterial bleeding that is usually more posteriorly sited and more severe.

EMI 2

Theme: Diagnosis

1. E   Atrophic rhinitis may be related to poor living conditions with atrophy of seromucinous glands in the nasal mucosa, although the exact cause is uncertain. It leads to excessive patency of the nasal airway with consequent drying of the mucosa, crusting and infection. Rarely, surgical removal of the inferior turbinates may cause this problem.

2. J   A rhinolith (stone in the nose) is a concretion of calcium and magnesium salts that can form around a foreign body in the nose if left for months or years.

3. I   Orbital cellulitis is an infection of the orbital contents, usually occurring by venous spread through the lamina papyracea from infection in the ethmoid sinuses. It mainly affects young children but can occur at any age.

CRQ answers

CRQ 1

a. Seasonal allergic rhinitis.

   Grass pollen.

Seasonal allergic rhinitis occurs only during the period when the allergen is in the air, as opposed to a perennial rhinitis, which is present all year. Seasonal rhinitis is caused by tree pollen in the spring, grass pollen in the summer, and moulds and spores in the autumn and winter.

b. Skin prick test.

   Radioallergosorbent test (RAST).

The skin prick test is a cheap and rapid method of demonstrating atopy. A standard battery of allergens is used consisting of a positive (histamine) and negative (saline) allergen, and dog, cat, grass and house dust mite allergens. Most atopic patients will react to one or more of these. The RAST is a blood test that measures the level of IgE circulating in the blood, which reacts with the various allergens tested against. It is more expensive but may be useful in testing for food allergies.

c. Antihistamines.

   Intranasal steroids.

Antihistamines are rapid acting and reduce nasal itch and discharge but are less effective at relieving nasal blockage. Intranasal steroids are slow acting but more effective at clearing the nose.

d. Asthma (or bronchial hyper-reactivity).

Provide a bronchodilator (e.g. sabutamol) and possibly an inhaled steroid.

Allergic asthma and allergic rhinitis have the same underlying causes and often coexist. Bronchodilators and inhaled steroids may be necessary to relieve bronchoconstriction.

e. Immunotherapy (desensitisation).

Immunotherapy involves injecting increasing amounts of an allergen subcutaneously until the patient becomes desensitised. It can offer extremely effective and long-lasting relief of symptoms.

CRQ 2

a. Nasal polyposis.

Inferior turbinate hypertrophy.

Septal deviation.

Nasal polyposis and non-allergic asthma often coexist, although the reason for this is not clear. Inferior turbinate hypertrophy may be the result of allergic rhinitis with swelling of the mucosa. Patients with turbinate hypertrophy often complain that the obstruction switches from side to side – this is the turbinate cycle. Deviation of the nasal septum is very common, even without a history of trauma, although it would not usually present at this age if there were no other factors involved. A minor septal deviation may not cause obstruction until there is a minor mucosal swelling. The combination may result in symptomatic obstruction.

b. Touch it with a blunt instrument.

Nasal polyps have no sensation. A swollen inferior turbinate may look quite like a polyp and they are often confused by the inexperienced. Touching a polyp will cause no pain but your patient will let you know if you touch a turbinate!

c. Intranasal steroids.

Intranasal steroids are the mainstay of the treatment of simple bilateral polyps. Occasionally, systemic steroids are required. Remember, unilateral polyps require urgent assessment and biopsy as they may be malignant. It is very rare for bilateral polyps to be malignant.

d. Simple nasal polypectomy.

Bilateral ethmoidectomies – either intranasal or external.

A simple nasal polypectomy may be performed under local or general anaesthesia, but the polyps are very likely to recur. Endoscopically controlled intranasal ethmoidectomies are now commonly performed and seem to lead to fewer recurrences of polyps (remember, the polyps arise in the ethmoid sinuses).

e. Haemorrhage.

Cerebrospinal fluid leak.

Damage to the orbit.

Recurrence of polyps.

Sense of smell may not return.

The area of the cribriform plate is very thin and can be traumatised when removing polyps. This may lead to a cerebrospinal fluid leak. The lamina papyracea is also thin and separates the orbit from the nose. If it is breached there will be bruising around the eye and occasionally damage to the globe or optic nerve. Any operation to treat polyps does not cure the problem, it simply debulks the volume of disease and improves the access for intranasal steroids. Polyps may therefore recur. The olfactory area in humans is very small and polyps or mucosal oedema will easily obstruct the passage of air to this narrow area. No guarantees can be given that smell will improve although, post-operatively, it sometimes does.

OSCE answers

OSCE 1

a. The nose has been packed.

A long gauze pack, impregnated with antiseptic, has been inserted to put pressure on the bleeding vessel and allow a clot to form within it.

b. Cautery.

Diathermy.

Arterial ligation.

Arterial embolisation.

Chemical cautery using a silver nitrate stick is often successful in stopping bleeding from the anterior septum. Bipolar diathermy can be used for more serious bleeds. The sphenopalatine artery can be clipped within the nose under endoscopic control. The internal maxillary artery can be clipped by exposing it behind the posterior wall of the maxilla, and the external carotid artery can be tied off in the neck. The anterior and posterior ethmoidal arteries can be clipped as they pass through the medial wall of the orbit.

c. Warfarin.

Aspirin.

Warfarin reduces the ability of the blood to clot, and aspirin inhibits the ability of platelets to aggregate. Both may cause bleeding to be prolonged.

d. Arteriosclerosis.

Arteriosclerotic changes in vessel walls reduce their ability to contract and close when damaged. Bleeding may therefore be prolonged.

e. Full blood count – to assess blood loss and give a baseline haemoglobin, and to measure platelet numbers.

Group and save/crossmatch blood – in case of further bleeding.

Coagulation screen/international normalised ratio – to detect abnormal clotting.

Liver function test – to estimate any liver dysfunction that may affect clotting.

Arterial blood gases – if respiration compromised by nasal packing.

A full blood count will give an estimate of the baseline haemoglobin but, if bleeding has been brisk, the patient will not have had time to haemodilute, so this must be treated with caution. An international normalised ratio should be requested if a patient is on warfarin, to ensure that their results are within the therapeutic range. Occasionally, warfarin may need to be stopped for a few days.

OSCE 2

a. Examine skull and cervical spine for injury.

Assess dental occlusion.

Feel for a step in the infraorbital rim.

Test sensation over the cheek.

A history of the nature of the injury should be obtained. Significant head and cervical spine injury must be excluded as a priority. The most likely associated injuries are those to the maxilla or zygoma. Problems with dental occlusion and a palpable step in the inferior orbital rim are features of a fracture of the maxilla. Loss of sensation over the cheek suggests damage to the infraorbital nerve, which is a feature of an orbital blow-out fracture where pressure on the eye has caused the floor of the orbit to fracture and orbital contents to prolapse into the maxillary sinus.

b. Cosmetic appearance.

Nasal obstruction.

The reasons for reducing any facial fracture are to achieve restoration of function and/or to improve cosmesis. If there is no significant deformity and the patient is able to breathe comfortably through both nostrils, reduction is unnecessary.

c. Approximately 2 weeks.

Fracture reduction should take place within 2 weeks of injury. The fractured nasal bones can be easily manipulated up to 10 days after injury but they become progressively more 'sticky' and, after 2 weeks, are virtually immobile.

d. Septorhinoplasty or rhinoplasty.

If reduction is delayed, definitive treatment usually involves a rhinoplasty, which entails osteotomies to refracture the nasal bones. They can then be manipulated into position.

Best of 5s answers

1. d. The type I hypersensitivity reaction seen in allergic rhinitis is mediated by IgE.

Multiple choice answers

1. a. **True.** Apical dental infections are usually caused by anaerobic organisms and the roots of the premolar and molar teeth may project into the antrum with minimal or absent bony covering.

   b. **False.** Epistaxis may be a feature of recurrent maxillary sinusitis but it is not a cause.

c. **False.** Otitis media, particularly in children, may be associated with sinus infections but it is not causative.

d. **True.** Deviations of the nasal septum may be sufficiently severe to cause impaired drainage of the maxillary sinus, resulting in recurrent infections.

e. **True.** Nasal foreign bodies are most common in children and the mentally ill and may result in obstruction of the maxillary sinus ostium producing chronic recurrent infections.

2. a. **True.** This results in degranulation of mast cells with release of histamine and other chemical mediators, which result in the classic symptoms of allergic rhinitis.

   b. **False.** The most appropriate treatment is avoidance of the allergen if possible. Topical nasal steroid sprays are the mainstay of treatment nowadays. Turbinate surgery should be limited to those patients in whom there is an irreversible turbinate hypertrophy.

   c. **False.** Mucosa tends to be swollen by oedema rather than by engorgement with blood.

   d. **False.** There is no association between allergic rhinitis and the development of nasal carcinoma.

   e. **False.** Allergic rhinitis tends to be less troublesome in the elderly. Symptoms tend to be maximal in the second and third decades of life.

The throat

EMI answers

EMI 1

Theme: Terminology

1. C Vocal abuse (shouting or other misuse of the voice) may cause trauma to the vocal cords and consequent formation of swelling or nodules presenting with hoarseness. These are called singer's nodules, or screamer's nodules in young children. Patients may also have laryngitis, but this is a diagnosis and not a symptom.

2. A Odynophagia is pain on swallowing. Dysphagia is difficulty swallowing.

3. D Stridor is caused by air flowing through a narrowed laryngeal or tracheal airway and is often louder on inspiration than on expiration. Stertor is caused by the vibration of tissues above the larynx, and snoring by the vibration of tissues in the oro- and nasopharynx. Wheeze arises in the bronchioles and is usually expiratory.

EMI 2

Theme: Diagnosis

1. A Paterson–Brown Kelly syndrome is usually seen in women in their 40s, often with a microcytic hypochromic anaemia. Such patients, who may

suffer from dysphagia, should have their haemoglobin checked and may require endoscopy and biopsy as it can be a premalignant condition.

2. H   Any condition that causes bilateral swelling of the tonsils or causes them to be pushed medially, as with bilateral quinsies, may cause obstruction of the airway. Epstein–Barr virus causes infectious mononucleosis (glandular fever).

3. E   A pharyngeal pouch is an outpouching of mucosa from the pharynx in which food and liquid may collect. This may later be regurgitated into the larynx and aspirated into the lungs causing pneumonia.

CRQ answers

CRQ 1

a. How often is he getting these attacks?

How long has he been having these problems?

How severe are the symptoms?

Can he eat and drink during an attack?

Does he get a fever?

Has he lost time from school?

Do the tonsils look any different during an attack?

It is important to determine how often the tonsillitis occurs and how severe the symptoms are, which can be measured by time lost from school, inability to eat and so on. The appearance of the tonsils during an attack confirms that the problem is indeed tonsillitis. It is by judging the severity of the problem that a decision can be made as to whether the risk of an operation is worthwhile.

b. Two to three times per year.

Five to six attacks in 1 year only, or three to four attacks over 2 or more years, are usually regarded as indications for tonsillectomy.

c. Reactionary haemorrhage.

Secondary haemorrhage.

Throat pain.

Ear pain.

Infection of tonsil bed.

Secondary tonsillar haemorrhage is common following tonsillectomy (5–10% of patients). Throat pain is universal and many patients complain of pain referred to the ear.

d. Obstructive sleep apnoea.

Recurrent quinsy (peritonsillar abscess).

Biopsy of tumour.

Airway management in glandular fever (rare).

Children suffering from obstructive sleep apnoea frequently benefit from removal of tonsils and adenoids to increase the potential airway. Following one peritonsillar abscess there is only a 20% chance of recurrence, therefore, tonsillectomy is not usually advised. A further abscess requires tonsillectomy as subsequent infection becomes much more likely. Tonsillitis may precipitate attacks of

nephritis and psoriasis in susceptible individuals or cause rheumatic fever. This is probably due to a common antigen on the streptococcus and the affected tissue, which is then attacked by the immune system.

CRQ 2

a. A barium swallow.

A barium swallow will often show a lesion in the pharynx or upper oesophagus. It can be used to make a diagnosis and to guide direct endoscopy.

b. Direct endoscopy under general anaesthesia with possible biopsy.

This patient requires an endoscopy to rule out malignancy. The web seen on barium swallow is often found to be a simple mucosal fold, but this may be difficult to identify. Direct endoscopy is, however, mandatory.

c. Yes, if it is minimal.

Correction of the anaemia with appropriate therapy (usually iron or vitamin B12, depending on the cause of the anaemia) will cause an early web to resolve.

d. That she may have developed a post-cricoid carcinoma.

Post-cricoid carcinoma is a potentially lethal condition that is associated with a post-cricoid web.

e. If limited, with radiotherapy.

If more extensive, by laryngo-pharyngo-oesophagectomy and stomach pull-up.

Early limited post-cricoid carcinoma may be successfully treated with radical radiotherapy. More extensive tumours require removal of the larynx, pharynx and oesophagus and replacement by pulling the stomach up through the chest and connecting it to the oropharynx.

OSCE answers

OSCE 1

a. Quinsy/peritonsillar abscess.

The photograph shows a right-sided peritonsillar swelling. Note that the tonsil itself looks normal but is pushed medially, i.e. the swelling is lateral to the tonsil, not in the tonsil itself. Approximately 4 ml of pus was drained from this abscess through a needle that was inserted through the anterior pillar. Some quinsies drain up to 10 ml of pus or more.

b. Unable to eat.

Unable to drink.

Severe pain.

If a patient can eat and drink, they can normally be managed with oral antibiotics as an outpatient. If they cannot drink because of pain and swelling, they require intravenous fluid therapy. They may also have marked trismus (limited mouth opening).

c. Intravenous fluids.

Intravenous antibiotics.

Drainage of abscess.

Analgesia.

A patient may put up with several days of pain and inablity to swallow before presenting and may, therefore, need fluid therapy. Drainage of the peritonsillar abscess usually results in rapid resolution of symptoms.

    d. If she has had a previous quinsy, she should have a tonsillectomy. Tonsillectomy is usually performed 6 weeks after the acute infection to allow inflammation to settle and to reduce bleeding during the procedure. Occasionally, the tonsils are removed during the acute episode to drain the pus.

After one quinsy, 80% of patients will not have a recurrence and, therefore, tonsillectomy is not usually indicated. A second quinsy means that the patient is at a higher risk of further recurrences and tonsillectomy should be performed. Tonsillectomy is only rarely performed during the acute infection because of the risk of increased bleeding, but may be necessary in patients who cannot tolerate drainage under local anaesthesia (particularly children, although quinsy is unusual in this group).

    e. At least 2 weeks off work.

    At least 7–10 days sore throat.

Many patients (and doctors!) underestimate the discomfort that they will suffer after tonsillectomy. Swallowing is painful for at least a week despite regular analgesia, and at least 14 days off work or school should be anticipated.

OSCE 2

    a. There are dips in the level of oxygen saturation.

The oxygen saturations can be seen to fall to below 70% on occasion. This is abnormal. Normal saturation levels never fall below 90%.

    b. The normal range is 95–100%.

The average oxygen saturation in this study is 92%; this is well below normal.

    c. Obstructive sleep apnoea.

Obstructive sleep apnoea suggests an abnormality in the airway. In children, this is usually due to enlarged tonsils and adenoids. Central sleep apnoea (when there is a reduced respiratory drive) is much less common. A full examination must be performed before surgery, however, to determine the site of any obstruction.

    d. Snoring.

       Daytime sleepiness.

       Poor concentration.

       Pulmonary hypertension.

       Failure to thrive.

       Bed wetting.

       Headache.

       Bagginess under eyes.

These children wake frequently throughout the night to improve their airway and, therefore, suffer from a very poor quality of sleep.

    e. Tonsillectomy.

       Adenoidectomy.

Removing the tonsils and adenoids should enlarge the airway sufficiently to cure the obstruction if preoperative examination has confirmed that this is the problem.

Best of 5s answers

1. c. All of these symptoms may be experienced except hoarseness. Otalgia (ear pain) is due to referred pain via the glossopharyngeal nerve, dysphagia (difficulty swallowing) by the swelling of the oropharynx, trismus (limitation of mouth opening) by inflammation in the medial pterygoid muscles and odynophagia (pain on swallowing) by the inflammatory process.

Multiple choice answers

1. a. **False.** The two conditions are quite distinct.
   b. **False.** Malignancy in hypopharyngeal diverticulum has been reported only extremely rarely.
   c. **False.** This disease tends to occur in people over the age of 50.
   d. **False.** The diverticulum tends to enlarge with time.
   e. **False.** The Plummer–Vinson syndrome, not hypopharyngeal diverticulum, is classically associated with iron-deficiency anaemia.

2. a. **True.** Subglottic narrowing may be congenital or acquired. Acquired cases usually result from prolonged endotracheal intubation. Most congenital cases are self-limiting as the child grows.
   b. **False.** Acute epiglottitis develops rapidly, usually in a period of hours. It would not cause symptoms for 2 months.
   c. **False.** Acute laryngotracheo-bronchitis develops rapidly and is associated with a characteristic cough.
   d. **False.** Tonsillar hypertrophy may cause airway obstruction producing stertor. Stridor results from narrowing of the laryngeal or tracheal airway.
   e. **True.** This is a common cause of stridor in this age group.

Head and neck neoplasia

EMI answers

EMI 1

Theme: Management

1. F A radical neck dissection involves removal of the sternocleidomastoid muscle and the internal jugular vein along with all the associated lymph nodes. Together with treatment of the primary tumour this may be curative, as head and neck tumours tend to metastasise late to the liver or lungs.

2. G The prefix gloss- refers to the tongue (as in glossopharyngeal, glossitis, etc).

3. E Many parotid tumours lie superficial to the facial nerve and, thus, only this part of the parotid gland has to be removed. If the tumour is deep to the nerve, a total parotidectomy is performed.

EMI 2

Theme: Disease processes

1. G Wegener's granulomatosis is a systemic vasculitis, which may present with crusting and bleeding from the nose. It is life threatening because of the necrotising glomerulonephritis that also occurs, leading to eventual renal failure, and because of lung involvement. Blood testing often shows a positive cANCA (antineutrophil cytoplasmic antibody). It is *not* a type of cancer.

2. E Pleomorphic adenoma is a benign parotid tumour, which makes up 80% of the tumours found in the gland. Warthin's tumour (monomorphic adenoma) is also benign but is much less common (8%). Adenoid cystic carcinoma is an aggressive malignant tumour that is fortunately unusual; 25% of patients present with a facial palsy as it often involves the facial nerve.

3. B Squamous cell carcinomas make up the vast majority of head and neck cancers. Adenocarcinoma is sometimes found in the ethmoid sinuses but usually occurs in people who work with hard woods, such as carpenters and cabinet makers.

CRQ answers

CRQ 1

a. The hypopharynx.

   The upper oesophagus.

   The larynx.

   The tonsil.

   The base of the tongue.

As he is complaining of ear pain, the area affected must be supplied by the glossopharyngeal or vagus nerves, which also send fibres to the ear (referred pain). Tumours involving the hypopharynx, tonsil and base of the tongue and the larynx are the most likely to cause ear pain.

b. Indirect or endoscopic examination of the larynx.

   Examination of the neck.

   Chest radiograph.

The immediate examination in outpatients is to see where his tumour is by examining the larynx, pharynx and mouth with an endoscope or a mirror. The neck is examined for enlarged cervical lymph nodes indicating possible spread of the tumour. The chest radiograph may show pulmonary metastases or a second primary lung tumour.

c. Barium swallow.

   CT of neck and chest (or MRI).

   Direct laryngoscopy, oesophagoscopy and bronchoscopy with biopsy.

A barium swallow allows a tumour in the oesophagus to be seen and CT of the neck and chest may show the extent of the tumour, involved lymph nodes and lung lesions. Direct endoscopy and biopsy are necessary for histological diagnosis.

d. Lung cancer.

As Colin is a heavy smoker he may have a second primary bronchial tumour.

e. Stenting of the tumour in the oesophagus.

   Palliative radiotherapy.

   Gastrostomy tube for feeding.

   Subcutaneous or rectal analgesia.

   Psychological support.

Palliative medicine is a specialty with its own experts, who should always be consulted when dealing with such patients. The type of palliative therapy that is appropriate depends on the clinical problem, but radiotherapy to shrink the tumour and enteral feeding are frequently used.

CRQ 2

a. Pleomorphic adenoma.

The mass involves the area of the right parotid gland. Over 80% of tumours in this area are pleomorphic adenomas. This is compatible with the age of the patient and the fact that the tumour has been enlarging slowly. Other salivary gland tumours are possible, as are tumours in adjacent structures, but a pleomorphic adenoma is the most likely in this area.

b. Fine needle aspiration cytology.

Fine needle aspiration cytology is the most accurate way of obtaining a tissue diagnosis without performing an open biopsy.

c. No, not if the tumour is benign.

It is very unusual for the facial nerve to be involved in a benign parotid tumour. Benign tumours grow slowly and the large motor fibres in the nerve can adapt to slowly increasing pressure. This is in contrast to malignant tumours, which invade the nerve early and may result in facial weakness or spasm when the tumour is relatively small.

d. Superficial parotidectomy.

In an otherwise healthy 60-year-old, superficial parotidectomy is the most appropriate treatment. Most of the tumours arise superficial to the facial nerve but, if left, will gradually enlarge. There is also a small risk of malignant change.

e. Possible damage to the facial nerve.

   Some loss of sensation in the side of the face postoperatively.

Frey syndrome.

Recurrence of tumour.

The main risk of superficial parotidectomy is damage to the facial nerve. In skilled hands this risk is small, but the course of the nerve is variable and the nerve is at risk even with small tumours. To remove the tumour, the great auricular nerve must be divided, which leads to a localised loss of sensation of the side of the face in the area of the ear lobe. Postoperatively, some patients become aware of sweating from the skin overlying the gland when eating or thinking of food (gustatory sweating). This results from aberrant innervation from nerve fibres that originally supplied the salivary gland tissue regrowing into the sweat glands of the overlying skin (Frey syndrome).

OSCE answers

OSCE 1

a. Tracheostomy.

This is a tracheostomy tube, which has been inserted into the trachea to create an airway as the normal airway has been obstructed (in this case, because of a carcinoma of the base of the tongue and supraglottis).

b. To create an airway if obstructed.

For ventilation.

To reduce dead space.

To allow suction of bronchial secretions.

Patients requiring ventilation in the intensive care unit often have a tracheostomy performed after 10 days or so to allow the oral endotracheal tube to be removed. This allows easier suction of secretions in the lungs, provides more comfort for the patient and prevents the formation of a subglottic stenosis, which may occur if an endotracheal tube is left in place for long periods. This is even more important in children.

c. Haemorrhage.

Displacement of the tube from the trachea and obstruction.

Crusting causing obstruction of the tube.

Pneumothorax (rarely).

Pulmonary oedema (very rarely).

Haemorrhage is a particular risk when performing a tracheostomy in a child as the innominate vein may lie high in the neck and be traumatised. The domes of the pleura may lie higher than usual in patients with lung disease such as emphysema and, if damaged, will lead to pneumothorax. Pulmonary oedema can occur in patients who have long-standing laryngeal or tracheal obstruction. The pressures needed to move air in these patients suddenly fall when a patent airway is created, and fluid may then leak into the lungs.

d. There is probably crusting in the tube or it has become displaced.

Remove the inner tube and clean it. If this is ineffective, remove and replace the entire tube. A tracheostomy is simply an opening into the trachea below the larynx. The normal airway remains, although it may be partially or totally obstructed. Following laryngectomy, the trachea is brought out onto the skin of the neck, the airway above it having been removed. These patients have no other route for breathing, a fact to be remembered if giving oxygen or nebulisers. Crusting of mucus within the tube is not uncommon and may not be noticed until the tube is almost occluded. Most long-term tracheostomy tubes have an inner cannula that can be removed and cleaned. After 3 weeks it should be possible to change the tube safely as a track will have formed. In the first week after tracheostomy this may be much more difficult.

e. Hoarseness.

Stridor.

Breathing difficulty (dyspnoea).

Dysphagia.

Haemoptysis.

Cervical node swelling.

Weight loss.

Otalgia.

Hoarseness is an early sign of glottic carcinoma (involving the vocal cords). Patients who have been hoarse for more than 3 weeks should have their larynx examined. Stridor occurs when the tumour starts to limit the airway and may be associated with dyspnoea – at first with exercise and then also at rest. Dysphagia and referred otalgia occur if the tumour is invading the hypopharynx. Haemoptysis may occur from the ulcerated surface of the tumour itself or from a second primary lung or oesophageal tumour. Enlargement of the cervical lymph nodes may suggest spread of the tumour to the lymphatic system, although sometimes nodes become enlarged because of infection on the surface of the tumour. Weight loss may occur because of dysphagia or wider metastatic spread.

OSCE 2

a. Gastrostomy.

A gastrostomy is an opening into the stomach. The tube can be placed further down the gastrointestinal tract into the duodenum or jejunum if required.

b. To allow feeding and drug administration.

The tube allows food and drugs to be given to the patient.

c. Dysphagia (or complete obstruction).

Odynophagia.

The ideal treatment for such a patient would be to allow food and drugs to be taken by mouth but, if this is not possible, a gastrostomy may be necessary.

d. Obstruction by tumour.

Mucositis caused by radiotherapy.

An obstructing tumour may not be resectable or amenable to stenting. Radiotherapy frequently causes a marked mucositis; therefore, during and after treatment, until the mucositis settles, a gastrostomy tube may be necessary to allow feeding and the administration of drugs. As the tumour shrinks and the mucositis settles, it may be possible to remove the tube.

e. A flexible endoscope is passed into the stomach. The light from the endoscope is seen through the anterior abdominal wall and the abdomen is punctured. The gastrostomy tube is then passed through.

Gastrostomy tubes are usually inserted endoscopically but, if the tumour is so extensive as to completely occlude the pharynx or oesophagus, an open approach through the abdomen may be necessary.

Best of 5s answers

1. a. Squamous carcinoma is the type of tumour that is found in over 90% of all head and neck malignancies although lymphoma can present in the tonsil or nasopharynx. Adenocarcinoma found in a neck lymph node is usually metastatic from elsewhere.

Multiple choice answers

1. a. **True.** Nasopharyngeal carcinoma is the most common malignant tumour in men from the Hong Kong area of China.

b. **False.** Pain is a late feature.

c. **False.** Radical radiotherapy is the mainstay of treatment.

d. **True.** Antibodies to specific parts of the Epstein–Barr virus are a sensitive measure of the presence of active tumour.

e. **False.** Overall survival in all series is much less than 90%.

2. a. **False.** Like most carcinomas of the mucosal surfaces of the head and neck, squamous cell carcinoma is the most common variant.

b. **True.** Involvement of the superior laryngeal branch of the vagus nerve results in otalgia.

c. **False.** Surgery and radiotherapy are the mainstays of treatment.

d. **False.** Early metastases are to the cervical lymph nodes. Widespread dissemination throughout the body is a late feature.

e. **False.** These tumours are commonly far advanced at the time of presentation and 5-year survival rates are generally less than 50%.

Index

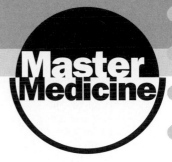